THE ENCYCLOPEDIA OF

WORK-RELATED ILLNESSES, INJURIES, AND HEALTH ISSUES

Disclaimer: The material in this book is not intended for application to specific medical or legal situations. Health or legal questions should be referred to personal physicians, occupational health care providers, industrial hygienists, attorneys, or other appropriate professionals. Information in this book and in references cited is intended to provide readers with a better understanding of workplace hazards, need for safety precautions, and major health issues in the workplace and is not intended to provoke tensions between employees and their employers.

THE ENCYCLOPEDIA OF

WORK-RELATED ILLNESSES, INJURIES, AND HEALTH ISSUES

Ada P. Kahn, Ph.D.
Foreword by Delbert H. Meyer, M.D.

Facts On File, Inc.

The Encyclopedia of Work-Related Illnesses, Injuries, and Health Issues

Copyright © 2004 by Ada P. Kahn, Ph.D.

Facts On File, Inc.
132 West 31st Street
New York NY 10001

Library of Congress Cataloging-in-Publication Data

Kahn, Ada P.
The encyclopedia of work-related illnesses, injuries, and health issues / Ada P. Kahn ;
foreword by Delbert H. Meyer, M.D.
p. cm.
ISBN 0-8160-4844-4 (HC : alk. paper)
1. Medicine, Industrial—Encyclopedias. 2. Occupational diseases—Encyclopedias. 3. Industrial accidents—Encyclopedias. 4. Industrial hygiene—Encyclopedias. I. Title.

RC963.A3K348 2003
616.9′.803′03   dc21—2003011484

Facts On File books are available at special discounts when purchased in bulk quantities for businesses, associations, institutions, or sales promotions. Please call our Special Sales Department in New York at (212) 967-8800 or (800) 322-8755.

You can find Facts On File on the World Wide Web at http://www.factsonfile.com

Text and cover design by Cathy Rincon
Illustrations by Dale Williams

Printed in the United States of America

VB FOF 10 9 8 7 6 5 4 3 2 1

CONTENTS

FOREWORD

Injuries are ubiquitous in work environments. When the field of industrial medicine began, the primary concern was to provide first aid after an accident, such as physical trauma or chemical body injury, and to diagnose occupational diseases, such as skin allergies, contact dermatitis, occupational asthma, or pneumoconiosis.

Today, industrial medicine encompasses a wide range of multidisciplinary specialists, ranging from orthopedists who treat the back injuries of construction workers, to plastic surgeons who treat burn injuries, to psychiatrists who treat people dealing with mental health issues. In addition, the field has gained the attention of epidemiologists and researchers interested in occupational-related allergies, toxic substances, mineral fibers, cancer, inhalation lung diseases, ergonomics, continual use of computers, and repetitive stress issues, just to name a few.

The *Journal of the American Medical Association* reports that 3.6 million Americans were treated at hospital emergency rooms for occupational injuries or illnesses in 1998. This translates to an overall occupational injury and illness rate of 2.9 per 100 full-time employees over age 15. Injury rates were highest in men and younger workers. The Occupational Safety and Health Administration (OSHA) reported that in 2000, occupational injury and illness rates dropped to their lowest level, 6.1 injuries per 200 workers, reflecting an eight-year downward trend since the United States began collecting this information.

Although we may think of external impact on the human body as a workplace injury, many injuries are subtler. I remember diagnosing a patient with ulnar neuropathy three months after she had been issued an expensive ergonomic chair with armrests. I suggested she either get rid of the chair or at least remove the armrests. Within two months after she removed the armrests, the ulnar neuropathy resolved. Physicians treat many work-related injuries that do not warrant loss of work. Consequently, there may be considerably more work-related injuries than the statistic would reflect.

Health maintenance organizations (HMOs) and their managed care organizations (MCOs) may have further skewed the data. Physicians forced to make decisions rapidly to comply with organization rules will not be able to explore all the possible causes of an illness. Empirical treatment will be less focused and thus less effective. Minor injuries that normally would not require time away from work may progress into something major and disabling.

A medical interview can reveal the true source of an injury. For example, a patient who attributes back pain to the work environment may come to realize that it occurred on the weekend while doing yard work, lifting heavy furniture, or moving an aquarium. These correlations take time. A physician complying with the HMO or MCO is expected to see a patient every 12 or 15 minutes and may be unable to evaluate the exact causation. Lack of interview and examination time could falsely inflate the number of workplace injuries.

A worker's lifestyle can make it difficult to correlate an illness to the work environment. A smoker with asbestosis will be more likely to develop lung cancer than either a smoker without asbestosis or a nonsmoker with asbestosis. It becomes difficult, however, to say with certainty that a smoker has developed lung cancer due to industrial asbestos exposure. This is the assessment that most worker compensation evaluations must address.

It is the responsibility of the working people of America to understand safety and health issues related to their work environment and to take the appropriate precautions. They should also understand their health and safety rights. Workers have the right to refuse a job if they think it will create a potentially unsafe workplace condition. If they are discriminated against for refusing, they can report this to OSHA. Many laws, including the OSHA Act of 1970 and the Asbestos Hazard Emergency Response Act, have whistleblower protections.

Ada P. Kahn makes an excellent selection of the injuries and illnesses that occur in the workplace. She covers a wide variety of occupations and outlines the hazards and injuries unique to those occupations. Psychosocial issues such as burnout, bullying, and stress, which affect a worker's well-being, are addressed. Kahn interconnects the stress of one worker to the diagnosis of a fellow worker. For instance, a patient with AIDS in the workplace is not considered infectious. However, coworkers may experience anxiety or panic attacks if they become aware of that diagnosis. These contempo-

rary issues are alphabetically tabulated for easy reference in this readable, user-friendly compendium of 600 entries. It describes many conditions that physicians see every day, including physical and emotional disorders. Preventive measures are also included in some instances.

This book is not intended to provide complete information on any one topic. Instead, this reference is designed for individuals who want an overview of work-related issues. Kahn's earlier books for Facts On File, *The Encyclopedia of Mental Health, The Encyclopedia of Phobias, Fears and Anxieties,* and *Stress A–Z,* have become popular among both professional and lay readers. *The Encyclopedia of Work-Related Illnesses, Injuries, and Health Issues* will also be an important volume for professionals in many fields, including health care, human resources, employee benefits, insurance carriers, employee assistance programs, librarians, and others. It gives the type of information employers and employees frequently need.

—Del Meyer, M.D.
HealthCareCommunication Network
Volunteer Clinical Faculty
UC Davis School of Medicine
Pulmonary Medicine
Sacramento, California

ACKNOWLEDGMENTS

Compilation of this encyclopedia was possible because of detailed information collected and made available by many government agencies, research centers and universities, health and trade associations, and journals in diverse fields, including industrial hygiene, safety, public health, health care, and human resources. Sources are appropriately cited in relevant entries.

Work on the book was facilitated by assistance from many skilled and knowledgeable reference librarians in the Evanston Public Library, Evanston, Illinois; the Skokie Public Library, Skokie, Illinois; the Winnetka-Northfield Public Library, Winnetka, Illinois; and the North Suburban Library System of Illinois.

Participation in this endeavor by Delbert H. Meyer, M.D., is appreciated.

—Ada P. Kahn, Ph.D.
Evanston, Illinois

INTRODUCTION

This encyclopedia emphasizes the need for worker safety in all fields and protection against health hazards wherever they may be. It underscores the economic consequences of health and safety issues that may be neglected in the workplace. Workplace injuries, illnesses, and health issues are a continuing public health concern. The World Health Organization (WHO) reports that each year, an estimated 160 million new cases of work-related diseases occur worldwide, and work-related injuries and illnesses kill an estimated 1.1 million people. According to a report in 2000, approximately 5,915 job-related injuries led to death, and other accidents produced approximately 13 million nonfatal injuries in the United States.

Costs of these workplace deaths, injuries, and illnesses are a tremendous financial drain on American industries, businesses, and insurers. Estimates are that the total direct and indirect costs associated with these workplace injuries and illnesses were $155.5 billion, or about 3 percent of the gross domestic product (GDP). Direct costs include expenses for health insurance, physicians, hospitals, and medications. For employees, direct costs involve lost wages and indirect costs include money spent on household services while the employee is incapacitated as well as transportation costs to medical and rehabilitative appointments. For employers, direct costs include additional labor charges and indirect costs include workplace disruption and downtime associated with the hiring and training of workers.

Contemporary issues in workplaces range from safety and ergonomic hazards to biological hazards, including the importance of hazard awareness, communicating hazard prevention, identifying dangerous materials, identifying and improving risk communication, improving indoor air quality, detecting toxic mold, increasing workplace security and prevention of violence, workplace ethics, confidentiality, screening for drug use, psychosocial issues, needs of special populations, and communicating with workers for whom English is not the first language.

Because a tremendous economic loss is associated with workplace injuries, illnesses, and lost time, there is increasing emphasis on safety and promoting good health among workers. Regulatory controls in the United States promulgated by many organizations, including the Occupational Health and Safety Administration (OSHA) and the National Institute of Safety and Health (NIOSH) have contributed considerably to increasing the safety of workers.

What characteristics are associated with job-related injuries and illnesses? The most frequent disabling injuries are to the back. Accidents involving heavy vehicles, industrial equipment, aircraft, boats and railroads contributed to about 40 percent of all work-related deaths. According to the study *Costs of Occupational Injuries and Illnesses* (University of Michigan Press, 2000), job experience correlated with disability injuries, as new employees experienced a disproportionately high number of injuries.

Who pays for workers' illnesses and injuries? Employers absorb some of this burden in high insurance costs and lower profits; workers absorb much of the costs in insurance premiums and lost wages. Additionally, costs are borne by insurers, including Workers' Compensations, Social Security, Medicare, and Medicaid, as well as other government entities. There can be significant cost savings to employers and workers from preventing injury and illness and from promoting workplace safety and well-being.

American society has evolved from a manufacturing economy to a service economy, and many workplace issues are different than those of 50 years ago. Many employees now work for small employers without updated safety programs. Among some employers, occupational health and safety activities are outsourced and reports do not include viewpoints and input from workers on the scene. One of the fastest growing sectors in employment today is temporary help. Often temporary agencies have poor control of safety practices in jobsites their workers are assigned to.

Workplaces have changed markedly in the last 50 years. Today many workplaces, particularly offices, look alike. For example, a reservations department in a hotel and an accounting office in a trucking business may look alike. Many people have similar work environments, with a cubicle, a desk and chair, and computer equipment, even though their job descriptions differ. Because of standardized processes in office work, people across many different industries can develop similar injuries, such as repetitive stress injuries and video display terminal difficulties.

There has been more outsourcing of jobs since the 1980s and 1990s, and no longer do many people have long relationships with one employer or group of coworkers. The support of coworkers is missing for many employees. Also, many people who work in home-based offices or in remote locations, away from their employer, have little opportunity for socialization or camaraderie with fellow employees.

Another change in today's workplace is demographics: Many workers are older. Baby boomers increasingly remain in the workforce, some taking a new career path in midlife. Healthy older workers provide employers with proven experience and track records of productivity. Still, there is age discrimination, as well as some concern about older workers' health, possibly their newness in the field of work, and possibility for injuries and ensuing health care costs.

Job descriptions according to gender have been legally replaced with descriptions according to ability to work. However, gender issues still abound in subtle and not-so-subtle ways in many of today's workplaces. Years ago, occupations such as heavy construction and roadwork were generally limited to men. Now, legal hiring practices in most instances demand equal opportunity for all. Gender issues include equal pay for equal work, concern for day care of children, and in some places, day care for elderly parents, and family leave. Employers vary in their approach to these issues.

Another contemporary workplace issue relates to ethics regarding employees' health information. Employees have a right to privacy concerning their medical information. There is concern that information from health records, pre-employment physicals, periodic screenings or health monitoring programs, or personnel files may be used for selective practices, such as in hiring or assigning work. At the same time, employers need information on working conditions and their employees' health to promote preventive measures and protect other employees exposed to the same risks in the workplace.

Boundaries between workplace life and private life are less clear today. This is because many worksite programs screen for drug use or HIV seropositivity and many programs provide assistance to employees with alcoholism or domestic violence situations. Employees may be concerned that their need for and obtaining of guidance from Employee Assistance Programs may become known to their employers and may be used against them in the future.

According to the International Code of Ethics for Occupational Health Professionals, "Occupational health professionals must always act, as a matter of priority, in the interests of the health and safety of the workers." While it is the right of the employee to be protected from hazards at work, an employer may experience a conflict between costs of improving safety and concern for the worker. To reduce such conflicts, governments, particularly in the United States and other Western nations, have established regulatory agencies that enforce laws regarding worker safety. However, not all worksite accidents and injuries are reported, and in some instances, hazards go unrelieved. Often, small businesses with few employees may be exempt from some regulations.

Laws in the United States protect workers against sexual harassment. Yet harassment is a source of stress that can threaten a worker's psychological integrity as well as physical security. The worker may have little control of the situation, and out of fear of retaliation, negative evaluation, or losing the job, may not report incidents.

Violence in the workplace ranges from verbal abuse by supervisors to shooting of coworkers. Factors contributing to violence at work range from low self-esteem, aggressive personalities, drug abuse, or domestic difficulties, to job dissatisfaction and unjust management or extremely unfavorable physical working conditions.

Gender issues, age of workers, and sexual harassment contribute to a psychosocial atmosphere in today's workplace that can cause stress for many. According to Herbert Benson, M.D., author of The *Relaxation Response,* approximately 80 percent of visits to physicians are stress-related. Reducing sources of stress in the workplace can contribute to healthier workers and reduce health care costs to employers.

Good health in the workplace includes a balance between mind, body, and spirit. Good workplace safety practices encourage good health because physical illness or injury influences mental health and workers' attitudes toward supervisors, coworkers, and jobs. This book includes many entries on mental health and complementary medicine, as well as entries on mind/body connections, tips for coping with stress, and useful relaxation techniques. Good mental health enables a worker to engage in productive activities, maintain fulfilling relationships, and cope with adversity and adapt to change. Mental health can directly affect physical health. Research has shown that an optimistic attitude can affect the immune system and contribute to good health. In contrast, depression can lower immune system activity and possibly invite physical illness.

Historically, in Western nations, there has been tremendous progress in protecting workers' health due to attitudes of social justice. However, substandard and unhealthful conditions still exist worldwide, even in overseas factories and facilities to which American companies send work. While investors focus on profits, human rights advocates look at workers' health and working conditions. More attention needs to be focused on improving conditions wherever people of all ages work.

A chart in the Appendix lists known carcinogens as identified by the National Institute of Occupational Safety and Health (NIOSH). Other government and national organizations have compiled similar listings, and not all are in agreement with each other. Readers will note that many entries refer to chemicals, carcinogens, and other hazards in the workplace that may cause illness or injury. However, just because such substances or hazards have been known to cause illness or injury in some instances, it often cannot be said with any degree of certainty that a worker's illness is directly related to an exposure in the workplace. Diverse factors contribute to most illnesses, such as lifestyle, a history of smoking, family history, use of drugs and alcohol, previous work exposures, gender, and age.

Statistics regarding health issues in the workplace are compiled by many sources, including government agencies, university researchers, trade associations, unions, and other organizations. Statistics cited in specific entries in the encyclopedia are often from a single source; diligent readers and researchers are advised to seek additional reports compiled from other perspectives. In that regard, the resource list in the Appendix may be helpful but is not, and cannot be, an exhaustive list of all the information that is presently available.

This book was compiled as a handy, easy-to-read reference for librarians, human resource departments, industrial hygiene departments, workers in a wide range of jobs, employers, and many other readers. Curious readers can use entries in this volume to orient themselves and perhaps explore certain areas further. To that end, we hope this book will provide a useful first step on the path toward understanding what some working individuals and their employers face. In the interest of producing a book of manageable size, many terms, occupations and industries were not included (particularly medical and legal aspects) because they are well described in other reference books and texts.

We encourage readers to utilize the extensive list of resources and the Bibliography in the Appen-dix at the end of this volume in search of information on various aspects of workplace safety, injuries, illnesses, and health issues.

—Ada P. Kahn, Ph.D.
Evanston, Ill.

absenteeism   Failure of employees to report for work when they are scheduled to work. Absenteeism affects productivity and incurs administrative costs. Frequent absence from work may be related to many factors, including:

- Serious accidents and illness
- Low morale, boredom
- Lack of job satisfaction
- Poor leadership or supervision
- Lack of recognition by superiors
- Role conflict (particularly with peers)
- Deadlines
- Job unsuitability
- Concerns about job security and career paths
- Poor health, poor nutrition, and poor physical fitness
- Transportation problems
- Stress
- Workload

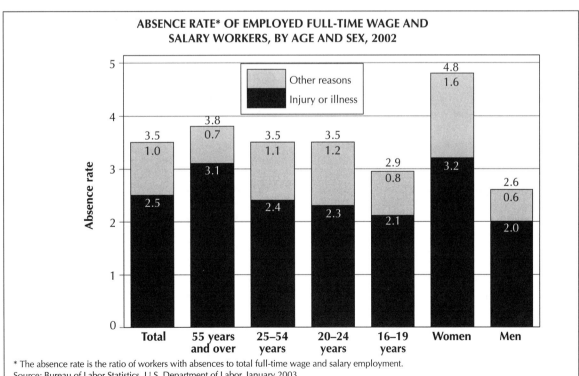

ABSENCE RATE* OF EMPLOYED FULL-TIME WAGE AND SALARY WORKERS, BY AGE AND SEX, 2002

* The absence rate is the ratio of workers with absences to total full-time wage and salary employment.
Source: Bureau of Labor Statistics, U.S. Department of Labor, January 2003

Costs of Absenteeism

A major cost of absenteeism is a decrease in productivity. With coworkers absent, others may be carrying an extra workload or supporting new or replacement staff. Employees may be required to train and give orientation to new or replacement workers. Staff morale and customer service may suffer.

Financial costs to the employer involve payment of overtime, cost of self-insured income protection plans, plus the costs of replacement employees. Premium costs may rise for insured plans. Administrative costs include staff time necessary to obtain replacement employees or to reassign the remaining employees.

Absenteeism Trends

According to the U.S. Department of Labor, in 1998 about 4 percent of full-time workers were absent from their job during an average workweek, meaning they worked less than 35 hours during the week because of injury, illness, or other reasons. About 5.1 percent of women were absent in the average week, compared with 2.7 percent of men. Among those absent, women were somewhat more likely to be absent for reasons other than injury or illness. One third of women's absences compared with less than one-quarter of men's absences were attributed to other reasons.

Absence rates vary somewhat by age. Younger workers are absent more frequently than older workers, but the latter are absent for longer periods of time.

Surveys have indicated that the higher the rate of pay and the greater the length of service of the employee, the fewer the absences. Women are absent more frequently than men, and single employees are absent more frequently than married employees.

Overcoming Absenteeism

Because poor health is a major cause of absenteeism, many corporations have established health promotion programs such as health examinations, health risk appraisals, and EMPLOYEE ASSISTANCE PROGRAMS (EAPs) and worksite wellness programs such as weight control, smoking cessation, exercise, and stress reduction.

See also DAY CARE; MENTAL HEALTH; STRESS; WORKING MOTHERS; WORKSITE WELLNESS PROGRAMS.

accidents Incidents caused by hazards in the workplace. Some types of accidents include:

- Machinery accidents
- Transportation accidents
- Overexertion or overstrenuous movements
- Falls (slips, trips on the level, from heights, from a moving vehicle)
- Falls of heavy objects, materials, wall collapses
- Stabs, cuts, amputations
- Striking against or being struck by objects (bone fractures, bruises)
- Stepping on objects
- Being caught in or between objects, including crushing and tearing accidents
- Pressure vessels, vacuum vessels (bursting, mechanical explosions or implosions)
- Burns and scalds (by hot or cold fluids or surfaces)
- Penetration by foreign particles in the eyes
- Drowning
- Acute injuries caused by animals (such as bites, scratches, kicks, squeezing and trampling, stings, and so on)

Chemical accidents include all acute injuries and effects related to accidental release, spillage, inhalation, swallowing of, or contact with chemical agents (except fire or explosions).

Electrical accidents include all injuries and effects related to electric current and static electricity.

Other accident hazards include fires and chemical explosions and radiation accidents involving accidental exposure due to high doses of ionizing and non-ionizing radiation, including laser beams and ultraviolet rays.

See also EYE INJURIES; FIRE/FIRE SAFETY PROTECTION; FOOT PROTECTION; HAND PROTECTION; NATIONAL SAFETY COUNCIL; PERSONAL PROTECTIVE EQUIPMENT.

acculturation   A process associated with getting acquainted with a new job or new situation, particularly for people who come from another culture. In situations where there are linguistic or cultural communication barriers or an individual's expectations are not congruent with what takes place, stress can increase. As reported in an editorial, "Physicians and Immigrant Patients," by Andrew Cave, et al, in *Canadian Family Physician* (Vol. 41: October 1995, pp. 1685–1690) the anxieties of the immigration experience are compounded particularly for individuals whose future working and residency status is in question.

There may be behavioral changes, such as increasing alcohol and tobacco consumption following immigration. When different family members become accustomed to the new culture at different rates, conflicts can arise between the generations, adding to the overall anxiety. Increasingly, mental health workers in the Western workplace see immigrant patients from ethnic backgrounds that do not use the Western medical model. Some of these patients see Western medicine as one of many healing systems. Cultural expectations can cause anxieties for both physicians and patients. For example, some East Indian women cannot allow pelvic examination by male physicians, even those from their own culture. Because such examination can be construed as grounds for divorce, the relatively simple procedure of a physical examination becomes both a cultural and a medical issue.

See also COMPLEMENTARY THERAPIES; MENTAL HEALTH; PERSONAL SPACE; STRESS.

Kahn, Ada P., and Jan Fawcett. *Encyclopedia of Mental Health.* 2d ed. New York: Facts On File, Inc., 2001.

Achilles injury/tendinitis   An inflammation of the largest tendon in the body. The Achilles tendon connects the gastrocnemius and soleus muscles to the heel and transfers the force of their contractions to lift the heel. Achilles tendinitis is an inflammation of the tendon and is a prime symptom of an overuse injury. The most common cause is excessive pronation of the ankle and foot, which cause the Achilles tendon to pull off-center. This condition may also be due to stress from frequent jumping, like that performed by basketball players. This group is often afflicted with Achilles tendinitis.

Achilles rupture, or rupture of the Achilles tendon, is often experienced by professional athletes. When the player steps or lunges and feels a snap at the back of the calf, the snap may sound like a bone breaking. A complete tear of the Achilles tendon is thought to be due to an accumulation of frequent small tears or inflammations that have weakened the tendon. Scar tissue may build up around the tendon, and swelling may be apparent above the heel.

See also BASKETBALL INJURIES; FOOT PROTECTION.

Levy, Allan M., and Mark L. Fuerst. *Sports Injury Handbook.* New York: John Wiley & Sons, 1993.

Acoustical Society of America (ASA)   An organization founded in 1929 of nearly 7,000 men and women who work in acoustics in the United States and abroad. Many fields related to sound are represented, including physics; nearly all engineering disciplines, including electrical-mechanical, civil, and aeronautical; robotics and computer science; biology and physiology; architecture; speech and hearing; music, noise and noise control and structural acoustics and vibration. Members have been involved since the society's inception with development of acoustical standards and criteria for determining the effects of noise and vibration. The society works closely with the AMERICAN NATIONAL STANDARDS INSTITUTE (ANSI).

The society publishes the *Journal of the Acoustical Society of America (JASA).* Additionally, it reprints out-of-print texts in acoustics.

For further information:

Acoustical Society of America (ASA)
2 Huntington Quadrangle
Suite 1NO1
Melville, NY 11747-4502
(516) 576-2360
www.asa.aip.org
(516) 576-2377 (fax)

See also HEARING LOSS; NOISE.

acquired immunodeficiency syndrome (AIDS)
AIDS is a debilitating disease caused by the human

immunodeficiency virus (HIV) that leads to many opportunistic infections, many types of cancer and in many cases, death. Since the early 1980s, more than 816,149 cases of AIDS and nearly 468,000 AIDS deaths have been reported to the U.S. Centers for Disease Control and Prevention. Of those, 666,026 cases have been in males and 141,048 in females. Between 650,000 and 900,000 Americans are currently living with HIV infection, while there are thought to be 40 million cases worldwide. Already an estimated 22 million worldwide have died from this disease. Each year, new therapies are developed, but as of 2003, there is no cure and no vaccine for prevention.

According to the American College of Occupational and Environmental Medicine, the population hardest hit is in the 25–49-year-old age bracket, indicating a substantial impact on the American workplace. HIV and AIDS continue to create sensitive medical, social, and political issues for the workplace. Employers and infected individuals face concerns while the afflicted try to remain occupationally productive. As more AIDS patients benefit from newer and more highly effective therapy, more are physically able to return to work.

Understanding AIDS

The word *acquired* sets AIDS apart from some similar conditions that are due to hereditary or genetic factors. AIDS is caused by a virus that has been given a number of names by scientists but is now officially known simply as HIV, for human immunodeficiency virus. The virus is found by blood testing, and a diagnosis of AIDS depends on test results plus specific evidence of associated illness. Evidence of infection with the virus may also be found in people who have no signs of illness and do not feel sick at all; these people are said to be HIV positive.

According to the American Lung Association, new antiviral drugs have been successful in controlling the infection. However, it is possible that most persons who are HIV positive will eventually develop AIDS. This process may take many years, during which the person may remain essentially productive, healthy and free of symptoms, although an HIV-positive person who is not ill can still pass the virus on to someone else.

Some viruses, such as those causing colds and influenza, are very contagious and easily given to another person. The AIDS virus is not. It is reassuring to fellow employees and employers to know that an individual can acquire HIV only by body fluids (such as semen or blood) from an infected person entering one's own body. AIDS cannot be caught from another person by working together, sharing a meal, or shaking hands.

If an employee is infected with AIDS, it is important for him or her to know it. The knowledge will help prevent the spread of AIDS, since the individual can take precautions against passing the virus on to others. Also, the person who is HIV positive can take steps to protect his or her own health, including using new treatments. Finally, while no cure for AIDS has yet been found, there are drugs that seem to slow down the virus and prolong life.

What Are Opportunistic Infections?

An opportunistic infection takes advantage of the fact that the body's normal defenses are down, giving it an opportunity to cause disease. *Opportunistic* describes an infection that probably would not occur if the individual were not infected with HIV (or suffering from some other condition that might cause lowered resistance to disease).

According to the American Lung Association, many disease-causing agents can trigger opportunistic infections in a susceptible person. While such agents are common in the environment, they generally do not cause disease because a healthy immune system disposes of them before they cause problems. One example often seen in AIDS patients is pneumocystic carinii pneumonia (PCP), a form of pneumonia that is otherwise extremely rare. An opportunistic infection may also be one that is present in latent form (not causing active disease), but that does not flare up into actual disease until the immune system is weakened. An example is TUBERCULOSIS (TB). Starting in the mid-1950s, the number of TB cases in the United States dropped steadily—until 1986, when the trend was reversed. It appears that the increase may have been due in part to the AIDS epidemic. Since the mid-1990s, there has been a downturn, probably because of new efforts at control.

Untreated active tuberculosis can be spread from person to person, and a person with or without AIDS can catch TB from someone who has untreated, active tuberculosis. Other pulmonary infections cannot be relayed from one person to another. For example, pneumocystic carinii pneumonia is not likely to be transmitted from person to person.

The American Lung Association recommends that a person who has AIDS or who is HIV positive be alert for respiratory symptoms such as coughing or shortness of breath, as well as any other symptoms (such as fever or chills) that may suggest active infection. A person experiencing such symptoms should seek medical care quickly.

Historical Background

The AIDS epidemic was recognized between 1981 and 1984. Many people discovered their illness for the first time in emergency rooms when AIDS-defining conditions were diagnosed. Before 1986 HIV testing was not generally available except to a few people enrolled in research studies. Then the picture changed somewhat. The drug AZT has been available since 1987. Other new and powerful treatments for opportunistic infections were subsequently approved. The treatment of infections became more sophisticated and more effective during the latter part of the 1980s and during the 1990s, giving persons with AIDS a more positive outlook.

How AIDS Can Affect Workers

Because people may be infected and not know it, and because symptoms may lie dormant for years, it is easy for a person to worry that he or she might have AIDS. Some individuals, especially hypochondriacs, homosexual men, and needle users, may experience ANXIETY or *panic attacks,* and even some minor, superficial symptoms that mimic AIDS. They may feel certain they are dying and become obsessed with details of the disease or the thought of having to face the stigma it continues to carry. Further, obsessive worries are common in populations at risk (which include women) and sometimes even more so in people not at risk who fear contracting the disease unknowingly.

People who fear AIDS may reduce their sexual contacts, have less interest in sexual activity, or have sexual difficulties, may stop participating in activities of the gay community, may feel depressed or anxious for no obvious reason, and may have sleeplessness, nightmares, or loss of appetite. To alleviate these fears, individuals should know that they are not alone with these fears, get a complete medical check-up, practice safe sex, and if they are drug users, be sure to use clean needles. Educational materials, available from health clinics and civic health departments, can also be helpful.

Because AIDS is transmitted through exchange of bodily fluids, including blood, drug users who share needles, persons receiving or donating blood, and health care workers are concerned about the disease. With proper precautions, risks to health care workers and persons receiving blood transfusions are minimal; risks to blood donors are virtually nonexistent.

Psychological Reactions to Diagnosis

Individuals may experience intense grief, heartbreak, and uncertainty when they learn that they have AIDS. They fear the loss of their jobs, loss of freedom to live each day without the threat of sudden illness, and loss of freedom to make plans for the future. Individuals may experience feelings of loss long before physical symptoms begin. In the early stages of disease, infected persons may wonder how long it will take to become ill, whether they will have to give up their jobs, whether they will experience pain, what treatments will be available for them, who will take care of them, and how they can maintain hope in the face of such great uncertainty.

ANGER is often a major reaction to the discovery that one is HIV positive. The anger may be directed at possible sources of infection, such as blood banks, past sexual partners, or needle-sharing friends, or it may be directed at oneself for perceived irresponsible behavior. However, anger can also contribute to a "fighting spirit" that some people with AIDS consider the explanation for their continued psychological and physical survival.

Family, Friends and Coworkers:
Disclosure and Support

For people who discover they are HIV positive through an antibody or blood test, there is usually no urgency about disclosure (except to sex- or needle-sharing partners). However, if one is hospitalized for an infection associated with AIDS, family, friends, and coworkers are likely to find out. Disclosure is usually a highly charged topic. When others learn about one's HIV status, they may react with varying degrees of shock and disbelief. Many people do not know how they should act or what they should say. Some people may avoid the infected person, or they may become overly solicitous. Usually coworkers need time to adjust to the news. Family and friends are understandably sad, angry, even distraught when they learn a loved one has HIV illness. However, it is important for coworkers and friends to express reassurance that the relationship will remain unchanged.

During acute illness, after hospital discharge, or when illness becomes chronic, the question of providing practical assistance arises. People may truly need help but do not want to acknowledge or accept it. Friends can be most helpful by making it clear that they are not "taking over," but merely doing whatever the ill person indicates is important to him or her. Friends or coworkers can let it be known that they are available for specific tasks, such as providing transportation for medical attention, shopping, delivering meals, or cooking.

An Employee's Relationship with Health Professionals

The primary doctor-patient relationship can provide constancy and comfort, as well as uncertainty. For people with AIDS, the association with a caring physician may become one of the patient's most enduring and emotionally intimate connections. Rabkin, Remien and Wilson, in their book *Good Doctors, Good Patients,* suggest that a successful relationship means shared expectations, good communication, and satisfaction about their collaboration at all stages of illness. Demands upon physicians and patients require flexibility, initiative, and courage to make difficult decisions.

Physicians and patients as well as employers have considerably different attitudes in the 2000s than in earlier years about prospects of survival and the possibilities for continuing to work after diagnosis. Before 1987 many patients were told that they had only six months to a year to live. In the

early 2000s an AIDS diagnosis no longer means imminent demise. Now, many infected persons lead reasonably healthy lives and continue to work when using medications.

Because occupational and environmental medicine physicians play a pivotal role in dealing with issues surrounding AIDS, the American College of Occupational And Environmental Medicine (ACOEM), an international medical society of more than 60,000 occupational and environmental physicians, developed the *HIV and AIDS in the Workplace Guideline.* The guideline addresses general issues and the role the OEM physician should play within the context of the Americans with Disabilities Act of 1990 and recommendations regarding issues specific to the health care industry, including infected health care workers, exposure prevention, and prophylactic therapy. "The OEM physician should be actively involved in developing institutional policies that address AIDS and HIV in the workplace," said Mark Russi, M.D., lead author and chair of the ACOEM Infectious Diseases Committee, which developed the guideline. "They should serve as a resource to provide advice as needed to both employers and employees and be prepared to respond to HIV- or AIDS-related medical problems with appropriate care."

The guideline also makes recommendations regarding the handling of sensitive medical information as well as the complexities of designing reasonable accommodations and evaluating the appropriateness of leaves under the Family and Medical Leave Act of 1993 (FMLA). Specifically, the guideline includes recommendations concerning the transmission of HIV from health care workers to patients, noting that accumulated evidence has found no basis to restrict the practice of HIV-infected health care workers who perform invasive procedures using appropriate precautions.

Worldwide Distribution of AIDS Patients

There is a growing gap between the developed and the developing world with respect to the scale of HIV spread as well as morbidity and mortality from AIDS. In North America, western Europe, Australia, and New Zealand, newly available antiretroviral drugs are reducing the speed at which

HIV-infected people develop AIDS. In most of these countries, substantial decreases in AIDS incidence have been observed since 1996. Additionally, early and targeted prevention programs were successful in reducing the number of HIV infections, especially in the high-risk groups in the mid- to late 1980s, further limiting the impact of the disease.

In less developed areas of the world, the number of new infections has reached dramatic levels and is still increasing in many regions. However, because of the long latency period between infection and the development of HIV-related diseases, the major impact of the disease is still to come, even if new infections could be reduced in the near future. Many HIV-infected persons in underdeveloped countries do not know about their HIV infection and very often do not have a chance to learn about it even if they would like to.

For information:

National AIDS Hotline (800) 342-2437
American College of Occupational and Environmental Medicine
American Lung Association

See also AIDS TREATMENT INFORMATION SERVICE; COMPLEMENTARY THERAPIES; ELISA TEST; HEALTH CARE WORKERS; HOSPITAL HAZARDS; HUMAN IMMUNODEFICIENCY VIRUS (HIV); LUNG DISEASES; NEEDLESTICK INJURIES.

Evans, Benjamin M. "Complementary Therapies and HIV Infection." *American Journal of Nursing* 99, no. 2, February 1999, pp. 42–45.
Kahn, Ada P., and Jan Fawcett. *Encyclopedia of Mental Health.* 2d ed. New York: Facts On File, Inc., 2001.
Over, Mead. "The Public Interest in a Private Disease: An Economic Perspective on the Government Role in STD and HIV Control." In King K. Holmes, Per-Anders Mardh, and P. Frederick Sparling, et al. *Sexually Transmitted Diseases.* 3d ed. New York: McGraw-Hill, 1999.
Rabkin, Judith G., Robert H. Remien, and Christopher R. Wilson. *Good Doctors, Good Patients: Partners in HIV Treatment.* New York: NCM Publishers, Inc., 1994.
Ungvarski, P. J., and J. H. Flaskerud. *HIV/AIDS: A Guide to Primary Care Management.* 4th ed. Philadelphia: Saunders, 1999.

actors   See PERFORMING ARTS MEDICINE.

acute beryllium disease   See BERYLLIUM.

acute solvent syndrome   See SOLVENTS.

addictions   Psychological dependence on a chemical substance or an activity. Some individuals develop addictions to alcohol, caffeine, tobacco, narcotics, or sedatives, many of which are prescribed by physicians. Other individuals develop addictions to gambling, stealing, or sexual activity. All of these addictions can interfere with an employee's health and productivity.

The term *substance abuse* (or *substance dependence*) has largely replaced the word *addiction* when referring to drug dependence. Employees suspected of substance dependence should be referred to an EMPLOYEE ASSISTANCE PROGRAM or other source for counseling.

Criteria for addiction include a compulsive craving leading to persistent use or repeated actions, a need to increase the dose or level or activity due to increasing tolerance, and possibly acute withdrawal symptoms if the drug is reduced or withdrawn abruptly, depending on the drug involved (alcohol, narcotics, barbiturates, and so on). Withdrawal symptoms alone do not necessarily imply addiction. However, physical dependence can develop with prolonged use of a drug, such as morphine for pain. Psychological dependence can involve a loss of control of the substance use and a tendency to orient behavior or life priorities toward obtaining the drug or pursuing the addictive behavior.

Addiction Severity Index

Mental health professionals gather information about an individual's social, legal, and mental health problems, employment, drug and alcohol use, and other habits. Using the Addiction Severity Index, health professionals can assess the worker's function in each dimension independently at the beginning of treatment and later after treatment interventions.

Kahn, Ada P., and Jan Fawcett. *Encyclopedia of Mental Health.* 2d ed. New York: Facts On File, Inc., 2001.

aerospace medicine   A subdivision of preventive and emergency medicine. Aerospace medicine incorporates life support, physicians, and medicine to protect workers and passengers involved in aviation and space operations. The field includes civil aviation and military aviation, and space flight, as well as ground support personnel such as air traffic controllers and maintenance workers. Aeromedical evacuations are common and aerospace physicians are often the first to arrive at a crash scene.

Aviation medicine, the forerunner of aerospace medicine, began in World War I. As the space age developed, the specialty broadened significantly and became aerospace medicine as practiced today. Most aerospace medicine specialists are affiliated with the Federal Aviation Administration (FAA), the National Aeronautics and Space Administration (NASA), the airlines, the military services, the aerospace industry, or are in private consulting.

Aircrew Clearance for Aviation Duties

Aircrews must sometimes be evaluated for their ability to fly. When aircrew members are found to have medical conditions that might impair their flying performance, authorities evaluate aviators individually. Supervising agencies include the FAA and its aerospace physicians, various branches of the armed forces, and private sector aviation organizations. Civilian and military aviators are required to report new medical problems to their respective aviation medical authorities.

Usually a flight physician can clear an aviator to fly if there is a question. Clearing an aviator for flying duties requires special training and authority, according to John Ogle, M.D., of the Department of Emergency Medicine at Stanford University Medical Center. Aviators' motor, sensory, and mental functioning must be optimal and there must be no increased risk of sudden incapacitation. Sudden loss of function can be caused by conditions such as vasovagal syndrome, seizures, hypoglycemia, and malignant arrhythmias. There should be no impairment of hearing or visual ability, including linear and distant vision, depth perception, night vision, and color visual field.

Air Quality in Flight Cabins

Many aircrew members as well as air passengers have registered a broad spectrum of complaints, including nausea, vomiting, headaches, dizziness, and fatigue. Many believe that their symptoms are due to poor air quality and recirculated air in aircraft cabins. According to Russell B. Rayman in an article for *Jacksonville Medicine,* there have been several studies of tuberculosis (TB) transmission from passenger to passenger and flight attendant to flight attendant. Two cases of TB transmission were attributed to being in a closed space and in proximity to the index case rather than to the aircraft ventilation system.

However, several in-flight studies of pollutants, such as carbon monoxide, carbon dioxide, oxygen, respiratory particulates, ozone, and volatile organic compounds, have consistently demonstrated levels well below those set by regulatory agencies.

Microgravity

Astronauts from the United States and cosmonauts from Russia have traveled to outer space for more than 40 years. Some have logged more than one year in space. Scientists and flight surgeons have defined the physiological effects of microgravity and readaptation upon return to Earth. Studies are underway concerning artificial gravity so that future astronauts can remain in space for longer durations.

Flying Physicians Association

Members of the Flying Physicians Association are dedicated to promoting safety, education, research, and human interest projects relating to aviation. Members strive to increase safety and to preserve health by providing basic information through example and teaching to the medical profession, aircrews, and the public. They work toward better utilization of aircraft for emergency services, better cooperation with state and federal aviation agencies, better qualified aviation medicine examiners, and more significant research.

For information:

Flying Physicians Association
P.O. Box 677427
Orlando, FL 32867
(407) 359-1423
(407) 359-1167
www.fpadrs.org

Ogle, John. "Aerospace Medicine"
Rayman, Russell B. "Issues in Aerospace Medicine." *Jacksonville Medicine* (June 1998): 229–231.

affective disorders   Feelings of extreme sadness or intense, unrealistic elation with corresponding disturbances in mood that are not due to any other physical or mental disorder. Severe mood changes in an employee noted by supervisors should be reported to the human resource department or an EMPLOYEE ASSISTANCE PROGRAM so that help can be obtained for the individual as soon as possible.

Affective disorders differ from thought disorders. Schizophrenic and paranoid disorders are primarily disturbances of thought, although individuals who have those disorders may also have some distortion of mood or affect.

The death rate for individuals with chronically depressed moods is about 30 times as high as that for the general population because of the higher incidence of suicide. Manic individuals also have a high risk of death which can be attributed to their tendencies to exhaust themselves physically, to neglect their health, and to have accidents (often alcohol related) at the workplace and at home.

Types of Affective Disorders

Affective disorders can be subcategorized as major depression and bipolar disorders. These disorders can be acute or chronic; both are indicated by changes in the biologic, psychological, and sociological functioning of the individual. In some individuals, bipolar disorders and DEPRESSION occur according to a seasonal pattern, with a regular cyclic relationship between the onset of the mood episodes and particular seasons.

Manic episodes are distinct periods during which the individuals experiences a predominant mood that is either elevated, expansive, or irritable. Such individuals may have inflated self-esteem, increased energy, accelerated and loud speech, flight of ideas, distractibility, grandiose delusions, and decreased need for sleep. The disturbance may cause marked impairment in working, social activities or relationships; an episode may require that the affected person be hospitalized to prevent his harming himself or others. There may be rapid shifts of mood, with sudden changes to depression or anger. The mean age for the onset of manic episodes is in the early 20s, but many new cases appear after age 50.

Hypomanic episodes are mood disturbances less severe than mania, but they may be severe enough to cause several symptoms: marked impairment in judgment; financial, social, or work activities associated with increased energy and business; exaggerated self-confidence; hypertalkativeness; euphoria or increased sense of humor. Often not recognized as illness by others, these behaviors are nevertheless associated with hypomanic episodes. Hypomanic episodes may be followed by depressions of moderate to great severity.

Major Depressive Episodes

Major depression affects approximately 10 percent of the adult population. A major depressive episode includes either depressed mood or loss of interest or pleasure in all, or almost all, activities for at least two weeks. Associated symptoms may include feelings of worthlessness or excessive or inappropriate guilt, difficulty in concentrating, restlessness, appetite disturbance, change in weight, sleep disturbance, decreased energy, an inability to sit still, pacing, hand-wringing, and recurrent thoughts of death or of attempting suicide.

Depressive episodes are more common among females than among males. The average age of onset of depressive episodes is the late 20s, but a major depressive episode may begin at any age.

Bipolar disorders (episodes of mania and depression) are equally common in males and females. Bipolar disorder seems to occur at much higher rates in first-degree biologic relatives of people with BIPOLAR DISORDER than in the general population.

Cyclothymia involves numerous periods of hypomanic episodes and numerous periods of depressed mood or loss of interest or pleasure that are not severe enough to meet the criteria for bipolar disorder or major depressive episode.

Dysthymia involves a history of a depressed mood for at least two years that is not severe enough to meet the criteria for a major depressive episode. This is a common form of depression, and the person who has this condition may have periods of major depressive episodes as well.

Causes of Affective Disorders

There are many explanations for affective disorders, including psychoanalytic, interpersonal, cognitive, behavioral, learned helplessness, biologic, and genetic theories.

All these theories have commonalities categorized as biological, psychosocial, and sociocultural. Personality characteristics of some individuals, such as lack of self-esteem and negative views of themselves and their future predispose them to affective disorders. A stressful life event can also activate previously dormant negative thoughts.

Individuals who become manic generally are ambitious, outgoing, energetic, care what others think about them, and are sociable before their episodes and after remission. However, depressive individuals appear to be more anxious, obsessive, and self-deprecatory. They often are prone to feelings of self-blame and guilt. Depressed individuals tend to interact with others differently from the way manics do. For example, some manic individuals dislike relying on others and try to establish social roles in which they can dominate others. On the other hand, depressed individuals may take on a role of dependency and look to others to provide support and care. Feelings of hopelessness and helplessness are central to most depressive reactions. In severe depression, LEARNED HELPLESSNESS may occur, in which the individual sees no hope and gives up trying to cope with his or her situation.

Incidence of affective disorders is higher among relatives of individuals with clinically diagnosed affective disorders than among the general population, indicating a hereditary predisposition.

Biologic factors also play an important role. Research during the 1970s and 1980s explored the view that depression and manic episodes both may arise from disruptions in the balance of levels of brain chemicals called biogenic amines. Biogenic amines serve as neural transmitters or modulators to regulate the movement of nerve impulses across the synapses from one neuron to the next. Two such amines involved in affective disorders are norepinephrine and 5-hydroxytryptamine (serotonin). Some drugs are known to have antidepressant properties and to biochemically increase concentrations of one or the other (or both) of these transmitters.

In many individuals, psychosocial and biochemical factors work together to cause affective disorders. For example, stress has been considered as a possible causative factor in many cases. Stress may also affect the biochemical balance in the brain, at least in some predisposed individuals. Some individuals experience mild depressions following significant life stresses, such as loss of a job or the death of a family member. Other major life events, especially those involving reduced self-esteem, physical disease or abnormality, or deteriorating physical condition, may precipitate changes in mood.

Treatment of Affective Disorders

A variety of treatments, including pharmaceutical medications and BEHAVIOR THERAPY, are used to treat affective disorders. Some behavioral approaches, known as cognitive and cognitive-behavioral therapies, include efforts to improve the thoughts and beliefs (implicit and explicit) that underlie the depressed state. Therapy includes attention to unusual stressors and unfavorable life situations, and observing recurrence of depression.

Prescription medications used to treat affective disorders include antidepressants, tranquilizers, and antianxiety drugs. Lithium carbonate, a simple mineral salt, is used to control manic episodes and is also in some cases of depression where the underlying disorder is basically bipolar. For many individuals, lithium therapy is often effective in preventing cycling from depressive to manic episodes.

Support groups for affected individuals as well as their families are available in many areas.

For further information:

National Depressive and Manic Depressive Association

See also MENTAL HEALTH; NATIONAL INSTITUTE OF MENTAL HEALTH; NATIONAL MENTAL HEALTH ASSOCIATION; SELF-ESTEEM; SELF-HELP GROUPS; SUPPORT GROUPS; SEASONAL AFFECTIVE DISORDER; STRESS.

Kahn, Ada P., and Jan Fawcett. *The Encyclopedia of Mental Health.* 2d ed. New York: Facts On File, Inc., 2001.

AFL-CIO See AMERICAN FEDERATION OF LABOR-CONGRESS OF INDUSTRIAL ORGANIZATIONS.

age discrimination Adults from 55 to 65 years (and older) are often the first workers to go in business downsizings and mergers and overlooked as potential employees when applying for new jobs. Both of these factors constitute age discrimination. Age discrimination is usually defined by negative stereotypes depicting older adults as less productive than younger workers and unable to be trained in new technology. According to Patricia O'Toole in the May 1992 issue of *Lear's* magazine, during 1990 and 1991 the ranks of unemployed U.S. men and women between the ages of 45 and 54 grew by more than 50 percent to almost 1 million. Too young to retire, they are finding that employers consider them too old and too expensive to hire.

Despite the fact that there has been much research to disprove the stereotypes attributed to aging, they continue to influence judgments made concerning employment. Statistics have shown that workers age 40 and older take less time off than any other age group and are less accident-prone than younger workers. This age group has also experienced more massive changes in technology over their lifetimes than any past generation and are no less—if no more—adept at learning and using technology than those who are younger.

Middle-aged, midcareer adults in the 40 to 55 year age range who lose their jobs experience loss of income and benefits at a time when their families may still be young and in need of their support and protection. They are often the most rooted in their communities and unwilling to move. Even when they are willing to leave, they can have the most difficulty in breaking even on heavily mortgaged homes.

For those older adults in the 55 to 65-year-and-older range, loss of work may mean loss of health insurance and/or pension benefits at a time when they need them most.

In *Coping with Job Loss,* authors Carrie R. Leana and Daniel C. Feldman report these comments of workers laid off from the aerospace industry:

"Age and salary had a great deal to do with my job loss. My job was not eliminated—myself, along with several others, were replaced by people half our age. Simple economics." "I felt tossed aside, like an old shoe." "Old age is most definitely a drawback in seeking employment, no matter what the law says."

Corporations that have ignored the stereotypes and made a point of hiring older workers have said it pays. Since the 1990s, Travelers Property Casualty, an insurance company, has operated an in-house temporary service staffed mainly by its retirees, who need little training and are highly productive because of their knowledge of the company. At Days Inns, the over-50 recruits stay longer and learn faster than younger workers, slashing the company's hiring costs. Many other companies report huge savings when employing older adults.

See also DISCRIMINATION; RETIREMENT.

ageism   Discrimination in the workplace against someone on the grounds of age, particularly older workers. Those individuals may experience stress and anxiety because of seemingly unwarranted behavior toward them.

See also AGE DISCRIMINATION; STRESS.

Agency for Toxic Substances and Disease Registry (ATSDR)   An agency of the U.S. Department of Health and Human Services. The mission of the ATSDR is to serve the public by using science, taking responsive public health actions, and providing health information to prevent harmful exposures and disease related to toxic substances.

Directed by congressional mandate, the ATSDR performs specific functions concerning the effect on public health of hazardous substances in the environment. These functions include assessments of waste sites, health consultations concerning specific hazardous substances, health surveillance and registries, response to emergency releases of hazardous substances, and education and training concerning hazardous substances.

For information:

Agency for Toxic Substances and Disease Registry (ATSDR)
Division of Toxicology
1600 Clifton Road NE
Atlanta, GA 30333
(888) 422-8737 (toll free)
(404) 498-0057 (fax)
www.atsdr.cdc.gov

See also WASTE INDUSTRY.

Agent Orange An herbicide used by U.S. forces during the Vietnam War to defoliate forested areas to find enemy guerrilla forces. It was sprayed between January 1965 and April 1970 to strip away dense jungle foliage. Exposure to the defoliant has been linked with many illnesses among service people who were there at the time. Illnesses reported include chemical acne, non-Hodgkin's lymphoma, Hodgkin's disease and soft-tissue sarcoma. Afflicted veterans brought a class action suit against manufacturers of Agent Orange, which was settled out of court; a fund was established to compensate veterans and their families for any disabilities. Estimates are that more than 105,000 Vietnam veterans or their survivors filed claims. Agent Orange contains varying amounts of dioxin.

In 1996 President Clinton broadened protection for Agent Orange victims by ordering disability benefits for Vietnam veterans who suffer from prostate cancer or a nerve disease, peripheral neuropathy. These two diseases were added to seven other diseases previously declared eligible for disability benefits owing to Agent Orange exposure. They are: chloracne, Hodgkin's disease, multiple myeloma, non-Hodgkin's lymphoma, porphyria cutanea tarda, respiratory cancers (of the lung, bronchus, larynx, and trachea), and soft-tissue sarcoma.

See also CHEMICAL TOXICITY; ENDOCRINE TOXICITY; IMMUNOTOXICITY.

aggression A general term for a variety of behaviors that appear outside the range of what is socially and culturally acceptable in the workplace or elsewhere. Aggression includes extreme assertiveness, social dominance to the point of producing resentment in others, and a tendency toward HOSTILITY. Individuals who show aggression in the workplace may do so for many reasons, such as FRUSTRATION or as a compensatory mechanism for low SELF-ESTEEM. Aggression may be motivated by ANGER or overcompetitiveness, or directed toward harming or defeating others.

An individual with an aggressive personality may behave unpredictably at times. For example, such an individual may start arguments inappropriately with coworkers, and may harangue them. The individual may write angry letters to government officials or others with whom he or she has some quarrel.

The opposite of aggression is passivity. The term *passive aggression* relates to behavior that seems to be compliant but in which errors, mistakes, or accidents for which no direct responsibility is assumed results in difficulties or harm to others. A pattern of behavior such as making "mistakes" that harm coworkers is considered passive aggressive.

See also VIOLENCE.

Kahn, Ada P., and Jan Fawcett. *Encyclopedia of Mental Health*. 2d ed. New York: Facts On File, Inc., 2001.

agriculture See DUST; FARMING; MIGRANT WORKERS; VIBRATION WHITE FINGER.

AIDS See ACQUIRED IMMUNODEFICIENCY SYNDROME; HUMAN IMMUNODEFICIENCY VIRUS.

AIDSinfo A free telephone reference service for human resource personnel, health care providers, and people living with HIV disease. Many people find relief from some of the stresses of living with HIV disease when they get answers to their questions and sources for further information.

AIDSinfo is sponsored by the Agency for Health Care Policy and Research, Centers for Disease Control and Prevention, Health Resources and Services Administration, National Institutes of Health, and the Substance Abuse and Mental Health Services Administration. The service is offered through the Center for Disease Control National AIDS Clearinghouse.

Reference specialists answer questions about the latest treatment options, provide customized database searches, and direct callers to other HIV/AIDS information resources. Through the service, callers can acquire copies of the latest federally approved treatment guidelines, including recommendations for HIV counseling and voluntary testing for pregnant women, guidelines for prevention of opportunistic infections in persons infected with HIV, and study results concerning anti-HIV therapy which lowers the risk of AIDS and death in patients with intermediate-stage HIV disease.

In late 1995 the treatment service developed the *Glossary of HIV/Aids-Related Terms* to help people understand the technical terms related to HIV, its associated treatments, and the medical management of related conditions.

For further information:

AIDSinfo
P.O. Box 6303
Rockville, MD 20849
(800) HIV-0440
www.aidsinfo.nih.gov
email: contactus@aidsinfo.nih.gov

See also HUMAN IMMUNODEFICIENCY VIRUS.

air conditioner's lung (hypersensitivity pneumonitis)   A lung disease incurred by workers with air conditioning equipment as a result of allergens produced by molds and fungi.

See also ALLERGIES; FUNGI.

air pollution   A term that covers many different types of pollution, such as acid rain, smoke, smog, the greenhouse effect, particulates, radionuclides, and ozone layer depletion. Air pollution is a concern to employers because they must protect workers inside their manufacturing plants or other industries and they must protect the general public from fumes emanating from their places of business.

One type of air pollution is the release of particulates into the air from burning fuel for energy. Diesel smoke is a good example of particulate matter. This type of pollution is sometimes referred to as "black carbon" pollution. The exhaust from burning fuels in industries and automobiles is a major source of pollution in the air.

Another type of pollution is the release of noxious gases, such as sulfur dioxide, carbon monoxide, nitrogen oxides, and chemical vapors. These can take part in further chemical reactions once they are in the atmosphere, forming smog and acid rain.

Biological pollutants, including molds, bacteria, viruses, pollen, dust mites, and animal dander promote poor indoor air quality and may be a major cause of days lost from work. In office buildings, heating, cooling, and ventilation systems are frequent sources of biological substances that are inhaled, leading to breathing problems.

Environmental tobacco smoke (ETS) also called "secondhand smoke," a major indoor air pollutant, contains about 4,000 chemicals, including 200 known poisons, such as FORMALDEHYDE and CARBON MONOXIDE, as well as 43 CARCINOGENS. ETS causes an estimated 3,000 lung cancer deaths and 35,000 to 50,000 heart disease deaths in nonsmokers.

Formaldehyde is a common chemical found primarily in adhesive or bonding agents for many materials used in offices, including carpets, upholstery, particle board, and plywood paneling. The release of formaldehyde into the air may cause such health problems as coughing, eye, nose, and throat irritation, skin rashes, headaches, and dizziness.

ASBESTOS fibers are flexible, light, and small enough to remain airborne. They can be inhaled into the lungs and cause asbestosis (scarring of the lung tissue), lung cancer, and mesothelioma, a relatively uncommon cancer of the lining of the lung or abdominal cavity. Many asbestos products are found in workplaces, including roofing and flooring materials, wall and pipe insulation, heating equipment and acoustic insulation. These products are a potential problem indoors only if the asbestos-containing material is disturbed and becomes airborne, or when it disintegrates with age.

Heating systems and other appliances using gas, fuel, or wood can produce several combustion products, of which the most dangerous are carbon monoxide and nitrogen dioxide. Carbon monoxide is an odorless, colorless gas that interferes with the distribution of oxygen to the body. Depending on the amount inhaled, this gas can impede coordination, worsen cardiovascular conditions, and produce fatigue, headaches, confusion, nausea, and dizziness. Very high levels can cause death. Nitrogen dioxide is a colorless, odorless gas that irritates the mucous membranes in the eye, nose, and throat and causes shortness of breath after exposure to high concentrations. Prolonged exposure to high levels of this gas can damage respiratory tissue and may lead to chronic bronchitis.

Cleaning agents, pesticides, paints, and SOLVENTS may be sources of hundreds of potentially harmful chemicals. Such components in products can cause dizziness, nausea, allergic reactions, eye/skin/respiratory tract irritation, and cancer.

Air pollution has short- and long-term effects on health. Workers who have health problems such as asthma or heart and lung disease may also suffer more when the air is polluted. The extent to which an individual is harmed by air pollution usually depends on the total exposure to the damaging chemicals, the duration of exposure, and the concentration of the chemicals.

Short-term effects include irritation to the eyes, nose, and throat, and upper respiratory infections such as bronchitis and pneumonia. Other symptoms can include headaches, nausea, and allergic reactions. Short-term air pollution can aggravate medical conditions of those who have asthma and emphysema.

Long-term effects can include chronic respiratory disease, lung cancer, heart disease, and damage to the brain, nerves, liver, or kidneys. Research into the health effects of air pollution is ongoing. Medical conditions arising from air pollution are expensive in terms of health care costs and lost productivity in the workplace.

For further information:

American Lung Association

See also AMERICAN LUNG ASSOCIATION; CHEMICAL TOXICITY; CLEAN AIR ACT OF 1990; DUST AND DEBRIS; ENVIRONMENTAL PROTECTION AGENCY; INDOOR ENVIRONMENT; PARTICULATE MATTER; SICK BUILDING SYNDROME.

air quality controls   See ENVIRONMENT; ENVIRONMENTAL PROTECTION AGENCY; INDOOR ENVIRONMENT.

alcohol dependency   Estimates indicate that there are approximately 5 million alcohol-dependent persons in the United States. According to the American Psychiatric Association's *Diagnostic and Statistical Manual of Mental Disorders, Fourth Edition,* as many as 90 percent of adults in the United States have had some experience with alcohol, and a substantial number (60 percent of males and 30 percent of females) have had one or more alcohol-related adverse life events, such as driving after consuming too much alcohol or missing school or work due to a hangover.

Factors that lead many individuals to alcohol dependence include stress at work, personality, environment, and the addictive nature of alcohol. Many people become dependent on alcohol for relief of symptoms ranging from loneliness to ANXIETY and PANIC ATTACKS. Some agoraphobics become alcoholic as a way of coping with their fears. Because agoraphobic individuals do not go out, it is fairly easy for them to conceal their habit.

The term *alcoholism* was coined by Magnus Huss, a Swedish scientist, in 1852, when he identified a condition involving abuse of alcohol and labeled it *alkoholismus chronicus.* However, references to the problem are found in earlier works of Benjamin Rush, an 18th-century American physician, considered the "father of American psychiatry," and the Roman philosopher Seneca. In 1956 the American Medical Association and the American Bar Association officially recognized alcoholism as a disease, an action that affected the legal status of alcoholics, alcoholism-related state and federal laws, program financing, insurance coverage, and hospital admissions.

How Alcohol Affects the Body

Contrary to popular belief, alcohol is a depressant, not a stimulant. The effects of alcohol are felt most noticeably in the central nervous system. As sensitivity is reduced in the nervous system, the higher functions of the brain are dulled, leading to impulsive actions, loud speech, and lack of physical control. The drinker's face may turn red or pale. While drinking, the alcoholic loses any sense of guilt or embarrassment, gains more self-confidence, and loses inhibitions as the alcohol deadens restraining influences of the brain. Large quantities impair physical reflexes, coordination, and mental acuteness.

Symptoms and Stages of Alcoholism

In the first phase of dependence on alcohol, the heavy social drinker may feel no effects from alcohol. In the second phase, the drinker experiences memory lapses relating to events that happen during drinking episodes. In the third phase, there is lack of control over alcohol and the drinker cannot be certain of discontinuing to drink by choice. The final phase begins with long binges of intoxication, and there are observable mental or physical complications.

Behavioral signs may include absenteeism, tardiness, frequent change of jobs, hiding bottles, aggressive or grandiose behavior, irritability, jealousy, uncontrolled anger, repeated promises to self and others to give up drinking, neglect of proper eating habits and personal appearance. Physical signs may include unsteadiness, confusion, poor memory, nausea, vomiting, shaking, weakness in the legs and hands, irregular pulse, and redness and enlarged capillaries in the face. Alcohol-dependent persons are more susceptible than others to a variety of physical and mental disorders.

Dr. Chapman Walsh and colleagues reported on 200 problem drinkers at a large New England manufacturing plant. The study participants' drinking problems were identified by the company's EMPLOYEE ASSISTANCE PROGRAM (EAP) between February 1, 1982, and June 20, 1987. Each subject was followed for two years. Mean age of the subjects was 32 years. Subjects were overwhelmingly male (96 percent) and white (90 percent). About half (51 percent) graduated high school, but not college; 47 percent had annual family incomes of less than $25,000. The authors wrote:

> Of the 200 seriously impaired workers in the sample, only 15 percent recalled warning that their abuse of alcohol might be compromising their health during the year before being identified on the job. Fully 74 percent (148) of the workers identified on the job had seen physicians in that year, but only 22 percent of them recalled health warnings. That the manifestations of alcohol abuse are overt enough to bring these heavy drinkers to the attention of intervention programs at work during the course of the year in which they have visited physicians lends further weight to the argument that many physicians are not sufficiently alert to their patients' alcohol use and abuse.

Treatment for Alcoholism

Medical help for alcohol dependence includes detoxification, or assistance in overcoming withdrawal symptoms, and psychological, social, and physical treatments. Psychotherapy is usually done in groups, using a variety of techniques. Therapists for alcohol-dependent persons may be psychiatrists, psychologists, or social workers. Social treatments involve family members in the treatment process. Many alcohol-dependent persons benefit from involvement in self-help groups such as Alcoholics Anonymous.

Life Expectancy May Increase with Abstinence

Life expectancy may be improved by alcoholics who go dry, according to a study published in the *Journal of the American Medical Association* on January 4, 1992. Results of a study supported the notion that achievement of stable abstinence reduces the risk of premature death among alcoholics. Kim D. Bullock, Psychiatry and Research Services, Veterans Affairs Medical Center, San Diego, and colleagues reported on 199 men who had histories of at least five years of drinking at alcoholic levels. All were current or former patients of the Veterans Administration Alcoholism Treatment Program and/or members of Alcoholics Anonymous. The men were recruited from 1976 to 1987. Follow-up on relapse and mortality revealed that 101 men had relapsed and 98 were abstinent. A control group of 92 nonalcoholics equated for age, education, and sex were also studied for mortality. There were 19 deaths among the relapsed alcoholics compared with the expected number of 3.83. Among abstinent alcoholics there were four deaths. Alcoholic men who achieved stable abstinence did not differ from nonalcoholic men in mortality. However, alcoholics who relapsed died at a rate 4.96 times that of an age-, sex-, and race-matched representative sample.

Alcoholics Anonymous and Self-help

Alcoholics Anonymous is an international organization founded in 1935 that is devoted to maintaining the sobriety of its members and helping them control the compulsive urge to drink through self-help, mutual support, fellowship, and understanding. Medical treatment is not used. The program includes the individual's admission that he or she cannot control drinking, the sharing of experiences, problems, and concerns at meetings, and helping others who are in need of support.

At the core of the program is the desire to stop drinking. Members follow a 12-step program that stresses faith, disavowal of personal responsibility, passivity in the hands of God or a higher power, confession of wrongdoing, and response to spiritual awakening by sharing with others.

See also ADDICTIONS; CODEPENDENCY; CONTROL; STRESS.

Allan, Carole A. "Alcohol Problems and Anxiety Disorders: A Critical Review." *Alcohol and Alcoholism* 30, no. 2 (1995): 145–151.

American Psychiatric Association. *Diagnostic and Statistical Manual of Mental Disorders.* 4th ed. Washington, D.C.: American Psychiatric Association, 1994.

Caldwell, Paul Elliott, and Henry S. Cutter. "Alcoholics Anonymous Affiliation During Early Recovery." *Journal of Substance Abuse Treatment* 15, no. 3 (May–June 1998): 221–228.

Alcoholics Anonymous   See ALCOHOL DEPENDENCY.

alcoholism   See ALCOHOL DEPENDENCY.

Alexander technique   Method of realigning body posture for relief of chronic pain, muscle tension, and stress, and to increase well-being and health. With instruction from trained teachers, individuals learn how to eliminate common habits such as hunching, slouching, and tensing the spine as they work that lead to back, neck, or shoulder pain. Some practitioners of PERFORMING ARTS MEDICINE refer performers to Alexander technique practitioners.

The Alexander technique has a long history of helping musicians and singers perform with less likelihood of injury. Musicians do some of the most complex and demanding physical movements of any profession. Musicians face the challenge of performing the same complex muscular actions over and over again, often leading to REPETITIVE STRESS INJURIES. By helping musicians improve the quality of the physical movements involved in playing an instrument or singing, the Alexander technique also helps improve the quality of the musical sound itself. For example, a violinist's stiff shoulders and arms will get in the way of a pleasing sound; a singer's tight neck or jaw will cause the voice to become less resonant. By helping musicians release undue tension in their bodies, the technique makes possible a more fluid and lively performance. The technique also appeals to people suffering from orthopedic or neurological problems, joint pain, headaches, and fatigue.

The technique is taught in music and drama colleges worldwide, and due to its positive influence on coordination, is seen as an essential element in a performer's training. Athletes learn it to give them the awareness in their chosen activities.

The technique was developed by Frederick Matthias Alexander (1869–1955), a Shakespearean actor. He was born in Australia, moved to England, and after the outbreak of World War I, divided his time between England the United States. He established his first school for the technique in England in 1924.

Teachers of the Alexander Technique work with individuals to develop mindful involvement so that they learn to move, sit, stand, or walk in new ways to prevent imbalances caused by automatic habits. The technique teaches that the misuse of the body begins in the brain, where thoughts of carrying out an activity cause an unconscious interference with the reflex mechanism by which the thought is translated into action. Interferences are learned behaviors that people pick up unconsciously and that then become automatic. For example, after years of slumping in front of the computer, or inefficient posture while practicing a musical instrument, faulty kinesthetic awareness signals the brain that all is correct. Customary behaviors feel right even if they are inefficient or out of balance.

See also COMPLEMENTARY THERAPIES; BODY THERAPIES; MUSICIANS' INJURIES.

De Alcantara, Pedro. *Indirect Procedures: A Musician's Guide to the Alexander Technique.* Oxford, U.K.: Clarendon Press, 1997.

Stevens, Chris. *The Alexander Technique.* Rutland, Vt.: Charles E. Tuttle Company, Inc., 1994.

allergic alveolitis   See HYPERSENSITIVITY PNEUMONITIS.

allergies   A variety of bodily reactions caused by reactions to stimuli to which the individual has been sensitized. Allergies occur when the respiratory system is exposed to particles of DUST AND DEBRIS or pollen, or many other substances encountered in industry and manufacturing, or when the skin touches certain substances. Allergies are exaggerated reactions of the immune system and occur only on second or subsequent exposures to the offending agent, after the first contact has sensitized the body.

ASTHMA is caused by an allergic reaction and affects the lungs. Asthma afflicts some 10 million Americans, many of whom contracted their disease in the workplace.

See also SKIN OR SENSE ORGAN TOXICITY.

ambulance driver   One who drives sick, injured, or convalescent persons. The driver may place patients on stretchers and load the stretcher into the ambulance, usually with the help of assistants. The driver takes sick or injured persons to hospitals, convalescent facilities, or home, using knowledge and skill to avoid sudden motions detrimental to patients. Further tasks of the driver may include changing soiled linen on the stretcher and administering first aid as needed.

Accident hazards, according to the fourth edition of the *Encyclopedia of Occupational Health and Safety,* include increased risk of road accidents due to high driving speeds under emergency conditions, crossing intersections during red traffic lights, SLIPS, TRIPS, AND FALLS while carrying stretchers or assisting patients, and sudden release of compressed gases, such as oxygen or anesthetic gases inside the ambulance.

The driver is exposed to high NOISE levels from the emergency horn, and may be exposed to radioactive isotopes in places where ambulances are used for transporting radioisotopes to hospitals. Further, the driver is exposed to contagious diseases from patients, and potential exposure to body fluids of patients, and may experience dermatitis caused by excessive use of rinsing, cleaning, and disinfecting agents. The driver may suffer back pain and other musculoskeletal problems as a result of overexertion and faulty postures during lifting and moving patients, driving over bumpy roads, and repairing the vehicle on the road.

Ambulance drivers experience psychological stress due to dangerous driving under time pressure, contact with accident victims, terminal patients, and dead bodies, unusual working schedules, and prolonged states of alertness.

See also BACK INJURIES, BACK PAIN; DERMATITIS; STRESS.

Mager-Stillman, Jeanne. *Encyclopaedia of Occupational Health and Safety.* 4th ed. Vol. 4. Geneva: International Labor Organization, 1998. p. 1035.

American Cancer Society   See CANCER.

American College of Occupational and Environmental Medicine (ACOEM)   An organization representing more than 6,000 physicians specializing in the field of occupational and environmental medicine. Founded in 1916, ACOEM is the nation's largest medical society dedicated to promoting the health of workers through preventive medicine, clinical care, research, and education. Specialists in a variety of medical specialties develop positions and policies on vital issues relevant to the practice of preventive medicine both within and outside the workplace.

The ACOEM periodically issues position papers and committee reports with guidelines for a variety of workplace/environmental settings. These papers and reports cover topics such as spirometry, radon, environmental tobacco smoke, genetic screening, multiple chemical sensitivities, workplace drug screening, confidentiality of medical information, workers' compensation reform, and reproductive hazards.

Each spring, the college cosponsors the annual American Occupational Health Conference, the largest U.S. conference of its kind. (The American Association of Occupational Health Nurses is a cosponsor.) ACOEM publishes the monthly *Journal of Occupational and Environmental Medicine* and other publications.

For further information:

American College of Occupational and Environmental Medicine
1114 N. Arlington Heights Road
Arlington Heights, IL 60004
(847) 818-1800 ext. 368
http://www.acoem.org

American Conference of Governmental Industrial Hygienists (ACGIH)   A member organization and community of more than 5,000 professionals who advance worker health and safety through education and the development and dissemination of scientific and technical knowledge. For more than 60 years, ACGIH has provided information to government, academia, and corporate facilities throughout

America, Canada, and countries abroad. Information is provided to members and others in the industry through a monthly peer-reviewed journal, *Applied Occupational and Environmental Hygiene,* many professional conferences and seminars, and more than 400 technical and scientific publications.

For information:

American Conference of Governmental Industrial
   Hygienists (ACGIH)
1330 Kemper Meadow Drive
Cincinnati, OH 45240
(513) 742-2020
www.acgih.org

See also AMERICAN INDUSTRIAL HYGIENE ASSOCIATION; HEALTH PROMOTION; INTERNATIONAL OCCUPATIONAL HYGIENE ASSOCIATION.

American Federation of Labor–Congress of Industrial Organizations (AFL–CIO)   A voluntary federation of 66 national and international labor unions. Workers and unions have joined together to improve the lives of America's working families, bring fairness and dignity to the workplace and secure social and economic equity. The AFL-CIO represents 13 million working men and women, including teachers, teamsters, musicians, miners, firefighters and farmworkers, bakers and bottlers, engineers and editors, pilots and public employees, painters, laborers, and more.

The AFL-CIO reports numerous accomplishments, including:

- Negotiated with employers for better wages, health and retirement benefits, and ways to improve the quality of the products and services provided

- Won and preserved laws to end child labor and sweatshops and to make workplaces safer and healthier

- Achieved fairer treatment for workers of color, working women, workers with disability, and gay and lesbian workers—on the job and in society

- Championed support for a stronger public education system, the right of all children to receive a quality education and opportunities for learning throughout adulthood

- Given skills, energy, blood, and money to help neighbors in need. On and after the September 11, 2001, terrorist attacks in New York and at the Pentagon, union members rescued victims, provided emergency medical care, put out fires, cleared away the rubble, counseled survivors, and began to repair the damage

- Worked to shape trade policies that do not allow corporate competition in the global economy to lower the living standards of working families in the United States and other countries

- Created important opportunities for working people to make their voices heard by government, to gain decision makers' recognition and respect for the needs of working families, and to hold elected leaders accountable for their votes.

For information:

American Federation of Labor–Congress of Industrial Organizations
815 16th Street, NW
Washington, DC 20006
(202) 637-5000
(202) 637-5058 (fax)
www.alfcio.org

See also CHILD LABOR; HEALTH INSURANCE; INTERNATIONAL BROTHERHOOD OF TEAMSTERS; RETIREMENT.

American Industrial Hygiene Association (AIHA)   AIHA, the world's largest association of occupational and environmental health professionals, in existence since 1939, is the most diverse professional association dedicated to improving the well-being of workers, the community, and the environment. Its 12,300 members come from government, labor, academia, and business. AIHA provides information for industrial hygienists, occupational and environmental health and safety professionals, and consumers. A 16-member board of directors governs AIHA. More than 30 technical committees dealing with health, safety, and environmental challenges facing workers report to the board.

For further information:

American Industrial Hygiene Association
2700 Prospect Avenue

Suite 250
Fairfax, VA 22031
(703) 849-8888
(703) 207-3561 (fax)
www.aiha.org
infonet@aiha.org

See also HEALTH PROMOTION; INTERNATIONAL OCCUPATIONAL HYGIENE ASSOCIATION.

American Lung Association (ALA) The oldest voluntary health organization in the United States, with a national office and affiliate associations around the country. Founded in 1904 to fight tuberculosis, ALA today fights lung disease in all its forms, with special emphasis on asthma, tobacco control, and environmental health. Contributions from the public, along with gifts and grants from corporations, foundations, and government agencies, fund ALA.

The American Lung Association has many programs and strategies for fighting lung disease in the workplace and elsewhere. These include asthma education, tobacco control, air pollution, and advocacy programs. The ALA played a major role in the passage of the landmark federal Clean Air Act of 1990, as well as the law prohibiting smoking on domestic passenger airline flights.

ALA emphasizes reaching minority communities with health education and other programs to prevent and control lung diseases, as well as on supporting research in aspects of lung disease afflicting particular populations.

For information:

American Lung Association
1740 Broadway
New York, NY 10019
(800) LUNG-USA or (212) 315-8700
(212) 315-8872 (fax)
www.lungusa.org

See also ALLERGIES; ASBESTOS; ASTHMA; LUNG CANCER; OCCUPATIONAL LUNG DISEASE.

American Meat Institute The national trade association representing packers and processors of 70 percent of U.S. beef, pork, lamb, veal, and turkey products and their suppliers. The institute provides legislative, regulatory, and public relations service, conducts scientific and economic research, offers marketing and technical assistance and sponsors educational programs. Membership is open to any North American company that engages in the packing or processing of animal proteins.

For further information contact:

American Meat Institute
1700 North Moore Street
Suite 1600
Arlington, VA 22209
(703) 841-2400
(703) 527-0938 (fax)
www.meatami.org

See also BUTCHERS, MEAT, POULTRY, AND FISH CUTTERS.

American National Standards Institute (ANSI)
A private, nonprofit membership organization representing more than 1,000 public and private organizations, businesses, and government agencies. The ANSI administers and coordinates the U.S. voluntary standardization and conformity assessment system. ANSI seeks to develop technical, political, and policy consensus among various groups. ANSI accredits qualified groups to develop standards in their areas of technical expertise. There are more than 14,000 ANSI-approved standards in use today. ANSI standards cover an extensive range of factors facing workers in varied occupations and workplaces, including:

- Hazardous industrial chemicals
- Materials safety data sheets
- First aid measures
- Firefighting measures
- Accidental release measures
- Handling and storage
- Exposure controls and personal protection
- Toxicological information
- Ecological information
- Disposal considerations
- Transport information

ANSI is the official U.S. representative to the International Organization for Standardization (ISO). There are several ANSI publications: *ANSI Reporter* (quarterly), *ANSI Insider* (monthly) *Standards Action* (biweekly).

For information:

American National Standards Institute
1819 L Street, NW
Suite 600
Washington, DC 20036
(212) 642-4900
www.ansi.org

American Society of Safety Engineers (ASSE)

The oldest and largest professional safety organization. More than 30,000 members manage, supervise, and consult on safety, health, and environmental issues in industry, insurance, government, and education. ASSE has 12 practice specialties, 150 chapters, 56 sections, and 64 student sections.

For further information:

American Society of Safety Engineers
1800 East Oakton Street
Des Plaines, IL 60018
(847) 699-2929
(847) 768-3434 (fax)
customerservice@asse.org

See also SAFETY.

Americans with Disabilities Act

A law protecting the rights of disabled persons that took effect in July 1992. Title I of the Americans with Disabilities Act of 1990 prohibits private employers, state and local governments, employment agencies, and labor unions from discriminating against qualified individuals with disabilities in job application procedures, hiring, firing, advancement, compensation, job training, and other terms, conditions, and privileges of employment. An individual with a disability is a person who:

• Has a physical or mental impairment that substantially limits one or more major life activities

• Has a record of such an impairment or

• Is regarded as having such an impairment

A qualified employee or applicant with a disability is an individual who, with or without reasonable accommodation, can perform the essential functions of the job in question. Reasonable accommodation may include, but is not limited to:

• Making existing facilities used by employees readily accessible to and usable by persons with disabilities

• Job restructuring, modifying work schedules, reassignment to a vacant position

• Acquiring or modifying equipment or devices, adjusting modifying examinations, training materials, or policies, and providing qualified readers or interpreters

An employer is required to make accommodation to the known disability of a qualified applicant or employee if it would not impose an "undue hardship" on the operation of the employer's business. Undue hardship is defined as an action requiring significant difficulty or expense when considered in light of factors such as an employer's size, financial resources, and the nature and structure of its operation. An employer is not required to lower quality or production standards to make an accommodation, nor is an employer obligated to provide personal use items such as glasses or hearing aids.

Inquiries About Disability

Employers may not ask job applicants about the existence, nature, or severity of a disability. Applicants may be asked about their ability to perform specific job functions. A job offer may be conditioned on the results of a medical examination, but only if the examination is required for all entering employees in similar jobs. Medical examinations of employees must be job-related and consistent with the employer's business needs.

Drug and Alcohol Abuse

Employees and applicants currently engaging in the illegal use of drugs are not covered by the ADA when an employer acts on the basis of such use. Tests for illegal drugs are not subject to the ADA's restrictions on medical examinations. Employers may hold illegal drug users and alcoholics to the same performance standards as other employees.

Enforcement of the ADA

The U.S. Equal Employment Opportunity Commission issued regulations to enforce the provisions of Title I of the ADA in July 1991. The provisions originally took effect in July 1992, and covered employers with 25 or more employees. In July 1994 the size threshold dropped to include employers with 15 or more employees.

For further information:

Equal Employment Opportunities Commission
1801 L Street, NW
Washington, DC 20507
(202) 663-4001
(202) 663-4110 (fax)
www.eeoc.gov

ammonia   A widely used refrigerant in many industrial facilities. Ammonia is considered a high health hazard to workers because it is corrosive to the skin, eyes, and lungs. Prolonged contact at concentrations greater than 300 ppm (parts per million) can cause permanent injury or death. Fortunately, ammonia has a low odor threshold (20 ppm), so most workers will seek relief at much lower concentrations.

Accidental releases of ammonia from refrigeration facilities have resulted in both injuries and deaths to employees of those facilities. These have resulted from contact with both liquid and vapor forms of ammonia. Because refrigeration systems operate at elevated pressures, additional care must be taken to maintain and operate these systems in order to prevent releases with potentially catastrophic consequences.

COMMON INDUSTRIES USING AMMONIA REFRIGERATION SYSTEMS

Meat, poultry, and fish processing facilities
Dairy and ice cream plants
Wineries and breweries
Fruit juice, vegetable juice, and soft drink processing facilities
Cold storage warehouses
Other food processing facilities
Petrochemical facilities

Source: U.S. Department of Labor, Occupational Safety & Health Administration

See also BREWING; EYE INJURIES/PROTECTION; SKIN OR SENSE ORGAN TOXICITY.

anger   An intense emotional state in which one feels a high level of displeasure and FRUSTRATION. It can be caused by workplace STRESS or can be a reaction to stress and is indicated by feelings ranging from slight irritation to explosive HOSTILITY that are directed to other people, objects, or oneself. Anger on the job can interfere with one's relationship with superiors and peers as well as one's productivity.

Physiological changes occur when one feels angry. For example, anger increases the heart rate, blood pressure, and flow of adrenaline. Suppressed anger may result in high blood pressure, skin rashes, and HEADACHES.

People who are angry often show characteristics including frowning, gritting the teeth, pacing, and wringing or clenching the hands. There may be changes in vocal tone. The person may yell or shout, or may speak in short, clipped sentences. During anger, one may attempt to gain CONTROL of a situation or clearly demonstrate that control has been lost.

Negative Anger

There are two attitudes—positive and negative—with regard to anger. On the negative side, anger can be destructive, leading to inappropriate or illegal behavior. Negative anger seems to be directly related to frustration and feelings of inferiority. Adults who express anger directly with physical violence or verbal abuse usually do so because they model their behavior on others in their environment or because there seems to be a reward for violent behavior. Since in most workplace situations it is unacceptable to express anger directly, many people react by becoming sulky or indifferent, or by adopting a superior, patronizing attitude toward the person or situation that angered them.

Positive Anger

Anger may be helpful and constructive. The coping mechanisms, such as physical exercise, that an individual chooses to use to work off anger may be helpful in other ways. Releasing an angry feeling sometimes brings with it a sense of pleasure. Some mental health professionals equate ambition and attempts to improve society with a healthy expression of anger.

Among athletes, anger can have a harmful effect on athletic performance. Anger drains energy and diverts attention from what must be done at the moment. However, professional athletes are trained to recover quickly from events that arouse anger. In some cases, anger may make a player more forceful and positive.

How to Overcome
Anger in the Workplace

An individual in psychotherapy who expresses extremely stressful and angry feelings might be given three goals: first, to identify the feelings of anger; second, to use constructive release of the energy of anger; and third, to identify thought and thought processes that lead to anger. For example, to identify feelings of anger, one might keep a diary of angry feelings at work and learn to recognize anger before losing control. The individual will learn to take responsibility for his or her own emotions and stop blaming others for arousing the anger. Also, with validation from a therapist, the individual will learn to accept that some anger is justified in certain situations. In learning to use constructive release of the energy of anger, the individual may benefit from assertiveness training, and learn to express anger verbally to the appropriate source. Assertive techniques will help the individual increase self-esteem, demonstrate internal control over behavior, and harness energy generated by the anger in a nondestructive manner.

Also, individuals can learn to expend energy through physical activity that involves the large muscles, such as running, walking, or playing a racket sport. Other techniques that are helpful in controlling anger are COMPLEMENTARY THERAPIES such as BIOFEEDBACK, GUIDED IMAGERY and MEDITATION.

See also AGGRESSION; ANXIETY; BODY LANGUAGE; DEPRESSION; TYPE A PERSONALITY; TYPE B PERSONALITY; TYPE C PERSONALITY.

Kahn, Ada P. *Stress A–Z: The Sourcebook for Coping with Everyday Challenges.* New York: Facts On File, Inc., 1998.

anhydrous ammonia   See AMMONIA.

animal handlers   Workers who perform any combination of duties to attend animals, such as cattle, pigs, mice, guinea pigs, dogs, and monkeys, on farms and in facilities such as kennels, pounds, hospitals, and laboratories. Handlers may be laboratory workers, agricultural handlers, or veterinarians or those who feed and water animals, clean and disinfect cages, pens, and yards, and sterilize laboratory equipment and surgical instruments. Duties of an animal handler may include examining animals for signs of illness and treating them accordingly and administering inoculations and anesthesia. Further, animal handlers may shave, bathe, clip, and groom animals.

Accident hazards for animal handlers, whether a veterinarian or a cage attendant in a zoo, include SLIPS, TRIPS, and FALLS on slippery surfaces, cuts caused by sharp objects, bites, goring and/or being attacked by domestic or wild animals, kicks, scratches, and stings caused by laboratory animals, road accidents while transporting animals, fire hazards at animal waste rendering plants, fires and explosions caused by inflammables and explosives, eye injuries caused by metallic splinters (in horseshoeing), electric shocks caused by defective or incorrectly operated electric equipment, and explosions of animal-feed dust-air mixtures.

Animal handlers also face exposure to ionizing radiation emitted by veterinary X-ray equipment and by laboratory animals investigated or treated with radioisotopes. Their skin and eyes are exposed to ultraviolet radiation used for sterilization and other purposes in laboratories and other settings, as well as to excessive noise. If the animal handlers work in mostly outdoor settings, they may encounter heat stress or frostbite.

Chemical and biological hazards are present in occupations involving animal handling, such as CHEMICAL TOXICITY and ALLERGIES, DERMATITIS, exposure to metallic, SOLVENTS and other fumes, and mercury poisoning in fur-processing workers. They face possibilities of infection from contact with sick or pathogen-carrying animals or exposure to airborne pathogens, resulting in development of any one of many communicable diseases such as blastomycosis, brucellosis, or cat-scratch fever. Many of pesticides and flea control products are cancer hazards. Also, animal handlers may experience musculoskeletal problems of the back and knees and job dissatisfaction because of the working conditions involving smells and dirt and the physical character of the work.

Finally, animal handlers may at times be exposed to protests and possible violence by animal rights groups, and danger of developing drug addiction because of the availability of medications.

See also ADDICTIONS; ANTHRAX; DUST AND DEBRIS; EYE INJURIES/PROTECTION; FIRE SAFETY/FIRE PROTECTION; ELECTRICITY RELATED INJURIES; NOISE; SKIN AND SENSE ORGAN TOXICITY; STRESS.

Encyclopaedia of Occupational Health and Safety. 4th ed. Vol. 4. Geneva: International Labor Organization, 1998, p. 103.6.

animal pelts and hair See ALLERGIES; ANIMAL HANDLERS; FUR PROCESSING.

anorexia See EATING DISORDERS.

anthraquinone dyes See SKIN OR SENSE ORGAN TOXICITY.

anthrax An infectious disease of animals that can be secondarily transmitted to humans. It is caused by a bacillus (*Bacillus anthracis*) that primarily affects sheep, horses, hogs, cattle, and goats and is almost always fatal in animals. Transmission to humans normally occurs through contact with infected animals but can also occur through breathing air laden with the spores of the bacilli.

The disease is almost entirely occupational, as it is usually restricted to individuals who handle hides of animals, such as farmers, butchers, and veterinarians, or workers who sort wool. However, in 2001 several humans contracted anthrax from an unknown source. Bioterrorism was suspected but never proven; nor was the perpetrator of the anthrax disseminations identified. Numerous post offices and other office buildings were closed for inspection because of detected anthrax spores. Many people who handled mail at work chose to wear gloves and face masks as protection against possibly anthrax-tainted letters.

There are different kinds of anthrax. The two kinds of anthrax reported in the news are skin anthrax and inhaled anthrax. In skin anthrax, spores enter the body through a cut or other opening in the skin. Inhaled anthrax comes from breathing in the spores and is more serious and requires hospitalization.

One cannot catch anthrax from someone else. Anthrax vaccine is available only to the military (as of 2002).

See also ANIMAL HANDLERS; BUTCHERS, MEAT, POULTRY, AND FISH CUTTERS; FARMERS.

antidepressant medications See DEPRESSION.

antimony A silvery-white metal found in the Earth's crust. Antimony ores are mined and then mixed with other metals to form antimony alloys or combined with oxygen to form antimony oxide.

Because antimony is found naturally in the environment, the general population is exposed to low levels of it every day, primarily in food, drinking water, and air. However, workers in industries that process it or use antimony ore may be exposed to higher levels. Antimony is found in air near industries that process or release it, such as smelters, coal-fired plants, and refuse incinerators.

When mixed into alloys, antimony is used in lead storage batteries, solder, sheet and pipe metal, bearings, castings, and pewter. Antimony oxide is added to textiles and plastics to prevent them from catching fire. It is also used in paints, ceramics, and fireworks, and as enamel for plastics, metal, and glass.

Exposure to antimony occurs in the workplace or from skin contact with soil at hazardous waste sites. Breathing high levels of antimony for a long time can irritate the eyes and lungs, and can cause problems with the lungs, heart, and stomach.

Tests are available to measure antimony levels in the body. Antimony can be measured in the urine, feces, and blood for several days after exposure. However, these tests cannot tell how much antimony one has been exposed to or whether one will experience any health effects.

The Environmental Protection Agency has set limits for antimony in drinking water and has regulations concerning reporting discharges or spills of antimony into the atmosphere. The Occupational Safety and Health Administration (OSHA) has set an occupational exposure limit of antimony for an eight-hour workday, 40-hour workweek. The American Conference of Governmental Industrial Hygienists (ACGIH) and the National Institute for Occupational Safety and Health (NIOSH) currently recommend the same guidelines for the workplace as OSHA.

For more information:

Agency for Toxic Substances and Disease Registry
Division of Toxicology
1600 Clifton Road NE
Mailstop E-29
Atlanta, GA 30333
(888) 422-8737
(404) 498-0057 (fax)

See also AMERICAN CONFERENCE OF GOVERNMEN-TAL INDUSTRIAL HYGIENISTS; CADMIUM; ENVIRONMEN-TAL PROTECTION AGENCY; OCCUPATIONAL SAFETY AND HEALTH ADMINISTRATION; WASTE INDUSTRY.

anxiety Unpleasant feelings of generalized fear and apprehension, often of unknown origin. The feeling may be triggered by one's environment (external), such as a difficult boss, or from one's own thoughts about an impending danger, such as speaking in front of coworkers (internal).

Anxiety and fear have similarities and differences. Fear is sometimes defined as a response to a consciously recognized and usually external threat. In general, fear is a response to a clear and present danger, whereas anxiety is a response to a situation, object, or person that the individual has come to fear through learning and experience, such as encountering a bully at work.

Anxiety, as noted by the existentialist philosopher Soren Kierkegaard, is the full experience of fear in the absence of a known threat. In both fear and anxiety, however, the body mobilizes itself to meet the threat, and certain physiological phenomena occur. Muscles become tense, breathing is faster, the heart beats more rapidly, and there may be sweating or diarrhea. There may be shakiness, increased breathing and heart rate, and acute sensitivity to environmental stimuli (for example, an intense startle reaction).

Anxiety is recognized as a major feature in many cases of depressive illness. Until 1980 anxiety was considered a one-dimensional condition. Since then, employee assistance workers and mental health professionals have come to understand that there are several specific symptom clusters, with unique causes, treatments, and outlook for improvement.

Following are several of the major categories described in the fourth edition of *The Diagnostic and Statistical Manual of Mental Disorders*, published in 1994:

- Generalized anxiety disorder
- Phobias: Specific phobia (formerly simple phobia), social phobia
- Agoraphobia
- Panic attacks and panic disorder
- Obsessive-compulsive disorder
- Post-traumatic stress disorder

However, according to Sheryle Gallant, Gwendolyn Keita, and Renée Royak-Schaler in *Healthcare for Women: Psychological, Social, and Behavioral Influences* (1997), the two most prevalent categories are generalized anxiety disorder and panic disorder. Primary care physicians have indicated that anxiety disorders are the most common mental health problems in their practice. These conditions can affect an employee's work performance because of distraction and attention to irrelevant matters.

In primary care settings, anxiety disorders often are underrecognized because anxious individuals often present with physical symptoms rather than psychological concerns.

See also ANXIETY DISORDERS; EMPLOYEE ASSIS-TANCE PROGRAMS; MENTAL HEALTH; PANIC ATTACKS AND PANIC DISORDER; PHOBIAS.

Kahn, Ada P., and Ronald M. Doctor. *Encyclopedia of Phobias, Fears, and Anxieties.* 2d ed. New York: Facts On File, Inc., 2000.

anxiety disorders A group of disorders in which anxiety is either the predominant characteristic or is experienced when a person confronts a dreaded object or situation or resists obsessions or compul-

CLINICAL SIGNS AND SYMPTOMS OF ANXIETY ATTACKS

Cognitive	Emotional	Perceptual	Physiological	Behavioral
Decreased concentration	Fear, tension, panic, dread	Blurred vision	Dizziness, sweating, dry mouth	Immobilized, agitated, and frantic
Impaired memory	Imminence of death	Paresthesias	Headache	Decrease in exercise tolerance
Indecisiveness	Feelings of helplessness	Numbness and tingling of lips and fingertips	Difficulty swallowing	Desperate for relief
Thought content fragmented with obsessive ruminations about symptomatology	Depression	Depersonalization, occasionally derealization	Insomnia, nightmares	Avoidance, escape
	Guilt		Increased urination, diarrhea	Dependence on others
Dreaded anticipation	Shame	Perceptual field narrowed	Chest discomfort, palpitations	Excessive worry
Catastrophic thinking	Anger	Ringing in ears	Dilated pupils, increase in blood pressure, pulse, respiratory rate	Superstitious behavior
Thoughts of going crazy	Loss of self-esteem	Tightness in throat		Anticipatory avoidance
Thoughts of physical catastrophe	Disengagement		Weakness	
Loss of control thoughts	Embarrassment		Perspiration	
Impending doom			Warmth	
			Shakiness, trembling	
			Hyperventilation, shortness of breath	
			Pain, cramps	
			Pallor or flushing	
			Nausea	
			Fatigue	

Source: Encyclopedia of Phobias, Fears, and Anxieties, 2nd ed.

sions. Individuals suffering from anxiety disorders are always apprehensive and worry, ruminate, and expect something bad to happen to themselves or loved ones. They feel on edge, impatient, and irritable, and are easily distracted. Some individuals have symptoms so severe that they are almost totally disabled and cannot work.

Following are several of the major categories described in the fourth edition of the *Diagnostic and Statistical Manual of Mental Disorders* (1994):

Phobias

Phobias afflict between 5.1 and 11.5 percent of all Americans, according to the American Psychiatric Association. People who suffer from phobias feel terror, dread, or panic when confronted with the feared object, situation, or activity. Many have such an overwhelming desire to avoid the source of this fear that it interferes with their job, family life, and social relationships. For example, they may lose their job because they fear traveling or taking an elevator to a meeting. Some become fearful of leaving their homes, live hermitlike existences, and cannot work outside the home.

Within the category of phobias are specific phobias, social phobias, and agoraphobia. Specific phobias are fears of specific objects or situations; examples are fear of flying or fear of closed spaces. Social phobias are fears of situations in which the individual can be watched by others, such as PUBLIC SPEAKING, or in which the individual behavior might prove embarrassing, such as eating in public. Agoraphobia, the fear of going outside, being in a public place, being in a place with no escape such as a train or plane, or being alone away from a place considered "safe" is the most disabling because sufferers can become housebound and unable to work.

Panic Disorders

Individuals who have panic disorders have intense, overwhelming terror for no apparent rational reason. Often people suffering a panic attack for the first time rush to the hospital, convinced they are having a heart attack. Sufferers cannot predict when the attacks will occur, although certain situations such as driving a car can become associated with them because it was in those situations where the first attack occurred.

Obsessive-Compulsive Disorders

Some individuals attempt to cope with their anxiety by associating it with obsessions, which are defined as repeated, unwanted thoughts, or compulsive behaviors, which are defined as rituals that themselves get out of control. Individuals who suffer from obsessive disorders do not automatically have compulsive behaviors. However, most people who have compulsive ritual behaviors also suffer from obsessions.

Individuals who have obsessive-compulsive disorders have involuntary, recurrent, and persistent thoughts or impulses that are distasteful to them. Examples are thoughts of violence or of becoming infected by shaking hands with others. These thoughts can be momentary or they can be long-lasting. The most common obsessions focus on hurting others or violating socially acceptable behavioral standards, such as cursing or making inappropriate sexual advances. They also can focus on religious or philosophical issues, which the individual never resolves.

Individuals who have compulsions go through repeated, involuntary ritualistic behaviors that are believed to prevent or produce an unrelated future event. Some people with this disorder also suffer from a complementary obsession, as in the case of worries over infection and compulsive handwashing.

Examples of compulsive rituals include cleaning; if the individual comes in contact with any dirt, he or she may spend hours washing, even to the point that the hands bleed. Another example is repetitious behavior, such as saying a loved one's name several times every time that person comes up in conversation. Compulsives also check and recheck that doors are locked or that electric switches or coffeepots are turned off. Others will retrace a route they have driven to check that they did not hit a pedestrian or cause an accident without knowing it.

Post-Traumatic Stress Disorder

This can occur in anyone who has survived a severe physical or mental trauma. For example, people who witnessed the September 11, 2001, attack on the World Trade Center in New York or survived a life-threatening crime may develop this illness. The severity of the disorder increases if the trauma was unanticipated. For that reason, not all war veterans develop post-traumatic stress disorder, despite prolonged and brutal combat. Soldiers expect a certain amount of violence, whereas rape victims, for instance, may be particularly affected by the unexpectedness of the attack.

Individuals who suffer from post-traumatic stress disorder reexperience the event that traumatized them through nightmares, night terrors, or flashbacks of the event. In rare cases, the person falls into a temporary dislocation from reality, in which he or she relives the trauma for a period of seconds or days. "Psychic numbing," or emotional anesthesia, may occur, in which victims have decreased interest in or involvement with people or activities they once enjoyed. They may have excessive alertness and a highly sharpened startle reaction. They may have general anxiety, depression, panic attacks, inability to sleep, memory loss, difficulty concentrating or completing tasks, and survivors' guilt.

Generalized Anxiety Disorder (GAD)

Diagnostically, generalized anxiety disorders consist of excessive, more or less chronic, persistent and relatively nonspecific anxiety and or worry that occurs over at least a six-month period of time. GAD includes excessive (unrealistic) worry and anxiety about two or more life circumstances that persist for at least six months. Impairment in occupational functioning is usually not greater than mild. The age of onset is commonly between 20 and 40 years of age. Onset sometimes follows a major depressive episode. This form of anxiety is not an anxiety or worry about having a panic attack (as found in panic disorder), being embarrassed in public (as might be found in social phobia), being contaminated (as in obsessive-compulsive disorder) or gaining weight (as in anorexia nervosa).

Causes of Anxiety Disorders

Probably no single situation or condition cause anxiety disorders. Instead, a combination of physical and environmental triggers may combine to create a particular anxiety illness. Recently, research has indicated that biochemical imbalances may be related to some anxiety disorders. According to this theory, medical treatment of biochemical imbal-

ances in the central nervous system should relieve anxiety. Studies have also indicated, conversely, that biochemical changes occur as a result of emotional, psychological, or behavioral changes.

Help for Employees with Anxiety Disorders

The first step may be referral to an EMPLOYEE ASSISTANCE PROGRAM (EAP) or mental health counselor. Anxiety disorders are usually treated with a combination of approaches. Phobias, agoraphobia, and obsessive-compulsive disorders often are treated by behavior therapy. This involves exposing the individual to the feared object or situation under controlled circumstances, until the level of fear is significantly reduced. Successfully treated with this method, many phobic individuals have long-term recovery and can be productive workers.

Medications can help reduce intense symptoms so that the individual can make better use of behavior therapy or other psychotherapy techniques. In addition to behavioral modification techniques and medication, psychotherapy can be an important component of treatment.

According to the American Psychiatric Association, 90 percent of the phobic and obsessive-compulsive individuals who cooperate with a therapist will recover with behavior therapy. Studies show that 70 percent of individuals who suffer from panic attacks improve with medication. Medication is effective for about half of those suffering from obsessive-compulsive disorder. However, medications by themselves are not considered adequate treatment for anxiety disorders.

See also BULLIES; DEPRESSION; *DIAGNOSTIC AND STATISTICAL MANUAL OF MENTAL DISORDERS;* MENTAL HEALTH; PERFORMANCE ANXIETY; PUBLIC SPEAKING.

American Psychiatric Association. *Diagnostic and Statistical Manual of Mental Disorders.* 4th ed. Washington, D.C.: American Psychiatric Association, 1994.

Gallant, Sheryle J., Gwendolyn Puryear Keita, and Renée Royak-Schaler, eds. *Health Care for Women: Psychological, Social, and Behavioral Influences.* Washington, D.C.: American Psychological Association, 1997.

Kahn, Ada P., and Jan Fawcett. *Encyclopedia of Mental Health.* 2d ed. New York: Facts On File, Inc., 2001.

Marks, Isaac. *Fears, Phobias, and Rituals: Panic, Anxiety and Their Disorders.* New York: Oxford University Press, 1987.

Applied Occupational and Environmental Hygiene The peer reviewed journal of the American Conference of Governmental Industrial Hygienists. It is a monthly resource aimed at enhancing the knowledge and practice of occupational and environmental hygiene. The journal presents original studies and reports conclusions that can be used by health and safety professionals in the prevention of occupational and environmental disease. Readers are professionals in the areas of general industrial hygiene, engineering control, occupational and environmental epidemiology, general occupational and environmental medicine, ergonomics and human factors, applied toxicology, and applied environmental chemistry.

For information:

Applied Occupational and Environmental Hygiene
Taylor & Francis, Inc.
Brunner-Routledge, Psychology Press
325 Chestnut Street
Suite 800
Philadelphia, PA 19106
(800) 354-1420
(215) 625-8914 (fax)

See also AMERICAN COLLEGE OF OCCUPATIONAL AND ENVIRONMENTAL MEDICINE (ACOEM); AMERICAN CONFERENCE OF GOVERNMENTAL INDUSTRIAL HYGIENISTS; AMERICAN INDUSTRIAL HYGIENE ASSOCIATION; ERGONOMICS.

arsenic An element found in the environment at low levels. Inorganic arsenic is found in many kinds of rock, especially those containing copper or lead. When these ores are heated in smelters to extract the copper or lead, most of the arsenic goes into the air as fine dust. Smelters collect this dust and purify the arsenic for several uses, chief of which is as a wood preservative to prevent rotting and decay. Arsenic is used to make several types of insecticides and herbicides, such as Ansar, Scorch, and Premix.

In addition, arsenic compounds are used in agriculture, pigment production, the manufacture of glass and enamels, textile printing, tanning, and taxidermy. They are used to control sludge formation in lubricating oils, as an alloying agent to harden lead base bearing materials, and with copper to improve its toughness and corrosion resistance.

Telecommunications cable splicers, outside plant technicians, or people who work on arsenic-treated telecommunications poles, as well as many who work in manufacturing and printing plants, are exposed to arsenic.

Exposure to high levels of inorganic arsenic occurs in the workplace or in areas with high natural levels. Health issues from arsenic exposure result after inhalation or ingestion of arsenic dust and fumes. Arsenic compounds are also a skin irritant, causing skin rashes or dermatitis. The mucous membranes of the body are most sensitive to the irritant action. Additionally, the skin, eyelids, angles of the ears, nose, mouth, and the respiratory membranes are also susceptible to the irritant effects.

The U.S. Department of Health and Human Services (DHHS) has determined that arsenic is a known carcinogen. Breathing it increases the risk of lung cancer. Ingesting inorganic arsenic increases the risk of skin cancer and tumors of the bladder, kidney, liver, and lung.

The Environmental Protection Agency (EPA) sets limits on the amount of arsenic that industrial sources can release. The Occupational Safety and Health Administration (OSHA) has established a maximum permissible exposure limit for workplaces. Arsenic has been found in at least 781 of 1,300 National Priorities List sites identified by the Environmental Protection Agency.

For more information:

Communications Workers of America
Occupational Safety and Health Department
501 Third Street, NW
Washington, DC 20001-2797
(202) 434-1160
www.cwa-union.org/osh

Agency for Toxic Substances and Disease Registry
1600 Clifton Road NE (E-60)
Atlanta, GA 30333
(888) 422-8737
(404) 498-9957 (fax)

See also AGENCY FOR TOXIC SUBSTANCES AND DISEASE REGISTRY; CARDIOVASCULAR OR BLOOD TOXICITY;

ELECTRICITY-RELATED INJURIES; GASTROINTESTINAL OR LIVER TOXICITY; TELECOMMUNICATIONS.

asbestos   A naturally occurring group of hydrated mineral silicates that can be identified only under a microscope. Synonyms and trade names include Actinolite, Amosite (cummingtonite-grunerite), Anthophyllite, Chrysotile, Crocidolite (Riebeckite), and Tremolite. Fibers released from these minerals, when used in many common building materials, cause irritation and inflammation of the lungs known as asbestosis. Workers in CONSTRUCTION, SHIP BUILDING, railroads, maintenance trades, and particularly those who have done plastering, fireproofing, or pipe or duct insulation, may have had heavy exposure to asbestos. Asbestos exposure, and the health risk, is also high for people who work in asbestos-contaminated buildings. Asbestosis, the disease caused by inhaling asbestos fibers, is a progressively crippling disease. It is not a cancer; it is caused by the scarring of the lung tissue from heavy exposure to asbestos fibers.

More than 3,000 products in use today contain asbestos. Most of these are materials used in heat or acoustic insulation, on boilers and steam pipes, in fireproofing or structural steel and decking, and/or sprayed or troweled on plaster material for acoustic, decorative, or other purposes on ceilings, walls, and other surfaces. Asbestos is often disturbed when workers enter crawl spaces or run electrical cables between floors. Building renovation work can also release asbestos fibers into the air.

According to the ENVIRONMENTAL PROTECTION AGENCY, about 20 percent of all public and commercial buildings in the United States contain some asbestos material. In about two-thirds of those buildings, at least some of the asbestos material is damaged, and almost half have significantly damaged asbestos. It is not possible to tell whether a building material contains asbestos by looking at it because asbestos and asbestos-substitute materials look very similar. The only way to tell for certain whether material contains asbestos is to have a small sample examined under a microscope by a specially trained laboratory technician. Results can usually be reported within 24 hours if necessary.

COMMON PRODUCTS THAT MAY CONTAIN ASBESTOS

Pipe and duct insulation
Building insulation
Carpet underlays
Roofing materials
Artificial fireplaces and materials
Patching and spackling compounds
Brake pads and linings
Pot holders and ironing board pads
Hair dryers
Floor tiles
Electrical wires
Textured paints
Cements
Toasters and other household appliances
Furnaces and furnace door gaskets

Source: American Lung Association

Some uses of asbestos have been banned: spraying of asbestos-containing materials (1973); certain pipe coverings (1975); certain patching compounds and artificial fireplace logs (1977); sprayed-on asbestos decorations (1978); and asbestos-containing hair dryers (1979).

Asbestos that is tightly bound or sealed into building material does not pose a health hazard. It is only when the asbestos material becomes "friable," or capable of becoming crumbled and releasing asbestos fibers into the air, that the danger of asbestos disease exists. This can happen when asbestos-containing material becomes damaged or deteriorated due to heat, water leaks, vibration, maintenance work, or renovation.

According to the Safety and Health Department of the International Brotherhood of Teamsters (IBT), another potential problem exists where asbestos fireproofing is exposed to airflow, when the air space between a ceiling and the floor above is used as part of the air conditioning system of a building. This air movement can pick up asbestos fibers and circulate them throughout the building. According to the American Lung Association, there is no known safe exposure to asbestos.

The OCCUPATIONAL SAFETY AND HEALTH ADMINISTRATION (OSHA) has separate standards governing worker exposure to asbestos in general industry and in construction. The construction asbestos standard covers asbestos removal, demolition, and renovation work. These standards are designed primarily for people who work directly with asbestos, not for people who work in asbestos-contaminated buildings.

Health Hazards of Inhaling Asbestos Fibers

The body attempts to neutralize the foreign fibers of asbestos in various ways, and some of these processes lead to further inflammation and cell damage. Eventually a fibrosis or scar tissue develops in the interstitial spaces around the small airways and alveoli. This thickening and scarring prevents oxygen and carbon dioxide from traveling between the alveoli and the blood cells, so breathing becomes more difficult.

Asbestosis affects both lungs and although it is mainly in the lower fields of the lungs, it is usually widespread. The condition is detected by X-ray findings. Symptoms typically include shortness of breath and coughing. It can be a progressive disease, worsening even after exposure to asbestos has stopped. In some cases it is fatal.

The condition is usually caused by heavy exposure to asbestos, such as sustained exposure over a period of years (for example, a longtime worker at an asbestos textile plant) and/or intense exposure during a shorter period (for example, a worker in the engine rooms of ships under construction in World War II).

Asbestos has been found to cause cancer. The most common asbestos-related cancer is LUNG CANCER. Asbestos also causes cancer of the mouth and throat areas, larynx, esophagus, stomach, colon, rectum, and kidneys. Asbestos is the only known cause of pleural mesothelioma, cancer of the lining of the lungs or the lining of the abdomen. Even a very small amount of asbestos exposure can lead to cancer. People who have worked with asbestos for only a few days and members of the families of asbestos-exposed workers have been known to contract asbestos-related cancer. According to the IBT, asbestos-related cancers usually do not show up until 20, 30, or more years after the person is first exposed.

There is currently no effective treatment or cure for asbestosis.

ASBESTOSIS: MOST FREQUENTLY RECORDED INDUSTRIES ON DEATH CERTIFICATE, SELECTED STATES, U.S. RESIDENTS AGE 15 AND OVER, 1991–1992

Industry	Number	Percent
Construction	149	25.8
Ship- and boatbuilding and repairing	50	8.7
Industrial and miscellaneous chemicals	23	4.0
Miscellaneous nonmetallic mineral stone products	23	4.0
Railroads	17	2.9
General government	17	2.9
Yam, thread, and fabric mills	11	1.9
Other rubber products, plastic footwear and belting	9	1.6
Not specified manufacturing industries	9	1.6
Trucking service	9	1.6
All other industries	244	42.2
Industry not reported	17	2.9
Total	578	100.0

Removing Asbestos

Buildings built before 1978 may have asbestos-containing substances. According to the American Lung Association, if the material is in good condition, it can be left alone. To be certain, however, materials should be inspected and if necessary, repaired or removed. Repair usually involves either sealing or covering asbestos material. Sealing (or encapsulation) involves coating materials so that asbestos is sealed in. This process is only effective for undamaged asbestos-containing substances. If materials are soft or crumbly or otherwise damaged, sealing is not appropriate. Covering involves placing something over or around the asbestos-containing material to prevent release of fibers.

The most permanent way to reduce or eliminate the hazard of asbestos is to remove it from a building. Asbestos removal is an expensive, complex, and hazardous process. It must be done by specially trained and equipped workers, following rigorous asbestos removal and handling procedures. If not, the asbestos removal may cause more exposure to people who use the building, and dangerous asbestos exposures to the people doing the work.

The IBT Safety and Health Department recommends the following procedures for worker safety involving asbestos removal:

- The work area should be completely sealed off with plastic sheeting and tape.

- All heating and ventilation openings into the work area should be sealed off.

- The work area should be kept under negative pressure, so no asbestos-contaminated air can escape. This is done with exhaust units equipped with special high-efficiency HEPA (high efficiency particulate air filters) filters.

- Air monitoring should be done outside the work area while the job is in progress, to make sure no asbestos fibers are escaping.

- Signs must be posted to warn unauthorized persons from entering the work area.

- Everyone who enters the work area must have a respirator and protective clothing to cover the entire body.

- Asbestos removal workers must leave their contaminated work clothes behind and shower before putting on their street clothes and leaving the work area.

- Asbestos material should be thoroughly wetted down before it is removed, and should be cleaned up and placed in sealed containers while still wet.

- All asbestos waste must be transported away from the work area in plastic bags or other sealed containers with warning labels.

- When removal is completed, the work area should receive a final cleaning with wet mops and special vacuum cleaners with high-efficiency "HEPA" filters.

- A final visual inspection followed by aggressive air monitoring, in which a purposeful effort is made to stir up any remaining dust, should be done when the job is completed, in order to make certain that no asbestos contamination remains.

For further information, see Appendix I.

See also AIR POLLUTION; AMERICAN LUNG ASSOCIATION; MESOTHELIOMA; OCCUPATIONAL LUNG DISEASES; INDOOR ENVIRONMENT (AIR QUALITY); INTERNATIONAL BROTHERHOOD OF TEAMSTERS; PARTICULATE MATTER; PERSONAL PROTECTIVE EQUIPMENT; PULMONARY REHABILITATION; SICK BUILDING SYNDROME.

asbestosis See ASBESTOS.

asphalt fumes More than a half-million workers are exposed to fumes from asphalt, a brownish-black substance used extensively in road paving, roofing, siding, and concrete work. Chemically, asphalt is a natural mixture of hydrocarbons. It varies in consistency from a solid to a semisolid, has great tenacity, melts when heated, and when ignited will burn with a smoky flame leaving very little or no ash.

Health effects from exposure to asphalt fumes include HEADACHE, skin rash, fatigue, reduced appetite, throat and eye irritation, cough, and skin cancer.

Asphalt is found in nature in deposits called asphalt lakes. Natural asphalt was probably formed by the evaporation of petroleum, and now is obtained as a residue in the distillation or refining of petroleum. It also occurs in asphalt rock, a natural mixture of asphalt with sand and limestone, which when crushed is used as road building material. Asphalt is also used in the manufacture of paints and varnishes, giving an intense black color.

See also CANCER; CONSTRUCTION; EYE INJURIES PROTECTION; SKIN OR SENSE ORGAN TOXICITY; PERSONAL PROTECTION EQUIPMENT.

assertiveness training A process through which one can change unwanted behaviors and communicate more effectively. People who are too inhibited or too anxious to act on their own wishes in workplace or social situations can benefit from assertiveness training, in which people learn to speak up whenever they believe an injustice is done. Assertiveness training helps reduce the ANXIETY felt in dealing with others as one learns to see himself or herself as an equal human being with rights regardless of role or title. Assertiveness training can help raise SELF-ESTEEM and help a person to see that choices in responses to others are available.

Assertive behavior is self-expressive, honest, direct, and firm. It respects the rights of others and allows one to take responsibility for his or her own feelings. Nonassertive behavior involves denying oneself, possibly wanting to assert oneself, but thinking of a proper response too late. In dealing with people, nonassertive individuals are uneasy and feel guilty because they do not assert themselves.

An example of the usefulness of assertiveness training is an employee who wants to ask for a raise but does not have the courage to do so. Assertiveness training teaches the individual to act upon his or her feelings in a manner that results in improving the specific situation.

Training sessions with a therapist (or self-help techniques) include rehearsals in how to act and what to say in common situations in which one is often taken advantage of, such as a demanding boss or a friend who takes advantage of generosity.

Assertiveness enables a person to act in his or her own best interests to make life decisions, take initiative, trust his or her judgment, set goals and work to achieve them, and ask for help from others when necessary. It enables a person to stand up for him- or herself without undue anxiety, to say no, set limits on time and energy, respond to criticism, put-downs, or ANGER, and express or defend a personal opinion. It allows one to express honest feelings comfortably, to agree or disagree with someone, to show anger, affection, and friendship, and to admit fear or anxiety. Assertiveness means that one is able to exercise personal rights, such as expressing opinions, and respond to violations of one's own rights or those of others. However, assertiveness also means allowing the rights of others without unfair criticism or hurtful behavior, manipulation, or undue control.

The Opposite of Assertive: Aggressive

The opposite of assertive behavior is aggressive behavior. An aggressive person does not respect the rights of others. If one is aggressive, one usually attains goals at the expense of others; this may even feel good. The aggressive person usually responds too vigorously and hurts others by making choices for them, thus minimizing their individual worth. The person put down by an aggressive individual feels hurt, defensive, humili-

ated, and even angry. Aggressive people put down nonassertive people in part because the nonassertive people let them behave this way.

Passive-aggressive individuals often achieve their goals by manipulation, covert hostility, and indirectness. If a passive-aggressive person cannot achieve his or her desired goals, he/she feels that others should not get theirs. People who interact with a passive-aggressive individual usually feel angry, hurt, or confused.

See also AGGRESSION; CONTROL; STRESS.

Kahn, Ada P. *Stress A–Z: A Sourcebook for Facing Everyday Challenges.* New York: Facts On File, Inc., 1998.

Association of Diving Contractors International
See COMMERCIAL DIVING.

Associated Landscape Contractors of America (ALCA)   This association, together with the National Aeronautical and Space Administration (NASA), in 2001 announced findings of a two-year study that suggests that common indoor plants may provide a natural way of helping combat SICK BUILDING SYNDROME.

Using common indoor plants for indoor air purification and revitalization, ALCA studied use of a dozen popular varieties of ornamental plants to determine their effectiveness in removing several key pollutants associated with indoor air pollution. NASA research on indoor plants found that living plants are so efficient at absorbing contaminants in the air that some will be launched into space as part of the biological life support system aboard future orbiting space stations.

Each plant was placed in a sealed Plexiglas chamber into which chemicals were injected. Philodendron, spider plant, and golden pothos were labeled the most effective in removing FORMALDEHYDE molecules. Flowering plants such as gerbera daisy and chrysanthemums were rated superior in removing BENZENE from the chamber atmosphere. Other good performers were *Dracaena massangeana,* spathiphyllum, and golden pothos. Researchers concluded that plants take substances and trace levels of toxic vapors out of the air through the tiny openings in their leaves.

See also AIR POLLUTION.

asthma, occupational A lung disease in which the airways overreact to dusts, vapors, gases, or fumes that exist in the workplace. When a worker inhales these irritants, airway inflammation begins, muscles in the airways tighten, the airway tissue swells, and too much mucus is produced. These changes make breathing difficult.

Symptoms of occupational asthma usually occur while the worker is exposed to a particular substance at work. Symptoms include wheezing, a tight feeling in the chest, coughing, and shortness of breath. A worker may have only a cough or any one of the other symptoms. In some cases, symptoms may develop several hours after the person leaves work, and then subside before the worker returns to the job the next day. In the early stages of the disease, symptoms usually decrease or disappear during weekends or vacations, only to recur upon return to work. In later stages of the disease, symptoms may occur away from work after exposure to common lung irritants.

Once the airways have a pattern of overreacting, many common substances such as cigarette smoke, house dust, or cold air may produce asthma-like symptoms.

Individuals Most Likely to Develop Asthma

According to the AMERICAN LUNG ASSOCIATION, workers in hundreds of occupations are exposed to substances in the air that may cause occupational asthma in susceptible people. Many of these substances are very common and not ordinarily considered hazardous. Only a small number of exposed workers develops occupational asthma. Those most likely to develop the disease are those with a personal or family history of allergies or asthma and frequent exposure to highly sensitizing substances. However, the disease also can develop in people with no known allergies.

Occupational asthma may be suspected when a worker begins to develop respiratory symptoms. It may take several years to develop. A thorough physical examination and medical history for a worker with asthma symptoms should include a detailed listing of his or her work history and workplace conditions.

Causes of Occupational Asthma

New substances and manufacturing processes are continually being identified. The following chart indicates some of the airborne substances and some related occupations known to be associated with the disease.

SUBSTANCES CAUSING ASTHMA AND RELATED OCCUPATIONS

Chemical dusts and vapors from plasticizers, polyurethane paints, insulation, foam mattresses and upholstery, and packaging materials used in manufacturing and processing operations. Among specific chemicals known to cause asthma are the isocynates, trimellitic anhydride, and phthalic anhydride.

Animal substances such as hair, dander, mites, small insects, and bacterial or protein dusts. Exposed workers at special risk include farmers, animal handlers, shepherds, grooms, jockeys, veterinarians, and kennel workers.

Organic dusts such as flour, cereals, grains, coffee and tea dust, Papuan dust from meat tenderizer. These substances cause asthma in millers, bakers, and other food processors.

Cotton, flax, and hemp dust inhaled by workers in cotton processing and textile industries.

Metals such as platinum, chromium, nickel sulfate, and soldering fumes. Workers are exposed to these in refining and manufacturing operations.

Smoking may make asthma more severe. Smoking also increases the chances of getting other complicating lung diseases, such as emphysema, chronic bronchitis, or lung cancer. Workers with occupational asthma who change their job environment and quit smoking are more likely to recover fully than a worker who changes jobs but continues to smoke. Secondhand smoke may also increase the symptoms of the worker who has occupational asthma.

Diagnosing and Treating Occupational Asthma

A physician will take a careful, detailed history to relate the occurrence of symptoms to work exposure. A physical examination of the chest is often normal if done several hours after exposure has taken place but is useful in ruling out other causes of shortness of breath. Pulmonary function tests given before and after work may detect narrowing of the airways. Laboratory tests on blood and sputum may be useful. Special studies can sometimes confirm the diagnosis but inhalation of a suspected agent (challenge test) may be necessary. A chest X ray is essential to exclude other lung disorders but has no direct role in diagnosing occupational asthma.

The best treatment is to completely avoid the substance causing the asthma. In some circumstances, where exposure is unavoidable or intermittent, drug treatment may be recommended. In advanced cases of occupational asthma with complications resulting in severely damaged airways, combined medical treatment including drugs, physical therapy, and breathing aids my be needed. Persons with occupational asthma should avoid exposure to gases such as sulfur dioxide, chlorine, or nitrogen dioxide. Breathing these irritating gases can make asthma symptoms worse.

For information:

American Lung Association
1740 Broadway
New York, NY 10019
(212) 315-8700
(212) 315-8872 (fax)
www.lungusa.org

See also ALLERGIES; CHEMICAL TOXICITY; EMPHYSEMA; LUNG CANCER; OCCUPATIONAL LUNG DISEASES; RESPIRATORY TOXICITY.

Adapted with permission from: "Occupational Asthma," April 9, 2001, American Lung Association.

auto body repair and refinishing   Workers in auto body shops can be exposed to a variety of chemical and physical hazards. Chemical hazards may include volatile organics from paints, fillers, and SOLVENTS, silica from sandblasting operations, dust from sanding, and metal fumes from WELDING and cutting. Physical hazards include repetitive stress and other ergonomic injuries, noise, cutting tools, and oil and grease on walking surfaces.

See also AUTOMOBILE MECHANICS; CHEMICAL TOXICITY; DUST AND DEBRIS; ERGONOMICS; NOISE; REPETITIVE STRESS INJURIES; SLIPS, TRIPS AND FALLS.

autoimmune disorders   Numerous disorders, including rheumatoid arthritis, insulin-dependent diabetes mellitus, systemic lupus erythematosus, and others, caused by a reaction of the immune system against the organs or tissues of the body. Workers who have allergic reactions to substances with which they work may have autoimmune disorders.

The function of the immune system is to respond to invading microorganisms, such as bacteria or viruses, by producing antibodies that will recognize and destroy the invaders. Autoimmune disorders occur when these reactions inexplicably take place against the body's own cells and tissues, producing a variety of disorders.

The disease-producing processes in autoimmunity are termed *hypersensitivity reactions.* Hypersensitivity reactions also occur in allergy. Both are inappropriate responses of the immune system; however, with allergy, the response is to substances from outside the body.

See ALLERGIES; COAL DUST; DUST AND DEBRIS; FARMING; GARDENERS; IMMUNOTOXICITY; LABORATORY WORKERS; MUSCULOSKELETAL TOXICITY.

Clayman, Charles B. *The American Medical Association Encyclopedia of Medicine.* New York: Random House, 1989.

automation   The transition to automated production systems wherein machines do the repetitive manual elements of the work process. As a result of automation, workers are displaced or left with mainly supervisory functions. Either of these situations can lead to STRESS.

Most industries, particularly manufacturing, have experienced displacement of workers as a result of automation of their production lines. Today, offices have been automated as well. It is estimated that office workers spend as much as 90 percent of their time at computers.

The advent of computers has also meant automation of the delivery of services. A good example is the automatic bank teller which not only dispenses cash and accepts deposit money, but can provide those services 24 hours a day.

Automation is generally considered a positive step if the worker is assisted by the machine but maintains some CONTROL over its services. However, if operator skills and knowledge are taken over by the machine, the resulting monotony, lack of control, and social isolation may result in stress. Even when automation requires high skills from process operators, the monitoring of machines can become monotonous. Skills are used only during a small percentage of the work hours. Mechanical breakdowns can mean loss of completed work if work flow is interrupted. All of these elements have been shown to constitute sources of stress at both the psychological and physiological level.

See also AUTONOMY; BOREDOM; MENTAL HEALTH.

automobile mechanics   Workers who repair, service, and overhaul automobiles and other motor vehicles. They examine vehicles to determine the nature, extent, and location of defects, dismantle engines, transmission, differential, and other parts requiring attention. They may rebuild parts of vehicles using lathes, shapers, welding equipment, and hand tools. They may do electrical and body repairs and spray painting.

Similar occupations with similar health hazards include bus mechanic, diesel engine mechanic, truck mechanic, and some garage workers.

Automobile mechanics face risk of injuries while working with mechanized equipment, such as lathes, drills, and boring machines, and various cutting and hand tools, such as wrenches, screwdrivers, chisels, and the like. Some mechanics experience injuries resulting from collapse, settling, or slipping of jacking, lifting, or hoisting equipment and falling vehicles. They may experience stabs and cuts caused by knives, sharp objects, and hand tools, banging on metal pieces or loose bolts during dismantling, repair, and assembly operations. They may experience SLIPS, TRIPS, AND FALLS on slippery or greasy surfaces, or from ladders, stairs, elevated platforms, and falls into inspection pits. Further, they may experience crushing of toes by heavy objects or burns as a result of contact with hot surfaces, hot exhaust pipes, or sudden release or hot water and steam from radiator and cooling system pipes, soldering, and welding operations. Further, they may experience eye injury from splinters and flying objects during grinding, machining, and similar operations or while operating compressed-air equipment for drum and brake cleaning.

Some accidents may occur due to bursting tires or poorly installed and inappropriately maintained steam and water pressure cleaners. Electrocution may be a result of defects, short circuits, or incorrect use of electromechanical equipment, or con-

tact with live wires (shocks from portable power tools). Another hazard is fire and explosion of flammable and explosive substances such as gasoline, solvents, and oils, or accumulating gas as a result of spills and leaks. Inspection pit workers face the hazard of CARBON MONOXIDE poisoning. Finally, mechanics may face road accidents during testing and driving of repaired vehicles.

Other hazards include hearing damage from NOISE while doing bodywork, development of vibration white finger (VWF) as a result of vibrating power-driven tools, exposure to low temperatures, and winds, particularly in open garages. Mechanics face the hazard of chronic poisoning as a result of exposure to many industrial chemicals, including brake fluids, detergents, lubricants, metal cleaners, and paint removers and thinners. Skin sensitization, dermatitis, eczema, and oil acne can be caused by adhesives, asbestos, antifreeze and brake fluids, epoxy resins, gasoline, oils, and other substances.

Eye irritations may be caused by contact with chemical irritants, dusts, and fumes. Eye and skin injuries can occur as a result of splashes of corrosive and reactive chemicals. Asbestosis and mesothelioma may be caused by asbestos dust from brake drum cleaning and processing operations. There may be blood changes during exposure to SOLVENTS, such as BENZENE, toluene, and xylene. During lifting and moving of heavy loads, many mechanics experience acute musculoskeletal problems caused by physical overexertion and incorrect lifting of heavy weights while working. Repetitive work over a long period of time may cause cumulative trauma disorders, including CARPAL TUNNEL SYNDROME.

Finally, according to the *Encyclopaedia of Occupational Health and Safety,* there is a danger of being attacked by dissatisfied customers in a workplace open to the public. The time pressure while working also can cause psychological stress.

See also ASBESTOS; AUTO BODY REPAIR AND REFINISHING; CHEMICAL TOXICITY; DERMATITIS; DUST; ELECTRICITY-RELATED INJURIES; REPETITIVE STRESS INJURIES; SKIN AND SENSE ORGAN TOXICITY; STRESS; VIBRATION WHITE FINGER; VIOLENCE.

Encyclopaedia of Occupational Health and Safety. 4th ed. Vol. 4. Geneva: International Labor Organization, 1998, pp. 103.8–103.9.

autonomy   A feeling of being in CONTROL associated with attitudes of independence and freedom that may take many forms in the workplace. An individual may express autonomy by making simple decisions on the job. For example, the ability to prioritize projects at work may give a feeling of autonomy. When one loses a sense of autonomy, one may experience anxieties, lose self-esteem, and become frustrated with the working situation.

In developing a sense of autonomy, peer groups play an important role. Young people with good peer relationships generally acquire good feelings about themselves and develop confidence that others will like them. They will also develop the ability to realize what others expect of them and to make choices about meeting those expectations in a flexible way without anxieties.

For some individuals, particularly teenage workers, peer groups may be destructive to autonomy. This may be the case with teenagers whose experiences with peers have not enabled them to develop self-confidence. Under these circumstances, anxieties and a desire for approval or acceptance may lead to drug abuse, cigarette smoking, or other destructive behaviors that seem to make the individual feel part of the group but may make them less effective if they have part-time or full-time jobs.

See also ANGER; FRUSTRATION; PEER GROUPS; SELF-ESTEEM; STRESS.

baby boomers The 76 million Americans born between 1946 and 1964. Baby boomers are products of the population explosion, or "baby boom," that began during World War II, peaked after the war, and lasted until the mid-1960s. The baby boom has been attributed to several factors, including wartime prosperity following the Great Depression, increased births as servicemen returned after the war, a lower marriage age than for previous generations, and a tendency to have children in quick succession early in marriage. At the beginning of the 2000s, many early baby boomers were approaching retirement or taking retirement benefits from their employment.

This generation has experienced many concerns during their working lives. Many baby boomers were influenced by the changing times in which they lived. Those who, as young adults, protested the Vietnam War may have been labeled hedonistic, rebellious, and undisciplined. Some fought for civil rights or were active in the women's movement. Improved birth control, more permissive sexual standards, and an emphasis on education for both sexes plunged young women of the baby boom generation into a world of choices. Resulting questions included pursuing careers, getting married, and having children.

A good job market and a rapidly expanding economy greeted baby boomers upon graduation from college. They were soon described as having tendencies toward materialism that included acquiring possessions at an early stage and "having it all." In reaction, baby boomers tended to become entrepreneurial and viewed a job as something that should be fulfilling and stimulating rather than simply a means to the end of supporting themselves and their families. However, the sheer numbers of the baby boom generation created a population bulge that increased competition for the remaining corporate and government positions. Challenges facing this generation in the 2000s include a changing economy, downsizing, the future of Social Security, rising heath care costs, and the need for RETIREMENT savings.

See also WORKING MOTHERS.

Light, Paul Charles. *Baby Boomers.* New York: Norton, 1988.
Mills, D. Quinn. *Not Like Our Parents: How the Baby Boom Generation Is Changing America.* New York: William Morrow, 1987.
Silver, Don. *Baby Boomer Retirement: 65 Simple Ways to Protect Your Future.* Los Angeles: Adams-Hall Publishers, 1994.

back injuries, back pain According to the Bureau of Labor Statistics (BLS), more than 1 million workers suffer back injuries each year, and back injuries account for one of every five workplace injuries or illnesses. Further, according to the BLS, one-fourth of all compensation indemnity claims involve back injuries, costing industry billions of dollars.

The National Institute for Occupational Safety and Health (NIOSH) reports that back injuries are the most common type of nonfatal occupational health injury involving lost work days. This category of injury resulted in nearly 800,000 cases in 1997. According to author Peter Greaney, 50 percent of the workforce experiences some type of back pain each year, from mild to severe. Employees who miss work due to more serious back injuries are away from work for an average of three months.

When a work-related back injury occurs, worker's compensation and medical costs may represent only a part of the costs the employer must bear. While the employee is recovering, the employer incurs indirect or "hidden" costs, including the loss of an experienced worker and the cost of training a replacement, downtime, lost productivity, and impaired quality control.

The BLS survey shows that four out of five of these injuries were to the lower back, and that three out of four occurred while the employee was lifting. Lifting, placing, carrying, holding, and lowering are involved in manual materials handling (the principal cause of compensable work injuries).

Overexertion is the most common cause of back sprains, strains, and tears, accounting for more than 50 percent of all cases. Overexertion injuries result from excessive lifting, pushing, pulling, holding, carrying, or throwing an object. These injuries, which involve the nerves, tendons, muscles, and supporting structures of the body, are considered musculoskeletal disorders (MSDs). Back strain occurs when the muscles, ligaments, and/or tendons in the back are damaged due to overstretching or overuse. Herniated disks are also a type of back injury found in workplace situations.

Common causes of low-back pain include:

- Improper and/or excessive methods of lifting, pulling, pushing, carrying, holding, or throwing an object
- Lowering, bending, or twisting
- Sudden slip or fall
- Cumulative trauma, or multiple micro-injuries sustained over a period of time

NIOSH examined the relationship between selected musculoskeletal disorders of the upper extremities and lower back, and exposure to physical factors at work. The review established strong evidence that lower back disorders are associated with work-related lifting and forceful movements. The review also cited strong evidence of a causal relationship between low back disorder and whole body vibration (WBV), which occurs when mechanical energy oscillations are transferred to the body as a whole. Typical exposures for WBV include driving automobiles or trucks and operating industrial vehicles. Other physical workplace factors found to have an association with back disorders include awkward posture and heavy physi-

cal work, although these risk estimates are more moderate than those for lifting and forceful movements. MSDs risk factors include intensity, frequency, and duration of the physical exposure.

Preventing Back Injuries

Because of the high cost of back injuries to employers and the pain and suffering experienced by employees, an increasing number of occupational health and safety managers are emphasizing back injury prevention programs. Many back injuries may be reduced by effective administrative and engineering control programs and better ergonomic design of work tasks.

To avoid workplace back injuries NIOSH recommends implementation of an ergonomics program focusing on redesigning the work environment and work tasks to reduce the hazards of lifting. A number of engineering and administrative components can minimize back injuries on the job. They include:

- Training in proper lifting techniques to reduce stress on the lower back
- Physical conditioning and stretching programs to reduce the risk of muscle strain
- Reducing the size of objects or materials being moved or lifted. Parameters of control should include maximum allowable weights for a given set of tasks, the compactness of a package, the presence of handles, and the stability of the package being handled
- Adjusting the height at which the object or materials are retrieved or deposited; adjusting the height of a pallet or shelf. Lifting that occurs below knee height or above shoulder height is more strenuous than lifting between these lines. Obstructions that prevent a worker's body contact with the object lifted also generally increase the risk of injury
- Implementing mechanical aids, such as hoists, pneumatic lifts, conveyors, adjusted lift tables, or automated materials handling equipment to reduce the need to bend, reach, and twist
- Evaluating workflow of production, storage, and display to reduce excessive reaching, bending, pushing, pulling, lifting, loading, and unloading

Training to Prevent Back Injuries

In jobs in which ergonomic stressors have the potential for injury, employees and their supervisors can receive ergonomic awareness and job-specific training in:

- Recognizing workplace risk factors and methods of control
- Identifying signs and symptoms of health effects of exposure to workplace risk factors
- Understanding the importance of early reporting
- Knowing the employer's medical management procedures
- Following corrective actions to be implemented; the role of each individual involved and how to participate in the process

The American Academy of Family Physicians offers tips on lifting safely to avoid back injuries. (See chart.)

TIPS TO HELP PREVENT BACK INJURIES

- Check every object before you lift by pushing the object lightly with your hands or feet to see how easily it moves. This tells you about how heavy it is. Remember, a small size does not always mean a light load.
- Make sure that the load you want to lift is packed right. Make sure that the weight is balanced and packed so it will not move around. Loose pieces inside a box can cause accidents if the box becomes unbalanced.
- Be sure you have a tight grip on the object before you lift it. Handles applied to the object may help you lift it safely.
- Consider how easy it is to reach the load. You can be injured if you arch your back when lifting a load over your head. To avoid hurting your back, use a ladder when you are lifting something over your head.
- When picking up an object, use slow and smooth movements. Hurried movements can strain the muscles in your back. Keep your body facing the object while you lift it. Twisting while lifting can hurt your back.
- Keep the load close to the body. Having to reach out to lift and carry an object may hurt your back.
- Lift "with your legs" only when you can straddle the load. To lift with your legs, bend your knees to pick up the load, not your back. Keep your back straight.
- Try to carry the load in the space between your shoulder and your waist. This puts less strain on your back muscles.

- Make sure you have enough room to lift safely. Clear a space around the object before lifting it.
- Look around before you lift and look around as you carry. Make sure you can see where you are walking. Know where you are going to put down the load.
- Avoid walking on slippery or uneven surfaces while carrying something.
- Get help before you try to lift a heavy load. Use a dolly or a forklift if you can.
- To avoid injury, pace yourself. Take small breaks between lifts if you are lifting a number of things.

Source: American Academy of Family Physicians

Back Safety for Health Care Workers

Lifting and moving patients is a large part of the job for nurses, occupational therapists, or physical therapists. Workers need to use proper technique to ensure their own and the patient's safety. The Arnot Ogden Medical Center in Elmira, New York, provides recommendations for HEALTH CARE WORKERS. (See chart.)

HEALTH CARE WORKERS: TIPS FOR PREVENTING BACK INJURIES

- When turning a patient over with a draw sheet (under the patient), position the patient's bed no higher than your thigh area. If the patient is safe enough, lower the bed rails. Place the patient's arms over chest and cross patient's legs. Place your knee on the bed near the patient's shoulder. Use the draw sheet and your whole body to turn the patient toward you, with your back in balance and your knees bent.
- When pulling the patient up from the bed, position the patient's bed below your waist. Stand alongside the bed with your knees bent, feet wide apart and face the direction in which you will move the patient. Reach under the back and shoulders to slide the patient up. An able patient can push against the mattress with elbows or feet to help you.
- When transferring the patient from the bed to a wheelchair, set the bed to its lowest height. Lock the wheels of the wheelchair. Use your knees to support the patient's weak knees. Keep your back balanced and your knees slightly bent. Rock the patient forward to a standing position. Bend your knees to turn and lower the patient into the wheelchair. The patient can hold onto your shoulder or waist, not your neck, for support.
- When transferring a patient from the bed to a gurney, get a partner to help. The bed and gurney must be next to each other, locked in place, and adjusted to the same height. To slide the patient more easily, place a plastic bag under the draw sheet.

- When transferring a patient from a wheelchair to a toilet, be prepared to prevent the patient from falling during the transfer. Lock the wheels of the wheelchair. If the patient is in a leg cast, have the patient use the wheelchair arm and the grab bar on the wall while you carefully lift the patient's leg cast.
- If you need to help a patient who is falling down, bend your knees as you help the patient gently to the floor. Keep close to the patient. Get help before lifting the patient from the floor.

Source: Arnot Ogden Medical Center

Preventing Back Injuries While Sitting at a Computer

If you spend most of your working hours at a computer terminal, you may experience backaches, minor muscle aches, and a stiff neck. There are steps you can take to help yourself. The Arnot Ogden Medical Center recommends that computer workers make adjustments to their work situations to protect their backs. Following are recommendations:

- Keep your feet flat on the floor, with knees slightly lower than your hips. Avoid crossing your legs. Place a folded towel or wedge-shaped cushion on the seat of your chair to tip your pelvis forward. This position reduces the strain on your lower back.

- Watch your posture. Slide your chair under your desk or workstation so that you do not have to lean into your work. Proper posture is key to maintaining a healthy back. Your spine is balanced with three natural curves that must be aligned to prevent strains and stress. The lower curve, called the lumbar curve, bears most of the strain when you are seated; it needs constant support. Position a lumber support or rolled-up towel in the small of your back to support your lumbar curve.

- Avoid slumping shoulders or a slouching spine. Shift your position frequently to eliminate strain. Take a brief walk around the office or do some simple stretching exercises to release the muscle tension caused by sitting.

- Use a document holder or other device to keep pages in an upright position. Move your computer screen so that the top of the screen is at forehead level.

Use of Industrial Back Belts

NIOSH reports an increase in the use of industrial back belts, although their effectiveness in preventing injuries has not been documented. The decision to wear a back belt is a personal choice; however, NIOSH advises that workers and employers should have the best available information to make their choice. Back belts, also called back supports are currently worn by various workers, including grocery store clerks, airline baggage handlers, and warehouse workers.

Back belts remind the wearer to lift properly, may reduce internal forces on the spine during forceful exertions of the back, may increase intra-abdominal pressure (which may counter the forces on the spine), and may stiffen the spine and decrease forces on the spine. However, there is currently inadequate scientific evidence that back belts reduce the risk of injury.

Back belts were initially used in medical settings. These belts, termed "orthoses," resembled corsets worn by 19th-century women and were typically used to provide additional back support during rehabilitation of injuries. Subsequently, athletes began using leather belts for weight lifting.

The industrial back belt has been used only in recent years. While there are more than 70 types of industrial back belts, the typical abdominal support used in workplaces today is a lightweight elastic belt worn around the lower back, sometimes held in place with suspenders.

For further information:

Arnot Ogden Medical Center
600 Roe Avenue
Elmira, NY 14905
(800) 952-2662 (toll free)
(607) 737-4499 (fax)
www.arnothealth.org

See also ERGONOMICS; LOST WORKDAYS; NATIONAL INSTITUTE OF OCCUPATIONAL SAFETY AND HEALTH; OCCUPATIONAL SAFETY AND HEALTH ADMINISTRATION.

Greaney, Peter P. "A Primer on Occupational Back Injuries and Safety Guidelines to Avoid Injury." *Work-Care Whitepaper Article,* March 30, 2001.

bakers   See FOOD SERVICE INDUSTRY.

baling machines   See DEATHS IN THE WORKPLACE.

barley itch   See BREWING.

barotrauma   See COMMERCIAL DIVING.

baseball injuries (professional)   Baseball is a popular recreational sport as well as a profession for some athletes. The playing field is their workplace and injuries can occur. Shoulder and elbow problems can result from excessive pitching or sliding into bases. Also, severe ankle sprains may occur while sliding into bases. Carpal tunnel syndrome can result from repeated bending of the wrist from throwing the ball. "Turf toe" is a sprain of the big toe that results from running on hard artificial turf.

Baseball Finger

Baseball finger is caused by a direct blow to the tip of the finger, which often happens to catchers going after foul tips. It can tear the extensor tendon in the finger or detach it from the bone. The job of the tendon is to straighten the tip of the finger. If it is injured, the player will not be able to fully extend the finger.

For further information:

American Academy of Orthopaedic Surgeons (AAOS)
6300 N. River Road
Rosemont, IL 60018-4262
(800) 346-AAOS (toll-free)
(847) 823-7186
(847) 823-8125 (fax)
http://aaos.org

See also CARPAL TUNNEL SYNDROME; SPORTS MEDICINE.

Levy, Allan M., and Mark L. Fuerst. *Sports Injury Handbook.* New York: John Wiley & Sons, Inc., 1993.

basketball injuries   Basketball is a popular sport as well as a profession for some athletes. Their workplace is the basketball court. There are many hazards to the players. As tall players try for rebounds, they make a great deal of contact. A player driving to the hoop may collide violently with an opponent, or if he is knocked off balance, fall on a hardwood floor. Additionally, as the game is played in a somewhat confined space, players may run into the pole holding the basket, the scorer's table, or the bench close to the court. Players can bang their heads going after loose balls, or a player can get an elbow blow to the head. Occasionally, a basketball player will be poked in the eye, resulting in a scratched cornea.

Overuse injuries are those caused by stressing an area repeatedly until it is damaged and begins to hurt. One such injury is patellar tendinitis, or "jumper's knee," which is characterized by pain in the tendon just below the kneecap.

Achilles tendinitis is another common overuse injury in basketball players. This injury of the tendon connecting the muscles in the back of the calf to the heel bone causes pain in the back of the leg just above the heel. Occasionally, the Achilles tendon can tear. Some basketball players overuse the tendons in their shoulders, resulting in an injury to the rotator cuff. The rotator cuff is composed of four muscles. The tendons that attach these muscles to the shoulder bones can become inflamed and painful, particularly when the player is doing a repetitive overhead motion, such as shooting the basketball.

Traumatic injuries are those caused by a sudden forceful injury. Common traumatic injuries in basketball are jammed fingers. The severity of a jammed finger can range from a minor injury of the ligaments, which connect bones, to a broken finger. Another type of traumatic injury is a muscle pull or tear. In basketball players, these injuries occur primarily in the large muscles of the legs.

Ankle Sprain in Basketball Players

The most common basketball injury is the ankle sprain, which often occurs when a player lands on another player's foot or the ankle rolls too far outward. When this happens, ligaments connecting bones and supporting the ankle are stretched and torn; ligaments can tear partially or completely.

Knee Injuries

A knee sprain is a small tear in the ligaments or joint capsules that is not severe enough to cause the knee to give way. If the player twists a knee, the meniscus can be torn; this is tissue that acts as a cushion between the bones of the upper and lower leg at the knee. A more severe injury is a complete tear of one or more of the ligaments supporting the knee. The anterior cruciate ligament is one of the more common torn ligaments in the knee; this ligament connects the upper and lower leg bones and helps hold the knee in place.

Physical fitness and adequate stretching before a basketball game helps professional players avoid injuries. According to authors A. M. Levy and M. L. Fuerst, tall people have long backs and need more muscle to stabilize the spine. A basketball player who comes down off balance from a rebound commonly strains a muscle and may even rupture a disc. All the jumping and twisting in basketball exerts tremendous torque on the back, and the muscles must be strong and well developed to absorb the shock.

See also FOOT PROTECTION; SPORTS MEDICINE.

Levy, Allan M., and Mark L. Fuerst. *Sports Injury Handbook.* New York: John Wiley & Sons, Inc., 1993.
O'Connell, Patrick. "Common Basketball Injuries: Keep Your Guard UP!" *Hughston Health Alert,* May 2002.

battered women   See DOMESTIC VIOLENCE.

battery manufacturing   See CADMIUM.

baton hazards   See CONDUCTORS (MUSICAL).

behavior therapy   A type of psychotherapy used to treat some mental health concerns that emphasizes learned responses. It is often used in conjunction with other types of therapies, including psychopharmacotherapy. Behavioral therapy is used to treat people who have a wide variety of issues, including alcoholism, anxieties, phobias, agoraphobia, obsessions, and compulsions. Many EMPLOYEE ASSISTANCE PROGRAMS employ or refer workers to therapists in this field.

Therapists strive to modify or alter undesirable or self-defeating behaviors, such as anxiety and avoidance, instead of working toward changing the personality by probing into the individual's unconscious. Behavior therapists work on the theory that behavior has a learned component (as well as a biologic component) and thus many unwanted behaviors and reactions can be replaced with more desirable behaviors and reactions.

Behavior therapy focuses on observable aspects of specific behaviors, such as the frequency or intensity of a physiological response (for instance, sweating as a reaction to anxiety) or obsessive hand washing. Reports by the patient and self-rating scales are also often used to describe details of behavior. Specific treatment techniques are tailored by each therapist to the particular needs of each individual.

Goals of treatment are determined by the therapist and the patient and often the patient's family as well. The patient in behavioral therapy views the therapist as a coach and usually makes choices about trying to learn new behaviors and responses. Usually the goal is for the patient to learn self-control of bad behaviors and increase the number of preferred behaviors.

Numerous learning techniques are used by behavioral therapists. These include classical conditioning, desensitization, flooding, operant conditioning, and modeling. In cases of social phobias, for example, therapists may use techniques in which the individual is gradually exposed to the fear-producing situations. The exposure may take place in the patient's imagination first and then in reality. Sometimes the reality never occurs (some situations are easy to imagine but difficult to simulate). However, the key to effective treatment is the gradualness of the exposure combined with the simultaneous use of relaxation training and new physiological and behavioral responses.

Exposure Therapy (Desensitization)

Exposure therapy refers to many behavioral techniques that involve the use of gradual exposure to an anxiety-producing situation. These techniques include systematic desensitization and exposure at full intensity (flooding and implosive therapy). In systematic desensitization, a technique used by behavioral therapists, patients learn to rank situations that cause anxiety and distress, as well as a variety of deep-muscle-relaxing techniques. For example, an individual who fears public speaking might place speaking at the top of the list of fear-producing activities and thinking about sitting with a date in a restaurant might rank at the bottom of the list.

The individual is trained in relaxation, both mental and physical. When these techniques are mastered, the person is asked to imagine, in as much detail as possible, the least fear-producing item from the list. When a comfort level is reached in imagining this item, the patient can move up through the hierarchy with success. However, when the individual has completed treatment and goes out in the real world to face fears, there may be slight regression down the list. For example, an individual who has learned to remain calm while speaking at a sales meeting may not be comfortable alone with a date. However, the individual will eventually be able to move from nonthreatening social events to more intimate settings.

Systematic desensitization was explained in 1958 by Joseph Wolpe (1915–97), an American psychiatrist. His first reports were on adults who had many mental health problems, including obsessive-compulsive disorder, reactive depression, and phobias. He adapted his technique from experiences gained in the 1920s when he worked with children in overcoming animal phobias.

Flooding and Implosive Therapy

Flooding is another technique used by behavioral therapists. The individual is asked to experience an anxiety-producing situation by imagination or in real life while experiencing the supportiveness of the therapist. Then the individual is directly exposed to an intense level of the anxiety-producing situation without benefit of a graduated approach, as is the case in the systematic desensitization technique. The therapist controls the content of scenes to be imagined and experiences that reoccur. The therapist describes scenes with great vividness, deliberately making them as disturbing as possible to the anxious individual, who has not been instructed to relax. Prolonged experience with these situations is planned to help the individual to experience "extinction" of the anxiety responses and thus overcome them.

Implosive therapy is a similar technique used by therapists. The individual is repeatedly encouraged to imagine anxiety-producing situations at maximum intensity and experience an intense anxiety reaction. The anxiety response is not reinforced and thus becomes gradually reduced.

Like desensitization, the techniques of flooding and implosion reduce anxieties and unwanted behavior in some persons (such as those with simple fears), but desensitization seems to be more effective and to have more permanent results.

Modeling

In modeling as a form of behavioral therapy, the individual watches another person—often of the same sex and age as the troubled person—successfully perform a particular feared action, such as entering a room full of strangers or going for a job interview. The fearful person experiences extinction of the feared responses in a vicarious way. The technique is really social learning or observational learning.

Modeling has another aspect; in "covert modeling," the anxious patient simply imagines that another person faces the same anxieties or concerns without unwanted physiological responses.

Hypnosis and Biofeedback

Hypnosis is considered a behavioral technique and is often used in conjunction with other techniques. Hypnosis can help the individual reach a trancelike state in which he or she becomes extremely receptive to suggestion. Then, through posthypnotic suggestions, the individual may learn to change patterns of behavior, such as having fearful reactions before a job interview. By itself, hypnosis is not considered an appropriate treatment for most mental health concerns. It is often used to modify specific unwanted behaviors, such as smoking cigarettes.

Biofeedback is often used in conjunction with relaxation training and to enhance possibilities for a person's response to treatments. In biofeedback, physiological reactions can be monitored electrically. An anxious person can learn to regulate certain processes, such as breathing or heart rate.

See also BIOFEEDBACK; COVERT REHEARSAL; DEPRESSION; MIND-BODY CONNECTIONS; PANIC ATTACKS

AND PANIC DISORDER; PHOBIAS; PSYCHOTHERAPIES; RELAXATION; SMOKING.

Hollandsworth, James G. *Physiology and Behavior Therapy: Conceptual Guidelines for the Clinician.* New York: Plenum Press, 1986.

Kaplan, Sheldon J. *The Private Practice of Behavior Therapy: A Guide for Behavioral Practitioners.* New York: Plenum Press, 1986.

Kahn, Ada P., and Jan Fawcett. *The Encyclopedia of Mental Health.* 2d ed. New York: Facts On File, Inc., 2001.

belting (vocal) injury   A type of injury incurred through very loud, brassy, "twangy" singing by popular, theatrical, and rock singers. Broadway theater music involves this type of singing, as does much ethnic music around the world. Voice teachers are asked to teach it, and apparently, there is no substitute. When it is good it can be very profitable to the singer, but if badly executed can be devastating for the vocal cords. According to author Jo Estill, physicians observe everything from reddened, vibratory margins of the vocal folds to polyps, nodes, and hemorrhagic blebs (blisters).

There are many demands on professional singers in all genres of music. While many belters can successfully imitate opera singers (often in comedy routines), many classical singers damage their voices by attempting the belting technique. According to Estill, there may be two different modes of voice production, and the physiology for each is distinctly unique. She also believes that it is more difficult to change the laryngeal posture and to increase the effort from less strenuous opera techniques to the new posture and effort of belting.

See also PERFORMING ARTS MEDICINE; MUSICIANS' INJURIES.

Estill, Jo. "Belting and Classic Voice Quality: Some Physiological Differences." *Medical Problems of Performing Artists* 3, no. 1 (March 1988): 37–43.

Benson, Herbert (1935–   )   Herbert Benson, M.D. is the founding president of the Mind/Body Medical Institute, the associate chief of the Division of Behavioral Medicine at Harvard Medical School, and the chief of the Division of Behavioral Medicine at New England Deaconess Hospital.

He is a cardiologist who discovered and described how the relaxation response is a protective mechanism against overreaction to stress and anxieties. He is the author or coauthor of several books relating to relaxation and stress, including *The Relaxation Response* and *The Mind/Body Effect;* hundreds of his articles have appeared in medical journals and popular magazines. His writings are often used in relaxation, meditation, and other stress reduction classes associated with EMPLOYEE ASSISTANCE PROGRAMS.

Dr. Benson discovered the relaxation response while studying people who practiced TRANSCENDENTAL MEDITATION. As a specialist in high blood pressure, Dr. Benson's particular interests have included how the relaxation response can help people with high blood pressure and other health concerns. He warns that people with high blood pressure should not just give up their medication. What MEDITATION and the relaxation response do, he maintains, is improve upon the benefit of the medication. He argues that "mindfulness" is needed to be healthy and productive.

For information:

Mind-Body Medical Institute
New Deaconess Hospital
Harvard Medical School
185 Pilgrim Road
Cambridge, MA 02215
(617) 632-9530

See also COMPLEMENTARY THERAPIES; RELAXATION.

Benson, Herbert. *The Relaxation Response.* New York: Avon Books, 1975.

———. *Beyond the Relaxation Response.* New York: Berkeley Press, 1985.

———. *The Mind/Body Effect: How Behavioral Medicine Can Show You the Way to Better Health.* New York: Simon and Schuster, 1979.

benzene   A colorless liquid with a sweet odor. Benzene evaporates into the air quickly, dissolves slightly in water, and is highly flammable. It is formed from both natural processes and human activities. Benzene ranks in the top 20 chemicals for production volume in the United States. Some industries use benzene to make other chemicals which are used to make plastics, resins, and nylon and other synthetic fibers. It is also used to make some types of rubbers, lubricants, dyes, detergents, drugs, and pesticides. Natural sources of benzene include volcanoes and forest fires. Benzene is also a natural part of crude oil, gasoline, and cigarette smoke.

People working in industries that make or use benzene may be exposed to the highest levels of it. Other people may be exposed to leakage from underground storage tanks or from hazardous waste sites containing benzene.

The major health effect from long-term exposure to benzene is on the blood. Benzene causes harmful effects on the bone marrow and causes a decrease in red blood cells, leading to anemia. It can also cause excessive bleeding and can affect the immune system, increasing the chance for infection.

Women who breathed high levels of benzene for many months had irregular menstrual periods and a decrease in the size of their ovaries. It is not known whether benzene exposure affects the developing fetus in pregnant women or fertility in men.

The Department of Health and Human Services (DHHS) has determined that benzene is a known human carcinogen. Long-term exposure to high levels of benzene in the air can cause leukemia, cancer of the blood-forming organs.

For further information:

Office of Policy and External Affairs
United States Agency for Toxic Substances and Disease Registry (ATSDR)
1600 Clifton Road NE (E-60)
Atlanta, GA 30333
(888) 422-8737 (toll-free)
(404) 498-0080
(404) 498-0057 (fax)
http://www.atsdr.cdc.gov

See also CHEMICAL TOXICITY; REPRODUCTIVE TOXICITY.

benzo[b]fluoranthene (B[b]F) One of several polycyclic aromatic hydrocarbon (PAH) compounds. It is formed when gasoline, garbage, or any animal or plant material burns, and is usually found in smoke and soot. Benzo[b]fluoranthene is found in the COAL TAR pitch used to join electrical parts together and in creosote, a chemical used to preserve wood.

Workers who handle or are involved in the manufacture of PAH-containing materials may be exposed to B[b]F. People who work in coal tar production plants, coking plants, asphalt production plants, coal-gasification sites, smokehouses, municipal trash incinerators, and facilities that burn wood, coal, or oil may be exposed to B[b]F in the workplace air.

Typically, exposure for workers and the general population is not to B[b]F alone but to a mixture of similar chemicals. Factories that produce coal tar also contribute small amounts of B[b]F into the air. People may come in contact with B[b]F from soil on or near a hazardous waste site, such as former gas-manufacturing sites or abandoned wood-treatment plants that used creosote.

The most common way B[b]F enters the body is through the lungs when a person breathes in air or smoke containing it. It also enters the body through the digestive system when substances containing it are swallowed.

The U.S Department of Health and Human Services has determined that B[b]F may reasonably be anticipated to be a carcinogen. B[b]F causes cancer in laboratory animals when applied to their skin. This finding suggests that it is likely that people exposed in the same manner could also develop cancer.

The National Institute for Occupational Safety and Health (NIOSH) has determined that workplace exposure to coal products can increase the risk of lung and skin cancer in workers and has suggested a workplace exposure limit. The OCCUPATIONAL SAFETY AND HEALTH ADMINISTRATION (OSHA) has set a legal limit of all PAHs per cubic meter of air.

For further information:

Office of Policy and External Affairs
Agency for Toxic Substances and Disease Registry (ATSDR)
1600 Clifton Road NE (E-60)
Atlanta, GA 30333
(888) 422-8737 (toll-free)

(404) 498-0080
(404) 498-0057 (fax)
http://www.atsdr.cdc.gov

See also BENZOPYRENE; CANCER; CHEMICAL TOXICITY; NATIONAL INSTITUTE FOR OCCUPATIONAL SAFETY AND HEALTH; POLYCYCLIC AROMATIC HYDROCARBONS; SKIN OR SENSE ORGAN TOXICITY.

benzo[a]pyrene (B[a]P) One of the polycyclic aromatic hydrocarbon (PAH) compounds formed when gasoline, garbage, or any animal or plant material burns. It is found in smoke and soot, in the COAL TAR pitch used to join electrical parts together, and in creosote, a chemical used to preserve wood.

People who work in coal tar production plants, coking plants, asphalt production plants, coal-gasification sites, smokehouses, municipal trash incinerators, and facilities that burn wood, coal, or oil may be exposed to B[a]P in their workplace air.

The most common way B[a]P enters the body is through the lungs when a person breathes in air or smoke containing it. It also enters the body through the digestive system when substances containing it are swallowed.

The U.S. Department of Health and Human Services has determined that B[a]P may reasonably be anticipated to be a carcinogen. B[a]P causes cancer in laboratory animals when applied to their skin. This finding suggests that it is likely that people exposed in the same manner could develop cancer.

The National Institute for Occupational Safety and Health (NIOSH) has determined that workplace exposure to coal products can increase the risk of lung and skin cancer in workers and has set legal limits for all PAHs in workplaces.

See also BENZOFLUORANTHENE; CANCER; CHEMICAL TOXICITY; OCCUPATIONAL SAFETY AND HEALTH ADMINISTRATION; NATIONAL INSTITUTE FOR OCCUPATIONAL SAFETY AND HEALTH; POLYCYCLIC AROMATIC HYDROCARBONS; SKIN OR SENSE ORGAN TOXICITY.

berylliosis See BERYLLIUM.

beryllium A brittle, steel-gray metal found as a component of coal, oil, certain rock minerals, volcanic dust, and soil. Elemental beryllium is the second lightest of all metals; beryllium is used as a metal alloy in such diverse areas as dental appliances, golf clubs, non-sparking tools, wheelchairs, and electronic gadgets. Although it was discovered in 1798, it was not widely used in industry until the 1940s and 1950s.

Other industrial applications of beryllium include use as a pure metal, mixed with other metals to form alloys, processed to salts that dissolve in water, and processed to form oxides and ceramic materials. The aerospace and defense industries have used beryllium in windshield frames and other structures in high-speed aircraft and space vehicles, aircraft and space shuttle brakes, satellite mirrors and space telescopes, inertial guidance systems and gyroscopes, neutron moderators or reflectors in nuclear reactors, X-ray windows, and nuclear weapons components.

Beryllium is a significant workplace hazard; in certain people it causes chronic beryllium disease, or CBD, an irreversible and sometimes fatal scarring of the lungs. The adverse health effects of beryllium exposure are caused by the body's immune system reacting with the metal, resulting in an allergic-type response.

Medical studies show that even small amounts of beryllium particles breathed deeply into the lungs may trigger an allergy-like sensitivity in 2 percent to 5 percent of people exposed. In studies of people in certain occupations where historically exposure to beryllium was greatest, such as machinists in beryllium operations, this number rose to as many as 10 percent to 14 percent.

Long-term or chronic health effects can take years to develop after the first exposure to beryllium and can affect people who were exposed to very small amounts of beryllium. In some cases, CBD has been diagnosed in former office workers and others who had only brief, incidental exposure to beryllium. The average time from first beryllium exposure to the development of symptoms of CBD is 10 to 15 years. Adverse health effects have appeared in some people a few months after exposure, but not for as long as 30 years in others.

More than 100 current and former employees of the Department of Energy (DOE) worksites have CBD. The percentage of people who were exposed and became ill is much larger than similar percentages known for other DOE workplace health hazards.

Dust control is the primary preventive measure. There is currently no widely available test to find out who is sensitive to beryllium before exposure occurs. CBD is treatable, but not curable.

Symptoms of chronic beryllium disease are very similar to those of other diseases, particularly sarcoidosis, that affect the lungs and sometimes other organs. In some cases, doctors have misdiagnosed what turned out to be CBD as sarcoidosis or another disease. CBD is primarily a lung disease, but it may also affect other organs, particularly the lymph nodes, skin, spleen, liver, kidneys, and heart.

SYMPTOMS OF CHRONIC BERYLLIUM DISEASE

Persistent coughing
Shortness of breath with physical exertion
Fatigue
Chest and joint pains
Blood in the sputum
Rapid heart rate
Loss of appetite
Fevers and night sweats

Treatment for CBD

After loss of lung function is detected, treatment may involve taking corticosteroids to reduce inflammation. If successful, treatment with steroids can slow the progress of CBD by reducing the buildup of scar tissue and delaying permanent lung damage. However, many individuals do not respond well to treatment or the side effects of long-term steroid treatment. Side effects from long-term use of steroids can include slower healing of infections, calcium loss from the bones, higher blood cholesterol, and fluid and salt retention, which worsen heart or kidney disease.

Individuals with insufficient levels of oxygen in their blood as a result of CBD may also need supplemental oxygen to help improve oxygen delivery to the body and to protect the heart from the damage that can be done by low oxygen levels. Individuals who cannot take steroids may continue to lose lung function and have a poorer quality of life; in some cases, they become invalids and their life span may be shortened.

Beryllium and Cancer

Beryllium has been classified as a human carcinogen by the International Agency for Research on Cancer. Studies suggest that beryllium metal and other beryllium compounds are carcinogenic by several routes of administration, including inhalation. A significantly elevated risk of lung cancer has been demonstrated among workers employed in several beryllium manufacturing facilities and also among individuals enrolled in the Beryllium Case Registry, who had either acute beryllium-related pneumonitis or CBD at the time of enrollment. The association between beryllium exposure and lung cancer in these studies was judged not to be compounded by cigarette smoking. There have been numerous lawsuits by employees who believe that they contracted illnesses while working with beryllium.

Acute Beryllium Disease

Acute beryllium disease (ABD) rarely occurs in modern industry because of improved industrial protective measures designed to reduce exposure levels. ABD is caused by breathing relatively high concentrations of beryllium in dust and metal fumes. High exposures may result in death or respiratory illness similar to pneumonia bronchitis. Symptoms of ABD present much more rapidly than those associated with CBD.

Both the Occupational Safety and Health Administration and the National Institute of Occupational Safety and Health have set limits for exposure to beryllium at many sites, including general industries, shipyards, and construction.

See also ALLERGIES; CANCER; CONSTRUCTION; DUST; LUNG CANCER; PERSONAL PROTECTION EQUIPMENT; RESPIRATORY TOXICITY.

Better Hearing Institute (BHI) A nonprofit educational organization, BHI informs persons with impaired hearing and the general public about hearing loss and available help through medicine, surgery, amplification, and other rehabilitation.

For information:

Better Hearing Institute (BHI)
P.O. Box 1840
Washington, DC 20013

(800) EAR-WELL
888-HEAR-HELP (Voice/TDD)
(703) 684-6048 (fax)
www.betterhearing.org

See also AMERICANS WITH DISABILITIES ACT; SELF-HELP FOR HARD OF HEARING PEOPLE; NOISE.

beverage industry   Workers in the beverage industry are exposed to many health hazards, including harsh cleaning agents used to clean and disinfect equipment. Skin and eye contact with the cleansers can cause severe dermatitis; inhalation of fumes or spray may cause damage to the lungs, nose, mouth, or throat. Slips and falls are common because of water in and around production areas.

High-speed filters, overhead conveyors, and glass containers can result in harm from flying and broken glass, making cuts and eye injuries common. While the shift to plastic and aluminum containers has reduced the use of glass, breakable containers are still used for wine and spirits.

Author Lance Ward reports that strains, sprains, and repetitive motion injuries are common. Large quantities of raw materials are moved in bags and barrels, and loads of empty bottles and cans and finished products in a variety of containers are moved. Repetitive motion injuries result from sorting and inspection of glass bottles and other packaging operations. Automation has taken over many operations in the beverage industry, but workers tempted to reach into a moving conveyor to put a bottle or can upright can be dragged into the mechanism; broken limbs can result from trying to clear a jammed machine. Noise levels are high and hearing loss can result. It occurs insidiously over time and is irreversible. While engineering controls to reduce noise levels are used, wearing the standard hearing protection is still the preferred method used.

CONFINED SPACES, such as tanks, casks, vats, wastewater pits, and storage or mixing vessels have the potential of causing catastrophic injuries. Ward reports that injuries involving forklifts and similar equipment often result in crushing injuries to pedestrian personnel or to the operator if the vehicle overturns. Cramped conditions are also conducive to accidents involving material-handling equipment.

Chemicals used in refrigeration systems include chlorine and liquid anhydrous ammonia; both are considered hazardous substances. Chlorine is often stored in pressurized metal cylinders. Injuries can occur during changeover from one cylinder to another or from a defective valve. Accidental release of anhydrous ammonia can cause burns of the skin and the respiratory system on contact. An uncontrolled release of anhydrous ammonia can result in air concentrations high enough to explode. Chlorine and anhydrous ammonia have strong, identifiable odors and are easily detectable in the air. Emergency systems to detect leaks, automatic ventilation and shutdown equipment, and evacuation and response procedures are essential.

See also AMMONIA; BREWING; CHEMICAL TOXICITY; FORKLIFT TRUCK INJURIES; PERSONAL PROTECTION EQUIPMENT; SKIN AND SENSE ORGAN TOXICITY; SLIPS, TRIPS, AND FALLS; WINE INDUSTRY.

Ward, Lance A. "Health and Environmental Concerns." *Encyclopaedia of Occupational Health and Safety.* Vol. 3. 4th ed. p. 65.14–65.15.

big box injuries   See FALLING MERCHANDISE.

biofeedback   A technique to monitor mental and physical events by electrical feedback. Biofeedback is useful in many approaches to therapy for mental health concerns such as anxieties and phobias. It provides an anxious or phobic individual with a basis for self-regulation of certain processes, such as autonomic system reactions to fear situations. It establishes a diagnostic baseline by noting physiological reactions to stressful events and enables therapists to relate this information to the individual's self-reports, fills gaps in the individual's history, and encourages relaxation in the part of the individual to whom the biofeedback equipment is applied. Relaxation training is often suggested to assist people in controlling anxiety reactions.

See also BEHAVIOR THERAPY; COMPLEMENTARY THERAPIES.

Doctor, Ronald M., and Ada P. Kahn. *The Encyclopedia of Phobias, Fears, and Anxieties.* 2d. ed. New York: Facts On File, Inc., 2000.

biological hazards   Threats to workers' health that include microorganisms and their toxic products, poisonous and allergenic plants, and exposure to animals which can lead to diseases and allergies.

See also ALLERGIES; ANIMAL HANDLERS; GARDENERS; HEALTHCARE WORKERS; LABORATORY WORKERS.

bipolar disorder   A group of mood disorders characterized by alternating mood swings of mania and severe depression. The fourth edition of the American Psychiatric Association's *Diagnostic and Statistical Manual of Mental Disorders* (1994) divides the bipolar disorders based on prevalence of symptoms.

During the manic phase, the individual may have an enormous amount of energy and may feel agitated, excited, and capable of any undertaking. There may be constant talking, inappropriate degrees of self-confidence, little need for sleep, irritability, aggressiveness, and impulsive behavior, such as excessive shopping and spending.

During the depressive phase, individuals suffer from any of the symptoms associated with major depression. They may feel sad, helpless, and hopeless.

Bipolar disorder may start in childhood or during the 40s and 50s. Often bipolar disorder is first noticed during adolescence. However, as moodiness and crises surrounding personal and school relationships often arise at this time, symptoms of bipolar disorder might be at first incorrectly attributed to normal adolescent problems.

Bipolar disorder often runs in families, and evidence from family and twin studies supports genetic transmission of the vulnerability. Evidence from biochemical and imaging studies using PET scanning, MRI, and CAT studies offers further support for the biological nature of this illness.

Additional problems of alcohol and substance abuse are common with bipolar disorder. This is called a "comorbid" condition. Early detection and finding the right medication is crucial in helping people recover. Many people are helped by taking lithium and/or one of many antidepressant medications as well as other drugs under the close supervision of their physician.

See also DEPRESSION; EMPLOYEE ASSISTANCE PROGRAMS; MENTAL HEALTH.

Fawcett, Jan, Nancy Rosenfeld, and Bernard Golden. *New Hope for People with Bipolar Disorder.* Roseville, Calif.: Prima, 2000.

Kahn, Ada P., and Jan Fawcett. *Encyclopedia of Mental Health.* 2d ed. New York: Facts On File, Inc., 2001.

bird fancier's lung   See HYPERSENSITIVITY PNEUMONITIS.

black lung disease (coal workers' pneumoconiosis)   Job-related diseases caused by continued exposure to excessive amounts of respirable coal dust. This dust becomes embedded in the lungs, causing them to harden, making breathing very difficult.

Silicosis is another job-related lung disease included in black lung. Miners develop silicosis when they are overexposed to dust containing silica. Respirable particles of silica embed in the lungs cause scar tissue to form, reducing the lungs' ability to extract oxygen from the air.

COAL WORKERS' PNEUMOCONIOSIS

Coal workers' pneumoconiosis: Most frequently recorded occupations on death certificate, residents age 15 and over, selected states and years, 1987–1996

Occupation	Number	Percent
Mining machine operators	3,811	70.0
Laborers, except construction	172	3.2
Managers and administrations, n.e.c.	73	1.3
Truck drivers	66	1.2
Janitors and cleaners	59	1.1
Electricians	55	1.0
Construction laborers	52	1.0
Carpenters	46	0.8
Machine operators, not specified	46	0.8
Farmers, except horticulture	45	0.8
All other occupations	801	14.7
Occupation not reported	221	4.1
Total	5,447	100.0

Source: National Center for Health Statistics

In the early stage of the illness, there may be no immediate symptoms. However, the later stages of the disease, known as progressive massive fibrosis or PMF, will cause shortness of breath, coughing, and pain during breathing. PMF may result in permanent disability and early death.

Black lung can be detected by X ray and pulmonary function tests. Every operator of an underground coal mine is required to have an X-ray plan approved by the National Institute for Occupational Safety and Health (NIOSH). At intervals not to exceed five years, X rays must be offered to employees at no cost. Results must be kept confidential.

To reduce the possibility of contracting the disease, workers should be familiar with the mine's ventilation plan and dust control provisions, make

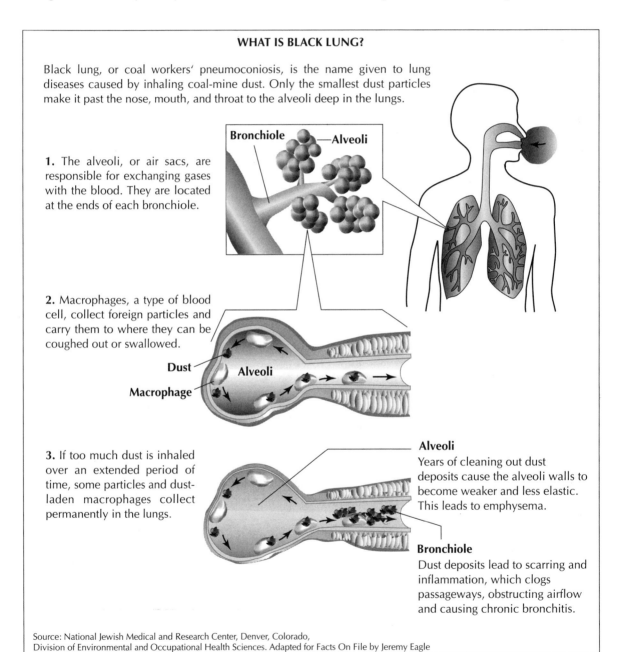

WHAT IS BLACK LUNG?

Black lung, or coal workers' pneumoconiosis, is the name given to lung diseases caused by inhaling coal-mine dust. Only the smallest dust particles make it past the nose, mouth, and throat to the alveoli deep in the lungs.

Bronchiole **Alveoli**

1. The alveoli, or air sacs, are responsible for exchanging gases with the blood. They are located at the ends of each bronchiole.

2. Macrophages, a type of blood cell, collect foreign particles and carry them to where they can be coughed out or swallowed.

Dust   **Alveoli**

Macrophage

3. If too much dust is inhaled over an extended period of time, some particles and dust-laden macrophages collect permanently in the lungs.

Alveoli
Years of cleaning out dust deposits cause the alveoli walls to become weaker and less elastic. This leads to emphysema.

Bronchiole
Dust deposits lead to scarring and inflammation, which clogs passageways, obstructing airflow and causing chronic bronchitis.

Source: National Jewish Medical and Research Center, Denver, Colorado,
Division of Environmental and Occupational Health Sciences. Adapted for Facts On File by Jeremy Eagle

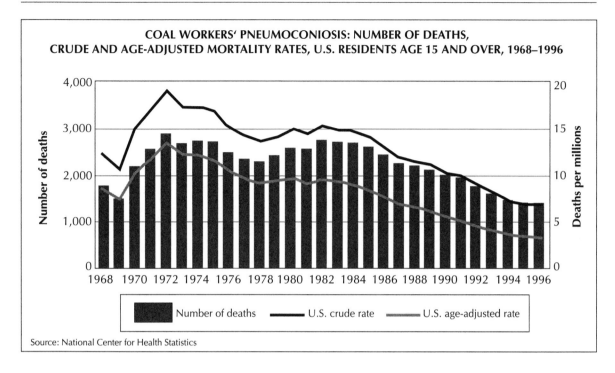

COAL WORKERS' PNEUMOCONIOSIS: NUMBER OF DEATHS, CRUDE AND AGE-ADJUSTED MORTALITY RATES, U.S. RESIDENTS AGE 15 AND OVER, 1968–1996

Source: National Center for Health Statistics

use of dust controls such as scrubbers and dry dust collectors, utilize respirators when necessary, and in underground coal mines, ensure that a respirable dust control on-shift examination is conducted.

The Federal Coal Mine Health and Safety Act of 1969 was enacted because of the tremendous number of fatal mine accidents and the epidemic of black lung disease then present in coal miners. Although the numbers of fatalities and incidence of the disease has been sharply reduced by safeguards, the disease continues.

See also OCCUPATIONAL LUNG DISEASE.

bloodborne pathogens   See HEALTH CARE WORKERS; LABORATORY WORKERS; NEEDLESTICK INJURIES AND PREVENTION.

blood toxicity   See CARDIOVASCULAR OR BLOOD TOXICITY.

body language   A form of COMMUNICATION through facial expression, posture, gestures, or movements, with or without words. Both the communicator and the listener may employ body language. It can be used to express emotion or a reaction to the meaning of communication in the workplace.

Body language may be an indicator of emotions the communicator and the listener are experiencing. According to Gay Turback in the *Rotarian* (April 1995), "Without uttering a syllable, it is possible to communicate love, hate, fear, rage, deceit, and virtually every other emotion in the human repertoire." The article goes on to describe how body signals have been around for more than 1 million years, with some researchers having catalogued 5,000 hand gestures and 1,000 postures, each with its own message. Turback says, "Although some body language is nearly universal, much of it is an accouterment of one culture or another. Certain actions may have one meaning in Mexico, a different meaning in the United States, and no relevance in Canada. Some examples that are common among North Americans are listed below.

EXAMPLES OF BODY LANGUAGE AS A MEANS OF COMMUNICATION ON THE JOB

Action	Meaning
Toes pointed outward	Confidence
Toes pointed inward	Submission
Jutting chin	Belligerence
Action	**Meaning**
Lip and nail biting	Disappointment
Lip licking	Nervousness
Foot tapping	Impatience
Leaning backward	Relaxation
Leaning forward	Interest
Open palms	Honesty
Rubbing hands together	Excitement

Kahn, Ada P., and Jan Fawcett. *Encyclopedia of Mental Health.* 2d ed. New York: Facts On File, Inc., 2001.

body therapies Body therapies encompass ancient Eastern traditions of spirituality and cosmology along with contemporary Western neuromuscular and myofascial systems of skeletostructural and neuroskeletal reorganization. They postulate that the body holds memory of trauma and that therapy must address body sensations. Many employers now include MASSAGE THERAPY as an employee benefit or make it available at the worksite as a way to relieve employees' stress.

Ancient disciplines in the category of body therapies include YOGA, T'AI CHI, Zen, Taoism, and Tantra. In the 20th century, Wilhelm Reich observed that patients with emotional disturbances all demonstrated severe postural distortions. This observation helped to uncover more connections between the body and the psyche and led to the development of the Reichian school of body therapy.

Another modern pioneer in the field was Moshe Feldenkrais, who postulated that the human organism began its process of growth and learning with one built-in response, the fear of falling. All other physical and emotional responses were learned as the human organism grew and explored. To attain the full potential of the body, mind, emotions, and spirit, there must be, according to Feldenkrais, "reeducation of the kinesthetic sense and resetting of it to the normal course of self-adjusting improvement of all muscular activ-

ity." This would "directly improve breathing, digestion, and the sympathetic and parasympathetic balance, as well as the sexual function, all linked together with the emotional experience." Feldenkrais believed that reeducation of the body and its functions was the essence of creating unity of the being. His method has helped many people with problems of back pain, whiplash, and lack of coordination. The Feldenkrais method is also used to help people who have temporomandibular joint syndrome (TMJ), which is a collection of symptoms, including pain, that affect the jaw, face, and head, often brought about by anxieties, stress, and tension.

Four Systems of Body Therapies

Although many systems overlap and encompass aspects of the others, body therapies can be divided into four general categories, based on their methods.

Physical manipulation systems include the connective tissue work of the Ida Rolf school (Rolfing) and the deep-tissue release systems such as myofascial release used by John Barnes, an American physical therapist.

Energy balancing systems include Chinese acupuncture and acupressure, polarity, and jin shin.

Emotional release systems include bioenergetics, primal therapy, and rebirthing.

Movement awareness systems include those of Aston, Feldenkrais, Trager, and Aguado.

For information:

Feldenkrais Guild of North America
c/o Ruth A. Hurst
3611 SW Hood Avenue
Suite 100
Portland, OR 97201
(800) 775-2118 (toll-free)
(503) 221-6612
(503) 221-6616 (fax)
http://www.feldenkrais.com

North American Society of Teachers of the Alexander Technique
P.O. Box 517
Urbana, IL 61801
(217) 367-6956

American Massage Therapy Association (AMTA)
820 Davis Street
Suite 100
Evanston, IL 60201-4444
(888) 843-2682 (toll-free)
(847) 864-0123
(847) 864-1178 (fax)
http://www.amtamassage.org

See also ALEXANDER TECHNIQUE; COMPLEMENTARY THERAPIES; EMPLOYEE ASSISTANCE PROGRAMS; MASSAGE THERAPY; MIND-BODY CONNECTION.

Eisner, Betty. "Body Work and Psychological Healing." *Advances* 13, no. 3 (Summer 1997): 64–66.
Feldenkrais, Moshe. *Awareness through Movement.* San Francisco: Harper & Row, 1972.
———. *Explorers of Humankind.* San Francisco: Harper & Row, 1979.
Feltman, John, ed. *Hands-On Healing.* Emmaus, Pa.: Rodale Press, 1989.

boredom   A subjective state of mind. Many working people seem bored with everything, while others are bored with nothing. Some working people enjoy jobs that many others think are boring. For some people, boredom is a self-imposed prison which keeps them from trying new things or having life-enriching experiences. Boredom often occurs in individuals who thrive on excessive stimulation and is a function not of their work or social causes but the reduction in stimulation.

Some people view things as boring because they really are afraid of failure. In his book *A New Guide to Rational Living,* Dr. Albert Ellis said: "Viewing failure with fear and horror, some people avoid activities that they would really like to engage in." The rationale of such people is: If life is boring, nothing is worth doing. Thus if nothing is worth doing, a person can hardly fail.

Overcoming Boredom

Overcoming boredom depends on whether people are bored because they cannot live without excitement or whether they are bored because they have chosen to remain in a shell of inaction. Life or work is not supposed to be thrilling all the time. If you crave continuous thrills, reduce your expectations for excitement. If you are encased by the stresses of boredom, try to face reality. Get out and do one new thing each day, such as talk to some new people at work, volunteer in your off-hours, or write letters. Boredom carried to the extreme can be a threat to mental health in that it can lead to depression and anxiety with lack of stimulation.

For further information:

The Boring Institute
P.O. Box 40
Maplewood, NJ 07040
(201) 763-6392

See also DEPRESSION; FRUSTRATION; GENERAL ADAPTATION SYNDROME; MENTAL HEALTH; SELYE, HANS.

Kahn, Ada P. *Stress A–Z: A Sourcebook for Facing Everyday Challenges.* New York: Facts On File, Inc., 2000.

bottling industry   Bottling plants that produce soft drinks and other beverages are now highly mechanized and efficient. In the 1960s, most bottlers produced beverages using machinery that ran at 150 bottles per minute. Now, with advances in production technology, filling lines are able to run in excess of 1,200 containers per minute. This automated environment has allowed bottlers to reduce the number of employees, but plant safety remains an essential consideration.

Soft drink bottling involves five major processes, each with its own safety issues: treating water, compounding ingredients, carbonating the product, filling the containers, and packaging. Hazards include lifting-related injuries, particularly to backs and shoulders. Through improved workstation design, lifting injuries can be minimized. Adjustable tables can be used to raise or lower material to waist level, for example, so that employees do not have to bend and lift as much.

Machine guarding is critical for safe beverage manufacturing. Equipment such as fillers and conveyors moves at high speeds, and if left unguarded, could snag an employee's clothing or body parts. Conveyors, pulleys, gears, and spindles must have appropriate covers to prevent employee contact. Overhead conveyors can create the additional hazard of falling cases.

In filling rooms, wet conditions are prevalent. Slip-resistant shoes can help prevent falls. All electrical equipment must be properly grounded and protected from any moisture. Appropriate LOCK-OUT/TAGOUT procedures must be followed during repairs.

While most of the chemicals present in bottling plants are not hazardous, every operation uses flammable substances, acids, caustics, corrosives, and oxidants. Safe handling is essential, and PERSONAL PROTECTIVE EQUIPMENT must be used. Training must cover the location and operation of emergency response equipment. Eyewash stations and showers can minimize injury to anyone who is exposed to unsafe levels of a hazardous chemical.

Chlorine, which is used in the water treatment area, could be hazardous in the event of an accidental release. Chlorine typically comes in steel cylinders, which should be stored in an isolated, well-ventilated area and secured from tipping. New chlorine compounds introduced in the late 1990s are gradually replacing the need for chlorine gas, and they are safer to handle than gas.

Ammonia is used as a refrigerant in bottling operations. In the event of a leak or spill, ammonia can create a health hazard. Carbon dioxide, used in filling operations, also can create a health hazard. Ventilation is essential and facilities should be monitored regularly for elevated carbon dioxide levels.

Forklift trucks are used throughout the bottling plants. Potential operators must be trained and safety inspections and programs followed.

See also AMMONIA; BREWING; FORKLIFT TRUCK INJURIES; SLIPS, TRIPS, AND FALLS; WINE INDUSTRY.

Stellman, Jean Mager, ed. *Encyclopaedia of Occupational Health and Safety.* Vol. 3. 4th ed. Geneva: International Labor Organization, 1999, p. 65.3–65.6.

boron A trace mineral, mined in California and other parts of the world. It is a dark powder used in compounds in many industries such as glass and detergent manufacture and in agriculture as a fertilizer ingredient. Pyrex glass is tough and heat resistant because of the boric acid used to make it. Boron is an essential mineral but can be toxic in excess.

Most reports of boron toxicity concern earlier use of borates as weak germicides. Now, aqueous solutions of borate are no longer used as antiseptic agents, nor is boric acid used in skin powders or ointments, because of the toxicity of these preparations. However, it is still possible to purchase boric acid.

Principal toxic effects of boron include possible irritation of the eyes and skin upon contact. There may be inflammation of the eyes, with redness, watering, and itching. Nausea, vomiting, and diarrhea are common, occurring shortly after ingestion. Skin effects characterized by itching, scaling, reddening, and, occasionally, blistering, are common following any route of exposure. Toxicity may be delayed for several hours following application to cut or severely abraded skin areas.

Precautions for Handling and Exposure

Precautions against exposure and personal protection include using engineering controls to keep airborne levels in industry below recommended exposure limits. Adequate local exhaust or general ventilation should be used to keep exposure to airborne contaminants below the exposure limits. The selection of PERSONAL PROTECTIVE EQUIPMENT varies, depending upon conditions of use. Appropriate respiratory protection for dust/mist should be used when ventilation is inadequate. A filtering dust mask is recommended for most applications if respiratory protection is needed. Where skin and eye contact may occur as a result of brief periodic exposures, wear long-sleeved clothing, coveralls, chemical resistant gloves, and safety glasses with side shields. A respiratory protection program that meets requirements of the Occupational Safety and Health Administration (OSHA) must be followed whenever workplace conditions warrant use of a respirator.

See also CHEMICAL TOXICITY; EYE INJURIES/PROTECTION; SKIN OR SENSE ORGAN TOXICITY.

Boyle's law See COMMERCIAL DIVING.

brainstorming A specialized approach to problem-solving by group or team effort. It is based on the concept that while a person alone may not be able to arrive at a solution to a problem because of a block in the thinking process or external distraction, several people working together will be more likely to reach a solution.

When properly conducted, brainstorming sessions can be an important management tool. Employees who take part in a brainstorming session feel like a part of the company. Furthermore, by making them part of the problem-solving process, they develop a feeling of *control* and ownership in what they do. As such, employee participation in brainstorming sessions may help to alleviate stress in the workplace.

In a typical brainstorming session, the coordinator, who is in charge of collecting the ideas, indicates that there should be a free flow of ideas, with no right or wrong answers or suggestions. All participants are encouraged to be a part of the process. However, if this brainstorming rule is not established, participants may feel self-conscious and may experience a great deal of stress and anxiety.

The basic proposition of brainstorming is that one idea can lead to another and thus increase the creative output. When successful, this approach generates enthusiasm and a large number of suggestions, as one person expands upon ideas of others. Often, brainstorming sessions backfire. Participants never see the results of a brainstorming session carried out. This leads to an increase of employee disappointment and the reduction of morale.

See also AUTONOMY; CREATIVITY.

brewing industry   Production of beer. Most of the injuries in breweries come from manual handling. Hands are bruised, cut, or punctured by jagged hoops, splinters of wood, and broken glass. Feet are bruised or crushed by falling or rolling barrels. Backs are injured due to lifting and carrying of barrels. Falls on wet and slippery floors are common.

Breweries are often hot. In some processes, such as cleaning out mash tuns, workers are exposed to hot and humid conditions. Cases of heat stroke and heat cramps can occur, particularly in new workers. These conditions can be prevented by increased salt intake, adequate rest periods, and provision and use of showers. Temperature and ventilation control, with attention to elimination of steam vapor and the use of PERSONAL PROTECTIVE EQUIPMENT (PPE), are important precautions against accident and injury and also against general hazards of high temperature and humidity.

Brewery workers also face a hazard in NOISE. Metal barrels have replaced wooden barrels. Wooden casks made little or no noise during loading, handling, or rolling, but empty metal casks increase noise. Also, automated bottling plants generate noise.

According to author J. F. Eustace, handling of grain used in brewing can produce barley itch, caused by a mite infesting the grain. Millworker's asthma, sometimes called malt fever, has been shown to be an allergic response to the grain weevil. Handling of hops can produce a dermatitis due to absorption of the resinous essences through broken or chapped skin.

Accidents with machinery occur in the brewing industry. Where there are walkways across or above conveyors, frequent stop buttons should be provided. In the filling process, serious cuts can be caused by bursting bottles. Adequate guards on the machines and face guards, rubber gloves, rubberized aprons, and nonslip boots for workers can help prevent injuries. There should be an effective LOCKOUT/TAGOUT program for maintenance and repair.

Electrical equipment needs special protection in brewing plants because of the usually damp conditions. Ground fault circuit interrupters should be installed where necessary. Wherever possible, low voltages should be used, particularly for portable inspection lamps. Steam is used, causing burns and scalds. Tagging and protection of pipes and safety locks on steam valves can prevent accidental release of scalding steam.

Carbon dioxide is formed during fermentation; concentrations of 10 percent, even if breathed for only a short time, can produce asphyxia, unconsciousness, and eventual death. Efficient ventilation is necessary in all fermentation rooms where open vats are used. There should be an acoustical warning system that will operate immediately if the ventilation system breaks down.

Accidental discharge of refrigerants also can produce serious toxic and irritant effects. Today AMMONIA is the most common refrigerant. In the past, chloromethane, bromomethane, and sulfur dioxide were used.

See also FOOT PROTECTION; HAND PROTECTION; SKIN AND SENSE ORGAN TOXICITY; SLIPS, TRIPS, AND FALLS; WINE INDUSTRY.

Eustace, J. F. "Brewing Industry." *Encyclopaedia of Occupational Health and Safety.* 4th ed. Vol. 3. Geneva: International Labor Organization, 1998, p. 65.12.

bricklayers, cement workers, and plasterers   In a survey reported in 1998 by John T. Joyce, retired president of the International Union of Bricklayers and Allied Craftworkers (BAC), 47 percent of members were worried about dangers of dust created by sawing, grinding, mixing, and demolition of masonry materials, and 36 percent of active members expressed concern about scaffolding.

In a survey of cement workers who had lost work because of on-the-job injuries, leading causes were bending, climbing, crawling, reaching or twisting, falling from a scaffold, and overexertion due to lifting. The most common types of injuries included back injuries, primarily ruptured or herniated disks, dislocations, back strains, strained muscles, and cuts and lacerations. When asked what health or safety issues they are most concerned about, exposure to masonry dust that may contain silica was on top. It is most commonly exposed through grinding, sawing, and cutting masonry products.

Workers classified as "masonry, stonework, and plastering" accounted for 11 percent of the 182,000 serious injuries and work-related illnesses among construction workers.

For information contact:

The International Union of Bricklayers and Allied Craftworkers
1776 I Street, NW
Washington, DC 20006
(202) 783-3788
www.bacweb.org

See also BACK INJURIES/BACK PAIN; CONSTRUCTION; SCAFFOLDING; SLIPS, TRIPS, AND FALLS.

bronchitis   Inflammation of the bronchi, the airways that connect the trachea (windpipe) to the lungs, resulting in a persistent cough that produces considerable quantities of sputum (phlegm). Bronchitis is more common in smokers and in areas with high atmospheric pollution. The disease is more prevalent in industrial cities and in manual and unskilled workers than among white-collar workers.

Bronchitis is considered chronic when sputum is coughed up on most days during at least three consecutive months in at least two consecutive years. The disease commonly results in widespread narrowing and obstruction of the airways in the lungs.

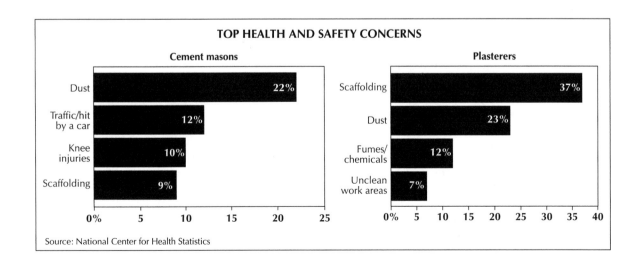

TOP HEALTH AND SAFETY CONCERNS

Cement masons

Dust	22%
Traffic/hit by a car	12%
Knee injuries	10%
Scaffolding	9%

Plasterers

Scaffolding	37%
Dust	23%
Fumes/chemicals	12%
Unclean work areas	7%

Source: National Center for Health Statistics

It often coexists with and may contribute to the development of emphysema, in which the alveoli (air sacs) in the lungs become distended. Chronic bronchitis and emphysema together are sometimes called CHRONIC OBSTRUCTIVE PULMONARY DISEASE (COPD).

Symptoms of chronic bronchitis are somewhat different than those of chronic asthma, in which wheezing and breathlessness vary in severity from hour to hour and day to day.

See also ASTHMA, OCCUPATIONAL.

Clayman, Charles B., ed. *American Medical Association Encyclopedia of Medicine.* New York: Random House, 1989.

brownfields Properties on which expansion, redevelopment, or reuse may be complicated by the presence of a hazardous substance, pollutant, or contaminant. They are called brownfields to distinguish them from undeveloped, pristine land in areas outside of the city (often called greenfields).

There are chemical, physical, and biological hazards to workers on brownfields. Chemical hazards include residues from former municipal and hazardous waste dumps, residues from former petroleum production and processing operations, residues from metal smelting and battery recycling operations, residues from railroad car repair and painting facilities, and contaminated soil from operations such as rocket fuel manufacturing and dry cleaning facilities. Physical hazards include working in confined spaces, electrical injuries, injuries from hand and power tools, heat stress, noise and hearing loss, trenching and excavation, slips, trips, and falls, welding, cutting and brazing. Biological hazards include bloodborne pathogens, municipal sewage treatment plant residues, fields fertilized with sewage plant sludge, molds and fungi in old wood structures, and biological waste dump sites.

The Occupational Safety and Health Administration (OSHA) has issued standards for identifying, evaluating and controlling employee exposures during investigations and cleanups.

See also BLOODBORNE PATHOGENS; CHEMICAL HAZARDS; CHEMICAL TOXICITY; CONFINED SPACES; ELECTRICITY-RELATED INJURIES; EMERGENCY RESPONSE; HAZARDOUS AND TOXIC SUBSTANCES; HAZARDOUS WASTE; NOISE; OCCUPATIONAL SAFETY AND HEALTH ADMINISTRATION; RESPIRATORY TOXICITY; SKIN OR SENSE ORGAN TOXICITY; PERMISSIBLE EXPOSURE LEVELS; WELDING.

brown lung disease See BYSSINOSIS.

bulimia See EATING DISORDERS.

bulimarexia See EATING DISORDERS.

bullies People who take on a type of intimidating, aggressive behavior that is of great concern in the workplace. Male bullies are more likely to use physical size and power to intimidate; female bullies are more likely to use verbal harassment.

Bullies have been thought to be compensating for anxieties or failure, but in actual fact they have been found to be self-confident people who look down on their victims and see violence as a positive way to solve problems. Many who show bullying behavior on the job were also bullies in school.

Employers should not ignore bullying incidents. Replacing people whom bullies drive away can cost up to three times their salaries, says Maria Korn of the international career services firm Lee Hecht Harrison. There are intangible costs, too, such as a bad reputation that makes it harder to replace victims of bullying.

TIPS ON DEALING WITH WORKPLACE BULLIES

- Do not procrastinate. Stand up to the bully or report the situation to your supervisor.
- Change your response to the bullying behavior.
- Learn negotiation techniques and communication skills.
- Plan in advance. Role play and know how you will respond before the bully next attacks.
- Exert self-control. Work on remaining calm but firm with any bully.
- Tell others what is happening. Most victims do not complain, letting the bully get away with it.
- Take notes. You may require legal help.
- Be sure your work performance is above reproach. Sort out the bully's legitimate requests from the illegitimate ones, so no one can say you are not doing your job.
- Arrive on time.
- Do not steal anything from the workplace (avoid accusations).

**TIPS ON DEALING WITH
WORKPLACE BULLIES** *(continued)*

- As a manager, monitor turnover and conduct frequent staff appraisals. The effects of being bullied can affect employees' performance and productivity.

According to author Melissa Gaskill, for employees, leaving is a common way of dealing with a workplace bully. Sometimes it is the only way, says Linda Dominguez, an executive coach in southern California. However, in uncertain economic times, she advises, when an otherwise good job could be hard to replace, quitting may not be an option.

"It will be better for your self-esteem if you try everything before you leave," says Michael Reggio, law-related education coordinator of the Oklahoma Bar Association.

WAYS TO CONFRONT BULLYING BOSSES

- Separate tactless putdowns from constructive criticism.
- Pick your conflict; raise only issues that really matter to you.
- Pick the right time and place for discussion.
- Address one issue at a time; do not get sidetracked.
- Be direct and use "I" statements. Example: "I felt embarrassed when . . ."
- Watch your body language; do not transmit cues of defensiveness or subservience.

See also BODY LANGUAGE; MENTAL HEALTH.

Gaskill, Melissa. "Bigger Bullies." *American Way,* August 1, 2001, p. 92–97.

Kahn, Ada P., and Jan Fawcett. *Encyclopedia of Mental Health.* 2d ed. New York: Facts On File, Inc., 2001.

Roberts, Wess. *It Takes More Than a Carrot and a Stick: Practical Ways for Getting Along with People You Can't Avoid at Work.* Kansas City, Mo.: Andrews McMeel, 2001.

bureaucracy An organization made up of rigid hierarchies bound up in structured procedures. Such organizations are often marked by delay or inaction. Examples of bureaucracies are government agencies, insurance companies, academia and higher education, banks, health care providers and hospitals, pharmaceutical and chemical companies, utilities, and most heavily-regulated industries. They have been criticized by modern management theorists as inflexible and easily co-opted by power structures to serve ends other than economic efficiency. In a bureaucracy, management's expectations for employees can be stressful.

Employees valued in bureaucracies play by the rules and are punctual and detail oriented. They do not question authority. They follow orders and procedures regardless of the consequences, and they spend long hours in meetings in which the most trivial as well as the most important decisions are made. They do not know if they are doing a good job until someone blames them for something. As a result, employees often suffer from the stress of covering for themselves regarding how the job was done rather than what the final outcome was.

Doing business with a bureaucracy as a citizen, client, or customer can be frustrating and stressful. Finding the person who knows the answer to questions or can give information and getting through to him or her, particularly when voice mail is giving directions, has become a major feat.

See also AUTONOMY; BOREDOM; CONTROL; STRESS.

Bureau of Labor Statistics (BLS) A U.S. government agency that since 1972 has issued annual reports on the number of workplace injuries, illnesses, and fatalities. Such information is useful in identifying industries with high rates or large numbers of injuries, illnesses, and fatalities, both nationwide and separately for states participating in this program.

With the 1992 survey, BLS began collecting additional information on the more seriously injured or ill workers in the form of worker and case characteristics. BLS also initiated the separate Census of Fatal Occupational Injuries to count these events more effectively than had been possible in the previous surveys.

The BLS safety and health statistics system presents three distinct types of data: (1) summary data, which reports on the number and rate of injuries and illnesses by industry; (2) case and demographic data, which provides additional details on the worker injured, the nature of the disabling condition, and the event and source of that condition for those cases that involve one or more days away from work; and (3) fatality data, which provides information on 28 separate data elements, including information on the worker, the fatal incident, and the machinery or equipment involved. Fatality data is described in greater detail below.

Fatality Data

The BLS Census of Fatal Occupational Injuries (CFOI) produces comprehensive and timely counts of fatal work injuries. CFOI is a federal-state cooperative program that has been implemented in all 50 states and the District of Columbia since 1992. The census uses multiple sources to identify, verify, profile, and count fatal worker injuries. Information about each workplace fatality, including occupation and other worker characteristics, equipment involved, and circumstances of the event, is obtained by cross-referencing the source records, such as death certificates, workers' compensation reports, and federal and state agency administrative reports.

Data compiled by the CFOI are issued annually for the preceding calendar year. Safety and health policy analysts and researchers use this data to help prevent fatal work injuries by informing workers of life-threatening hazards associated with various jobs; to promote safer work practices through improved job safety training; to assess and improve workplace safety standards; and to identify new areas of safety research.

For further information:

U.S. Bureau of Labor Statistics
OCWC/OSH
Suite 3180
2 Massachusetts Avenue, NE
Washington, DC 20212-0001
www.bls.gov
Nonfatal injuries and illnesses questions: osh-staff@bls.gov
Fatalities questions: cfoistaff@bls.gov

burnout   A progressive loss of energy, purpose, and idealism resulting from overexposure to job or other stimuli that leads to stress, stagnation, FRUS-TRATION, and BOREDOM. It may result from chronic stress at work and it is a cause of stress for the sufferer as well as his or her coworkers.

According to Beverly Potter, in her book *Beating Job Burnout: How to Transform Work Pressure into Productivity,* burnout is a destruction of motivation caused by feelings of powerlessness. Power, the ability to influence and accomplish, is essential for well-being and ongoing motivation.

Burnout can strike anyone, from top executives, surgeons, defense attorneys, and airline pilots to assembly-line workers and postal employees. Burnout has no relationship to intelligence, money, or social position.

Burnout victims are often high achievers, workaholics, idealists, and competent, self-sufficient, and overly conscientious individuals. This common denominator is the assumption that the real world will be in harmony with their ideals. They often hold unrealistic expectations of themselves, their employers and society, and often have a vague definition of personal accomplishment.

Burnout begins slowly and progresses gradually over weeks, months, and years to become cumulative and pervasive. Physical symptoms of burnout include excessive sleeping, eating, or drinking, physical exhaustion, loss of libido, frequent colds, headaches, backaches, neck aches, and bowel disorders. The burnout victim desires to be alone, is irritable, impatient, and withdrawn, and complains of boredom, difficulty concentrating, and burdensome work. Fellow workers may notice indecisiveness, indifference, impaired performance, and high absenteeism. Intellectual curiosity declines and interpersonal relationships deteriorate. "Overloaded," "tired of thinking," and "I don't know what I'm doing anymore," are some phrases that express the feelings of burnout sufferers.

**TIPS FOR COPING WITH
BURNOUT IN THE WORKPLACE**

- Recognize that no one job (or personal relationship) is a total solution for life. Strive for variety in work; avoid routine.
- Put priorities into perspective; stop trying to be all things to all people.
- Take responsibility for change.
- Set personal goals by answering these vital questions: "Where am I going?," "What do I want to achieve?" and "How am I going to achieve this?"
- Learn a new skill to enhance your optimism.
- Create an "outside life," interest and activities unrelated to your work.
- Develop a support system, people you can turn for help in problem solving.
- Consider switching careers.

**TIPS FOR COPING WITH
BURNOUT IN THE WORKPLACE**
(continued)

- Learn how to manage your personal time.
- Take breaks during the workday; go out for lunch, take walks, and so on.
- Establish an exercise program and do it at least three times a week.
- Look into alternative therapies such as relaxation techniques.
- Take mini-vacations.

See also ABSENTEEISM; AUTONOMY; CHRONIC FATIGUE SYNDROME; CONTROL; DEPRESSION; RELAXATION; STRESS.

Kahn, Ada P., and Jan Fawcett. *The Encyclopedia of Mental Health.* 2d ed. New York: Facts On File, Inc., 2001.
Potter, Beverly. *Beating Job Burnout: How to Transform Work Pressure into Productivity.* Berkeley, Calif.: Ronin Publishing, Inc., 1994.
Stevens, Paul. *Beating Job Burnout: How to Turn Your Work into Your Passion.* Lincolnwood, Ill.: NTC Publishing Group, 1995.

bursitis   Inflammation of a bursa (pillowlike sac of fluid) causing it to swell and be painful. Bursitis usually is the result of pressure, friction, or a slight injury to the membrane surrounding the joint. *Bursitis* usually refers to pain in the shoulder, but it can occur elsewhere in the body. Overuse of the shoulder through lifting or repetitive motion may result in bursitis. Bursitis is fairly common among construction workers, welders, electrical workers, and plumbers.

Tibial tubercle bursitis (known as clergyman's knee) results from kneeling on a hard surface.

See also OVERLOAD INJURIES; REPETITIVE STRESS INJURIES.

butchers and meat, poultry, and fish cutters
According to the Bureau of Labor Statistics, workers in meatpacking plants have among the highest incidences of injury and illness of all workers. In 1999, more than one-quarter of nearly 150,000 meatpacking workers suffered a job-related injury or illness. The industry also has the highest rate of lost workdays of all occupations.

As many as 40,000 meatpacking workers are injured on the job every year, according to the Bureau of Labor Statistics. This figure may be inaccurate because many injuries go unreported. The industry's rate of serious injuries is five times the national average, while the rate of cumulative trauma injuries is 33 times the national average. Meat, poultry, and fish cutters commonly work in meatpacking or fish and poultry processing plants, while butchers are usually employed at the retail level. As a result of this distinction, the nature of these jobs and the rate of injury varies.

In meatpacking plants, meat cutters slaughter cattle, hogs, goats, and sheep and cut the carcasses into large wholesale cuts, such as rounds, loins, ribs, and chucks, to facilitate handling, distribution, and marketing. In some of these plants, meatcutters also further process these parts into retail-ready cuts. These workers also produce hamburger meat and meat trimmings, such as that used to prepare sausages, luncheon meats, and other fabricated meat products.

Meat cutters usually work on assembly lines, with each individual responsible for only a few of the many cuts needed to process a carcass. Depending on the type of cut, they use knives, cleavers, meat saws, bandsaws, or other, often dangerous equipment.

In wholesale establishments and grocery stores that supply meat to restaurants and institutional food service facilities, butchers separate wholesale cuts of meat into retail cuts or individual servings. They cut meat into steaks and chops, shape and tie roasts, and grind beef for sale as chopped meat. Boneless cuts are prepared using knives, slicers, or power cutters, while bandsaws are required to carve bone-in pieces. Butchers in retail food stores may also weigh, wrap, and label the cuts of meat, arrange them in refrigerated cases for display, and prepare special cuts of meat to fill special orders.

Poultry cutters slaughter and cut up chickens, turkeys, and other types of poultry. Although the poultry processing industry is becoming increasingly automated, many jobs, such as trimming, packing, and deboning, are still done manually. As in meatpacking, most poultry cutters perform routine cuts on poultry as it moves along production lines.

Fish cutters may be employed in manufacturing or retail establishments. These workers primarily cut, scale, and dress fish by removing the head, scales, and other inedible portions and cutting the fish into steaks or boneless fillets. In retail markets, they may also wait on customers and clean fish to order.

Meat, poultry, and fish cutters also prepare ready-to-heat foods. This often entails filleting meat or fish or cutting it into bite-sized pieces, preparing and adding vegetables, or applying sauces or breading.

The Hazard of Production Line Speed

One of the crucial determinants of profitability for a slaughterhouse is also responsible for many of its greatest dangers: the speed of the production line. Once a plant is fully staffed and running, the more head of cattle slaughtered per hour, the less it costs to process each one. If the production line stops for any reason, costs go up. The typical line speed in an American slaughterhouse 25 years ago was about 175 cattle per hour. Some line speeds now approach 400 cattle per hour, according to an article by Eric Schlosser in *Mother Jones* (July-August 2001).

Plants in which cattle are slaughtered may be the most dangerous. Poultry slaughterhouses are somewhat safer because they are more highly mechanized. Chickens are bred to reach a uniform size at maturity; cattle, however, vary in size, shape, and weight when they arrive at a slaughter-house. As a result, most of the work at a modern beef plant is still performed by hand, and the most important tool is a very sharp knife.

While technological advances are responsible for some of the increase in injuries, pressure on work-ers explains the rest. When hundreds of workers stand closely together on a single line, wielding sharp knives, accidents happen. The most common meat industry accident is a laceration. Workers accidentally stab themselves or stab someone near them. They struggle to keep up with the pace as carcasses rapidly swing toward them, hung on hooks from a moving overhead chain. Accidents involving power tools, saws, knives, conveyor belts, slippery floors, and falling carcasses become more likely when the chain moves fast.

Working Conditions

In meatpacking plants and large retail food stores, butchers and meat cutters work in large rooms equipped with power machines and conveyors. In small retail markets, the butcher or fish cleaner may work in a space behind the meat counter. Butchers and meat, poultry, and fish cutters often work in rooms that are refrigerated to prevent meat from spoiling and are damp because meat cutting generates large amounts of blood, conden-sation, and other substances. Cool, damp floors increase the likelihood of slips and falls. The com-bination of low temperature, standing for long periods of time, and strenuous physical tasks, makes the work tiring. As a result, butchers and meat, poultry, and fish cutters are more susceptible to injury than most workers.

Injuries include cuts, and even amputations, that occur when knives, cleavers, and power tools are used improperly. Also, repetitive slicing and lifting often lead to cumulative trauma injuries, such as carpal tunnel syndrome.

Cumulative Trauma Injuries

The rate of cumulative trauma injuries in meat-packing is the highest of any American industry. It is about 33 times higher than the national average. According to federal statistics, nearly one out of every 10 meatpacking workers suffers a cumulative trauma injury every year. The regimentation and division of labor in slaughterhouses means that workers must repeat the same motions again and again throughout their shift. The cumulative trauma injuries that meatpacking workers rou-tinely suffer may cause lifelong impairments. Mak-ing the same knife cut 10,000 times a day or lifting the same weight every few seconds can cause seri-ous injuries to a worker's back, shoulders, or hands. Some workers have disc problems, tendini-tis, and "trigger finger" (a syndrome in which a fin-ger becomes stuck in a curled position), which can permanently limit their ability to work produc-tively. To reduce the incidence of cumulative trauma disorders, some employers have reduced workloads, redesigned jobs and tools, and increased awareness of early warning signs. How-ever, workers in this occupation continue to face the serious threat of disabling injuries.

Improvements in Safety

The American Meat Institute outlined an agenda of steps for improving plant safety in testimony before the U.S. Congress in 1987. For example, the institute cited mesh safety gloves and enforcement of glove usage as contributing to fewer knife cuts. They also pointed to increased use of new flooring materials and cleaning compounds as well as better-designed work boots to reduce slip and fall hazards.

Ongoing work on safety and health, will focus on the field of ergonomics, or the study of equipment design to reduce fatigue and discomfort. The American Meat Institute developed an illustrated ergonomics manual on strains and sprains, largely in response to the extensive exposure of industry workers to injuries. Ongoing activities also include a review of knives, knife handles, and such alternatives to knives as lasers; meetings with equipment and tool manufacturers; and a reevaluation of assembly line speeds and the use of "micro" breaks or exercise. Safety and health hazards may improve with controls such as these.

See also AMERICAN MEAT INSTITUTE; FORKLIFT TRUCK ACCIDENTS; LOST WORKDAYS; MACHINE ACCIDENTS; TENDINITIS.

byssinosis (brown lung disease) An industrial lung disease caused by allergy to an unknown agent in the dust produced during the processing of flax, cotton, hemp, or sisal. It produces a feeling of tightness in the chest and shortness of breath that may become chronic. In the United States, preventive measures in the textile industry have reduced the incidence of the disease, but it is common in many developing countries.

Symptoms may be most noticeable at the beginning of the workweek but gradually they become troublesome on every working day. In chronic byssinosis (the risk of which is increased by smoking), the sufferer is short of breath even when away from work. Respiratory failure may eventually develop when lung damage becomes extensive.

Although the disease is treated with drugs used to treat asthma, such as bronchodilators, prevention is the key to avoiding the disease. Treating raw textiles before processing reduces dust levels. Also, face masks can be worn.

According to the American Medical Association, workers who suffer from byssinosis have a statutory right to compensation by the government.

See also ALLERGIES; ASTHMA; DUST AND DEBRIS; PERSONAL PROTECTIVE EQUIPMENT; RESPIRATORY TOXICITY; OCCUPATIONAL LUNG DISEASE.

Clayman, Charles B., ed. *American Medical Association Encyclopedia of Medicine.* New York: Random House, 1989.

cadmium   A natural element in the Earth's crust, usually found as a mineral combined with other elements such as oxygen, chlorine, or sulfur. Cadmium has many uses, particularly in industry and consumer products, for batteries, pigments, metal coatings, and plastics.

Some individuals breathe workplace air contaminated by cadmium (battery manufacturing, metal soldering, or welding), breathe contaminated air near the burning of fossil fuels or municipal waste, or breathe cadmium in cigarette smoke. Breathing high levels of cadmium severely damages the lungs and can cause death. Long-term exposure to lower levels of cadmium in air, food, or water leads to a buildup of cadmium in the kidneys and possible kidney disease. Other potential long-term effects are lung damage and fragile bones.

The Department of Health and Human Services (DHHS) has determined that cadmium and cadmium compounds may reasonably be anticipated to be carcinogens. This is based on weak evidence of increased lung cancer in humans from breathing cadmium and on strong evidence from animal studies.

The National Institute for Occupational Safety and Health (NIOSH) currently recommends that workers breathe as little cadmium as possible.

See also AGENCY FOR TOXIC SUBSTANCES AND DISEASE REGISTRY; AIR POLLUTION; CARCINOGENS; NATIONAL INSTITUTE FOR OCCUPATIONAL SAFETY AND HEALTH.

caffeine   One of several stimulants affecting the central nervous system by causing a rise in heart rate, blood pressure, and muscular tension. When under stress, many workers reach for a cup of coffee. Doing so, however, may actually increase their stress level because within a few minutes of consuming caffeine-containing drinks, there is a stimulant effect on all organs and tissues. Peak blood levels are reached in about 30 minutes.

Caffeine acts directly on individual cells by affecting the chemical reactions within them. It acts indirectly by increasing the release, from the adrenal glands into the circulation, of epinephrine (adrenaline) and norepinephrine (noradrenaline), hormones that stimulate cell activity.

Caffeine in small amounts stimulates brain cells, helping reduce drowsiness and fatigue. Concentration is improved and reactions are speeded up. However, large amounts cause overstimulation, anxiety, irritability, and restlessness.

In small amounts, caffeine stimulates the heart muscle, augmenting its pumping action. This causes the blood to circulate faster and blood pressure to increase for a short time. However, too much caffeine results in overstimulation of the heart muscle and can result in palpitations.

People consume caffeine primarily in coffee and tea but also in cola drinks, cocoa, certain headache pills, diet pills, and over-the-counter medications such as NoDoz and Vivarin. Regular use of more than 600 milligrams a day (approximately eight cups of percolated coffee) may lead to chronic ANXIETY and DEPRESSION, and stomach upset.

Additional Effects of Caffeine

While caffeine in moderate doses may increase alertness and decrease fatigue for some individuals, regular use of 350 milligrams or more a day may result in a form of physical dependence. (Coffee contains 100 to 150 milligrams of caffeine per cup; tea contains about 50–75 milligrams, and cola about 30–50 milligrams.) Interruption of this pattern of use can result in withdrawal symptoms, the most noticeable of which may be severe headache, which can be relieved by taking caffeine. Many people who drink large amounts of coffee on weekdays at work have headaches on weekends because of a sudden drop in the amount of caffeine they are consuming.

Caffeine has been known to produce panic attacks in susceptible individuals. About half of those who suffer from panic disorder have panic experiences after consuming caffeine equivalent to four to five cups of coffee. Research may determine whether caffeine has a direct or causative effect on panic or simply alters the body state, triggering a panic cycle as perceived by the individual. It may be that caffeine produces its effects by blocking the action of a brain chemical known an adenosine, a naturally occurring sedative.

Caffeinism

Caffeinism is a disorder caused by recent consumption of more than 250 milligrams of caffeine. Symptoms of caffeinism may include restlessness, increased anxiety, increases in phobic reactions in phobic individuals, nervousness, excitement, insomnia, frequent and increased urination, gastrointestinal complaints, rambling thought and speech, and cardiac arrhythmia. These symptoms may be recognized by supervisors and employees and should be referred to an EMPLOYEE ASSISTANCE PROGRAM or other appropriate counseling services.

See also PANIC ATTACKS AND PANIC DISORDER.

Kahn, Ada P. *Stress A–Z: A Sourcebook for Facing Everyday Challenges.* New York: Facts On File, Inc., 1998.

cancer   A group of diseases having signs that are due to unrestrained growth of cells in one or more of the body organs or tissues. Malignant tumors commonly develop in major organs, such as the lungs, breasts, intestines, skin, stomach, or pancreas, but also may develop in the nasal sinuses, testes or ovaries, lips, or tongue. Cancers may also develop in the blood-cell-forming tissues of the bone marrow (leukemia) and the lymphatic system, muscles, or bones.

According to the National Institute for Occupational Safety and Health (NIOSH), based on well-documented associations between occupational exposures and cancer, it is estimated that approximately 20,000 cancer deaths and 40,000 new cases

of cancer each year in the United States are attributable to occupation. Millions of U.S. workers are exposed to substances that have tested as carcinogens in animal studies. Occupationally induced cancers are not new—in 1775 cancer of the scrotum was linked to chimney sweeping occupational exposure.

According to author Howard Frumkin, occupational exposure occurs most frequently through direct contact with carcinogenic agents, with any of their active metabolites during absorption through the skin or respiratory tract, or during excretion (urinary tract). A carcinogen is a substance that causes cancer. Carcinogens can be chemicals, physical agents such as ionizing radiation, or biologic agents such as viruses or aflatoxin. Frumkin reports that in some cases, such as in parts of the rubber industry, elevated rates of cancer have been detected but a specific carcinogen has not been identified. The mechanisms by which chemicals cause cancer are not fully understood, nor is there complete understanding of why some chemicals are carcinogenic and others are not.

It may take only a few years to as long as 40 years for a cancer to develop after exposure to a carcinogen. The time period between exposure and detection is called the latency period. Because of the latency period, by the time symptoms are noticed, workers may have been exposed to more than one carcinogen, may have changed jobs, and may not have been aware of their exposure(s). It is difficult for workers to fully know the occupational origin of cancer, if there is an occupational origin.

NIOSH Carcinogen List

NIOSH has compiled a list of substances considered to be potential occupational carcinogens. A number of the carcinogen classifications deal with groups of substances: anilines and homologies, chromates, dinitrotoluenes, arsenic and inorganic arsenic compounds, beryllium and beryllium compounds, cadmium compounds, nickel compounds, and crystalline forms of silica. There are also substances of variable or unclear chemical composition that are considered carcinogens, such as coal tar pitch volatiles, coke oven emissions, diesel exhaust, and environmental tobacco smoke (secondhand smoke). NIOSH may reevaluate some of the potential carcinogens the agency has identified as new data become available. Recommendations regarding the status of potential occupational carcinogens or appropriate recommended exposure limits may change. (See the NIOSH carcinogen list in Appendix III.)

Risk Factors for Cancer

According to the American Cancer Society (ACS), a risk factor is anything that increases a person's chance of getting a disease. Some risk factors can be changed and others cannot. A person's risk of developing a particular cancer is influenced by a combination of factors that interact in ways that are not fully understood. Risk factors for cancer include age, sex, and family medical history, as well as cancer-causing factors in the environment. Other risk factors relate to lifestyle choices such as tobacco and alcohol use, diet, and exposure to the Sun.

Different kinds of cancer have different risk factors. For example, cancers of the lung, mouth, larynx, bladder, kidney, cervix, esophagus, and pancreas are related to tobacco use, including cigarettes, cigars, chewing tobacco, and snuff. Smoking causes one-third of all cancer deaths, according to the ACS. Skin cancer is related to unprotected exposure to strong sunlight. Breast cancer risk factors include age, change in hormone levels throughout life, such as age at first menstruation, number of pregnancies, and age at menopause; obesity; and physical activity. Some studies have also shown a connection between alcohol consumption and an increased risk of breast cancer. Also, women with a mother or sister who have had breast cancer are more likely to develop the disease themselves. While all men are at risk for prostate cancer, several factors can increase the chances of developing the disease, such as age, race, and diet. The chance of getting prostate cancer goes up with age. Prostate cancer is more common among African-American men than among white men. According to the ACS, reasons for the difference are unknown. A high-fat diet may be a factor in causing prostate cancer. Also, men with a father or brother who have had prostate cancer are more likely to get prostate cancer themselves.

According to NIOSH, in many cases various risk factors may act together or in sequence to cause cancer.

Cancer Survival and Continuing to Work

According to Cancer Care, Inc., early detection of cancer, advances in cancer treatment survival rates, and management of side effects during radiation and chemotherapy have enabled more people with cancer to continue working. Despite various laws protecting rights of workers who suffer from a chronic disease such as cancer, those continuing to work during treatment or reentering the workplace after cancer may face challenges. Employers may think they are a poor risk for promotion or that they cannot do their previous tasks. If a worker's family member has cancer, and caregiving responsibilities fall on the worker's shoulders, the employer may make the same assumption.

Common forms of discrimination relating to cancer patients include refusal to hire, demotion or denial of promotion, not allowing time off for medical appointments, or suggesting that the person with cancer might be better off not continuing to work.

Those reentering the work force after absence due to cancer can rebuild confidence in themselves by attending classes or seminars to refresh skills in their particular area. Focus on skills, expertise, and experience rather than chronology when writing a resumé. Do not volunteer your history of cancer during an interview. Wait until you have been offered the job to ask about health benefits, but be truthful about your medical history. Focus on your current health, abilities, and skills.

The Americans with Disabilities Act (ADA) prohibits all types of discrimination based on actual disability, *perceived* history of a disability, or actual history of a disability. Also, the Family Medical Leave Act of 1993 (FMLA) guarantees the right to take time off due to illness or caring for an ill dependent without the risk of losing a job.

Prevention of Occupationally Related Cancers

The Occupational Safety and Health Administration (OSHA) sets limits for air contaminants and has adopted many separate standards for chemicals and minerals, some of which are potential occupational carcinogens. These standards require use of engineering control, work practices, and PERSONAL PROTECTIVE EQUIPMENT (PPE), including respirators, as well as other requirements. While comprehensive health standards have greatly reduced worker risk of exposure to some substances, there is still significant risk to exposed workers because of the need to make standards economically and technologically feasible.

The National Institute for Occupational Safety and Health (NIOSH) has not identified thresholds for carcinogens that will protect 100 percent of workers. NIOSH usually recommends that exposures be limited to the lowest feasible concentration and recommends use of the most reliable and protective equipment.

The American Cancer Society

The American Cancer Society is a nationwide community-based voluntary health organization dedicated to eliminating cancer as a major health problems by preventing cancer, saving lives and diminishing suffering from cancer through research, education, advocacy, and service. It is one of the oldest and largest voluntary health agencies in the United States, with more than 2 million Americans involved in research, education, patient advocacy, and rehabilitation. The American Cancer Society provides current, accurate, and unbiased information on research, news, and other cancer-related issues.

For information:

American Cancer Society
Public Information Department
1599 Clifton Road, NE
Atlanta, GA 30329
(800) 227-2345
(404) 315-9348 (fax)
www.cancer.org

See also AMERICANS WITH DISABILITIES ACT; ARSENIC; ASBESTOS; BERYLLIUM; CADMIUM; CARCINOGENS; CAREGIVERS; CHEMICAL TOXICITY; COAL TAR PITCH VOLATILES; DIESEL EXHAUST; FAMILY AND MEDICAL LEAVE ACT OF 1993; LUNG CANCER; NATIONAL INSTITUTE FOR OCCUPATIONAL SAFETY AND HEALTH; *NIOSH POCKET GUIDE TO CHEMICAL HAZARDS*; RECOMMENDED EXPOSURE LIMITS; SKIN OR SENSE ORGAN TOXICITY.

American Cancer Society, Inc. "What is Cancer?" Cancer Information Data Base, August 2001.
Frumkin, Howard. "Cancer Epidemiology and the Workplace." *Salud Pública de México* (1997): 356–369.

carbon monoxide   A colorless, odorless, poisonous gas, produced by incomplete burning of carbon-based fuels, including gasoline, oil, and wood. Carbon dioxide is also produced from incomplete combustion of many natural and synthetic products. Cigarette smoke contains carbon monoxide. When carbon monoxide gets into the body, the carbon monoxide combines with chemicals in the blood and prevents the blood from bringing oxygen to cells, tissues, and organs. The body needs oxygen for energy; high exposures to carbon monoxide can cause serious health effects, with death possible from massive exposures.

Symptoms of exposure to carbon monoxide can include vision problems, reduced alertness, and general reduction in mental and physical functions. According to the U.S. Environmental Protection Agency, carbon monoxide exposures are especially harmful to people with heart, lung and circulatory system diseases.

See also AIR POLLUTION; AUTO BODY REPAIR AND REFINISHING; CARDIOVASCULAR OR BLOOD TOXICITY; COMBUSTION POLLUTANTS; INDOOR ENVIRONMENT.

carbon tetrachloride   A chemical used widely in the DRY CLEANING industry which can be toxic to workers.

See also GASTROINTESTINAL OR LIVER TOXICITY.

carcinogens   Agents that can cause CANCER. In industry, there are many potential exposures to carcinogens. According to the OCCUPATIONAL SAFETY AND HEALTH ADMINISTRATION (OSHA), workplace exposures are considered to be at higher levels than for public exposures. MATERIAL SAFETY DATA SHEETS (MSDSs) should always contain an indication of carcinogenic potential.

Carcinogen exposure should be controlled primarily by using engineering and process control. Personal protective equipment should only be used as a supplement to these measures. Many substances with OSHA standards are classified as carcinogens or potential carcinogens by the National Toxicity Program.

See also AIR POLLUTION; ARSENIC; ASBESTOS; BENZENE; CADMIUM; CHEMICAL TOXICITY; CLEAN AIR ACT OF 1990; ETHYLENE OXIDE; FORMALDEHYDE; HAZ-

ARDOUS AIR POLLUTANTS; HAZARDOUS AND TOXIC SUBSTANCES; PERSONAL PROTECTIVE EQUIPMENT; REPRODUCTIVE HAZARDS; VINYL CHLORIDE; WOOD DUST.

cardiovascular or blood toxicity Adverse effects on the cardiovascular or hematopoietic systems that result from exposure to chemical substances. The cardiovascular system is composed of the heart and blood vessels; the hematopoietic system is composed of various blood cell types: erythrocytes (red blood cells), leukocytes (white blood cells), and platelets. Exposure to cardiovascular toxicants can contribute to a variety of diseases, including hypertension (elevated blood pressure), arteriosclerosis (hardening of the arteries), cardiac arrhythmia (abnormal heartbeat), and coronary ischemia (decreased blood flow to the heart). Exposure to hematopoietic toxicants can reduce the oxygen-carrying capacity of red blood cells, disrupt important immunological processes carried out by white blood cells, and induce cancer.

Adverse effects resulting from exposure to chemicals can occur in a variety of ways. Toxicants can contribute to cardiovascular disease by directly damaging cardiac and blood vessel tissue, initiating arteriosclerotic plaque formation, stimulating the inflammatory response, or causing kidney-related hypertension. Lead, carbon disulfide, arsenic, cadmium, ozone, and vinyl chloride have been implicated in the causes of cardiovascular disease. These chemicals may produce functional changes, such as cardiac arrhythmias, that can have serious and often lethal consequences. They can also induce hypertension, a major cause of cardiac hypertrophy and heart failure. Several toxicants have been found to aggravate preexisting cardiovascular disease. Carbon disulfide and arsenic can irreversibly accelerate coronary heart disease.

The blood cells of the hematopoietic system can also be severely affected by chemical substances. For example, benzene, a component of motor fuel, is a hematopoietic toxin. Chronic exposure to benzene vapors leads to the decreased production of all types of blood cells (pancytopenia). The long-term effect of exposure to benzene is leukemia, a cancerous proliferation of white blood cells.

See also ARSENIC; BENZENE; CADMIUM; VINYL CHLORIDE.

Smith, R. "Toxic Responses of the Blood." Chap. 8 in *Casarret and Doull's Toxicology,* C. Klassen, M. Amdur, and J. Doull, eds. New York: Pergamon Press, 1996.

Taylor, A. E. "Cardiovascular Effects of Environmental Chemicals." *Otolaryngology, Head and Neck Surgery* 114, no. 2 (1996): 209–211.

caregivers Individuals who are health care professionals, social workers, friends or family members of a child, elderly, ill, or disabled person who cannot completely care for him- or herself.

Caregiving has become a workplace health issue because many people, particularly women, are caregivers for an elderly parent, spouse, or child, and may be absent from work for prolonged periods of time or very frequently. Within families, the caregiver responsibility has usually fallen heavily on women. This tendency has not changed even though other institutional options are available. Some 75 percent of care of the elderly is still provided by a family member.

Now other social forces are making the responsibility particularly difficult. Social mobility and shrinking family size may make some women solely responsible for care of both their own and their husbands' aging parents. At the same time, women are moving into highly responsible professional positions at about the time in life that their parents need care. The Older Women's League in Washington, D.C., has determined that at least one-third of all women over age 18 can expect to be continuously in the caregiver role from the birth of their first child to the death of their parents.

According to the American Association of Retired Persons, some women are pressured to turn down promotions, avoid traveling, and even take early retirement to care for aging parents.

The caregiver role can be extremely draining of both physical and mental energy. Caregivers may feel powerless and depressed in the face of the suffering of a loved one.

See also DAY CARE.

carpal tunnel syndrome A chronic condition characterized by numbness, tingling, and pain in the thumb, index, and middle fingers. It may affect one or both hands and is sometimes accompanied by weakness in the thumb. This syndrome results from pressure on the median nerve where it passes into the hand via a gap (the "carpal tunnel," under a ligament at the front of the wrist). The median nerve carries sensory messages from the thumb and some fingers and also motor stimuli to the muscles in the hand. Damage to the nerve results in sensory disturbances, particularly the numbness or tingling sensations.

This syndrome is sometimes referred to as repetitive stress injury (RSI) because it is common to certain occupations in which the wrist is subjected to repetitive stresses and strains, particularly those involving gripping or pinching with the wrist held flexed. For example, computer operators, checkout clerks, typists, carpenters, factory workers, meat cutters (meat cleaver's elbow), violinists, and even hobbyists such as golfers or canoers may also develop carpal tunnel syndrome.

These injuries are stressful for many sufferers because they may experience confusion over continuing or quitting the job that contributes to their discomfort.

Claims for RSI cost employers some $100 billion annually, according to industry estimates in 1995. The number of workers with disorders caused by repeated trauma on the job increased from 22,600 in 1982 to 302,000 in 1993. Some severely injured carpal tunnel victims qualify for help under the Americans for Disabilities Act of 1990. This measure extended civil rights protections to an estimated 43 million Americans with physical and mental impairments. Repetitive stress injury sufferers may qualify as disabled if they can demonstrate that their impairment is permanent and substantially limits major life activities. Proof of the source injury may be difficult in some cases, as two people may be doing the identical job and only one of them develops carpal tunnel syndrome.

Treatment

With appropriate treatment, the pain can be relieved and there may be no permanent damage to the wrist or hand. Resting the affected hand at night in a splint may alleviate symptoms. If symptoms persist, a physician may inject a small quantity of a corticosteroid drug under the ligament in the wrist. If this does not help, surgical cutting of

the ligament may be performed to relieve pressure on the nerve.

For further information:

American Physical Therapy Association
1111 North Fairfax Street
Alexandria, VA 22314
(703) 684-2782
(703) 684-7343 (fax)
http://www.apta.org

Association for Repetitive Motion Syndrome
Box 471973
Aurora, CO 80047
(303) 369-0803 (fax)
http.www/.certifiedpst.com/arms

See also AMERICANS WITH DISABILITIES ACT; MUSICIANS' INJURIES; REPETITIVE STRESS INJURIES; VIDEO DISPLAY TERMINALS; WOMEN AND JOB-RELATED INJURIES AND DEATHS.

Kahn, Ada P. *Stress A–Z: A Sourcebook for Facing Everyday Challenges.* New York: Facts On File, Inc., 1998.

carpenters Carpenters are workers in a variety of fields, including construction, who join pieces of wood together and attach wood and many types of wood products to other building materials. They may work indoors or outdoors, in small settings or on large construction projects.

Working conditions of carpenters can lead to injuries and illnesses. They are often exposed to hazardous equipment, such as power saws, may be exposed to working in high places, such as when climbing on roofs or LADDERS, exposed to CONFINED SPACES that require getting into awkward positions, and may be exposed to very hot or very cold temperatures while working outdoors.

Physical demands of carpentry include using muscles repetitively for extended periods, lifting, stretching, twisting, kneeling, or crawling.

Researchers Lipscomb, Dement, Loomis, et al. reported on an analysis of work-related musculoskeletal injuries (WRMIs) among union carpenters. The highest rates of claims were for back sprains, neck and back sprains, and knee sprains. Older carpenters had a higher risk of foot fractures than younger workers. Female workers had a higher risk of sprains or strains and nerve disorders of the wrist or forearm. Light commercial and dry-wall work was a significant risk factor for injuries to the axial skeleton. Being a member of the union for at least four years was associated with a lower risk for most of the WRMIs.

The United Brotherhood of Carpenters and Joiners of America, with 500,000 members in the United States and Canada, provides information on Occupational Safety and Health Administration (OSHA) standards and other data relating to the field of carpentry.

For further information:

The United Brotherhood of Carpenters and Joiners
   of America
101 Constitution Avenue NW
Washington, DC 20001
(202) 546-6206
(202) 543-5724 (fax)
http://www.carpenters.org

See also ASBESTOS; BACK INJURIES/BACK PAIN; COLD ENVIRONMENTS; CONSTRUCTION; DUST AND DEBRIS; ELECTRICITY-RELATED INJURIES; EYE IN-JURIES/PROTECTION; HAND PROTECTION; FOOT PROTEC-TION; PERSONAL PROTECTIVE EQUIPMENT; REPETITIVE STRESS INJURIES; SLIPS, TRIPS, AND FALLS; WOOD DUST.

Lipscomb, H. J., J. M. Dement, D. P. Loomis, et al. "Surveillance of Work Related Musculoskeletal Injuries Among Union Carpenters." *American Journal of Industrial Medicine* 32, no. 6 (19): 629–640.

catering and food service   One of the main occupational risks in these industries is occupational DERMATITIS. Workers of all ages in food service industries represent a high-risk group with regard to occupational dermatitis. Those most at risk are chefs, cooks, kitchen and serving personnel, and counter people. Others at risk include waiters and waitresses, bar staff, and cleaners. In food manufacturing, those at risk include bakers, confectioners, meat, poultry, and fish handlers, and fruit and vegetable handlers.

In food preparation and catering, it is usually the hands and forearms which are affected. If the condition gets worse, the skin can crack and bleed. It can be extremely painful and enough to keep peo-ple off work and serious enough to force them to change jobs.

How quickly dermatitis is developed depends on the substance, its strength or potency, and how long and how often it touches the skin. Sometimes it can be caused by a combination of things, for example, using detergents at work means that hands are likely to be in water much of the time. Over a period of time the combination of the wet-ness and the detergents can cause dermatitis.

Contact with Foods and Other Causes of Dermatitis

A wide variety of foods have been shown to cause dermatitis among employees in the catering and food service industries. These include sugar, flour/dough, citrus fruits and their peels, other fruits, vegetables, spices, herbs and seasonings (such as horseradish, mustard, and garlic), fish and seafoods, meat, and poultry.

Other cases of dermatitis are due to contact with nickel (coins) and rubber, including rubber gloves, chemicals, and cleaners. Some alcohol-based hand sanitizers may also cause dermatitis. Such sanitizers that are applied to and rubbed between the hands after washing can contain as much as 30 percent to 70 percent concentration of isopropyl alcohol, which can be a source of allergy or cause dermatitis.

See also BAKERS, CHEFS, AND COOKS; BUTCHERS AND MEAT, POULTRY, AND FISH CUTTERS; CHEMICAL TOXICITY; DERMATITIS; SKIN OR SENSE ORGAN TOXICITY.

cattle, sheep, and goat workers   Raising cattle, sheep and goats includes milking and disposing of livestock waste, feeding, parasite and disease control, hair clipping and fleece shearing. The main occupational hazards involved in dealing with these animals include injuries, respiratory problems, and zoonotic diseases.

According to a 1997 survey of farmworkers in the United States, incidents caused by handling livestock represented 26 percent of lost-time injuries. This percentage was higher than any other farm activity. Injuries from cattle usually occur in or near the farm buildings. Cattle inflict injuries when they kick or step on workers or crush them against a hard surface, such as the side of a pen.

Workers may fall when working with cattle, sheep, and goats. Bulls inflict the most serious injuries. Most of the people injured are family members rather than hired workers. Fatigue can reduce judgment, and thus increase the chance of injury.

According to the *Encyclopaedia of Occupational Health and Safety,* livestock exhibits can be hazardous to workers. Cattle and sheep have strong herding instincts, and imposed limits such as isolation or overcrowding can lead to escape attempts. Territorialism is another predictable animal behavior. When an animal is removed from its normal quarters and placed in a confined environment, it may struggle to escape. Animals restrained by chutes for loading onto trucks or trailers often become agitated, making them difficult to handle.

Production facilities for cattle, sheep, and goats are hazardous for workers because of slippery floors, corrals, dusty feed areas, silos, mechanized feeding equipment, and animal confinement buildings. Confinement buildings may have manure storage pits, which can emit lethal gases.

Heavy physical labor, heat, high humidity, and dehydration from lack of drinking water contribute to the hazards of heat exhaustion and stroke among workers.

Respiratory illness from exposure to inhaled dusts is another hazard for livestock handlers. A common illness is organic dust toxic syndrome, which may follow exposures to heavy concentrations of organic dusts contaminated with microorganisms.

Sheep shearers face hazards of cuts and abrasions during the shearing operation as well as blows from animal hoofs and horns. Slips and falls are also common. Power for the shears is sometimes transferred by belts, and belt guards must be maintained to prevent electricity-related injuries. Shearers also face postural hazards, especially to the back, as a result of catching and tipping the sheep. Shearers restrain the animals between their legs, which may strain the back, and twisting movements are common.

Control of insects on cattle, sheep, and goats with pesticide can expose workers to pesticides. Sheep dips submerge animals in a pesticide bath, and handling the animal or contact with the bath solution or contaminated wool can also expose workers to the pesticide.

Prevention of Injuries to Workers

Prevention of injuries from working with animals includes maintaining stairways and keeping floors even to reduce fall hazards. Maintenance of guards on belts, mechanical screws, and shear sharpening equipment is essential. All electrical equipment must be in good condition to prevent electrical shock. Ventilation should be checked wherever internal combustion engines are used in barns. Facilities should be designed so that workers do not have to enter small or enclosed areas with animals.

Reducing spoilage of feed to minimize potential fungal spore exposure can minimize risks of organic dust exposure. Mechanized equipment can be used to move decaying materials. Respirators should be worn when organic dust exposure cannot be avoided.

To prevent zoonoses, livestock facilities must be clean, animals must be vaccinated, and sick animals should be quarantined to avoid exposure to others. Rubber gloves should be worn when treating sick animals to avoid exposure through cuts in the hands. Common zoonoses include rabies, brucellosis, bovine tuberculosis, trichinosis, salmonella, leptospirosis, ringworm, and tapeworm. Diseases that may be contracted while working with hair and fleece include tetanus, salmonellosis from tagging and crutching, leptospirosis, anthrax, and parasitic diseases. Animal feces and urine also can be infectious for workers. Cattle can transmit cryptosporidosis to humans through the fecal-oral route. Schistosomiasis, an infection by blood flukes, is found in cattle and other animals in several parts of the world. Penetration can occur while workers are wading in water.

See also ANIMAL HANDLERS; ELECTRICITY-RELATED INJURIES; ERGONOMICS AND ERGONOMIC REGULATIONS; FARMING; SLIPS, TRIPS AND FALLS.

Stellman, Jeanne Mager, ed. *Encyclopaedia of Occupational Health and Safety.* Vol. 3. 4th ed. Geneva: International Labor Organization, p. 70.20–70.22.

cement workers   See BRICKLAYERS, CEMENT WORKERS AND PLASTERERS; CONSTRUCTION.

Census of Fatal Occupational Injuries (CFOI)   A
study of fatal work injuries conducted by the

Bureau of Labor Statistics (BLS) of the U.S. Department of Labor. The census is part of the BLS occupational safety and health statistics program; it provides the most complete count of fatal work injuries available. The program uses diverse state and federal data sources to identify, verify, and profile fatal work injuries. The 2001 report is the ninth year for which the fatality census has been conducted in all 50 states and the District of Columbia. The BLS fatality census is a federal/state cooperative venture in which costs are shared equally.

Fatal Work Injuries: 2000

A total of 5,915 fatal work injuries were recorded in 2000, a decline of about 2 percent from 1999, according to the census. The decline occurred even though overall employment increased in 2000. The number of job-related deaths from highway incidents, the most frequent fatal work injury, declined for the first time since the fatality census was first conducted in 1992. According to the census, fatalities resulting from electrocutions, fires, explosions, and contact with equipment also were down in 2000. Fatal job-related falls and homicides both increased.

Deaths resulting from on-the-job-falls increased slightly to 734 in 2000, the largest annual total recorded by the fatality census. Falls to a lower level increased in 2000 and accounted for 659 of the 734 falls. Fatalities resulting from falls off ladders and from nonmoving vehicles were both higher in 2000, though falls from scaffolds, building girders, and roofs decreased. Falls on the same level declined from 70 to 56 in 2000.

The number of job-related homicides increased for the first time in six years, from 651 in 1999 to 677 in 2000. However, the total number of workplace homicides in 2000 was still 37 percent lower than the high of 1,080 homicides reported in 1994. For those workplace homicides in which the motive could be ascertained, homicides in which robbery was the initial motive increased from 255 cases in 1999 to 291 cases in 2000.

According to the report released in August 2001, fewer workers were killed by electrocution than in any year since the fatality census was first conducted. The number of fatal injuries resulting from fires or explosions in 2000 fell from its highest

annual total in 1999 to its lowest annual total since 1992. The number of workers who were fatally injured through contact with objects or equipment also was down from the previous year, but still accounted for nearly one out of every six fatal work injuries in 2000.

CONSTRUCTION recorded the highest number of total work injuries by any industry, although the total for the industry was down about 3 percent in 2000, the first decline for construction since 1996. Fatal work injuries in MANUFACTURING (down 7 percent) and in agriculture, forestry, and FISHING reached the lowest levels recorded for those industries. The decrease in agriculture, forestry, and fishing occurred despite an increase in the number of fatal work injuries in landscape and horticultural services. The number of total work injuries in the mining industry, however, was higher in 2000, led by an increase in fatal injuries in the oil and gas extraction industry. Fatalities were also higher in retail trade, largely as a result of the increase in workplace homicides.

The census report indicated that fatal work injuries in the service industries increased about 4 percent in 2000. Fatalities in business services increased, led by a rise in work-related deaths in personnel supply services. Educational services and membership organizations were some of the other industry groups in services recording increases in 2000. Health services, personal services (such as laundry services and beauty shops), and amusement/recreation services were among the service industries recording lower fatal work injury counts.

In 2000, rates of fatal work injuries were highest in the mining, agriculture, construction, and transportation industries. The mining industry recorded a rate of 30.0 fatal work injuries per 100,000 workers in 2000, the highest of any industry and about seven times the rate for all workers. Agriculture recorded the second-highest rate in 2000 (20.9 fatalities per 100,000 workers). Despite an increase in the number of incidents in the services industry and in retail trade, the rates for both these industries remained relatively low (2.0 for services and 2.7 for retail trade).

Fatal Work Injuries by Occupation

Operators, fabricators, and laborers recorded the largest number of fatal work injuries of any occupational group in 2000, accounting for more than one out of every three fatalities. However, the number of fatalities for this group was down 4 percent from 1999, and fatal work injuries involving transportation and material moving occupations were down 4 percent. Service occupation fatalities also were lower in 2000, despite an increase in fatalities involving police and detectives. Fatal work injuries involving FARMING, forestry, and fishing occupations were down sharply, from 904 in 1999 to 806 in 2000, a decline of 11 percent. Two other occupational groups, managerial and professional specialty occupations and technical, sales, and administrative support occupations, recorded increases in 2000.

Truck drivers were fatally injured on the job more than any other individual occupation, although fatal work injuries for this occupation declined 5 percent in 2000. Fatalities involving airplane pilots and navigators rose from 94 in 1999 to 130 in 2000. The fatality rate for this occupation (100.8 for every 100,000 employed) was exceeded only by timber cutters (122.1) and fishers (108.3). (See Appendix).

Fatal Work Injuries: Demographic Characteristics

According to the census report, the numbers of fatal work injuries among white (non-Hispanic) and black (non-Hispanic) workers were lower in 2000, but fatal injuries among Hispanic or Latino workers were up sharply, from 730 in 1999 to 815 in 2000. This increase in Hispanic worker fatalities was led by a 24 percent jump in construction fatalities involving Hispanic workers. Nationally, Hispanic employment was up 6 percent in 2000.

Fatal work injuries to men were down nearly 3 percent, and fatalities to women increased slightly in 2000. There was an increase in self-employed workers fatally injured in the job (up 3 percent in 2000). Self-employed workers, who constitute only 7 percent of employment, accounted for 20 percent of the fatality total. On average, about 16 workers were fatally injured each day during 2000. There were 214 multiple-fatality incidents (incidents that resulted in two or more workers' deaths), resulting in 531 job-related deaths. The multiple-fatality count for 2000 represents a sub-stantial decrease over the 1999 count, when 235 multiple-fatality events were reported, involving 617 job-related deaths.

For further information:

Bureau of Labor Statistics
U.S. Department of Labor
Washington, DC 20212
(202) 691-6175 (Technical information)
(202) 691-5902 (Media Information)
http://stats.bls.gov/oshhome.htm

See also ELECTRICITY-RELATED INJURIES; SLIPS, TRIPS AND FALLS; TRUCK DRIVERS; SURVEY OF OCCUPATIONAL INJURIES AND ILLNESSES.

Bureau of Labor Statistics, Washington, D.C., August 14, 2001.

central nervous system (CNS)   Anatomical term for the brain and the spinal cord. The CNS works together with the peripheral nervous system (PNS) which consists of all the nerves that carry signals between the CNS and the rest of the body. The overall role of the CNS is to receive sensory information from such organs as the eyes, ears, and receptors within the body, analyze this information, and initiate an appropriate motor response, for example, moving muscles.

Some chemicals and other fumes in the workplace can cause neurotoxicity. Injury or disease to the CNS can cause death or serious disability.

See also NEUROTOXICITY.

CERCLA   See COMPREHENSIVE ENVIRONMENTAL RESPONSE, COMPENSATION AND LIABILITY ACT.

chain saws/chain saw injuries   High-powered cutting machines used in the lumber (treefelling) industry and others. Chain saws expose operators to high levels of noise and hand-arm vibration, which can lead to hearing loss and conditions such as VIBRATION WHITE FINGER. These risks can be controlled by good practices, including use of low-noise/low-vibration chain saws, wearing suitable hearing protection, properly maintaining chain saws, wearing protective equipment, and being informed and trained on the health risks associated with chain saws.

Personal protective equipment should always be worn, no matter how small the job. Protective equipment for chain saw operators includes safety helmet, hearing protection, eye protection, upper body protection, gloves, leg protection and chain saw boots.

Checking the Worksite to Avoid Accidents

A worker should check the worksite thoroughly to identify any potential hazards before beginning the job. This is particularly important when undertaking felling or demolition work. For any work with a chain saw, potential risks must be assessed and controlled. The operator must be competent to do the job, must wear appropriate protection, and either stop the engine or apply the chain brake when not cutting with the saw.

Avoiding Kickback Injuries

Kickback is the sudden uncontrolled upward and backward movement of the chain and guide bar towards the operator. This can occur when the saw chain at the nose of the guide bar hits an object. Kickback is responsible for a significant proportion of chain saw accidents, many of which are to the face and parts of the upper body where it is difficult to provide adequate protection. A properly maintained chain brake and use of low-kickback chains (safety chains) reduces the effect, but cannot entirely prevent it.

Other Safety Precautions

Chain saw workers should avoid working alone. However, where this is not possible, there should be an established procedure to get help if needed. Such procedures may include:

- Regular contact with others using either a radio or telephone
- Someone regularly visiting the worksite
- Carrying a whistle to call for help
- An automatic signaling device that sends a signal at a preset time unless prevented from doing so
- Checks to assure operators return to base or home at an agreed time.

Workers on chain saws should be trained in emergency first aid and know how to control major bleeding and to deal with crush injuries. In remote sites, people who have been injured may also be at risk of hypothermia. Operators should carry a personal first-aid kit (including a large wound dressing) and have reasonable access to a more comprehensive kit.

See also CONSTRUCTION; LOGGING; VIBRATION (HAND, ARM).

Health and Safety Executive Information Services, Suffolk, England.

chauffeurs Workers who drive an automobile to transport individuals to and from airports, appointments, and social occasions, and office personnel and visitors to commercial or industrial establishments. They may perform miscellaneous errands for their employers, may make extended trips requiring irregular hours and may clean the vehicle and make minor repairs. Chauffeurs are sometimes called limousine drivers.

Accident hazards for chauffeurs include an increased risk of road accidents as a result of overnight drives and extended trips during irregular hours, SLIPS, TRIPS, AND FALLS while carrying luggage and packages, and injuries while changing a tire or repairing the vehicle.

Chauffeurs are potentially exposed to infectious diseases while transporting sick passengers. They may suffer eyestrain because of driving in the dark for long hours, and low back pain and pains in the arms and leg joints due to extended driving, sometimes over bumpy roads. Further, they may suffer psychological stress and job dissatisfaction as a result of performing a subordinate role and a need to cater to unexpected demands of passengers. In the case of fulfilling an additional duty as a bodyguard, the chauffeur will face hazards typical for this function.

See also TRUCK DRIVERS; STRESS.

Stillman, Jeanne Mager, ed. *Encyclopaedia of Occupational Health and Safety*. Vol. 4. 4th ed. Geneva: International Labor Organization, 1998, p. 103.11.

cheesemaker's lung See WHEEZING.

chefs See FOOD SERVICE INDUSTRY.

chemical dependency See ADDICTIONS.

chemical hazards Substances in the workplace or the working environment that contribute to allergic reactions or illness. The Occupational Safety and Health Administration (OSHA) defines hazards as those chemicals present in the workplace which are capable of causing harm. In this definition, the term CHEMICALS includes dusts, mixtures, and such common materials as paints, fuels, and solvents. OSHA currently regulates exposure to approximately 400 substances, including allergies due to contact with or inhaling FORMALDEHYDE vapors and other synthetic or natural allergenic substances; exposure to metallic, solvent, and other fumes; exposure to various carcinogenic, mutagenic, and teratogenic agents; mercury poisoning; and skin irritations due to contact with such chemicals as SOLVENTS, pesticides, herbicides, detergents, and disinfecting agents.

Additionally, chemical hazards include exposure to anesthetic gases administered to patients, lead poisoning, blood changes as a result of exposure to solvents such as benzene, and toluene. Chronic poisoning may be a result of exposure to many industrial chemicals, including heavy metals, paint removers, and thinners. Chemical hazards also include CHEMICAL SPILLS.

See also CHEMICAL TOXICITY.

chemical sensitivity See CHEMICAL HAZARDS; CHEMICAL TOXICITY; EXPOSURE ASSESSMENT; HAZARDOUS AND TOXIC SUBSTANCES; SKIN OR SENSE ORGAN TOXICITY.

chemical spills Accidental release of hazardous materials. Chemicals are often transported through densely populated centers and bodies of water, and spills can occur en route. Natural disasters such as floods and earthquake might also result in chemical spills. Businesses that use hazardous materials include hospitals, metal plating and finishing plants, the aircraft industry, public utilities, cold storage companies, fuel industries, the communication industry, chemical distributors, and high-tech firms. All are required to maintain plans for warning, notification, evacuation, and site security in case of spills under various regulations.

Many spills involve petroleum products, but a significant number involve extremely hazardous materials such as ammonia, chlorine, or sulfuric acid.

Two major governmental agencies, the National Oceanic and Atmospheric Administration and the Environmental Protection Agency, have jointly developed a system to help public safety agencies deal with the thousands of chemicals that can harm people or the environment.

For information:

National Oceanic and Atmospheric Administration
U.S. Department of Commerce
14th Street and Constitution Avenue NW
Room 6013
Washington, DC 20230
(202) 482-6090
(202) 482-3154 (fax)
http://www.noaa.gov

See also CHEMICAL HAZARDS; CHEMICAL TOXICITY; HAZARD COMMUNICATION; ENVIRONMENTAL PROTECTION AGENCY; HAZARDOUS AND TOXIC SUBSTANCES; MATERIAL SAFETY DATA SHEETS; SKIN OR SENSE ORGAN TOXICITY.

chemical toxicity A measure of the poisoning strength of a chemical. All chemicals can be toxic. Chemicals that are only weakly toxic require large doses to cause poisoning. Stronger chemicals only need small doses to cause poisoning. It is the amount that enters the body that determines whether or not they will cause poisoning.

Several factors can influence the degree of poisoning from a chemical. They include how they enter the body, amount or dose entering the body, toxicity of the chemical, removal from the body, and individual differences between workers.

Breathing contaminated air is the most common way that chemicals enter the body. Some chemicals, when contacted, can enter the skin. Less commonly, workplace chemicals may be eaten if hands or food are contaminated. Small quantities of chemicals may enter through the eyes.

Results of *acute toxicity* sometimes are seen within minutes or hours after a sudden exposure to a chemical. For example, inhalation of high concentrations of acid vapors might cause burns of the mouth and airways leading to the lungs. Skin contact with substantial amounts of certain substances absorbed through the skin may cause dizziness and nausea. Inhalation of dusts can cause irritation of the respiratory tract and the throat, and coughing. However, in some instances high-level exposure causes delayed effects. For example, symptoms from exposures to certain pesticides may not appear for several days.

Chronic toxicity usually appears after occupational exposure to a chemical for many years. For example, repeated exposure to dusts containing quartz can cause damage to the lungs, leading to severe and permanent lung damage. Repeated exposure to certain chemicals for long periods of time may cause CANCER. Some examples of types of chemicals in various workplaces that may cause toxicity include:

Acids: Acids are corrosive substances widely used throughout the electronics industry and others for cleaning and etching and may be in liquid or powder form; they are acutely hazardous, particularly when concentrated. Acids can penetrate clothing rapidly, causing serious burns and damage to tissues under the skin.

Cyanides: In the electronics industry, cyanides are used for cleaning, plating, and metallizing. As a group, they are highly irritating and rapidly acting poisons. Cyanide is quickly absorbed through the skin and lungs. It prevents the body tissues from taking up oxygen and may cause sudden death by asphyxiation. Repeated low-level exposure can cause severe dermatitis, thyroid disease, and lack of muscle coordination. Isocyanates are another highly reactive and poisonous group of chemicals.

Oxidizers: Oxidizers are used to clean or remove corrosion from a metal surface. During oxidation, oxygen combines with a metal or semiconductor surface to form a protective oxide layer. Some oxidizers have strong corrosive action and workers must protect their eyes, skin, and lungs from exposure. Examples of oxidizers include chlorine, hydrogen peroxide, nitrous oxide, and silver nitrate.

Resins: Resins include plastics, epoxies, glues, paints, waxes, synthetic rubber, and some synthetic fibers. Resins are used in many applications throughout industry, and also used as wire coatings and a variety of other electrical insulation materials. Resins can produce a wide variety of highly toxic vapors and gases when heated or burning. Fires caused by burning plastic are sometimes difficult to control.

Solvents: Solvents are used primarily for cleaning and degreasing, and for thinning plastics, resins, glues, inks, paints, and waxes. Some are very toxic and others only mildly toxic. The aromatic compounds and the chlorinated hydrocarbons may be the most dangerous groups of solvents, as many are known to cause cancer and other serious illnesses.

Many forms of chemical toxicity can be prevented by appropriate use of personal protective equipment.

See also CARCINOGENS; DUST AND DEBRIS; GASTROINTESTINAL OR LIVER TOXICITY; GENOTOXICITY; GLUERS; HAZARDOUS AND TOXIC SUBSTANCES; IMMUNOTOXICITY; ISOCYANATES; KIDNEY TOXICITY; PEROXIDES; PEST CONTROL WORKERS; SKIN OR SENSE ORGAN TOXICITY; SOLVENTS.

child care   See DAY CARE; WORKING MOTHERS.

child labor   The 1990 census documented more than 20 million working young people aged 12 through 17. At any given time during the year, it is estimated that some 5.5 million of them are working, and that does not include those under 12 years old who work illegally. More than half of the 16- and 17-year-olds and more than a quarter of all 15-year-olds are part of the nation's workforce.

The U.S. Department of Labor Bureau of Labor Statistics reports that almost four out of five young workers aged 16 through 19 are concentrated in three types of employment: retail sales and service (particularly food service), administrative support staff, and laborers and handlers.

Types of Injuries
Sustained by Young People at Work

Occupationally-related accidents and injuries among young people have increased in recent years. The National Institute of Occupational Safety and Health (NIOSH) estimates that each year more than 64,000 teenagers are treated in emergency rooms for their occupational injuries, exclusive of agricultural injuries. Adolescents suffer an estimated occupational injury rate of up to 16 per 100 full-time employees, compared with the adult rate of less than nine per 100 full-time employees. The most common youth injuries at the workplace are cuts and lacerations, usually of the fingers and hands, followed by bruises and contusions, and strains and sprains. However, these injuries result from inexperience, not age. A large proportion of workplace injuries, some 30 percent, occur to workers in their first year of work, regardless of their age.

Child Labor Laws Vary by States

Child labor laws are regulations by federal and state governments concerning conditions under which minors may work, as well as hours and wages. Historically, child labor laws evolved out of the movement toward avoiding exploitation and endangerment of children. Now, exploitative child labor is defined (by the Child Labor Coalition) as employment in the formal or informal sector, or unpaid, that is coerced, forced, bonded, slavery, or otherwise known to be unfair in wages, injurious to the health and safety of children, and/or obstructs a child's access to education or impairs educational attainment.

Now child labor laws are important because more teenagers are working at more types of jobs, during more weeks of the year for longer weekly hours than has even been true in the past.

On a national level, the federal law, the FAIR LABOR STANDARDS ACT of 1938 (FLSA), as amended, is administrated by the U.S. Department of Labor's Wage and Hour Division. It is applicable in most instances in every state. According to estimates by the U.S. Department or Labor, more than 90 percent of all nonagricultural businesses are covered by the FLSA's child labor laws.

Additionally, each state has its own child labor laws that vary widely. Some were enacted nearly 150 years ago and address virtually every type of labor and many working conditions, from corn detasseling to seasonal fish processing. Other states enacted minimal child labor provisions. However, in any particular state, when both the FLSA and that state's child labor laws regulate the same activity or conduct and their rules conflict, the labor standard that applies is the one that is stricter. For example, according to Mississippi child labor laws, youngsters can work in mills, canneries, workshops, factories, and manufacturing establishments at the age of 14. However, the FLSA does not permit any manufacturing, workshop, or processing work until age 16. Because the federal law is stricter, Mississippi complies and the minimum age for milling, canning, workshop occupations, and other types of manufacturing is 16.

Generally, 14 is the minimum lawful working age for specified nonagricultural employment. For those under 16, work activities are highly circumscribed and the hours of work and times of day and week are strictly limited. In agriculture, children are usually permitted to work at any age on their parents' farm, and they are usually either unregulated or permitted to work at age 12 in commercial farming.

States have their own enforcement personnel as well as codes of violations and penalties. States vary widely in use of resources and political motivation. Maryland, for example, according to the National Consumers League, has had no child labor law enforcement for several years and refers complaints and inquiries to federal labor enforcement offices in their states. New York state employs more than 100 labor investigators, many of them assigned to specialized units devoted to seeking child labor violations in the garment industry, agriculture, or retail trades.

The more common form of enforcement is the "complaint method," in which state labor investigators respond to complaints received by letter or telephone. Investigating complaints helps assure that young people are safe, legal, and healthy on their jobs.

The National Consumers League reported results of a survey conducted by the Child Labor Coalition in 1997 with 46 states reporting. This represented a 92 percent response rate. Nonrespondents were Florida, Ohio, Pennsylvania, Vermont, and the District of Columbia.

The survey reported details about specific provisions in state child labor laws:

Eighteen of the responding states have no minimum age for children who work as migrant and seasonal farmworkers. Sixteen states have minimum ages between eight and 12 years old.

- 28 responding states reported state restrictions for occupational driving for 16- and 17-year-olds.

- 22 responding states reported companies specializing in door-to-door sales by children (such as candy or magazine subscriptions) active in their state during 1996.

- 13 states (59 percent of the 22 states that reported door-to-door companies at work in the state took action against the companies in 1996.

- Four states instituted new child labor regulations or passed child labor laws in 1996.

The following summarized the state child labor enforcement personnel in 1996 as found by the Child Labor Coalition's survey:

- 8.5 compliance officers are responsible for investigating child labor compliance/violations exclusively in 46 states.

- 26 of responding states have a total number of 10 or fewer compliance officers who are responsible for enforcing labor laws in the state, including child labor laws.

- Eight of responding states have a total number of 25 or more compliance officers who are responsible for enforcing labor laws in the state, including child labor laws.

The Child Labor Coalition's survey also summarized the number of inspections conducted by states in which child labor compliance was an issue:

- Three states conducted no inspections

- 12 states conducted 100 or fewer inspections

- 24 states conducted more than 100 inspections

- 16 percent of the inspections resulted in finding child labor violations

- 6,229 employers were found to be in violation of child labor laws in 33 states

- 7,577 minors were found to be illegally employed in 29 states

- Only seven states of the 38 respondents conducted any inspections in 1996 in which child labor compliance in agriculture was targeted.

Only three of the seven conducted a significant number of inspections. Thirty-one employers were found to be in violation of child labor laws and 91 children were found illegally employed.

- 45 responding states assessed in total $2,469,016 for child labor violations in 1996.

For information:

National Consumers League
1701 K Street, NW 1200
Washington, DC 20006
(202) 835-3323
(202) 835-0747 (fax)
http://www.nclnet.org

See also CHILD LABOR COALITION; NATIONAL CONSUMERS LEAGUE; NATIONAL RESEARCH AND DISSEMINATION CENTERS FOR CAREER AND TECHNICAL EDUCATION.

National Consumers League; National Center for Research in Vocational Education

Child Labor Coalition (CLC) A national network for the exchange of information about child labor. The CLC also provides a forum and a unified voice on protecting working minors and ending child labor exploitation. CLC also develops informational outreach to the public and private sectors to combat child labor abuses and promote progressive initiatives and legislation.

The CLC formed in 1989 as concerned groups mobilized following a Washington forum, "Exploitation of Children in the Workplace." Objectives of the CLC include:

- Influencing public policy on child labor issues through an increased understanding of the impact of work on children's health, the quality of their lives, and their ability to produce effectively in jobs as adults, as well as increase recognition of how child labor exploitation reinforces and promotes poverty, adult unemployment, poor living standards, low literacy rates, and lax enforcement of labor regulations.

- Working for strengthened protections, guarding youth from excessive, inappropriate, and hazardous labor.

- Advocating for better enforcement of child labor laws and regulations, including devising and encouraging innovative ways to ensure employer compliance.

- Educating the public, business, and governments to broaden awareness and understanding about the nature of child labor exploitation in the United States and other countries, and how it differs from legitimate and positive youth employment.

Activities of the CLC include:

- Testifying before state and federal legislatures and agencies on child labor
- Presenting comments in response to regulatory initiatives
- Hosting conferences, forums, and briefings
- Creating and distributing educational and public awareness materials
- Initiating research
- Conducting campaigns and media events.

For information:

The Child Labor Coalition
1701 K Street, NW
Suite 1200
Washington, DC 20006
(202) 835-3323
(202) 835-0747 (fax)
http://www.nclnet.org/child

See also CHILD LABOR; FAIR LABOR STANDARDS ACT.

child labor laws See CHILD LABOR; CHILD LABOR COALITION; FAIR LABOR STANDARDS ACT; TEENAGE WORKERS.

children See CHILD LABOR; DAY CARE; TEENAGE WORKERS; WORKING MOTHERS.

chiropractic medicine Chiropractic medicine deals with the relationship between the articulations of the skeleton and the nervous system and the role of this relationship in restoring and main-

taining health. Many employees visit chiropractors to relieve physical discomforts caused by workplace actions or environment, such as faulty chairs and work stations.

According to chiropractic philosophy, the body is a self-healing organism and all bodily function is controlled by the nervous system. Abnormal bodily function may be caused by interference with nerve transmission and expression. This interference can be caused by pressure, strain, or tension on the spinal cord, spinal nerves, or peripheral nerves as a result of a displacement of the spinal segments or other skeletal structures.

The art of the chiropractic practitioner pertains to the skill and judgment necessary for detecting, locating, controlling, reducing, and correcting of primarily the vertebral subluxation complex. A subluxation refers to a slight dislocation or biochemical malfunctioning of the vertebrae (bones of the spine). According to the International Chiropractors Association, subluxation can irritate nerve roots and blood vessels which branch off from the spinal cord between each vertebrae. The irritation causes pain and dysfunction in muscle, lymphatic, and organ tissue as well as imbalance in normal body processes.

Causes of subluxation include falls, injury, trauma, inherited spinal weaknesses, poor posture, poor lifting habits, obesity, lack of rest, and exercise.

Chiropractors restore misaligned vertebrae to their proper position in the spinal cord through procedures known as "spinal adjustments," or manipulation. The adjustment itself does not actually heal the body. It is the alignment of misaligned spinal vertebrae that restores balance so that the body can function more optimally.

Chiropractic is often chosen as therapy for temporomandibular joint dysfunction, headache, whiplash, and bursitis. It may not be the treatment of choice for all medical problems or conditions.

Choosing a Chiropractor

Before choosing a chiropractor, ask him or her to fully explain the benefits, risk, and costs of all diagnostic and treatment options. Interview more than one doctor of chiropractic before making a decision on the practitioner.

See also COMPLEMENTARY THERAPIES; BACK INJURIES, BACK PAIN.

chloracne   An acne-like eruption of comedones, cysts, and pustules, usually on the face; cysts are frequently filled with straw-colored fluid. Chloracne develops in association with a history of being exposed to herbicides or being exposed to chlorinated chemicals.

Chloracne is the one human effect universally linked to dioxin exposure. The presence of chloracne is considered a clinical sign of exposure. The severity and abrupt onset of chloracne follows a dose-response curve. The lesions are remarkably persistent and resistant to usual acne treatment regimens.

See also AGENT ORANGE; CHEMICAL TOXICITY; SKIN OR SENSE ORGAN TOXICITY.

chlordecone   The generic name for a chlorinated insecticide commercially sold under the trade name Kepone. The compound, first introduced in 1958, was used as an insecticide on tobacco, ornamental shrubs, bananas, and citrus tress, against leaf-eating insects, ants and cockroaches, as a larvicide against flies, and in roach traps. According to the Agency for Toxic Substances and Disease Registry, chlordecone has not been manufactured or used in the United States since 1978.

Workers who were exposed to high levels of chlordecone over a long period (more than one year) showed harmful effects on the nervous system, skin, liver, and male reproductive system. These workers were probably exposed mainly through touching chlordecone, although they may have inhaled or ingested some as well.

According to the World Health Organization Program on Chemical Safety, a large number of cases of occupational poisoning were reported in a manufacturing plant where work hygiene and safety precautions were insufficient. Neurological symptoms, especially nervousness and tremors, together with oligospermia, (low sperm count) and joint pains were reported.

On the basis of findings in mice and rats, this chemical should be considered potentially carcinogenic for human beings.

For more information:

Agency for Toxic Substances and Disease Registry
Division of Toxicology

1600 Clifton Road, NE
Mailstop E-29
Atlanta, GA 30333
(888) 422-8737
(404) 498-0057 (fax)
www.atsdr.cdc.gov

See REPRODUCTIVE TOXICITY; SKIN OR SENSE ORGAN TOXICITY.

chlorine   See ASTHMA, OCCUPATIONAL.

chloroethene   See VINYL CHLORIDE.

chloroethylene   See VINYL CHLORIDE.

chlorofluorocarbons (CFCs)   A group of chemicals used in large quantities in industry for refrigeration and air conditioning, and in consumer products. When released into the air, CFCs rise into the stratosphere, a layer of the atmosphere high above the Earth. In the stratosphere, CFCs are part of chemical reactions that reduce the stratospheric ozone layer, which protects the Earth's surface from harmful effects of radiation from the sun. The CLEAN AIR ACT of 1990 includes provisions for reducing emissions and eliminating production and use of these ozone-destroying chemicals.

See also AIR POLLUTION.

chloroform   A colorless liquid with a nonirritating odor. In the past, chloroform was used as an inhaled anesthetic during surgery. Today, chloroform is used to make other chemicals and can also be formed in small amounts when chlorine is added to water. Other names for chloroform are trichloromethane and methyltrichloride.

According to the Occupational Safety and Health Administration (OSHA), many industrial operations may involve chloroform and result in worker exposure. They include manufacture of fluorocarbons for refrigerants and aerosol propellants, fire extinguishers to lower the freezing temperature of carbon tetrachloride, fluorocarbon resins, plastics, and artificial silk, floor polishes, dyes, and pesticides. Further, chloroform is used as an extractant solvent in the manufacture of rubber, essential oils, sterols and alkaloids, and resins, and in photographic processing. It is used as a general solvent of lacquers, plastics, dyes, adhesives, and waxes, and in the rubber cleaning and dry cleaning industries.

Exposure to chloroform can occur when breathing contaminated air or when drinking or touching the substance or water containing it. Breathing chloroform can cause dizziness, fatigue, and headaches. Breathing chloroform or ingesting it over long periods of time may damage the liver and kidneys. It can cause sores if large amounts touch the skin.

Toxic gases and vapors such as hydrogen chloride, chlorine, phosgene, and carbon monoxide may be released in a fire involving chloroform.

The Department of Health and Human Services (DHHS) has determined that chloroform may reasonably be anticipated to be a carcinogen. The Environmental Protection Agency (EPA) requires that spills or accidental release of 10 pounds or more of chloroform into the environment be reported to the EPA. OSHA has set maximum allowable concentrations of chloroform in workroom air during an eight-hour workday in a 40-hour workweek at 50 parts per million (ppm).

See also CARCINOGENS; CENTRAL NERVOUS SYSTEM; CHEMICAL TOXICITY; GASTROINTESTINAL OR LIVER TOXICITY; HAZARD COMMUNICATION; HAZARDOUS AIR POLLUTANTS; PERSONAL PROTECTIVE EQUIPMENT.

Chopra, Deepak (1947–) Indian-born physician whose philosophy of healing, books, tapes, lectures, and clinics in the United States are based on the Indian holistic system called ayurveda. He was once a disciple of Maharishi Mahesh Yogi, but formed his own organization in 1993. Among his books are the best-selling *Ageless Body, Timeless Mind: The Quantum Alternative to Growing Old* (1993) and a fiction work, *The Return of Merlin* (1995). Many of Chopra's philosophies and writings are incorporated into employee wellness and RELAXATION programs.

Chopra's philosophy advocates that awareness of the mind/body connection can facilitate healing, lead to inner peace, and even reverse the aging process. Chopra's mind/body programs incorporate massage, yoga, meditation, herbal supplements, nutritional guidelines, and exercise regimens. Chopra advocates minimizing negative stress but also maximizing positive stress. He recommends doing something that brings joy and concentrating fully on that activity while practicing it, reducing distractions at work, and finding inner satisfaction in daily tasks.

In one chapter on longevity in *Ageless Body, Timeless Mind,* Chopra outlines 10 keys to active mastery. They may be useful guidelines to those wishing to reduce stress in their workplace and personal lives. In brief, they are:

- Listen to your body's wisdom
- Live in the present
- Take time to be silent, to meditate, to quiet the internal dialogue
- Relinquish your need for external approval
- When you find yourself reacting with anger or opposition to any person or circumstance, realize that you are only struggling with yourself
- Know that the world "out there" reflects your reality "in here"
- Shed the burden of judgment
- Do not contaminate your body with toxins
- Replace fear-motivated behavior with love-motivated behavior
- Understand that the physical world is just a mirror of a deeper intelligence

See also COMPLEMENTARY THERAPIES; HEALTH PROMOTION PROGRAMS; MEDITATION; MIND-BODY CONNECTIONS.

chromated copper arsenic See ARSENIC.

chronic beryllium disease (CBD) See BERYLLIUM.

chronic fatigue syndrome (CFS) Chronic fatigue syndrome is an illness characterized by fatigue that starts suddenly, improves, and relapses, bringing on debilitating tiredness or easy fatigability in an individual who has no apparent reason for feeling this way. There is profound weakness that does not go away with a few good nights of sleep but instead steals a person's vigor over months and years.

It is particularly difficult for an employed person who has the syndrome because employers may not understand the illness and believe that the employee is malingering. Because many individuals who have CFS experience frustration before being diagnosed, and again over the fact that there is no cure, many develop DEPRESSION, which also interferes with good workplace performance. Many sufferers feel that others do not take their suffering seriously. Some friends, family members, or coworkers may fear that CFS is contagious, and try to maintain a distance from the sufferer. (Medical opinion seems to indicate that CFS is not contagious.)

Diagnosing CFS is difficult because many of the symptoms are like those of other disorders. For example, CFS is not infectious mononucleosis, although profound fatigue is common in both disorders. It is not Alzheimer's disease, although there is memory loss and periodic confusion associated with both disorders. While there are immune system abnormalities, just as there are in AIDS, it is not AIDS. It has also been confused with rheumatoid arthritis, Hodgkin's disease, multiple sclerosis, and lupus.

While the illness strikes children, teenagers, and people in their 50s, 60s, and 70s, it is most likely to strike adults from their mid-20s to their late 40s, many of whom are in the prime of their working careers. Women are afflicted twice to three times as often as men; the vast majority of patients are white.

Because of the age group most afflicted, during the 1980s the name "yuppie flu" was attached to CFS. However, sufferers regarded the new name as tending to trivialize their illness.

Criteria for Diagnosis

In 1988, the Centers for Disease Control (CDC) published an official definition of chronic fatigue syndrome. A case of CFS must fulfill two major criteria:

1. New onset of persistent or relapsing debilitating fatigue or easy fatigability in a person who has no previous history of similar symptoms. The fatigue does not resolve with bed rest and is severe enough to reduce or impair average daily activity below 50 percent of the individual's customary level for at least six months.

2. Other clinical conditions that may produce similar symptoms must be excluded by thorough evaluation, based on a medical history, physical examination, and appropriate laboratory tests. Conditions specifically mentioned by the CDC include malignancy; autoimmune diseases; localized infection; chronic or subacute bacterial, fungal, or parasite disease (such as Lyme disease, tuberculosis, toxoplasmosis, amebas, or giardia); AIDS, AIDS-related condition (ARC), or any other HIV-related infection; chronic psychiatric disease (such as depression, neurosis, schizophrenia; chronic use of tranquilizers, drug dependency or abuse; side effects of medication or a toxic agent (such as a chemical solvent or a pesticide); chronic inflammatory disease; neuromuscular disease, such as multiple sclerosis or myasthenia gravis; endocrine disease, such as hypothyroidism or diabetes; any other known chronic pulmonary, renal, cardiac, hepatic (relating to the liver), or hematologic (relating to the blood or blood-forming tissues) disease.

According to the National Institutes of Health, CFS leaves many people bedridden, or with headaches, muscular and joint pain, sore throat, balance disorders, sensitivity to light, an inability to concentrate, and inexplicable body aches. Symptoms wax and wane in severity and linger for months and sometimes years, causing the individual to retreat from work and social obligations. Some individuals have been helped with some treatments. Some individuals do recover while others must function at a reduced level for years.

The course of CFS from onset to recovery varies greatly from one individual to another. However, for all sufferers, the cumulative effect is the same, namely, transforming ordinary activities into tremendous challenges. Sufferers cannot tolerate the least bit of exercise, and often their cognitive functions become impaired and memory, verbal fluency, response time, and abilities to perform calculations and to reason abstractly suffer.

Depression versus CFS

There are some commonalties between CFS and depression. However, the symptoms of CFS do not fit the description of *exogenous* depression, which is depression precipitated by external factors. Also, in CFS there usually is no evidence in the recent personal or family history to support a diagnosis of primary depression. Instead, the CFS-related depression seems to be *endogenous*, meaning that it has physiological origins within the body. Secondary depression, which follows from disease, rather than causes it, is just as disabling. However, knowing that there is a chemical basis for mood swings and that they are directly related to illness can be reassuring to many individuals.

Sleep and CFS

Despite constant exhaustion and desire for sleep, sufferers rarely sleep uninterruptedly and do not wake feeling refreshed. Some have severe insomnia, while others have difficulty maintaining sleep once they have gone to sleep. There is often not enough rapid-eye-movement sleep (REM), which is considered necessary for a good night's rest; REM usually takes up about one-fifth of the average night's sleep.

There is a cyclical relationship between CFS symptoms of pain, depression, and anxiety and difficulty sleeping soundly. All symptoms seem to be exacerbated by the others and add to the cycle of stress for the sufferer.

Vestibular disorders and CFS

Many CFS sufferers experience disorders of balance, or of the vestibular system, which is modulated by the inner ear. Any event that causes chemical changes in the brain, such as emotional stress or trauma, can influence the vestibular system. Those with balance disorders sometimes feel dizziness, lightheaded, or nauseous. According to the Dizziness and Balance Disorders Association of America, severe balance problems are "periods of violent, whirling sensations where the world is spinning out of control" (vertigo). Sometimes even walking is difficult, with sufferers tilting off balance or stumbling for no apparent reason. Some individuals who have balance disorders develop phobias, such as a fear of falling.

Therapies for CFS

Many therapies have been tried on CFS sufferers. Usually a plan is devised for each patient, depending on symptoms. Pharmacological therapies include use of antidepressant drugs, pain relieving drugs, and muscle-relaxing drugs.

Other therapies that have been tried include deep relaxation, YOGA, BIOFEEDBACK, and visualization therapy to relieve stress and chronic pain. Nutritional therapies that have been tried include emphasizing certain vitamins, such as vitamins A, B_6, B_{12}, C, and E, as well as zinc, folic acid, and selenium, all of which are said to have immuneboosting potential.

Role of Support Groups and Self-help

Several nationwide organizations encourage research and political advocacy and also provide lists of local support groups. EMPLOYEE ASSISTANCE PROGRAMS can help direct employees to local branches of these groups. CFS sufferers may find some relief with practical and emotional needs through such organizations.

Chronic Fatigue and Immune Dysfunction Syndrome Association (CFIDS)
P.O. Box 220398
Charlotte, NC 28222
(800) 442-3437 (toll-free)
(704) 362-CFID
(704) 365-9755 (fax)
http://www.cfids.org

National Chronic Fatigue Syndrome and Fibromyalgia Association (NCFSFA)
P.O. Box 18426
Kansas City, MO 64133
(816) 313-2000
(816) 524-6782 (fax)
http://www.ncfsfa.org

See also DEPRESSION; SUPPORT GROUPS.

chronic obstructive pulmonary disease The combination of chronic bronchitis and emphysema in which there is persistent disruption of airflow into or out of the lungs. The lungs of many workers are continuously exposed to airborne particles, such as bacteria, virus, and allergens, all of which can cause lung disorders.

For further information:

American Lung Association
1740 Broadway

New York, NY 10019
(212) 315-8700
(212) 315-8872 (fax)
www.lungusa.org

See also AIR POLLUTION; ASTHMA; BRONCHITIS; CHEMICAL TOXICITY; EMPHYSEMA; INDOOR ENVIRONMENT; LUNG DISEASE.

circadian rhythms Circadian rhythms are coordinated by an inherent timing mechanism known as a biological clock. Alertness and mental capability seems to be most available to us when we follow our internal clocks. Most people's "clocks" are synchronized to the Sun's 24-hour cycle. For example, sunrise means waking and working, while sundown means dinner and sleep. However, individuals who do SHIFT WORK find that their "day" is reversed. Most shift workers go home to sleep during the day, when their bodies want to be awake, and they have to work at night, when their bodies want to sleep, according to Charmane I. Eastman, Ph.D., associate professor of psychology and social sciences and director of the Biological Rhythms Research Laboratory at Rush-Presbyterian-St. Luke's Medical Center, Chicago.

The circadian rhythm of body temperature is a marker for internal clocks. Body temperature rises and falls in cycles parallel to alertness and performance efficiency. When body temperature is high, which it usually is during the day, alertness and performance peak, but sleep is difficult. A lower temperature (generally during the night) promotes sleep, but hinders alertness and performance.

Kahn, Ada P. *Stress A–Z: A Sourcebook for Facing Everyday Challenges.* New York: Facts On File, Inc., 1998.

clarinetist's cheilitis Drooling of saliva or formation of beads of perspiration under the lower lip can result in this discomfort on the border of the lower lip. Contact dermatitis also occurs on the lip from prolonged contact with a metal alloy mouthpiece, particularly from sensitivity to nickel or chromium. Clarinetists may also experience acne mechanica or localized acneiform eruptions of the lips as a result of friction, rubbing, or repetitive mechanical pressure.

See also ALLERGIES; DERMATITIS; FLUTIST'S CHIN; PERFORMING ARTS MEDICINE.

Sataloff, Robert Thayer, Alice G. Brandfonbrener, and Richard J. Lederman, eds. *Textbook of Performing Arts Medicine.* New York: Raven Press, 1991.

Clean Air Act of 1990 A federal law designed to make sure that all Americans have safe air to breathe. While public health protection is the primary goal, the law also seeks to protect the environment from damage caused by AIR POLLUTION. Congress passed the core provisions of the Clean Air Act in 1970, then amended the act in 1977 and again in 1990 to specify new strategies for cleaning up the air.

Under this law, the ENVIRONMENTAL PROTECTION AGENCY (EPA) sets limits on how much of a pollutant can be in the air anywhere in the United States. The law allows individual states to have stronger pollution controls, but states are not allowed to have weaker pollution controls than those set for the whole country. The EPA assists states by providing scientific research, expert studies, engineering designs, and money to support clean air programs that help employers to comply with the law.

The EPA enforces the law and has the power to fine companies and employers for violating the act.

For further information:

Clean Air Trust
1625 K Street, NW
#790
Washington, DC 20006
(202) 785-9625
www.cleanairtrust.org

See also ACID RAIN; CARBON MONOXIDE; CHLOROFLUOROCARBONS; HAZARDOUS AIR POLLUTANTS; INDOOR ENVIRONMENT; NITROGEN OXIDES; PARTICULATE MATTER; SULFUR DIOXIDE; VOLATILE ORGANIC COMPOUNDS.

U.S. Environmental Protection Agency

clergyman's knee See BURSITIS.

clinical depression See DEPRESSION; MENTAL HEALTH.

coal dust   An odorless, dark brown to black dust created by crushing, grinding, or pulverizing coal. Workers involved in the mining and transportation of coal, and use of coal during operations involving grinding, crushing, or pulverizing, may be at risk.

Coal dust often contains 5 percent or more free silica. Exposure to coal dust can occur through inhalation, ingestion, and eye contact. Signs and symptoms of acute exposure include coughing, wheezing, and shortness of breath. Chronic exposure to coal dust may result in symptoms of bronchitis and emphysema. Coal dust causes coal workers' pneumoconiosis, bronchitis, and emphysema in exposed workers.

The National Fire Protection Association has not assigned a flammability rating to coal dust. However, other sources rate coal dust as a fire hazard and consider the airborne dust an explosion hazard when exposed to heat or open flame.

See also BLACK LUNG DISEASE; BRONCHITIS; EYE INJURIES/PROTECTION; MINE SAFETY AND HEALTH; SKIN OR SENSE ORGAN TOXICITY.

U.S. Department of Labor, Occupational Safety and Health Administration

coal miners   See EXTRACTIVE INDUSTRIES.

coal tar   See COAL TAR PITCH VOLATILES.

coal tar pitch volatiles (CTPVs)   Materials composed of various chemical vapors that become airborne during the heating of coal tar pitch. Coal tar pitch is usually a thick, black or dark-brown liquid or semisolid that has a smoky odor. Other terms for coal tar pitch volatiles include *coal tar pitch, pitch, pitch oil, topped coal tar,* and *creosote.*

Coal tar pitch volatiles (CTPVs) are found in industry when coal tar or coal tar pitch is heated. Once the pitch is heated, chemicals vaporize and become available for inhalation by workers. Industries in which workers may be exposed to CTPVs include coking, roofing, road paving, aluminum smelting, wood preserving, and any others where coal tar is used.

The severest health hazards of being exposed to CTPVs are cancer of the skin, lungs, and bladder. Other health effects include dizzy spells, shortness of breath, nose soreness and bleeding, loss of appetite, irritability, and reproductive effects. With repeated exposure, skin pigmentation may change or severe rashes may form.

The main chemicals of concern in CTPVs are POLYCYCLIC AROMATIC HYDROCARBONS (PAHs), which are also known as polynuclear aromatic hydrocarbons (PNAs).

CTPVs are measured by passing workplace air through a sampling device and then analyzing the sample for the compounds of interest. To control exposure to CTPVs, engineering controls include ventilation, isolating processes involving the use of CTPVs, and where possible, automated handing of open coal tar products. Respirators may also be worn by workers exposed to CTPVs, and PERSONAL PROTECTIVE EQUIPMENT may be used to prevent contact with products containing CTPVs.

See also CARCINOGENS; POLYCYCLIC AROMATIC HYDROCARBONS; RESPIRATORY TOXICITY; SKIN OR SENSE ORGAN TOXICITY.

U.S. Department of Labor, Occupational Safety and Health Administration

coal workers' pneumoconiosis   See BLACK LUNG DISEASE.

COBRA (Consolidated Omnibus Budget Reconciliation Act)   This law, enacted in 1986, enables workers to keep their health coverage during times of voluntary or involuntary job loss, reduction in hours worked, transition between jobs, and in certain other cases.

COBRA generally requires that group health plans sponsored by employers with 20 or more employees in their prior year offer employees and their families the opportunity for a temporary extension of health coverage (called continuation coverage) in certain instances where coverage under the plan would otherwise end. Events that can cause workers and their family members to lose group health coverage may result in the right to COBRA coverage. These include:

- Voluntary or involuntary termination of the covered employee's employment for reasons other than gross misconduct

- Reduced hours of work for the covered employee
- Covered employee becoming entitled to Medicare
- Divorce or legal separation of a covered employee
- Death of a covered employee
- Loss of status as a "dependent child" under plan rules

Coverage under COBRA may be for 18 or 36 months, depending on circumstances. Qualified individuals may be required to pay the entire premium for coverage up to 102 percent of the cost of the plan. Premiums may be higher for persons exercising the disability provisions of COBRA. Premiums may be increased by the plan; however, premiums generally must be set in advance of each 12-month premium cycle. Individuals subject to COBRA coverage may be responsible for paying all costs related to deductibles, and may be subject to catastrophic and other benefit limits.

See also HEALTH INSURANCE; HEALTH MAINTENANCE ORGANIZATIONS.

cocaine An addictive drug that stimulates the central nervous system and induces feelings of euphoria. Use of cocaine becomes a workplace health issue because the use and addiction interferes with productivity.

Different users react to the drug in different ways. However, many experience an instant feeling of enormous pleasure known as a "rush." It also initially may make the user feel energetic and self-confident. However, the pleasurable feelings produced by cocaine are followed by depression and fatigue, known as a "crash." To avoid the crash, users take more cocaine, establishing an expensive cycle of use and dependency which is extremely difficult to end and often requires lengthy treatment.

Use of cocaine can lead to severe psychological and physical dependence. It can increase the pulse, blood pressure, body temperature, and respiratory rate. Paranoid psychosis, hallucinations, and other problems can result from cocaine use. Cocaine use

also causes bleeding and other damage to nasal passages. Cocaine-related heart and respiratory failure can lead to death.

Cocaine is most often used in the form of white powder, and is typically ingested by inhaling, or "snorting," usually through a straw or other tube in the nose. It can also be injected into the veins. After conversion to its base form, cocaine can be smoked, which is known as "freebasing." *Crack* is the street name given to tiny chunks or "rocks" of freebase cocaine in smokeable form. Crack is even more rapidly physically and psychologically addicting than powdered cocaine. Cocaine powder breaks down with heat and so cannot be effectively self-administered by smoking. In contrast, base cocaine or "freebase," which has been chemically "freed" from its hydrochloride salt, readily vaporizes into smoke by heat. Inhalation of the smoke gets the cocaine rapidly into the bloodstream through the lungs, faster than if powder cocaine is snorted.

Cocaine is sometimes used with other drugs. The cocaine/heroin combination has been known as "speedball" and the cocaine/PCP mixture has been known as "space base."

Employees suspected of being cocaine users should be referred to their EMPLOYEE ASSISTANCE PROGRAM.

See also ADDICTIONS; DRUG TESTING.

codependency A relationship in which participants have a strong need to be needed as well as to create mutual needs in a detrimental, weakening manner in order to preserve the dependent relationship. Codependent relationships are extremely destructive for one or both of the partners and can interfere with an individual's workplace performance.

An example of a codependent relationship is one in which a husband covers up his wife's alcoholism. He may be absent from his job because he does the household chores, drives the children to their activities, and explains her problem as an "illness." He is an "enabler," because he makes it possible for her to continue with her addiction. Another example of a codependent relationship is a parent who continues to support an adult child who should be responsible for himself because the parent enjoys the feeling of the child's dependence. Many alcoholics and drug addicts also have enablers.

When parents continue to compensate for or cover up a child's difficulties in school or with the law, thinking that they are protecting the child, that too is a codependent relationship. It is often interpreted that this behavior persists because preserving the child's flaws and immature behavior will keep him or her forever dependent on the parent. Since codependency is viewed as a type of addiction, advocates of the codependent theory feel that these tendencies can be overcome with a process similar to the recovery process used by Alcoholics Anonymous. In many cases, an individual would like to eliminate the difficulties caused by the codependent relationship but is too "addicted" to the situation to change.

Employers who believe that an employee is in a detrimental codependent relationship may wish to advise the employee to seek help from an EMPLOYEE ASSISTANCE PROGRAM.

See also ADDICTIONS; ALCOHOL DEPENDENCY.

coffee　Coffee is considered by many workers as a source of relief from stress. This may be because having a cup of coffee is also a social experience and an opportunity for individuals to sit together and relax for a few moments of conversation.

However, coffee is primarily a stimulant, as it contains CAFFEINE. Some individuals enjoy the feeling of instant energy that caffeine produces and use coffee to help wake themselves up or recharge themselves throughout the day. This is because caffeine affects the central nervous system, increasing the heart action in rate and strength. There is also increased activity of the kidneys and brain centers.

Individuals tolerate differing levels of caffeine in coffee. Some people are overly sensitive to caffeine, while others overdose themselves, developing ANXIETY, insomnia, or irritability, which are symptoms of "caffeinism."

Those who believe they consume too much coffee each day in an effort to relieve stress may benefit from learning techniques to reduce stress such as relaxation therapy, MEDITATION, or GUIDED IMAGERY.

coffee worker's lung　See WHEEZING.

cognitive therapy　A therapeutic approach based on the concept that ANXIETY results from patterns of thinking and distorted attitudes toward oneself and others and that one can alter one's behavior by changing one's thinking. Cognitive therapy is used to treat depressed individuals and others who have anxieties and PHOBIAS. One innovator during the late 1970s was Aaron Beck (born 1921), an American psychiatrist. Earlier forms of cognitive therapy were introduced by Albert Ellis in the late 1960s under the name Rational Emotive Therapy (RET).

Individuals with mental health concerns may be referred by an EMPLOYEE ASSISTANCE PROGRAM for cognitive therapy, which has the goal of helping the individual change his or her unwanted behavior. It emphasizes the importance of the individual's thoughts, feelings, imagery, attitudes, and hope and their causative relationship to behaviors.

See also AGGRESSION; DEPRESSION; MENTAL HEALTH.

cold environments　Workers in cold winter months face the occupational hazard of exposure to the cold. Prolonged exposure to freezing temperatures can result in health problems such as trench foot, frostbite, and hypothermia. Workers in industries as construction, commercial fishing, and agriculture need to be aware of the weather, its effects on the body, proper protective techniques, and treatment of cold-related disorders.

MAJOR RISK FACTORS WHEN WORKING IN COLD ENVIRONMENTS

- Wearing inadequate or wet clothing increases the effects of cold on the body
- Taking certain drugs or medications such as alcohol, nicotine, caffeine, and medication that inhibits the body's response to the cold or impairs judgment
- Having a cold or certain diseases, such as diabetes, heart, vascular, and thyroid problems, may make a person more susceptible to the winter elements
- Becoming exhausted or immobilized, especially due to injury or entrapment, may speed up the effects of cold weather
- Aging: the elderly are more vulnerable to the effects of harsh cold weather

Source: Occupational Health and Safety Administration

Trench Foot, Frostbite, and Hypothermia

Trench foot is caused by long, continuous exposure to a wet, cold environment, or actual immersion in water. This is a hazard for commercial fishermen, who experience these types of cold, wet environments daily. Frostbite occurs when the skin tissue actually freezes, causing ice crystals to form between cells and draw water from them, which leads to cellular dehydration. Although this typically occurs at temperatures below 30° F (–1° C), wind chill effects can cause frostbite at temperatures above freezing. This is a hazard for workers on roads or in construction. General hypothermia occurs when body temperature falls to a level at which normal muscular and cerebral functions are impaired. While hypothermia is generally associated with freezing temperatures, it may occur in any climate where a person's body temperature falls below normal; this can occur during construction or mining.

Preventing Cold-Related Disorders

Engineering controls in the workplace through a variety of practices help reduce the risk of cold-related injuries. Air jets or radiant heaters can be an on-site source of heat. Work areas can be shielded from drafty or windy conditions. A heated shelter can be provided for employees who experience prolonged exposure to low temperatures. Thermal insulating material can be used on equipment handles in cold weather.

Safe work practices, such as changes in work schedules, are necessary to combat the effects of very cold weather. A period of adjustment to the cold should be allowed before embarking on a full work schedule. Employees should be permitted to set their own pace and take extra work breaks when needed. The number of activities performed outdoors should be reduced as much as possible. When employees must work in a cold atmosphere, select the warmest hours of the day and minimize activities that reduce circulation. Employees should be well hydrated; there should be a buddy system for working outdoors. Finally, employees should be educated regarding the symptoms of cold-related stresses, such as heavy shivering, uncomfortable coldness, severe fatigue, drowsiness, or euphoria. Quiet symptoms of potentially deadly cold-related ailments often go undetected until the worker's health is endangered.

PREVENTING COLD-RELATED INJURIES

- Wear at least three layers of clothing: an outer layer to break the wind and allow some ventilation and a middle layer of wool or synthetic fabric to absorb sweat and retain insulation in a damp environment (down is a useful lightweight insulator; however, it is ineffective when it becomes wet); an inner layer of cotton or synthetic weave to allow ventilation
- Protect your hands, feet, face and head
- Footgear should be insulated to protect against cold and dampness

Source: Occupational Safety and Health Administration

---

combustion pollutants   Gases or particles that come from burning materials. Many workers are exposed to combustion pollutants from both indoor and outdoor sources. After secondhand smoke, the major combustion pollutants present in workplaces (as well as homes) are carbon monoxide, nitrogen dioxide, and sulfur dioxide.

Carbon monoxide is a poisonous gas that is difficult to detect, as it is colorless, odorless, and tasteless. It has toxic effects when absorbed through the lungs into the bloodstream, where it inhibits the oxygen-carrying abilities of blood.

Nitrogen dioxide can irritate and damage the respiratory system, particularly after prolonged exposure.

Sulfur dioxide is produced when sulfur-containing fuels are burned, as in kerosene heaters. It causes impaired breathing.

Elevated levels of combustion pollutants are present in buildings with improperly vented oil or gas hot water heaters and furnaces, gas clothes dryers, and gas ranges and stoves. Wood-burning or coal stoves and kerosene heaters also produce combustion pollutants, which contribute to indoor pollution levels if they are not vented properly.

Automobiles and trucks produce carbon monoxide and nitrogen dioxide. If a building has an attached or underground garage, or a loading dock located near air intake vents, these combustion pollutants can be drawn into the ventilation system and distributed throughout the building.

Many problems can be avoided by careful attention to operation and maintenance of appliances and ventilation systems.

Health Effects of Combustion Pollutants

Health effects range from headaches and breathing difficulties to death. Carbon monoxide in indoor air can cause headaches, dizziness, nausea, vomiting, fatigue, decreased hearing, heart palpitations, and loss of appetite. Older people, pregnant women, and people with a history of heart disease are particularly sensitive to carbon monoxide exposure. Continued exposure to high levels can cause collapse, unconsciousness, and in extreme cases, death.

Nitrogen dioxide can cause eye, nose, throat, and respiratory tract irritation. Prolonged exposure may lower resistance to respiratory infection and can be damaging to respiratory tissue.

Sulfur dioxide is particularly threatening to people with asthma, in whom it can constrict the airways leading to and from the lungs, making breathing difficult. People with lung disease and allergies may also have adverse reactions to sulfur dioxide fumes. Sulfur dioxide can cause irritation of skin and eyes.

See also AIR POLLUTION; ASTHMA; CHEMICAL TOXICITY; HAZARDOUS AND TOXIC SUBSTANCES; HEADACHES; INDOOR ENVIRONMENT; SKIN OR SENSE ORGAN TOXICITY.

American Lung Association

commercial diving   Workers who dive as part of their job assignment, whether classified as commercial divers or not, are exposed to underwater hazards. Divers are exposed not only to the possibility of drowning but also to such occupational safety and health hazards as respiratory and circulatory risks, hypothermia, low visibility, and physical injury from the operation of heavy equipment underwater. The type of dive, length and frequency of dive, and the type of operation increase the already high risk of this work. Additional hazards associated with the work include underwater cutting and welding, materials handling, hull scrubbing, and other types of work utilizing hands and power tools.

Adverse Health Effects: Dysbarism

Dysbarism is a generic term applicable to any adverse health effect due to a difference between ambient pressure and the total gas pressure in tissues, fluids, or cavities in the body. Increased gas pressure underwater is called hyperbaric pressure. Most dysbarisms are predictable using some combination of Boyle's law, Dalton's law, and/or Henry's Law. Boyle's law applies to expansion and contraction of gases within the body because of external pressure changes due to depth. Dalton's law states that in a mixture of gases, the partial pressure of each gas is proportional to the molar fraction of each gas that makes up the total, and can be used to determine how much nitrogen, oxygen, or carbon dioxide is in the ambient air at any hyperbaric pressure underwater. Henry's law states that a gas will dissolve into a liquid in proportion to its partial pressure in the air and its solubility in the liquid, and can predict the body's absorption of inert gases into and back from the body at any pressure or depth.

Unique Health Hazards

Divers face many unique health hazards. Gas narcosis is caused by nitrogen in normal air dissolving into nervous tissue during dives of more than 120 feet. Helium, substituted for nitrogen in "mixed gas diving," can cause an effect called high pressure nervous syndrome.

Gas toxicities are caused by oxygen and carbon dioxide. Damage to the lungs and brain varies with partial pressure and time of exposure.

Pain due to expanding or contracting trapped gases can lead to barotrauma, an acute symptom from which potential damage can occur either during ascent or descent and can be most severe when gases are expanding. The most common sites of pain from trapped gases are the digestive tract, sinuses, teeth, middle ear, and lungs. Blockage of sinus passages due to nasal congestion or a head cold can cause pain during either ascent or descent. Sinus pain during descent is known as "sinus squeeze." Divers should be trained to detect blocked sinuses and not dive with a cold or an allergic inflammation. The most common source or pain on descent is from the contraction of air in the middle ear if the eustachian tubes are inflamed or blocked. Divers should be trained to clear their ears every two feet and to stop and rise back up a few feet before attempting to clear a blockage.

Decompression sickness (DCS) is due to the evolution of inert gas bubbles. DCS is sometimes referred to as "evolved gas dysbarism," "compressed air sickness," or "caisson worker's syndrome." Acute symptoms of DCS can occur during a decrease in pressure, but they occur most commonly soon after the ascent has been completed.

Dysbaric osteonecrosis is bone lesions, most commonly on the body's long bones—the humerus, femur, or tibia. This chronic disease may be related to the evolution of gas bubbles that may or may not be diagnosed as a decompression sickness.

Other hazards divers face include microbes and parasites, noise, fire, and chemicals used during underwater cleanup operations.

The Occupational Safety and Health Administration (OSHA) has set standards covering a wide range of commercial diving applications, including boat captains, marine terminals, scuba training and construction.

The Association of Diving Contractors, Inc., is a nonprofit group representing more than 300 companies organized to promote commercial diving, establish uniform safety standards for commercial divers, and encourage industry-wide observance of these standards.

For information:

Association of Diving Contractors International
5206 FM 1960
Suite 202
Houston, TX 77069-4406
(281) 893-8388
(281) 893-5118 (fax)
http://www.adc-usa.org

See also CHEMICAL TOXICITY; NEUROTOXICITY; NOISE.

communication Process through which meanings are exchanged between individuals, whether in the workplace or in personal life. When individuals feel understood, they are communicating effectively. They are in control of events, other people trust and respect them, and they feel valued in work settings. Communicating effectively enhances health and self-esteem, nurtures relationships, and helps people cope with the stresses inherent in all workplaces.

Failure to Communicate in the Workplace

When individuals do not communicate well with their superiors or subordinates, they may feel misunderstood, frustrated, distressed, defensive, and often hostile. Faults and flaws in communication habits, or communication gaps, cause stress for many people. People who do not communicate effectively are more vulnerable to disease; they can be hostile and confrontational and are at increased risk for heart disease. People who feel misunderstood report more depression and more mood disorders of the kind shown to weaken their immune function. When communication breaks down, heart rate speeds up, cholesterol and blood sugar levels rise, headaches and digestive problems are more common, and people are more sensitive to pain. In work settings, communication gaps can reduce productivity, make workers irritable, and even increase the risk of accidents.

Differences in Male-Female Communication Styles

According to Bee Reinthaler, a personnel communications specialist, in business, differences between communication styles of male and female managers can cause problems in efficiency and in accomplishing goals. Males in the corporate world often use a complex combination of business, sports, and military jargon. Their behavior is action-oriented and competitive. On the other hand, women generally are more demonstrative and express their feelings. Many women frame their speech with qualifiers, questions, and questioning intonations. They express doubts and uncertainties more frequently than men.

According to Reinthaler, when women wait for men to speak first, they create an image of incompetence. "Men may then fall into the stereotypical role of treating women as incompetent and the stereotypical interaction continues in a destructive way. It would be more effective if both genders of managers would 'speak the same' language."

"Many women attempt to crack the male communication code in the workplace until something happens that shows they have underestimated its complexities," says Candiss Rinker, an expert in the science and practice of change management. She explains that women have been socialized from childhood to avoid direct communication about difficult issues, so they often use a sugar-coated approach that other women understand, but men do not.

Deborah Tannen, a linguistics professor, says gender differences put women in a double bind at work that is not as evident in personal relationships. "Workplace communication norms were developed by men, for men, at a time when there were very few women present. The situation is aggravated when women hold positions of authority. If they talk in ways expected of women, they may not be respected; if they talk in ways expected of men, they may not be liked," says Tannen, author of *Talking From 9 to 5: How Women's and Men's Conversational Styles Affect Who Gets Heard, Who Gets Credit, and What Gets Done at Work* (1994).

Removing the Stress from Your Workplace Communication Style

Individuals should apply the old "golden rule" in communicating with superiors, coworkers, and employees. They should speak the way in which they would like to be spoken to and listen to others the way they hope others will listen to them. It is important that they learn to express their likes and dislikes in a tactful and diplomatic way. They will find that when they are more direct, other people will be more responsive.

IMPROVE WORKPLACE PRODUCTIVITY: AVOID COMMUNICATION GAPS

---

* ***Learn to cope with criticism.*** Receiving criticism causes stress. The impact on our mood and body depends more on how we describe the negative feedback to ourselves. Ask yourself: Does this seem reasonable? Is it fact or opinion? Are there others who might confirm or dispute this view? How would others have behaved?
* ***Learn to listen.*** Listening is an active process requiring openness and receptivity. Keep your mind free of distracting reactions, responses, judgments, and questions and answers.
* ***Observe your own body language.*** Research shows that more than half of what we communicate is conveyed by body language. Smiling, frowning, sighing, touch-

ing, or drumming fingers give out strong messages. Women tend to smile more than men, nod their heads, and maintain more continuous eye contact while listening and speaking than men. Under stress or in new situations, this tendency becomes even more pronounced.
* ***Recognize and respect differences in conversational styles.*** Styles of conversing play a major role in triggering misunderstanding. For example, women tend to ask more personal questions than men. Men more often give opinions and make declarations of fact.
* ***Become more assertive.*** Speak and act from choice and stand up for your rights without being aggressive.
* ***Learn to say no when you want to.*** Avoid feeling resentful, frustrated or guilty. Take time before you respond to a request. You need not give lengthy explanations for saying no.
* ***Try to resolve conflicts when you recognize them.*** Use "I" statements whenever possible, rather than attacking the other person with a "you" statement. Make sure you understand each other's concerns, positions, or feelings by summarizing what you heard.

See also ASSERTIVENESS TRAINING; BODY LANGUAGE; CONFLICT RESOLUTION; CRITICISM; FRUSTRATION; IMMUNE SYSTEM; RELATIONSHIPS; SELF-ESTEEM; STRESS.

Kahn, Ada P. *Stress A–Z: A Sourcebook for Coping with Everyday Challenges.* New York: Facts On File, Inc., 1998.

Reardon, Kathleen Kelley. *They Don't Get It, Do They?: Communication in the Workplace—Closing the Gap Between Women and Men.* New York: Little, Brown, 1995.

Reinthaler, Bee. "Verbal Communications." *The Professional Communicator,* Fall 1991.

Sobel, David S. "Rx: Prescriptions for Improving Communication." *Mental Medicine Update* III, no. 2, 1994.

Tannen, Deborah. *Talking from 9 to 5: How Women's and Men's Conversational Styles Affect Who Gets Heard, Who Gets Credit, and What Gets Done at Work.* New York: William Morrow, 1994.

Tingley, Judith C. *Genderflex: Men and Women Speaking Each Other's Language at Work.* New York: Amacom, 1995.

commuting   See WORK RELATIONSHIP CRITERIA.

compactors   See DEATHS IN THE WORKPLACE.

competition   One of the many dichotomies present in American workplaces today that induces

STRESS. It encourages individual achievement and the need to win. As such, it is the extreme opposite of another American workplace concept—teamwork—which teaches us to respect others, appreciate their strengths and weaknesses, share our skills and knowledge, and help others meet their goals.

Early in life, children on the playing field experience the contradiction of competition and teamwork. Thus begins a source of stress we carry through much of our adulthood and working careers. Competition encourages comparisons between ourselves and others, both on a job category and economic level; this in turn affects our feeling of self-esteem and may interfere with work productivity and good health.

See also AUTONOMY; CONTROL; FRUSTRATION; SELF-ESTEEM; TYPE A PERSONALITY.

Kahn, Ada P. *Stress A–Z: A Sourcebook for Facing Everyday Challenges*. New York: Facts On File, Inc., 1998.

complementary therapies   A set of practices that, depending on the viewpoint, either complement or compete with conventional Western medicine in the prevention and treatment of stress-related disorders as well as other diseases. These practices are increasingly being covered by insurance in the workplace and being embraced by an increasing number of people. Complementary therapies are sometimes referred to as "alternative" therapies.

According to David Edelberg, M.D., writing in *The Internist* (September 1994), the term *complementary* commonly refers to anything that is not conventionally practiced or taught in medical school. In 1994 there were more than 200 fields of complementary medicine. Complementary fields can be divided into four broad categories: traditional medicine, such as Chinese or Native American; hands-on bodywork; psychological or psychospiritual medicine; and many holdovers from the 19th century, such as chiropractic medicine and homeopathy.

Complementary therapies for dealing with anxieties and healing mind as well as body include emotional release therapies with or without body manipulation, emotional control or self-regulating therapies, religious or inspirational therapies, cognitive-emotional therapies, and emotional expression through creative therapies. Some of these have been known by such names as *encounter groups, gestalt therapy, primal therapy, EST, bioenergetic psychotherapy,* ROLFING, TRANSCENDENTAL MEDITATION, and BIOFEEDBACK.

Complementary therapies are not subject to scientific scrutiny through controlled efficacy studies with placebo or comparison of treatments. They are accepted and promoted as helping on the basis of "anecdotal evidence" stemming from individual reports of success. Some may be truly helpful while others may be useless or ineffectual.

Many individuals find relief for anxiety-induced conditions from one or a combination of complementary therapies either along with or after seeking traditional care. For example, mental imagery is rated one of the six most commonly used alternative treatments among cancer patients and is believed by physicians as well as patients to reduce both the pain and distress of symptoms. However, as with other medical conditions, individuals should not overlook traditional psychiatric or medical treatments in favor of alternative therapies because they may be robbing themselves of valuable time as their condition progresses.

Complementary vs. Conventional Care

Conventional medical practitioners adhere to scientific models and methodologies that many complementary medical practitioners believe focus too exclusively on reductionist and physiochemical explanations of biological phenomena. Proponents of alternative medicine suggest that this approach shows limited understanding of health and disease and, in particular, of interactions between mind-body connections, psychological, social, and biological factors that influence coping with stress and disease processes.

Advocates of complementary approaches, in recent decades known also as "holistic" (or "wholistic") medicine, regard the influence of psychological factors and cognitive processes as equal to, if not more powerful than, the insights and methods of conventional medicine in coping with stress and disease and improving clinical outcomes.

For most of the 20th century, the generally accepted model for understanding biological phenomena and intervening therapeutically was the allopathic method. It achieved scientific, economic, and political primacy over the competing models such as osteopathic medicine, homeopathy, and chiropractic, as well as other alternative approaches. However, the public's interest in complementary therapies has grown tremendously during the last two decades.

In a survey reported by Harvard Medical School researchers, more than a quarter of the people they interviewed saw a physician regularly but were also employing another treatment, usually with their doctor's knowledge. One in 10 respondents were relying on nontraditional treatments exclusively. The study emphasized the widespread acceptance of "alternative medicine," a variety of unrelated practices from acupuncture to yoga that are promoted as having healing benefits. The common factor between them is that they have not yet been subjected to scientific review, the process most of the Western world uses to determine whether a treatment is safe and effective.

Herbal and "Folk" Therapies

In many cultures, herbs and other natural and botanical products are used to relieve anxiety-induced health conditions instead of modern diagnostic techniques and pharmacological treatments. Herbs are used to cure specific illnesses, improve health, lengthen life, and increase sexual vigor and fertility.

Increasing Interest
by Government and Insurers

In 1991 the Office of Alternative Medicine (OAM) was created within the National Institutes of Health. In the later 1990s it was renamed the Office of Complementary and Alternative Medicine. The goal of the OCAM is to research and evaluate many alternative or unconventional medical treatments.

Increasingly, some health insurers are paying for complementary therapies, removing some of the financial stress involved in seeking these treatments. A study reported in the *Journal of Health Care Marketing* (spring 1995, vol. 15, no. 1) included insurers from government, third-party insurance companies, and HMOs; results indicated the mechanisms through which each of three complementary therapies (chiropractic, acupuncture, and biofeedback) gained some credibility and acceptance by insurers. Results indicated that these

therapies have each achieved at least moderate success in obtaining third-party reimbursement.

For information:

National Center for Complementary and Alternative Medicine
National Institutes of Health (NIH)
31 Center Drive
Building 31
#2B11, MSC 2182
Bethesda, MD 20892-2182
(301) 435-5042
(301) 435-6549 (fax)
http://www.nccam.nih.gov

See also CHIROPRACTIC MEDICINE; CHOPRA, DEEPAK; CROSS-CULTURAL INFLUENCES; GUIDED IMAGERY; MEDITATION; MIND-BODY CONNECTIONS.

Burton Group. *Alternative Medicine: The Definitive Guide.* Puyallup, Wash.: Future Medicine Publishing, 1993.
Eisenberg, D., et al. "Unconventional Medicine in the United States: Prevalence, Costs, and Patterns of Use." *New England Journal of Medicine* 328 (1993): 246–252.
Goldfinger, Stephen E., ed. "Alternative Medicine: Insurers Cover New Ground." *Harvard Health Letter* 22, no. 2 (December 1996).
Goleman, Daniel, and Joel Gurin, eds. *Mind Body Medicine: How to Use Your Mind for Better Health.* Yonkers, NY: Consumer Reports Books, 1993.
Roach, Mary. "My Quest for Qi." *Health,* March 1997.
Weil, Andrew. *Eight Weeks to Optimum Health: Proven Program for Taking Full Advantage of Your Body's Healing Power.* New York: Knopf, 1997.

Comprehensive Environmental Response, Compensation, and Liability Act (CERCLA) Commonly known as Superfund, this law was enacted by Congress in 1980 and amended in 1986. The law created a tax on the chemical and petroleum industries and provided broad federal authority to respond directly to releases or threatened releases of hazardous substances that may endanger workers, the environment, or public health. Over five years, $1.6 billion was collected and the tax went to a trust fund for cleaning up abandoned or uncontrolled hazardous waste sites.

CERCLA established prohibitions and requirements concerning closed and abandoned hazardous waste sites, provided for liability of persons responsible for releases of hazardous waste at these sites, and established a trust fund to provide for cleanup when no responsible party could be identified.

The law authorizes short-term removals, where actions may be taken to address releases or threatened releases requiring prompt response. Additionally, the law requires long-term remedial response actions that permanently and significantly reduce the dangers associated with releases or threats of releases of hazardous substances that are serious, but not immediately life threatening. These actions can be conducted only at sites listed on the Environmental Protection Agency's NATIONAL PRIORITIES LIST (NPL).

See also HAZARDOUS WASTE; ENVIRONMENTAL PROTECTION AGENCY.

compressed gas and equipment Hazards associated with use of compressed gases include oxygen displacement, fires, explosions, and toxic effects. There are also physical hazards associated with pressurized systems. Special storage, use, and handling precautions are essential to control these hazards.

Compressed gas equipment is used in many industries, notably commercial diving, process safety management, hand and power tools, pulp, paper, and paperboard manufacturing, welding, cutting, and brazing.

The Compressed Gas Association (CGA) is dedicated to the development and promotion of safety standards and safe practices in the industrial gas industry. CGA develops and publishes technical information, standards, and recommendations for safe and environmentally responsible practices in the manufacture, storage, transportation, distribution, and use of industrial gases.

For information contact:

Compressed Gas Association (CGA)
4221 Walney Road
5th Floor
Chantilly, VA 20151-2923
(703) 788-2700
(703) 961-1831 (fax)

See also COMMERCIAL DIVING; PULP, PAPER, AND PAPERBOARD MILLS; WELDING.

computer workstations Computer technology has changed the workplaces of America, and use of computers continues to increase. In 1984 only 25 percent of the U.S. population used computers at work. According to the OCCUPATIONAL SAFETY AND HEALTH ADMINISTRATION, in 1993 this increased to 45 percent. Since then the numbers have grown tremendously. More than 18 million workers are in jobs that require intensive keying. Along with this expanding use of computers have come reports of adverse health effects to computer operators.

A computer consists of display screen, a keyboard, and a central processing unit. Many business machines and typewriters have been replaced by computers. This technology enables workers to accomplish in a matter of seconds or minutes what may have formerly required several hours.

The growth in computer use has raised many concerns about their potential health effects. Complaints include excessive fatigue, eyestrain and eye irritation, blurred vision, headaches, stress, and neck, back, and arm pain. Research has shown that these symptoms can result from problems with the equipment, workstations, office environment, or job design, or from a combination of these factors. Concerns about potential exposure to electromagnetic fields also have been raised.

The *display screen,* or video display terminal (VDT), is the output device that shows what the computer is processing. Display screens can be monochrome (green, white, or orange on a black background), or full color.

The *keyboard* is the input device that allows the user to send information to the "brain" of the computer. Keyboards are commonly used for data entry and inquiry. The keyboard is designed after a standard typewriter keyboard but with additional special keys and functions.

The *central processing unit,* or CPU, is the "brain," or center of operation for the computer. It performs calculations and organizes the flow of information into and out of the system.

Computers operate at high voltage, but the power supplies generating the voltage produce very little current. All data processing equipment must meet stringent international safety standards in this regard.

Visual Problems

Eyestrain and eye irritation are among the most frequent complaints of computer operators. Symptoms can result from improper lighting, glare from the screen, or poor positioning of the screen. These problems usually can be corrected by adjusting the physical setting. For example, workstations and lighting should be arranged to avoid direct and reflected glare anywhere in the field of sight, from the display screen, or surrounding surfaces.

Many computer jobs require long sessions in front of a VDT. Consequently, some people may need corrective lenses to avoid eyestrain and headaches. Vision examinations should therefore be conducted to assure early detection and correction of poor vision. Eye care specialists should be informed of computer use.

Computer users also can reduce eyestrain by taking rest breaks after each hour or so of work. The National Institute for Occupational Safety and Health (NIOSH) recommends a 10-minute rest break after two hours of continuous work for operators under moderate visual demands, and a 15-minute rest break after one hour of continuous work where there is a high visual demand or repetitive task.

Changing focus is another way to give eye muscles a chance to relax. The employee needs only to glance across the room or out the window from time to time and look at an object at least 20 feet away.

Fatigue and Musculoskeletal Problems

Workers at VDTs may sit still for considerable time and usually use small frequent movements of the eyes, head, arms, and fingers. Retaining a fixed posture over long periods of time causes muscle fatigue and, if this practice is consistent, can eventually lead to muscle pain and injury.

Computer operators also are subject to a risk of developing various musculoskeletal disorders, such as CARPAL TUNNEL SYNDROME and TENDINITIS. Musculoskeletal disorders are injuries to the muscles, joints, tendons, or nerves that are caused or made worse by work-related risk factors. Early symptoms of musculoskeletal disorders include pain and swelling, numbness and tingling (hands falling asleep), loss of strength, and reduced range of motion. These symptoms should be reported to a doctor as soon as possible. If not treated early, these symptoms can result in loss of strength in affected areas, chronic pain, or permanent disability.

Radiation

Another concern for the computer user is whether the emissions from radiation, such as X-ray or electromagnetic fields in the radio frequency and extreme low frequency ranges, pose a health risk. Some workers, including pregnant women, are concerned that their health could be affected by electromagnetic fields emitted from VDTs. The threat of X-ray exposure is low because of the very low emission levels. The radio frequency and extreme low-frequency electromagnetic fields are still an issue despite the low emission levels. To date, however, according to the U.S. Department of Labor there is no conclusive evidence that the low levels of radiation emitted from VDTs pose a health risk to computer users. Some workplace designs, however, have incorporated changes, such as increasing the distance between the operator and the terminal and between workstations to reduce potential exposures to electromagnetic fields.

For more information:

Prevent Blindness America
500 E. Remington Road
Schaumburg, IL 60173
(800) 331-2020
(847) 843-2020 (fax)
http://www.preventblindness.org

See also ERGONOMICS AND ERGONOMICS REGULATIONS; INDOOR ENVIRONMENT; REPETITIVE STRESS INJURIES.

U.S. Department of Labor, Occupational Safety and Health Administration, OSCH 3092, 1997 (Revised).

conductors (musical)   Those who conduct musical performances, usually from a podium, are at risk of falls from the podium. Many, particularly those in their later years, use a guardrail around part of the podium. The famed conductor Arturo Toscanini used such protection.

Some conductors also may encounter musculoskeletal problems. Inflammation of the shoulder and neck, back strains, and sprains are fairly common. Some conductors sit on high stools during rehearsals or for rest periods during long sessions. If conductors keep time with their heels they may develop plantar fasciitis.

The conductor's baton is also a hazard to the conductor, musicians, and audience, as it may fly out of the conductor's hand in a grandiose gesture. Injuries to the vocal cords also can occur, as conductors often shout instructions to their musicians over loud playing.

See also FOOT INJURIES; MUSCULOSKELETAL INJURIES; PERFORMING ARTS MEDICINE.

Sataloff, Robert Thayer, Alice G. Brandfonbrener, and Richard J. Lederman, eds. *Textbook of Performing Arts Medicine*. New York: Raven Press, 1991.

confined spaces   In assessing workplace hazards, attention should be given to any area where it might be possible for a person to become trapped, such as walk-in freezers, elevators or where there is a possibility of anything collapsing or overturning. Action must be taken to prevent this from happening. The first preventive step is having a system of work that averts the need for entry to a confined space.

Low-ceilinged areas such as cellars and mezzanines should be identified and appropriate precautions taken to prevent risk of injury to persons entering these areas. If there is no alternative to work in a confined space, it is essential that the persons carrying out such work be properly trained, competent, and physically capable of doing so. Lone working is not recommended in such situations. If this cannot be avoided, a means of communication must be available and safe system of work assured.

Where there is a possibility of oxygen deficiency or a contaminated atmosphere, suitable breathing apparatus must be used and at least one other person who is trained and equipped to carry out rescue procedures and sound an alarm for help in case of an accident must be present.

conflict resolution   The ability of people to come out of a workplace encounter respecting and liking each other. This is a win-win situation in which the stress of ANGER and confrontation are minimized, and those involved are able to be heard, to express their position and articulate their needs.

HOW TO USE CONFLICT RESOLUTION IN THE WORKPLACE

- Think before speaking.
- Say what you mean and mean what you say.
- Listen carefully to the other person.
- Do not put words in the other person's mouth.
- Stick to the problem at hand.
- Refrain from faultfinding.
- Apply the same rules to handling business and personal conflicts.

See also COMMUNICATION.

Kahn, Ada P., and Jan Fawcett. *Encyclopedia of Mental Health*. 2d ed. New York: Facts On File, Inc., 2001.

Consolidated Omnibus Budget Reconciliation Act   See COBRA.

construction   According to the National Institute of Safety and Health (NIOSH), more than 7 million people work in the construction industry, which is about 6 percent of the U.S. labor force. The majority of construction companies employ fewer than 20 workers each and require formal safety and health programs. NIOSH says that falls are the leading cause of fatal injury in the construction industry nationwide. Most construction falls are from buildings and other structures, scaffolds, and ladders.

"Struck-by" Accidents

The second highest cause of construction-related deaths is being struck by an object. Approximately 78 percent of struck-by fatalities involve heavy equipment such as trucks or cranes. According to the Occupational Safety and Health Administration (OSHA), the number of workers fatally struck by a vehicle was at a seven-year high in 1998.

Safety and health programs must consider the many ways struck-by accidents can occur. The hazards that cause the most struck-by injuries are vehicles, falling or flying objects, and constructing masonry walls.

If vehicle safety practices are not observed at a site, workers are at risk of being pinned between construction vehicles and walls, struck by swinging backhoes, crushed beneath overturned vehicles, or involved in other similar accidents. Work near public roadways carries a risk of being struck by trucks or cars.

Struck-by accidents also occur from falling or flying objects. A worker is at risk from falling objects when working beneath cranes or scaffolds or where overhead work is being performed. There is a danger from flying objects when power tools or activities like pushing, pulling, or prying may cause objects to become airborne. Injuries can range from minor abrasions to concussions, blindness, or death.

Using Cranes and Hoists

To protect themselves, workers should avoid working underneath loads being moved. Barricade haz-

ard areas and post warning signs. Inspect cranes and hoists to see that all components, such as wire ropes, lifting hooks, and chains are in good condition. The lifting capacity of the cranes or hoists should not be exceeded.

**TIPS: AVOID HAZARDS OF
STRUCK-BY ACCIDENTS DURING CONSTRUCTION**

- Wear hard hats.
- Wear seat belts that meet OSHA standards, except on equipment that is designed only for standup operation, or that has no rollover protective structure.
- Check vehicles before each shift to assure that all parts and accessories are in safe operating condition.
- Do not drive a vehicle in reverse gear with an obstructed rear view, unless it has an audible reverse alarm or another worker signals that it is safe.
- Drive vehicles or equipment only on roadways or grades that are safely constructed and maintained.
- Be sure that you and other personnel are in the clear before using dumping or lifting devices.

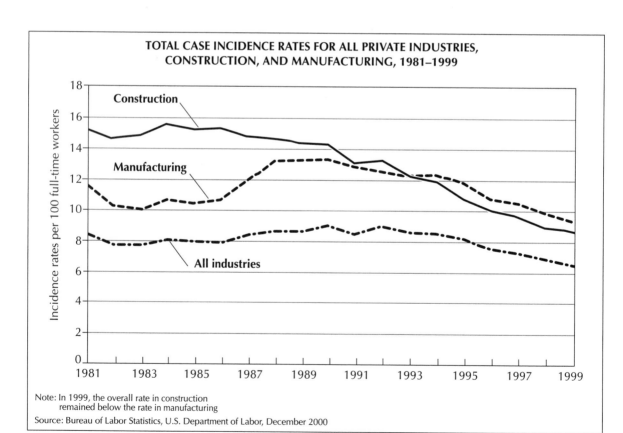

TOTAL CASE INCIDENCE RATES FOR ALL PRIVATE INDUSTRIES, CONSTRUCTION, AND MANUFACTURING, 1981–1999

Note: In 1999, the overall rate in construction remained below the rate in manufacturing

Source: Bureau of Labor Statistics, U.S. Department of Labor, December 2000

- Lower or block bulldozer and scraper blades, end-loader buckets, and dump bodies when not in use, and leave all controls in neutral position.
- Set parking brakes when vehicles and equipment are parked and chock the wheels if they are on an incline.
- All vehicles must have adequate braking systems and other safety devices.
- Haulage vehicles that are loaded by cranes, power shovels, loaders, and the like must have a cab shield or canopy that protects the driver from falling materials.
- Do not exceed a vehicle's rated load or lift capacity.
- Do not carry personnel unless there is a safe place to ride.
- Use traffic signs, barricades, or flaggers when construction takes place near public roadways.
- Be highly visible in all levels of light. Warning clothing, such as red or orange vests, is required. If worn for night work, vests must be of reflective material.
- Stack materials to prevent sliding, falling, or collapse.
- Use safety glasses, goggles, or face shields where machines or tools may cause flying particles.

Source: Occupational Safety and Health Administration

Trenching and Excavation

All excavations are hazardous because they are inherently unstable. According to the OSHA, cave-ins are perhaps the most feared trenching hazard. Other potentially fatal hazards include asphyxiation due to lack of oxygen in a CONFINED SPACE, inhalation of toxic fumes, and drowning. If protective systems or equipment are not used while working in trenches or excavations, there is a danger of suffocating, inhaling toxic materials, fire, drowning, or being crushed by a cave-in. Also, pre-job planning is vital to accident-free trenching. Safety cannot be improvised as work progresses. Here are some guidelines to be addressed by a competent person:

- Evaluate soil conditions.

- Construct protective systems in accordance with the standard.

- Contact utilities (gas, electric) to locate underground lines, plan for traffic control if necessary, and determine proximity to structures that could affect choice or protective system.

- Test for low oxygen, hazardous fumes, and toxic gases, especially when gasoline-engine-driven equipment is running, or the dirt has been contaminated by leaking lines or storage tanks. Insure adequate ventilation or respiration protection if necessary.

- Provide safe access into and out of the excavation.

- Provide appropriate protections if water accumulation is a problem.

- Inspect the site daily at the start of each shift, following a rainstorm, or after any other hazard-increasing event.

- Keep excavations open the minimum amount of time needed to complete operations.

OSHA requires that workers in trenches and excavations be protected, and that safety and health programs address the variety of hazards they face. Most trenching and excavation injuries occur due to lack of a protective system, failure to inspect trench and protective systems, unsafe spoil-pile placement, and unsafe access or egress.

Constructing Masonry Walls

Constructing concrete and masonry walls is particularly dangerous because of the tremendous loads that need to be supported. There are risks of major accidents, and even death, when jacks or lifting equipment are used to position slabs and walls, or when shoring is required until structures can support themselves. The following charts offer some tips from OSHA:

**AVOID HAZARDS:
CONSTRUCTION OF MASONRY WALLS**

- Do not place construction loads on a concrete structure until a qualified person indicates that it can support the load.
- Adequately shore or brace structures until permanent supporting elements are in place, or concrete has been tested to assure sufficient strength.
- Allow only those who are essential to and actively engaged in construction or lifting operations to enter the work area.
- Take measures to prevent unrolled wire mesh from recoiling, such as securing each end or turning the roll over.
- Do not load lifting devices beyond their capacity.
- Use automatic holding devices to support forms in case a lifting mechanism fails.

INDIRECT COSTS TO AN EMPLOYER OF AN INJURY ON A CONSTRUCTION SITE

- Lost productivity
- Job shutdown at the time of the injury
- The injured worker at the time of the injury
- The injured worker's reduced capacity upon return to work
- Coworkers at the time of the injury: watching and helping the injured
- Coworkers who are shorthanded following the injury
- Coworkers who must train a replacement worker
- Supervisor/management time hiring or retraining a temporary or permanent replacement worker
- Management time investigating and reporting on the incident
- Fines
- Production delays
- Damaged equipment and the costs of repairing or replacing it
- Lawsuits
- Damage to the company image and reduced company competitiveness
- Higher workers' compensation premiums
- Reduced worker morale

Source: Electronic Library of Construction, Occupational Safety and Health Administration

contact urticaria   See DERMATITIS.

control   Having a feeling of control over one's life means directing the outcomes of everyday events. While work and other aspects of life are going well, most people do not consciously think about their level of control. However, when that sense of control is threatened, they become aware and this loss of control leads to STRESS, ANGER, and FRUSTRATION.

Some people are stressed in their jobs because they work hard but have no control over their work environment, which may be displeasing, or the pace of the work, which may be unpredictable. Other people do not recognize their own options for decisions and feel trapped by invisible forces. An example of this type of stress is experienced by one who always tries to please others in an effort to gain validation and self-esteem.

Issues of personal control involve situations in which people who could help themselves do not do so. They may have lost their motivation because of previous experiences with failure or may be experiencing what researchers call "learned helplessness." They feel that whatever they do will not make any difference. An example is a person in an organization who is given little opportunity to initiate change or who feels that things are being done to or for him or her. They learn not to even try, but continue to feel anger, frustration, and hostility, which may lead to physical symptoms.

See also BIOFEEDBACK; DECISION-MAKING; HOSTILITY; MENTAL HEALTH; RELAXATION.

cooks   People who prepare food in restaurants and other food service establishments usually withstand the pressure and STRESS of working in close quarters, standing for hours at a time, lifting heavy pots and kettles, and working near hot ovens and grills. Job hazards include SLIPS, TRIPS, AND FALLS, cuts, and burns, but injuries are seldom serious. Work hours for chefs, cooks, and other kitchen workers may include early mornings, late evenings, holidays, and weekends, which may take a toll on a worker's personal life.

See also CATERING AND FOOD SERVICE.

coping   The psychological as well as practical solutions that people must find for extremely distressing as well as everyday situations in the workplace. Examples of these situations are job change, downsizing, layoffs, dealing with a difficult superior, having to terminate an employee, or random nuisances. Different individuals develop different ways of coping and learn to adapt their responses to reduce their level of stress.

Authors Arthur Stone and Laura Porter, writing in *Mind/Body Medicine* (March 1995), defined *coping* as "constantly changing cognitive and behavioral efforts to manage specific external and/or internal demands that are appraised as taxing or exceeding the resources of the person."

To some, *coping* means getting on with life and letting things happen as they may. To others, it is consciously using the skills they have learned in the past when facing problems. Coping can mean anticipating situations, or it can mean meeting problems head on. For example, managers who are able to handle employees in everyday situations may become nervous and jittery just anticipating giving a speech to a group. In a serious medical crisis, some people cannot cope with their own illness but manage to muster strength when they need to provide support for a staff member.

Individuals can learn new coping skills from psychotherapists as well as those who practice alternative or complementary therapies such as meditation and RELAXATION training. Relaxation and deep breathing techniques can help overcome the stress involved in a difficult situation.

Better Coping for
Better Health and Productivity

Hans Selye (1907–82), an Austrian-born Canadian endocrinologist and psychologist, in his landmark book *The Stress of Life* (1956) described the GENERAL ADAPTATION SYNDROME. The secret of health, he said, was in successful adjustment to everchanging conditions.

Research studies have shown that people who cope well with life's stresses are healthier than those who have maladaptive coping mechanisms. In his book *Adaptation to Life,* George Valliant, a Harvard psychologist, summarized some insights about relationships between good coping skills and health. He found that individuals who typically handle the trials and pressures of life in an immature way also tend to become ill four times as often as those who cope well.

Stone and Porter reported that coping efforts may have direct effects on symptom perception and may have indirect effects on physiological changes and disease processes, as well as mood changes, compliance with physician's instructions, and physician-patient communication.

See also COMPLEMENTARY THERAPIES; BEHAVIOR THERAPY; COMMUNICATION; EXERCISE; HARDINESS; MEDITATION.

Kahn, Ada P. *Stress A–Z: A Sourcebook for Coping with Everyday Challenges.* New York: Facts On File, Inc., 1998.
Selye, Hans. *The Stress of Life.* New York: McGraw-Hill, 1956.
———. *Stress without Distress.* Philadelphia: J. B. Lippincott Company, 1974.
Stone, Arthur A., and Laura S. Porter. "Psychological Coping: Its Importance for Treating Medical Problems," *Mind/Body Medicine* 1, no. 1 (March 1995).

copper   See GASTROINTESTINAL OR LIVER TOXICITY.

corporate buyout   The purchase of a controlling interest in a company by either the employees or another company. The term originated in the mid-1970s when there was a marked increase in company takeovers and tender offers. When corporate buyouts occur, stresses and health issues often result for all employees concerned during reorganization.

See also DOWNSIZING, LAYOFFS; STRESS.

cortisol   See DEPRESSION.

cotton dust and textile industry   BYSSINOSIS, a disabling lung disease commonly known as brown lung disease, is caused by cotton dust exposure. In 1978 approximately 12,000 textile workers suffered from brown lung disease. At the end of the 1990s, that number was reduced to approximately 700. The Occupational Safety and Health Administration (OSHA) attributes that reduction to the Cotton Dust Standard. OSHA's review of the standard in 2000 showed that it not only helps save lives and reduce illness, but is also cost effective for industry. The purpose of the Cotton Dust Standard is to greatly reduce the significant risk of byssinosis. Before adoption of the standard, more than 50,000 cotton textile workers suffered from the disease at any one time.

The Cotton Dust Standard sets maximum permissible exposure limits (PELs) for cotton dust that vary by operation. It includes requirements for monitoring, medical surveillance, work practices and other requirements. The major impact of the Cotton Dust Standard is on certain firms in the cotton-using sectors of the textile industry. These are firms that open and process raw cotton, spin that cotton into cotton and cotton-blend yard and thread, and turn that yarn and thread into cotton and cotton-blend fabrics. It is estimated that there are approximately 466 cotton-using establishments in these textile sectors. It is also estimated that between 70,000 and 105,000 employees work in these establishments. Certain sections of the industry, such as knitting, are partially or completely exempt from the standard because those sections do not present significant risk of byssinosis.

Washing cotton according to certain protocols reduces the bioactivity of cotton and its ability to cause byssinosis. Not all washing processes reduce the bioactivity, and cotton washed by certain processes cannot be spun and woven into quality textiles. The industry, government, union Task Force for Byssinosis Prevention sponsors research to develop techniques that reduce bioactivity and create processable cotton.

The Cotton Dust Standard does not conflict with other federal or state rules. Most of the cotton textile industry is located in states with their own state OSHAs. Those states have adopted cotton dust standards that are virtually identical to the federal standard (they must adopt standards that are at least as effective as the federal standard), and those states enforce their state standards.

See also ASTHMA; LUNG DISEASES, OCCUPATIONAL.

counseling   The term *counseling* includes many varied professional services available to individuals seeking help in some area of their life, including job-related concerns. These services may range from those of a trained social worker to a psychiatrist. They may be provided through EMPLOYEE ASSISTANCE PROGRAMS, in local hospitals, or in community centers.

To seek counseling, talk to your human resource department, call a local hospital, or look in the yellow pages of the telephone directory under "psychologists" or "psychiatrists." Some listings have the heading "counselors." There are also many community self-help and support groups in which participants share experiences. For participants in these groups, sharing means they are not alone with their problems, and they learn from one another to solve problems.

Before beginning therapy with any counselor, ask what his or her credentials are and whether they are certified by any state agency or professional board. As with any other professional, some may meet an individual's needs better than others. Individuals should not be afraid to change counselors if needs are not being met.

See also BEHAVIOR THERAPY; MENTAL HEALTH; PSYCHOTHERAPIES; SELF-HELP GROUPS; SUPPORT GROUPS.

covert modeling   Imagining or observing another person performing a behavior or action and then imagining the particular consequences. For example, an employee who feels extremely anxious about speaking at a sales meeting can imagine another person getting up on the stage, delivering a talk, answering questions, and feeling successful about the situation. The next step in the concept is when the individual imagines himself or herself doing the same thing at a reduced stress level.

See also BEHAVIOR THERAPY; COVERT REHEARSAL; MENTAL HEALTH; PSYCHOTHERAPIES.

covert rehearsal   An imagery technique in which an individual in therapy is asked to imagine himself or herself effectively doing a stressful task, such as going for a job interview. The individual may repeat the visualization many times, and consider different alternatives. This procedure often follows COVERT MODELING. The goal of the technique is to help the individual do the task at a reduced level of stress.

See also BEHAVIOR THERAPY; COVERT REINFORCEMENT; MENTAL HEALTH; PSYCHOTHERAPIES.

covert reinforcement   A technique used in psychotherapy in which the individual imagines two responses to an action or situation, one stressful and another less stressful. For example, the person who first imagines seeing another give a public speech (covert modeling) and then practices covert rehearsal (imagining giving the speech), now imagines that the speech has been given, and that there was a favorable audience response without an undue level of stress.

See also BEHAVIOR THERAPY; COUNSELING; COVERT MODELING; COVERT REHEARSAL; MENTAL HEALTH; PSYCHOTHERAPIES.

coworkers   Relationships at work can contribute to stress on the job. Colleagues who do not pull their own weight and complain constantly can make work life miserable. Backstabbers, gossips, and tattletales damage reputations and innocent people's careers.

DEALING EFFECTIVELY
WITH TROUBLESOME COWORKERS

- Tell them, in a nonconfrontational manner, how their actions affect your work.
- Avoid providing the complainer with an audience and the bully with a target.
- Consider talking to your supervisor about the problem, but be prepared for possible negative results.
- Remember that you cannot change someone else's behavior but you can change how you react to that behavior.

One of the stresses unemployed workers face is lack of companionship. The day-to-day interactions with coworkers are gone and the unemployed worker may become withdrawn, spending less and less time with peers. On the other side of the coin are the coworkers who are left in the corporation after downsizing or layoffs have occurred. Research has shown that their productivity is reduced, they develop poor work attitudes, and they often seek new positions. Factors influencing these reactions include: when the layoff is seen as unnecessary, when workers receive information about termination in a degrading or unfair way, when criteria used to select workers in a lay-off is perceived as politically motivated or biased in any way, and when termination benefits and compensation are not considered adequate.

See also CORPORATE BUYOUT; DOWNSIZING; LAY-OFFS; STRESS.

Kahn, Ada P. *Stress A–Z: A Sourcebook for Coping with Everyday Challenges.* New York: Facts On File, Inc., 1998.

crane, derrick, and hoist safety   See CONSTRUCTION.

creativity   Unusual association of ideas or words and ingenious methods of problem solving on the job or in personal life. It may involve using everyday objects or processes in original ways or ways that involve using an imaginative skill to bring about new thoughts and ideas. Some creative ideas are ahead of their time and may never be appreciated or are not appreciated until after their creator's death. On the other hand, there are those who overestimate their creativity and feel stress from thinking they are undervalued and underappreciated.

Creativity and the Workplace

While creativity is strongly associated with the arts, it is equally important in fields such as science, business, or manufacturing. People who try to be creative and cannot, feel stressed. This is particularly true of people who were hired because of their creativity. Fortunately, in corporations today, a free and voluminous flow of ideas is thought to be an important part of the creative process even though many of the ideas may not be truly creative. Techniques such as BRAINSTORMING and other group strategies, encourage the flow of ideas. These techniques bring in new people who have never been a part of the creative process and encourage fresh viewpoints.

The Creative Process

Biographers and researchers of creative individuals have identified certain stages in the creative process. Often the scientist or artist identifies an area of work or project but after approaching it feels dissatisfied and returns to less creative endeavors. Suddenly during this incubation period, a solution or artistic concept emerges. It then must be elaborated or tested.

Creativity has been found to correlate with certain personality and intellectual characteristics. Although intelligence and creativity are thought to be separate mental gifts (and not all intelligent people are creative), intelligence does seem to be necessary for creativity. Creative people have been found to be leaders and independent thinkers. They are self-assured, unconventional, and have a wide range of interests. Since they are frequently involved in their own thoughts and inner life, they tend to be introverted and uninterested in social life or group activities. Passion for their field of work and a sense that what they do will eventually be recognized and make a difference are also qualities that support creativity.

Mental health professionals have been interested in creativity for years. For example, J. P. Guilford (1897–1987), who explored this area in the 1960s, described two areas of thinking: convergent or narrow, focused thinking, and divergent thinking, which allows the individual to let the mind roam and explore a broad spectrum of ideas. Guilford felt that divergent thinking was most creatively productive. Under his direction, the Torrance Tests of Creative Thinking were developed at the University of Southern California.

Stimulation to increase creativity also is of interest to researchers. It has been found that people's creativity may increase or decrease according to their environment and work habits. For example, certain people can be more or less productive at work depending on the atmosphere, the time of day, and even the clothing they wear.

See also BRAINSTORMING; WRITER'S BLOCK.

Kahn, Ada P. *Stress A–Z: The Sourcebook for Coping with Everyday Challenges.* New York: Facts On File, Inc., 1998.

Weisberg, Robert. *Creativity, Genius and Other Myths.* New York: W. H. Freeman and Company, 1986.

Wilmer, Harry A. *Creativity: Paradoxes and Reflections.* Wilmette, Ill.: Chiron Publications, 1991.

creosote   See BENZO[B]FLUORANTHENE; SKIN and SENSE ORGAN TOXICITY.

cresol   A chemical that causes many health hazards and presents a fire and explosion hazard to workers, particularly if there are spills or releases. It is used as a SOLVENT, fumigant, or disinfectant and in the synthesis of phenolic resins. It is toxic by all routes, including inhalation, ingestion, and absorption by the skin. Effects from exposure may include serious burns to the skin and eyes (sometimes causing blindness), weakness, HEADACHE, dizziness, unconsciousness, and death from cardiac or pulmonary failure, or damage to the kidney or liver.

Airborne levels of cresol should be controlled through the use of local exhaust ventilation. In emergencies, a self-contained breathing apparatus should be worn. Skin exposure presents the most common hazard and should be protected against by wearing a face shield, rubber gloves and boots, and chemical protective clothing that is specifically recommended by the cresol shipper or producer.

While cresol does not ignite easily, it can burn, emitting highly toxic fumes. Also, containers may explode in the heat of a fire. Cresol may be shipped via air, rail, road, or water in containers bearing the label "poison." Small spills of cresol may be taken up with sand or other noncombustible absorbent and placed in containers for later disposal.

See also CHEMICAL SPILLS; CHEMICAL TOXICITY; FIRE SAFETY/FIRE PROTECTION; HAND PROTECTION; KIDNEY TOXICITY; PERSONAL PROTECTIVE EQUIPMENT.

crowding   A large mass of people or animals. In Hans Selye's landmark book, *The Stress of Life* (1956), he suggested that in humans, crowding may make men more competitive, somewhat more severe, and like each other less, whereas women tend to be more cooperative and lenient and like each other more. Crowding in the workplace takes the form of cubicles and many people in one large room.

Selye speculated that crowding in itself does not produce psychological or physical symptoms of stress and anxiety. In fact, under certain conditions, interpersonal contact is supportive, as long as the people know they have the space to get away from each other when they want to. His studies, however, did not reflect later 20th-century anxieties from heavy traffic, high-rise buildings, air pollution, noise, and so on, associated with contemporary urban life.

See also AUTONOMY; CONTROL; GENERAL ADAPTATION SYNDROME; MENTAL HEALTH; PERSONAL SPACE; SELYE, HANS; STRESS.

Kahn, Ada P. *Stress A–Z: The Sourcebook for Facing Everyday Challenges.* New York: Facts On File, Inc., 2000.

crisis   A turning point for better or worse in an emotionally significant event or radical change in a person's life. The change may be loss of a job or relocation, loss of a loved one, or being the victim of a crime. The physical and mental stress involved in such a situation may result from a combination of the individual's perception of an event as well as his or her ability or inability to cope with it. Some people cope with a crisis better than others.

Crisis intervention is often necessary to provide immediate help, advice, or therapy for employees or workers with acute psychological or medical problems. Crisis intervention is often provided at the workplace by trained counselors after a disaster such as a shooting or bombing.

The goal of crisis intervention is to restore the individual's equilibrium to the same level of functioning as before the crisis, or to improve it. Such help may last from a few days to a few weeks. A wide variety of therapists and self-help groups provide crisis intervention. Therapy may include talking to the individual and appropriate family members, or short-term use of appropriate prescription drugs. Crisis intervention is not a substitute for longer-term therapy. In crisis intervention the individual may learn to immediately modify certain environmental factors as well as interpersonal aspects of the situation causing the crisis. There is emphasis on reducing anxiety, promoting self-reliance, and focusing on the here-and-now. In many cases of crisis intervention, longer-term therapy is recommended after the individual has regained some degree of composure and coping skills.

Often crisis intervention centers for suicide prevention utilize telephone counseling. In some cases, a rape victim's first step toward seeking professional assistance is a call to a rape crisis hot line. In a case of a mass shooting in a restaurant or school, or a bombing of a public building, crisis intervention services are provided for witnesses. In many cases, crisis intervention may prevent the onset or ameliorate POST-TRAUMATIC STRESS DISORDER (PTSD).

See also COUNSELING; EMPLOYEE ASSISTANCE PROGRAMS.

crisis intervention   See CRISIS.

criticism   Comments directed to another regarding behavior, appearance, performance, quality of work, or other personal characteristics. Criticism may be favorable, but usually is regarded as the opposite of praise.

Receiving criticism in the workplace may lower one's SELF-ESTEEM and even make one reluctant to make changes. For example, when an employee makes suggestions that are never followed, he or she may become reluctant to suggest innovations.

Criticism usually is not pleasant for the one being criticized and is often unpleasant for the critic. In work situations, some supervisors find it difficult to offer criticism to employees. Some supervisors avoid direct criticism, which may actually make problems worse. Putting criticism in writing is a way to avoid direct confrontation, but may seem harsher than intended and gives the employee no immediate opportunity to respond. Writing a memo to a group criticizing acts that only a few have committed is another way of avoiding confrontation, but usually offends the innocent and makes the guilty feel that what they are doing is a common practice. Employers may also have a tendency to mix praise and blame in such a way that the employee takes neither seriously.

Some supervisors may have a tendency to scrutinize the employee too closely and make general comments about his or her behavior in addition to what is needed to resolve the situation. Any criticism of an employee that fails to get to the heart of the problem and to deal with elements of the problem that may recur is counterproductive. A supervisor should expect that criticism of an employee should be a learning experience for the supervisor as well.

Kahn, Ada P. *Stress A–Z: A Sourcebook for Facing Everyday Challenges*. New York: Facts On File, Inc., 1998.

cryosurgery   See DENTISTRY.

cultural difference (in overwork)   See *KAROSHI*.

cumulative trauma disorders   See CARPAL TUNNEL SYNDROME; ERGONOMICS; REPETITIVE STRESS DISORDER.

Dalton's law See COMMERCIAL DIVING.

dancers (professional) A wide range of individuals call themselves dancers, among them professional ballet, modern, jazz, tap and ethnic dancers. All encounter similar injuries and health concerns. Because of extreme physical demands, most dancers are chronically fatigued and often display highly irregular eating and sleeping patterns. According to authors Sataloff, Brandfondbrener, and Lederman, constant impact and unnatural positions, especially of the lower extremities, can lead to sprains, fractures, tendinitis, arthritis, ligament and muscle injuries, nerve injuries as well as other problems. Dance positions lead to foot and ankle injuries. In many cases, injuries can be prevented by proper training and equipment, especially appropriate shoes and dancing surfaces.

Many young dancers may develop eating disorders such as anorexia in an effort to remain thin. Some young women have delayed menarche (onset of menstrual periods) and some suffer the consequences of later infertility problems.

The dancer's career is often short and many are forced into retirement by age 35 or 40 due to declining physical abilities. However, many performers turn to coaching and teaching to continue their careers in the field. Performance anxiety and stress are frequent symptoms among dancers, as well as other performing artists.

See also PERFORMANCE ANXIETY; PERFORMING ARTS MEDICINE; STRESS.

Sataloff, Robert Thayer, Alice G. Brandfondbrener, and Richard J. Lederman, eds. *Textbook of Performing Arts Medicine.* New York: Raven Press, 1991.

day care A system of caring for children or other dependents in other people's homes, in churches, and other community centers while parents work. Changes in the economy, employment, and family patterns have made day care an important issue for many people. Some employers have set up day care centers for their employees' young children.

Today, when both parents need or want to work, they are faced with the dilemma of seeking day care. Some parents, traditionally the mother, feel some degree of guilt about seeking day care for their children. However, as a practical matter, it has become more difficult to support a family on one income. Additionally, some wives and mothers who are not forced to work for financial reasons have been encouraged by contemporary media to believe the position of housewife and mother is not rewarding. Still others, faced with the specter of a high divorce rate, may want to keep up their skills and have their own employment benefits "just in case." For the single working parent with small children, some type of child care is a necessity.

Many children whose parents work are cared for by a relative or sitter in their own home; however, the day care alternative does offer certain benefits. In day care children learn to socialize with their peers before entering school. Centers may offer educational programs, toys, and equipment. Legitimate day care centers are licensed and run by professionals.

Social mobility has also increased the need for some type of daytime child care. At one time, stay-at-home mothers depended on grandmothers when they needed child care. Now grandmothers may be hundreds of miles away and may be working themselves.

To meet the needs of sick children, some day care centers have separate areas. Also, some day care centers specifically for sick children have been set up either independently or in pediatric wards of hospitals.

Among some employers, day care has become a corporate responsibility. A day care center in the mother's or father's place of employment solves transportation problems and allows the parent to visit with the child during the day. The Stride Rite Corporation in Cambridge, Massachusetts, is an example of a company that started a program which combines both care for small children and elderly dependents of employees in the same facility.

Studies of the effect of day care on children have not shown that children suffer any real difficulties from participation in day care and that, in some cases, children from deprived backgrounds benefit from day care. However, putting children in the hands of caregivers may lessen the extent to which parents can influence their child with their own values and standards.

Day Care for Elderly

A trend in day care has been the establishment of facilities for care of elderly persons whose condition does not necessitate institutional care, but who need assistance that their family cannot provide during the day. Caregiving for the elderly usually falls upon the woman in the family. Women with high-level executive and professional jobs may suffer a loss of income and advancement if they take time off frequently to care for the elderly parent. Day care for the elder permits them to move forward in their careers without undue absenteeism.

Although many midlife children experience guilt about placing an elderly parent in day care, they understand that there are benefits for the older individual. For example, day care for the older person offers socialization, learning opportunities, and encouragement of better nutritional patterns for the midday meal.

See also CAREGIVERS; WORKING MOTHERS.

Edmundson, Brad. "Where's the Day Care?" *American Demographics* (July 1990): 17–19.
Gallo, Nick. "Too Sick for School?" *Better Homes and Gardens,* September 1990, pp. 62–65.

Kahn, Ada P. *Stress A–Z: A Sourcebook for Facing Everyday Challenges.* New York: Facts On File, Inc., 1998.
Kantrowitz, Barbara. "Day Care Bridging the Generation Gap." *Newsweek,* July 16, 1990, p. 52.

deadlines   A date or time at which something must be done. Deadlines are common in many workplaces, such as publication offices and manufacturing plants. Deadlines may be for the entire workforce, such as in a manufacturing plant, or for one individual, such as for a writer.

Deadlines become a health issue because once people have fallen behind, it is difficult to catch up. They find that rushing tends to add to the stress and decrease effectiveness. Ineffectiveness leads to FRUSTRATION. Some people become moody and blame themselves or others for the deadline failure.

The key to avoiding the stress produced by deadlines is setting realistic time schedules, enlisting the help needed when deadlines go awry, and negotiating new deadlines when it appears that for one reason or another, deadlines are going to be missed. For individuals to keep a positive outlook, they should break deadlines down to a series of small steps. As each step is completed, they will feel a sense of success, and that success, in turn, will keep them motivated toward their final goal.

See also AUTONOMY; CONTROL.

deaths in the workplace   Workplace deaths in the United States have dropped by nearly half since 1980, according to a Centers for Disease Control (CDC) report in April 2001. The drop was attributed to new technology, stricter safety regulations, and a shift in the economy toward service-industry jobs that may be safer than manufacturing jobs.

According to the report, 5,285 workers died from on-the-job-injuries in 1997, the latest year for which figures are available. That is a rate of 4.1 deaths per 100,000 workers, down 45 percent from 1980, when it was 7.4.

Car crashes have accounted for one in four on-the-job-deaths since 1980. Homicides accounted for 14 percent and machinery accidents 13 percent. Mining appeared to be the most dangerous sector, with 30 deaths per 100,000 workers over the two decades. Agriculture and forestry followed at 19 per 100,000. Men accounted for 93 percent of all workplace deaths since 1980.

The government also issued a warning about baling machines and compactors, which were tied to 34 work-related deaths from 1992 to 1998.

In a separate report, the CDC said that U.S. workers were treated in emergency rooms for 3.6 million work-related injuries in 1998. Hands and fingers were most commonly treated.

See also CENSUS OF FATAL OCCUPATIONAL INJURIES (CFOI); FATAL INJURIES; MACHINE ACCIDENTS; NONFATAL OCCUPATIONAL ILLNESS; WOMEN AND JOB-RELATED INJURIES AND DEATHS.

decision making   Some decisions in the workplace are made easily, while others are arrived at after considerable struggle. Decision making is stressful because it involves addressing alternatives, options, and possibilities for reassessment at a later time. Decision making may involve job change, promotion, or relocation.

Information used in making decisions is extremely important. How people perceive a situation, past experiences with like situations, as well as their own background and culture, play a large part in the decision making process. Problems may occur when complete information is not gathered or not carefully analyzed in terms of where it has come from.

Decisions outside of the workplace can affect work performance. For example, important decisions may focus on health and well-being or large amounts of money. Decisions require risk-taking. Because many people are uncomfortable taking risks, doing so may generate stress and in turn, that stress can interfere with making the best decisions.

See also COPING; GENERAL ADAPTATION SYNDROME.

decompression sickness   See COMMERCIAL DIVING.

defense mechanisms   Part of an unconscious mental process that individuals use to reach compromise solutions with stressful problems. Individuals have a wide variety of defense mechanisms ranging from projection, which is blaming someone else for one's situation, to rationalization, which is justifying questionable behavior by defending its propriety. Denial is another defense mechanism. The presence of pathological denial (for example, of a drinking problem) is often seen in people with alcoholism or substance abuse problems. Defense mechanisms are often used by employees when facing confrontations with employees or subordinates. While defense mechanisms can be helpful in coping with daily situations at the workplace, excessive use of such devices and dependence on them can lead to high levels of stress for the individual.

See also COPING; GENERAL ADAPTATION SYNDROME; HUMOR; STRESS.

demolition   Work that involves many of the hazards associated with CONSTRUCTION. However, demolition incurs additional hazards due to unknown factors such as deviations from the design of the structure introduced during construction, approved or unapproved modifications that altered the original design, material hidden within structural members, and unknown strength or weaknesses of construction materials. Workers must be aware of these types of hazards and the safety precautions to take to control the hazards.

See also ASBESTOS; COLD ENVIRONMENTS; CONFINED SPACES; CONSTRUCTION; DUST AND DEBRIS; FIRE SAFETY/FIRE PROTECTION; HOT ENVIRONMENTS; NOISE; PERSONAL PROTECTIVE EQUIPMENT; SCAFFOLDING, WELDING.

Occupational Safety and Health Administration

dental problems (performing artists)   See PERFORMING ARTS MEDICINE.

dentistry   Professionals who work with teeth and mouth disorders and restorations. They are at risk for exposure to numerous biological, chemical, environmental, physical, and psychological workplace hazards. These hazards include but are not limited to bloodborne pathogens, pharmaceuticals and other chemical agents, ergonomic hazards, noise, vibration, and workplace violence.

Dentists and dental employees are exposed to waste anesthetic gases and vapors that leak out and into the surrounding room during dental procedures. The waste anesthetic gases and vapors of concern are nitrous oxide and halogenated agents (vapors) such as halothane, enflurane, methoxyflurane, trichloroethylene, and CHLOROFORM. Some potential effects of exposure to waste anesthetic gases are nausea, dizziness, headaches, fatigue, and irritability, as well as sterility, miscarriages, birth defects, cancer, and liver and kidney disease among dental staff and/or their spouses (in the case of miscarriages and birth defects). Employers and employees should be aware of the potential effects of waste anesthetic gases and be advised to take appropriate precautions.

Chronic beryllium disease is a serious and even fatal lung disease that can occur in dental laboratory technicians as they work with dental alloys that contain beryllium.

See also BERYLLIUM; BLOODBORNE PATHOGENS; CHEMICAL TOXICITY; ERGONOMICS AND ERGONOMICS REGULATIONS; HEALTH CARE WORKERS; NEEDLESTICK INJURIES AND PREVENTION; VIOLENCE.

Occupational Safety and Health Administration

depression   A mood or affective disorder characterized by sadness, hopelessness, despair, personal devaluation, and helplessness. (An affective disorder refers to a condition involving the external expression of an internal state [mood or emotion]). Some depressions are marked by anxiety, withdrawal from others, loss of sleep or excessive need for sleep, constant fatigue, loss of appetite or compulsive eating, loss of sexual desire, lethargy or agitation, and an inability to concentrate and make decisions, and possibly exaggerated guilt feelings or thoughts. When depression is observed in an employee, a referral is often made to an EMPLOYEE ASSISTANCE PROGRAM.

The term *depression* applies to a condition of varying severity. It can be a temporary mood fluctuation, a symptom associated with a number of mental and physical disorders, or a clinical syndrome such as major depression or dysthymic disorder encompassing many symptoms. When psychological, physical, or interpersonal functioning is affected for more than two weeks because of depression, it can be considered a mental health problem. Depression is the most common and most treatable of all mental health problems. On the other hand, it has been shown to be second only to

severe heart disease in days of work lost, and in its more severe forms, carries a 15 percent lifetime risk of suicide.

Depression can appear at any age, although major depressive episodes peak at age 55 to 70 in men and 20 to 45 in women. Recent studies have shown a trend for earlier onset of depression, especially in females. About 20 percent of major depressions last two years or more, with an average duration of eight months. About half of those experiencing a major depression will have a recurrence within two years.

Some sufferers of depression have episodes that are separated by several years, and others suffer clusters of episodes over a short time span. Between episodes, such individuals function normally. However, 20 to 35 percent of sufferers have chronic depression that prevents them from responsibly holding a job and functioning normally.

Estimates are that 2 to 3 percent of men and 4 to 9 percent of women suffer a major depression at any given time in the United States. The lifetime risk may be as high as 10 percent for men and 25 percent for women. About 66 percent of those who suffer from depression fail to recognize the illness and do not get treatment for it.

Clinical depression refers to a depression that lasts for more than a few weeks or includes symptoms that interfere with job performance and the ability to handle everyday decisions and routine situations. Clinical depression is a term that overlaps with the terms *major depression, dysthymia, unipolar depression,* and *endogenous depression.*

Seasonal mood disorder (seasonal affective disorder) is a condition marked by mood symptoms related to changes of season, with depression occurring most frequently during winter months and improvement in the spring. Many sufferers experience periods of increased energy, productivity, and even euphoria in the spring and summer months. This type of depression often responds well to light therapy, or phototherapy.

Melancholia is a severe form of depression that may originate without any precipitating factors. This is in contrast to a reactive, or exogenous depression which occurs after some major life-changing event such as loss of a job or divorce.

Symptoms

Depressed individuals usually have pervasive feelings of sadness, hopelessness, helplessness, and irritability. Often they withdraw from human contact but do not admit to symptoms. They may also experience noticeable change of appetite, either significant weight loss without dieting or weight gain; change in sleeping patterns, such as fitful sleep, inability to fall asleep, or sleeping too much; loss of interest in activities formerly enjoyed; feelings of worthlessness; fatigue; inability to concentrate; feelings of inappropriate guilt; indecisiveness; recurring thoughts of death or suicide or even attempting suicide. Persistence by family, friends and coworkers is essential, because in many cases, depression is the illness that underlies suicide.

SIGNS AND SYMPTOMS OF DEPRESSION IN EMPLOYEES

Psychological
- Loss of interest
- Unexplained anxiety
- Inappropriate feelings of guilt
- Loss of self-esteem
- Worthlessness
- Hopelessness
- Thoughts of death and suicide
- Tearfulness, irritability, brooding

Physical
- Headache, vague aches and pains
- Changes in appetite and changes in weight
- Sleep disturbances
- Loss of energy
- Psychomotor agitation or retardation
- Loss of libido
- Gastrointestinal disturbances

Intellectual
- Slowed thinking
- Indecisiveness
- Poor concentration
- Impaired memory

Causes

There is no single cause of depression. It is related to many factors, including a family history of depression, psychosocial stressors, diseases, alcohol, drugs, gender, and age. Depression occurs in mood disorders, anxiety disorders, psychotic disorders, adjustment disorders, and psychoactive substance use disorders, including alcoholism. Individuals who have personality disorders, especially obsessive-compulsive, dependent, avoidant, and borderline personality disorders, are susceptible to depression.

Psychosocial factors An individual's lack of confidence in his or her interpersonal skills and personality traits such as overdependency on others as a source of support and self-esteem, perfectionism and unrealistic expectations work together with psychosocial stressors to cause depression. Such psychosocial events include death of a spouse, loss of a job, and for some, urban living.

Social learning theory Some psychologists say that stress disrupts involvement with others, resulting in a reduction in degree and quality of positive reinforcement. This leads to more negative self-evaluation and a poor outlook for the future. Depressed people view themselves and their world negatively, which leads to a further sense of low self-worth, feelings of rejection, alienation, dependency, helplessness, and hopelessness.

Cognitive theory Often unrecognized negative attitudes toward oneself, the future, and the world can result in feelings of failure, helplessness, and depression. These distorted attitudes may activate a prolonged and deepening depressive state, especially under stress. Learning what they are, understanding their negative distortion and challenging those hopeless and negative thoughts in real life can reverse both depression and a tendency for future depression.

Psychoanalytic theory A psychoanalytical position regarding depression is that a loss, or a real or perceived withdrawal of affection in childhood, may be a predeterminant for depression in later life. Sigmund Freud and Karl Abraham mentioned the role of ambivalence toward the lost love object, identification with the lost object and subsequent anger turned inward.

Later theories suggested an unrealistic expectation of self and others and loss of self-esteem as essential components leading to depression. Depression that arises following a loss may result from failure to work through the loss.

Interpersonal theory This theory emphasizes the importance of social connections for effective functioning. An individual develops adaptive responses to the psychosocial environment at an early age. When early attachment bonds are disrupted or impaired, the individual may be vulnerable later on to more interpersonal and social problems that lead to depression.

Genetic factors   Some individuals may be biologically predisposed to develop depression, based on genetic factors that researchers do not yet fully understand. There are genetic markers which indicate susceptibility to manic-depressive illness, and considerable research has been underway since the 1970s toward understanding the biochemical reactions controlled by these genes.

There is considerable evidence that depression runs in families. For example, if one identical twin suffers from depression or manic-depression, the other twin has a 70 percent chance of also having the illness. Research studies looking at the rate of depression among adopted children supported this finding. Depressive illnesses among children's adoptive families had little effect on their risk for the disorder; however, among adopted children whose biological relatives suffered depression, the disorder is three times more common than the norm. Among more severe depressives, family history is more often a significant factor.

Neurotransmitter theory   Recent research indicates that people suffering from depression have imbalances of neurotransmitters, natural biochemicals that enable brain cells to communicate with one another. Three biochemicals that often are out of balance in depressed people are serotonin, norepinephrine, and dopamine. An imbalance of serotonin may cause the ANXIETY, sleep problems, and irritability that many depressed people experience. An inadequate supply of norepinephrine, which regulates alertness and arousal, may contribute to fatigue and lack of motivation. Dopamine imbalances may relate to a loss of sexual interest and an inability to experience pleasure. Several neurotransmitter imbalances may be involved, and research is finding other neurotransmitters that may be important in clinical depression.

Role of cortisol   Another body chemical that may be out of balance in depressed people is cortisol, a hormone produced by the body in response to extreme cold, fear, or anger. In most people, cortisol levels in the blood peak in the morning, then decreases later in the day. In depressed people, however, cortisol peaks early in the morning and does not level off or decrease in the afternoon or evening. Recent research in animals suggests that abnormal elevations of cortisol sustained over three months may cause changes in brain structure.

Environmental influences   Environment plays an important role, although researchers view depression as the result of interaction of environmental as well as biologic factors. Historically, depression has been viewed as either internally caused (endogenous depression) or related to environmental events (exogenous or reactional influences). Major changes in the individual's environment (such as a move or job change) or any major loss (such as a divorce or death of a loved one) can bring on depression. Feeling depressed in response to these changes is normal, but if it becomes a severe long-term condition (lasting more than one month) and interferes with effective functioning, treatment can be helpful.

Some environmental factors relating to depression include being unemployed, elderly and alone, poor, single, and a working mother of young children. However, depression exaggerates the negative aspects of ordinary life, leading to feelings of being hopeless, helpless, and overwhelmed.

Illness   Psychological stressors caused by physiological dysfunctions can lead to depression. For example, a debilitating disease can severely restrict usual lifestyle, resulting in depression. Any illness that impinges on cerebral functioning and impairs blood flow to the brain can produce depression. Such illnesses may include adrenal cortex, thyroid, and parathyroid dysfunctions, and many neurologic, metabolic, and nutritional disorders, as well as infectious diseases.

Medications   Some medications have been known to cause depression. For example, during the 1950s doctors learned that some people taking reserpine, a medication for high blood pressure, suffered from depression. Since then, depression has been noted as a side effect of some tranquilizers, hormones, and a number of medications. However, alcohol is more likely to cause depression than any medication.

Treatments

A variety of therapies and medications help people of all ages who have depression. Estimates are that between 80 and 90 percent of all depressed people can be effectively treated. In general, therapists use "talk" treatment to try to understand the disturbed personal and social relationships that may have caused or contributed to the depression. Depression, in turn, may make these relationships more difficult. A therapist can help an individual understand his or her illness and the relationship of depression and particular interpersonal conflicts. If psychotherapy is not helpful or the depression is so severe that there is a loss of work or function, or persistent and increasing suicidal ideation over one to three months, medications may be needed to lift the depression in conjunction with therapy.

Psychoanalysis. Treatment of depression with psychoanalysis is based on the theory that depression results from past conflicts pushed into the unconscious. Psychoanalysts work to identify and resolve the individual's past conflicts that have led to depression in later years.

Short-term psychotherapy. In the mid-1980s researchers reported effective results of short-term psychotherapy in treating depression. They noted that cognitive/behavior therapy and interpersonal therapy were as effective as medications for some depressed patients. Medications relieved patients' symptoms more quickly, but patients who received psychotherapy instead of medication had as much relief from symptoms after 16 weeks, and their gains may last longer. Data from this and other studies may help researchers better identify which depressed patients will do best with psychotherapy alone and which may require medications.

Behavior and cognitive therapy. This therapy is based on the understanding that people's emotions are controlled by their views and opinions of themselves and their world. Depression results when individuals constantly berate themselves, expect to fail, make inaccurate assessments of what others think of them, catastrophize, and have negative attitudes toward the world and their futures. Therapists use techniques of talk therapy to help the individual replace negative beliefs and thought patterns.

Electroconvulsive therapy (ECT). Use of ECT to treat depression declined in the last two decades of the 20th century as more effective medications were developed. However, ECT is still used for some individuals who cannot take medications because of their physical condition or who do not respond to antidepressant medication. ECT is considered as a treatment when all other therapies have failed or when a person is suicidal.

Pharmaceutical approach to treating depression

Effectiveness of medication depends on an overall health, metabolism, and other unique characteristics. Results are usually not evident right away; antidepressant medications usually become fully effective about 10 to 20 days after an individual begins taking them. Approximately 70 percent of patients will improve or recover while taking antidepressant medications, but some may need to continue medication over a six-month or year-long period to prevent relapse or recurrence.

The major types of medications used to treat depression are tricyclic antidepressants, monoamine oxidase inhibitors (MAOIs), lithium, and serotonin reuptake inhibitors (SRIs).

Tricyclic antidepressants are often prescribed for individuals whose depressions are marked by feelings of hopelessness, helplessness, fatigue, inability to experience pleasure, and loss of appetite and resulting weight loss.

Monoamine oxidase inhibitors (MAOIs) are often prescribed for individuals whose depressions are characterized by anxiety, phobic and obsessive-compulsive symptoms, increased appetite, and excessive sleepiness, or those who fail to improve on other antidepressant medications.

Lithium is sometimes prescribed for people who have manic-depressive illness (a severe affective disorder characterized by a predominant mood of elation or depression, and in some cases an alternation between the two states). Sometimes it is prescribed for people who suffer from depression without mania. Those most likely to respond to treatment with lithium are depressed individuals whose family members have manic-depression or whose depression is recurrent rather than constant.

Serotonin reuptake inhibitors. During the 1990s, more specifically active antidepressant drugs with fewer propensities for side effects were developed.

Serotonin reuptake inhibitors (SRIs)—for example, fluoxetine (Prozac) and sertraline (Zoloft)—are one class; buproprion (Wellbutrin) is another. Many other medications are under development to treat depression.

Anticonvulsants as antidepressants. For patients with manic-depressive illness (bipolar disorder) in whom lithium is not effective, drugs used to prevent temporal lobe seizures are sometimes used.

Side effects of antidepressant medications. Some people experience side effects from antidepressant medications. Common side effects include dry mouth, constipation, drowsiness, and weight gain; these effects usually diminish somewhat or disappear as the body makes adjustments. Those more recently developed SRIs have a lower incidence of those side effects.

Self-help

Many depressed individuals in self-help groups share ideas for effective coping and self-care for depression. These include regular exercise, more contact with other people (for example, in special interest groups), coping with exaggerated thoughts (such as self-deprecation), catastrophizing by introducing more realistic thoughts and supporting them.

The National Depressive and Manic-Depressive Association is a national self-help organization formed in the 1980s. Chapters throughout the country meet locally to help members cope effectively with depression.

The Depression and Related Affective Disorders Association (DRADA) is a nonprofit organization focusing on manic-depressive illness and depression. DRADA distributes information, conducts educational meetings, and runs an outreach program for high school counselors and nurses. DRADA helps organize support groups and provides leadership training programs and consultation for those groups.

For information:

Depression and Related Affective Disorders Association (DRADA)
Johns Hopkins Hospital (Meyer 3-181)
600 N. Wolfe Street
Baltimore, MD 21287
(410) 955-4647

(410) 614-3241 (fax)
www.med.jhu.edu/drada

National Alliance for the Mentally Ill
2101 Wilson Boulevard
Suite 302
Arlington, VA 22201
(703) 524-7600
(703) 524-9094 (fax)
www.nami.org

National Depressive and Manic Depressive Association
730 N. Franklin Street
Suite 501
Chicago, IL 60610-3526
(800) 826-3632 (toll-free)
(312) 642-0049
(312) 642-7243 (fax)
www.ndmda.org

National Institute of Mental Health (NIMH)
6001 Executive Boulevard
Room 8184
Bethesda, MD 20892-9663
(800) 421-4211 (toll-free)
(301) 443-4513
(301) 443-4279 (fax)
www.nimh.nih.gov

National Mental Health Association
1021 Prince Street
Alexandria, VA 22314-2971
(800) 969-6642 (toll-free)
(703) 684-7722
(703) 684-5968 (fax)
http://www.nmha.org

See also COPING; DEFENSE MECHANISMS; MENTAL HEALTH.

Greist, John H., and James W. Jefferson. *Depression and Its Treatment: Help for the Nation's #1 Mental Problem.*

Washington, D.C.: American Psychiatric Press, Inc., 1984.

————. *Depression and Its Treatment*. New York: Warner Books, 1994.

Kahn, Ada P., and Jan Fawcett. *The Encyclopedia of Mental Health*. 2d ed. New York: Facts On File, Inc., 2000.

Karp, David Allen. *Speaking of Sadness: Depression, Disconnection, and the Meanings of Illness*. New York: Oxford University Press, 1996.

Robs-Nicholson, Celeste. "Depression." *Harvard Women's Health Watch*. March 1995, pp. 2–3.

DeQuervain's syndrome   See MUSICIANS' INJURIES; PERFORMING ARTS MEDICINE.

dermatitis (occupational)   An inflammation of the skin, caused by the skin coming into contact with certain substances at work. It is also known as occupational contact dermatitis. It is not infectious and cannot be passed from one person to another.

Dermatitis can result in painful itching and extreme discomfort. For some individuals, if the itching persists, dermatitis leads to a feeling of helplessness and DEPRESSION. People in many occupations experience dermatitis, from manicurists to leather workers.

How quickly a worker gets it depends on a number of things, such as the substance, its strength or potency, and how long and how often it touches the skin. Some substances might affect a worker almost the first day using them, and some might take weeks, months, or even years.

BUSINESS SECTORS WITH THE HIGHEST RISK OF WORK-RELATED SKIN DISEASE

Hairdressing/beauty care
Catering and food processing
Cleaning
Construction
Engineering
Printing
Chemical
Health care
Agriculture/horticulture
Rubber
Offshore

Dermatitis usually affects the hands or forearms, the places most likely to touch the substance. However, it can also occur on the face, neck, or chest from certain types of dusts, liquids, or fumes. Dermatitis can even spread to parts of the body that have not been in contact with the substance.

While dermatitis can affect people working in all sectors, some job categories are more susceptible than others.

In some jobs there is little to do to stop contact with substances that cause dermatitis. However, there are many precautions a worker can take.

PROTECTION AGAINST DERMATITIS AT WORK

Wear the right type of gloves. If you cannot wear gloves all the time, wear them when you are handling substances that can cause dermatitis and change them frequently.

Use a moisturizing cream before and after work. This will help replace the natural oils your skin loses when you wash or when you come into contact with detergents and solvents.

Wear a face shield or full-face mask, and protective coveralls if you do a job where liquids, fumes, or dust that can cause dermatitis might get onto you face and neck.

Make sure your protective clothes are clean and intact.

If you use diluted chemicals, make sure they are diluted to the correct strength. If they are over strength, they are more likely to cause dermatitis.

See also ALLERGIES; CATERING AND FOOD SERVICE; CHEMICAL TOXICITY; SKIN OR SENSE ORGAN TOXICITY.

detective/protective services   See VIOLENCE.

detoxification   See ALCOHOL DEFENDENCY.

developmental toxicity   Adverse effects on the developing child that result from exposure to chemical substances. While developmental toxicity usually results from prenatal exposures to toxicants experienced by the mother, it can also result from paternal exposure, or from postnatal exposures experienced by a developing child. Maternal exposure to toxic chemicals during pregnancy can disrupt the development of or even cause the death of the fetus. Exposure of pregnant women to the developmental toxicant MERCURY, for example, has been shown to lower the birth weights of and cause severe brain damage in their children. Among the adverse effects associated with maternal exposure to toluene are central nervous system dysfunction, craniofacial and limb anomalies, and developmental delay. Dark brown pigmentation, shorter gestation time, and lower birth weight have been found in the children of women exposed to POLYCHLORINATED BIPHENYLS (PCBs) during their pregnancies.

Paternal exposure to toxicants can cause male reproductive toxicity, such as sterility, and may contribute to early fetal loss or birth defects. An example is VINYL CHLORIDE, which has been associated with increased rates of spontaneous abortion.

Also called teratogens, developmental toxicants include agents that induce structural malformations and other birth defects, low birth weight, metabolic or biological dysfunction, and psychological or behavioral deficits that become evident as the child grows older. Developmental toxicity is sometimes considered as a subcategory of REPRODUCTIVE TOXICITY, but is treated as a distinct health endpoint.

Manson, J. "Teratogens." Chap. 7 in *Casarett and Doull's Toxicology,* edited by C. Klaasen, M. Amdur, and J. Doull. New York: Pergamon Press, 1996.

Diagnostic and Statistical Manual of Mental Disorders (DSM-IV)

A categorical guide, revised periodically, for classification of mental disorders. The fourth edition was published by the American Psychiatric Association in 1994. Counselors in EMPLOYEE ASSISTANCE PROGRAMS may refer to it in describing an employee's condition. The DSM-IV groups mental health disorders into 16 major diagnostic classes. The book is used for clinical, research, and educational purposes by psychiatrists, other physicians, psychologists, social workers, nurses, occupational and rehabilitation therapists, and other health and mental health professionals who wish to base a diagnosis of mental disorders, including anxieties and phobias, on standardized criteria.

American Psychiatric Association. *Diagnostic and Statistical Manual of Mental Disorders.* 4th ed. Washington, D.C.: American Psychiatric Association, 1994.

dieldrin See IMMUNOTOXICITY.

diesel exhaust A pervasive airborne contaminant in workplaces where diesel-powered equipment is used. More than 1 million workers in the United States are exposed to diesel exhaust and face the risk of adverse health effects, ranging from HEADACHES and nausea to CANCER and respiratory disease. These workers include mine workers, bridge and tunnel workers, railroad workers, loading dock workers, truck drivers, material handling machine operators, farmworkers, longshoring employees, and auto, truck, and bus maintenance garage workers.

Diesel fuel is a complex mixture of petroleum compounds. When combusted, this fuel produces thousands of chemical compounds that are released into the atmosphere as the exhaust. The major components are water, carbon dioxide, nitrogen, and carbon (soot).

The major mechanisms for the control of diesel emission is proper operation of the engines, so the training of maintenance personnel in their care and adjustment is critical. All personnel involved in engine maintenance should thoroughly understand maintenance procedures recommended by the engine manufacturer and follow all preventive and maintenance schedules.

See also AUTO BODY REPAIR AND REFINISHING; FARMING; HAZARD COMMUNICATION; TRUCK DRIVERS.

Occupational Safety and Health Administration.

dieting Following a special or modified diet for the purpose of losing weight. Motivation to be as thin as models unrealistically motivates many people, particularly women, to begin dieting. Losing weight is not easy; it means setting realistic goals. It requires time—often a year for positive results—for some people; it means hard work, both in losing the weight and in keeping it off. It is also stressful because many people perceive themselves as overweight, whether this is the case of not. To help employees control weight, some health promotion programs in business and industry make weight control activities available to employees.

Some dieting approaches involve extensive behavior modification. These programs offer SUPPORT GROUPS and education about good nutrition and exercise. Most importantly, they offer help in altering the individual's behavior in order to limit food intake, increase physical activity, and reduce the stress of the current social pressures to be thin.

Individuals who believe they are overweight should have a physical examination from their family physician to determine whether they are actually overweight or are weight-, shape-, or food-obsessed. If overweight, further assessment is necessary; if not overweight, they need supportive strategies to help them feel better about themselves and referral to workplace or community resources to help them with their concern.

For information:

American Dietetic Association
216 W. Jackson Boulevard
Suite 800
Chicago, IL 60606
(800) 877-1600 (toll-free)
(312) 899-1979 (fax)
http://www.eatright.org

Food and Nutrition Information Center
National Agricultural Library Building
Room 105
10301 Baltimore Avenue
Beltsville, MD 20705-2351
(301) 504-5719
(301) 504-6409 (fax)
http://www.nal.usda.gov/fnic

See also EATING DISORDERS; OBESITY; SELF-ESTEEM.

Kahn, Ada P. *Stress A–Z: A Sourcebook for Facing Everyday Challenges.* New York: Facts On File, Inc., 1998.

dioxin See AGENT ORANGE: ENDOCRINE TOXICITY; IMMUNOTOXICITY.

disabilities Temporary or permanent loss of faculty. The term may refer to physical disabilities such as loss of a leg or of hearing, or mental capabilities, such as retardation or autism. COPING with a disability causes stress for the one who has the disability and also for coworkers and employers.

Persons who become disabled often struggle with the anxiety of trying to be like everyone else. Because of their disability they may feel a loss of SELF-ESTEEM compounded, in many cases, by the limitations of the working situations which they encounter.

For information:

Architectural and Transportation Barriers Compliance Board
1331 F Street, NW
Suite 1000
Washington, DC 20530
(202) 272-5434 or (800) 8972-2253 or (800) USA-ABLE

Mobility International, U.S.A.
P.O. Box 3551
Eugene, OR 97403
(503) 343-1284

See also AMERICANS WITH DISABILITIES ACT; GENERAL ADAPTATION SYNDROME.

Disaster Unemployment Assistance A program administered by U.S. states as agents of the federal government that provides financial assistance to individuals whose employment or self-employment has been lost or interrupted as a direct result of a major disaster declared by the president. Before an individual can be determined eligible for disaster unemployment assistance, it must be established that the individual is not eligible for regular unemployment insurance benefits, either state or federal.

discrimination Making distinctions, differentiation, or showing favoritism or acting on the basis of prejudice or bias. Federal laws prohibit discrimination in the workplace, but in subtle ways, some employees may still notice effects of discrimination. For example, there may be a preference to hire a man or woman in a particular job, or a preference for a younger worker rather than an older worker. When layoffs occur, preference may be given to retaining younger workers who receive lower salaries than more tenured workers. In some circumstances, employees have rights that can be appealed.

Types of discrimination covered by federal laws include race/color, national origin, pregnancy, religious, disabilities, sexual orientation, status as a parent, marital status, political affiliation, and medical information.

Age discrimination is a fast-growing category of discrimination claims filed with the U.S. Equal Employment Opportunity Commission (EEOC). In 2001, 17,405 EEOC age discrimination claims were filed, up from 16,008 in 2000, the highest number of claims since 1995.

The U.S. Equal Employment Opportunity Commission (EEOC) began in 1965. The EEOC enforces the principal federal statutes prohibiting employment discrimination.

See also AGE DISCRIMINATION; AGEISM; DIVERSITY; NURSING MOTHERS IN THE WORKPLACE; WORKING MOTHERS.

For information:

U.S. Equal Employment Opportunity Commission
Publications Information Center
P.O. Box 12549
Cincinnati, OH 45212-0549
(800) 669-3362 (toll-free)
(800) 800-3302 (TDD)
(513) 791-2954 (fax)

dis-stress Hans Selye (1907–82), an Austrian-born Canadian endocrinologist, differentiated between the unpleasant or harmful variety of stress, called *dis-stress,* from the Latin *dis* (bad, as in dissonance, disagreement), and eustress, from the Greek *eu* (good, as in *euphonia, euphoria*). During both distress and eustress the body undergoes virtually the same nonspecific responses to various stimuli acting upon it. However, certain emotional factors, such as frustration and hostility, are particularly likely to turn stress into dis-stress. Many people experience dis-stress in the workplace, which leads to FRUSTRATION and BURNOUT.

See also COPING; EUSTRESS; GENERAL ADAPTATION SYNDROME; SELYE, HANS; STRESS.

Selye, Hans. *Stress without Distress.* New York: Lippincott, 1974.
———. *The Stress of Life.* Rev. ed. New York: McGraw-Hill, 1978.

diversity The condition of being diverse; the term relates to any group of people, such as an employee group, that is mixed in terms of race, religion, ethnicity, and gender. Respect for, and understanding of differences can make diversity a successful concept in the workplace.

It is effective for businesses to have diversity in their workforces because no business can afford to ignore any population segment. Companies dependent on direct sales to customers must pay attention to the differing cultures in their marketplace. Additionally, the business management process can benefit from the imagination and creativity generated from diverse viewpoints.

Conducting diversity awareness workshops is one way companies have introduced the idea of valuing personal differences. However, these workshops are only a first step in creating an environment in which previous prejudices are erased and a true sensitivity to diverse employee needs prevails.

See also ACCULTURATION; COMMUNICATION.

diving See COMMERCIAL DIVING.

domestic violence Abuse of spouses, children, or parents, in the home. This may take the form of wife-battering, child abuse, incest, elder abuse. Domestic violence affects an estimated 6.2 million American women each year and claims the lives of an average of four women each day. Domestic violence is not something that occurs only at home; it spills over into the workplace because a batterer often knows the victim's routine and how to find her on the job.

According to the New York State Safe Work Coalition, as many as 74 percent of working battered women are harassed by their abusive partners on the job. Of them, each year, 54 percent miss at least three full days a of work a month; 56 percent are late for work on at least 60 days, and 28 percent leave early on at least 60 days. Another study found that 20 percent of working battered women lose their jobs altogether. Battered women consistently identify the lack of financial resources as a primary obstacle to separating from their abusive partners. For working women, battering can further weaken their financial security by compromising their ability to perform and keep their jobs.

Domestic violence happens in all strata of society, and there are many more cases than records of employers or officials indicate because it is a subject often covered up out of fear and shame. Characteristics of persons who are victims of family violence include ANXIETY, powerlessness, GUILT, and lack of SELF-ESTEEM.

Professionals who treat victims of family violence are concerned with getting the victims, usually women or children, away from the abuser and into therapy before the abuse becomes too severe. Some perpetrators as well as victims of family violence compound their difficulties with use of alcohol of drugs.

Protecting the health and safety of all employees is in the interest of both employer and employee. It can reduce unnecessary turnover and abuse-related costs to the victim and coworkers and enhance employee well-being and productivity. According to the New York State Safe Work Coalition, many employers, both public and private, deal with effects of domestic violence whether they know it or not.

Having well-defined responses to domestic violence in the workplace will also better protect employers from potential liability. Workers in many EMPLOYEE ASSISTANCE PROGRAMS are trained to offer help to victims of domestic violence, both men and women.

Battered Women

Battered women are victims of physical assault by husbands, boyfriends, or lovers. Battering may include physical abuse sometimes for purposes of sexual gratification, such as breaking bones, burning, whipping, mutilation, and other sadistic acts. Generally, however, battering is considered part of a syndrome of abusive behavior that has very little to do with sexual issues. Drug- and alcohol-related problems are more common among families with battering behaviors. Women who select and choose to remain in abusive relationships were also abused as children. Many women stay in such relationships without reporting the abuse and without seeking counseling. Batterers often were abused themselves as children.

Help for battered women is available. First, physical protection, often provided by women's shelters within the community, must be assured for the woman and her children. Second, social support services must provide economic protection, since women often stay in abusive relationships due to lack of practical economic alternatives. Finally, psychotherapeutic intervention should be aimed at both batterer and victim to trace antecedents of the violent behavior, correct substance abuse problems, and substitute positive coping mechanisms for violent behavior patterns.

Most abused women do not seek help until beatings become severe and have occurred over a period of time, often two to three years. Some women are too embarrassed or believe that if they report the beating to police they will not be taken seriously. The majority of women who seek help because of family violence are between age 20 and 60. In 75 percent of households in which abuse takes place, the husband or boyfriend is an alcoholic or on drugs.

**HELP FOR FEMALE VICTIMS
OF DOMESTIC VIOLENCE**

- Leave the home when the abuser is absent to eliminate confrontation.
- Leave the scene of the abuse; stay with a friend or family member who will be supportive emotionally and provide a safe haven so that you can go to work as usual.
- Take bank records, children's birth certificates, cash and other important documents, along with clothing and personal items.
- If possible, photograph or videotape any consequences of abuse, such as injuries to yourself or damage to the home. These could be important for possible later court proceedings.
- Call the police and file a police report. Obtain an order of protection as soon as possible.
- Seek counseling for yourself and your children, join a support group with others who have been victims of family violence.
- Talk with counselors in your employers' employee assistance program, if one is available.

Legal Rights of Domestic Violence Victims

Until the later years of the 20th century, police and the legal system often viewed domestic violence as a private matter and not a crime. Now, in many states, the police may arrest a batterer if there is evidence of abuse. Civil actions might include legal separation, child custody, child support, and divorce. One common civil action in cases of domestic violence is the temporary restraining order, which involves making a complaint and going to a hearing to obtain a legal document that limits how close an abuser may come to a woman and her children.

A criminal complaint can be filed in addition to or instead of civil actions. A criminal complaint involves a police investigation, and if enough evidence is found, may lead to an arrest and involvement of the judicial system.

For further information:

New York State Safe Work Coalition
Website: www.safeatworkcoalition.org

See also ADDICTION; AGGRESSION; COPING; CODEPENDENCY; SUPPORT GROUPS; VIOLENCE; WOMEN AND JOB RELATED INJURIES.

Kahn, Ada P., and Jan Fawcett. *Encyclopedia of Mental Health.* 2d ed. New York: Facts On File, Inc., 2001.

dopamine   See DEPRESSION.

dose-response assessment/relationship   The amount of a chemical that a person is exposed to is called the dose, and the severity of the effect of that exposure is called the response. A dose-response assessment is a scientific study to determine the relationship between dose and response, and how much dose is correlated with how much response.

See also CHEMICAL TOXICITY.

downsizing   Employee layoffs in positions that will not be refilled. Downsizing is stressful for the managers who make the decision who will go and who will stay and for the employees who are asked to leave.

In many cases, the stress involved in downsizing leaves workers with ANGER and is a possible trigger for DEPRESSION. To help workers avoid and/or handle anger, such issues as job category, seniority, and performance must be addressed. Equally important issues include treatment of dismissed employees, positive employee recommendations, and dealing with remaining employees.

Most companies now consider downsizing or employee cutbacks as a routine part of business. As they become more and more common, the very idea of downsizing brings stress to many workers.

With downsizing, workers at all levels are affected, no matter how long they may have worked for the organization, no matter how well they perform their job or how effectively they have managed their budget and staff.

Signs of impending downsizing include a hiring freeze, pessimistic budget projections, closed-door meetings, decreasing sales, and consolidation of operations. Middle managers should be particularly alert to requests for department justification and works plans based on budget reductions.

See also JOB CHANGE; LAYOFFS.

Kahn, Ada P. *Stress A–Z: A Sourcebook for Facing Everyday Challenges.* New York: Facts On File, Inc., 1998.
Meyer, G. J. *Executive Blues: Down and Out in Corporate America.* New York: Franklin Square Press, 1995.

drowning   See CONSTRUCTION; FISHING.

drug testing   A method of identifying employees or candidates for employment who use illicit drugs. An increasing number of employers are instituting drug testing programs. Drug testing may include tests for alcohol, cocaine, heroin, inhalants, LSD (acid), marijuana, MDMA (Ecstasy), methamphetamine, nicotine, and anabolic steroids.

Testing is usually carried out by independent testing organizations. A variety of tests may be used. Breathalyzers can be used to detect alcohol, and urinalysis can detect many drugs present in the body. Hair, blood, saliva, and brain waves are also used for testing.

Testing may be before employment, after accidents, done randomly or periodically, or when the employer believes there are reasonable grounds for testing. In many cases, drug testing is carried out as part of the preemployment physical examination.

According to author Tyle D. Hartwell, et al., the incidence of testing is partially based on the type of worksite, characteristics of employees, and policies of the company. Drug testing has increased since the mid-1980s. Programs that test for illicit drugs are more than twice as prevalent as those that test for alcohol use. Programs are most prevalent in large worksites, industries affected by drug testing legislation, and those employing high-risk or unionized workers. At many locations drug testing is part of the EMPLOYEE ASSISTANCE PROGRAM.

The American Civil Liberties Union (ACLU) opposes indiscriminate urine testing. The ACLU claims that urine tests do not determine when a drug was used; they only detect metabolites, or inactive, leftover traces or previously ingested substances. Also, the ACLU asserts that drug screens used by many companies are not reliable and many tests yield false positive results 10 percent to 30 percent of the time.

For further information:

American Civil Liberties Union (ACLU)
125 Broad Street
18th Floor
New York, NY 10004
(212) 549-2500
(202) 549-2649 (fax)
http://www.aclu.org

See also ADDICTIONS; ALCOHOL DEPENDENCY; COCAINE; CODEPENDENCY; WORKSITE WELLNESS PROGRAMS.

Hartwell, Tyler D., Paul D. Steele, Michael T. French, Nathaniel F. Rodman. "Prevalence of Drug Testing in the Workplace." *Monthly Labor Review,* November 1996, pp. 35–46.

dry cleaning In the United States, the commercial dry cleaning industry consists of approximately 36,000 shops. Most of these shops are small businesses, with fewer than 10 employees. Approximately 85 percent of dry cleaning shops in the United States use perchloroethylene as their primary solvent.

National Institute for Occupational Safety and Health (NIOSH) researchers have conducted numerous studies of the commercial dry cleaning industry. Some of these studies have evaluated a variety of health and safety hazards; however, the greatest emphasis has been placed on worker exposure to perchloroethylene. NIOSH research in this industry has involved exposure assessment, engineering control evolutions, and epidemiological studies.

Many hazards are associated with dry cleaning processes, including chemical, fire, and ergonomic hazards. Exposure to hazardous chemicals commonly used in dry cleaning shops can occur through skin absorption, eye contact, or inhalation of the vapors. Perchloroethylene (PERC), a potential human carcinogen, is the most commonly used dry cleaning solvent. Symptoms associated with exposure include depression of the central nervous system, damage to the liver and kidneys, impaired memory, confusion, dizziness, headache, drowsiness, and eye, nose, and throat irritation. Repeated dermal exposure may result in dermatitis.

Many hazardous chemicals are commonly used in dry cleaning shops to remove garment stains. Workers performing stain removal may be exposed to these toxic chemicals through skin absorption, eye contact, or inhalation of vapors. The primary hazards is dermatitis from chronic or acute exposure. Dilute hydrofluoric acid, found in some products that remove rust stains, may cause severe chemical burns with deep tissue destruction that may not be evident until several hours after prolonged contact.

Dry cleaning shops contain all elements necessary for uncontrolled fires, including fuels, ignition sources, and oxygen. Potential combustible materials include furniture, garments, lint, and portions of the building. The greatest risk of fire and explosion exists if the dry cleaning shop uses a petroleum-based solvent in dry cleaning machines. Approximately 10 percent of dry cleaning shops in the United States use these highly flammable solvents. Ignition can be triggered by a burning or smoldering cigarette, heated equipment such as a press, a frictional spark inside the solvent reclaimer cage, or even static electricity within the reclaimer.

Ergonomic risks occur during garment transfer, pressing, and bagging. These activities, combined with a high work rate and frequency, may cause physical discomfort and musculoskeletal problems for workers. Disorders can include damage to tendons, muscles, nerves, and ligaments of the hand, wrist, arm, shoulder, neck, and back. Musculoskeletal disorders are caused by repetitive motions, awkward postures, excessive reaching, and precision gripping.

To reduce exposure to dry cleaning solvents, NIOSH recommends that a comprehensive control approach be followed involving engineering measures, work practices, and personal protection. Engineering measures are preferred as the most effective means of control and should generally be considered first.

In 1999 a report was published in the *American Journal of Industrial Medicine* reporting results of a qualitative study involving two owner and four worker focus groups. Findings suggested that overall, health and safety issues were not of great concern. Owners were primarily concerned with the economic impact of regulations. Workers did express some anxiety about SOLVENT exposure and burns, but most felt that these hazards were "just part of the job." Also, other than the installation of air-conditioning in the shops and the provision of health benefits, workers could not think of ways health and safety on the job could be improved.

See also CHEMICAL TOXICITY; DERMATITIS; ERGONOMICS; FIRE SAFETY/FIRE PROTECTION; HEADACHES; KIDNEY TOXICITY; SKIN AND SENSE ORGAN TOXICITY.

dust and debris   A mixture of very fine particles. In the case of the aftermath of the burning and collapse of the World Trade Center on September 11, 2001, dust and debris was from the materials that originally made up the buildings and the aircraft that struck them. These particles differ depending on what material the dust came from, how the dust was created, and what happened to the dust after it was released.

Intense exposure to dust and smoke causes eye, nose, throat, and lung irritation, triggering coughing and sneezing. These short-term symptoms are the body's way of removing foreign material. Short-duration, high-intensity exposures to dust and smoke are more likely to result in short-term and reversible effects. Asthma and symptoms such as wheezing and difficulty breathing are occasionally caused by exposure to a high dose of an irritant.

The U.S. Department of Health and Human Services (DHHS) advises persons entering areas covered with dust and debris to avoid prolonged exposure. Individuals entering these areas should avoid inhaling the dust or entering visibly dusty areas.

Precautions for Workers in Dusty Areas

The DHHS advises avoidance of dry sweeping of dust and other dust-clearing procedures that disturb settled dust. A limited dampening of settled dust with a fine water mist can reduce the amount of dust raised during cleanup. Excessive wetting may create a slip-and-fall hazard. Slip-resistant shoes or boots may be helpful. People who have been covered in dust that potentially contains asbestos should avoid taking the dust into their cars or homes (on clothes, skin, and hair), where others might be exposed. It is best to remove dusty clothing while wearing respiratory protection. A person should then shower completely and change into fresh clothing before going home. Dusty clothing should be handled without shaking, and should be placed in bags. Potentially contaminated clothing should be laundered separately.

Use of protective dust masks and dust-filtering respirators can effectively remove dust from inhaled air. Exposure can be reduced by wearing well-fitted dust masks. Dust-filtering masks are effective only against dust and provide no protection against toxic fumes or suffocation from lack of air. Firefighters and other emergency responders with potential for intense exposures often need air-supplied respirators for such special situations.

Additionally, the DHHS advises that one can protect eyes by wearing appropriate goggles, protect skin by wearing gloves, shoes, and clothing designed to keep dust away, wash face and hands often and always before eating and drinking, rinse hair, hands, and face with water before leaving the dusty area.

See also CONSTRUCTION; DEMOLITION; FIREFIGHTERS; PERSONAL PROTECTIVE EQUIPMENT; SLIPS, TRIPS, AND FALLS.

dysbarism   See COMMERCIAL DIVING.

dysthymia   See AFFECTIVE DISORDERS; DEPRESSION.

eating disorders Compulsive misuse of food to achieve some desired physical and/or mental state. Eating disorders are characterized by an intense fear of being fat and severe weight loss and may result in ill health, psychological impairments, and workplace impairment. Supervisors who suspect that an employee has an eating disorder should refer that person to the EMPLOYEE ASSISTANCE PROGRAM or other counseling program.

People with eating disorders may be experiencing stress in some aspect of their lives which they think will be improved by dieting in excess. There is low SELF-ESTEEM and a mortal fear of fatness. Sufferers typically hide their illness; when coworkers, family, or friends discover their illness, they try to help. Typically, people with eating disorders feel they do not deserve to be helped, and this creates a great deal of stress for all concerned.

Eating disorders share common addictive features with alcohol and drug abuse, but unlike alcohol and drugs, food is essential to human life, and proper use of food is a central element of recovery.

Estimates indicate that there are 8 million reported victims of eating disorders in the United States—7 million of them women (although the number of males is increasing) between the ages of 15 and 30. Eating disorders can be cured when the sufferer accepts treatment; an estimated 6 percent of all reported patients die.

Anorexia Nervosa

Anorexia nervosa is a syndrome of self-starvation in which people willfully restrict intake of food out of fear of becoming fat, resulting in life-threatening weight loss. Anorexics (people who suffer from anorexia nervosa) "feel fat" even when they are at normal weight or when emaciated, deny their illness, and develop an active disgust for food. Deaths from anorexia nervosa are higher than from any other psychiatric illness.

Causes of anorexia vary widely. Many anorexics are part of a close family and have special relationships with their parents. They are highly conforming, eager to please, and may be obsessional in their habits. There is speculation that young girls who refrain from eating wish to remain "thin as a boy" in an effort to escape the burdens of growing up and assuming a female sexual and marital role. Another contribution to the increase in anorexia is contemporary society's emphasis on slimness as beauty. This is particularly prevalent in the fashion industry with its overly thin models. Most women diet at some time, particularly athletes and dancers, who seem more prone to the disorder than other women. In some cases, anorexia nervosa is a symptom of depression, personality disorder, or ever schizophrenia.

Symptoms include severe weight loss, wasting (cachexia), food preoccupation and rituals, amenorrhea (cessation of the menstrual period), and hyperactivity (constant exercising to lose weight). The anorexic may suffer from tiredness and fatigue, sensitivity to cold, and complain of falling hair.

Eating disorders sometimes result in other mental health disorders as well as DEPRESSION. Individuals may suffer from withdrawal, mood swings and feelings of shame and guilt. Both anorexics and bulimics develop rituals regarding eating and exercise. They often are perfectionists in habits, such as their jobs, clothes, and personal appearance, and have an "all or nothing" attitude about life.

Bulimia

Bulimia is characterized by recurrent episodes of binge eating followed by self-induced vomiting, vigorous exercise, and/or laxative and diuretic abuse to prevent weight gain. Most people view vomiting as a disagreeable experience, but to a bulimic, it is a means toward a desired goal.

Another eating disorder is bulimarexia, which is characterized by features of both anorexia nervosa and bulimia. Some individuals vacillate between anorexic and bulimic behaviors. After months and perhaps years of eating sparsely, the anorexic may crave food and begin to binge, but the fear of becoming overly fat leads her/him to vomit.

Bulimics may be of normal weight, slightly underweight, or extremely thin. Bingeing and vomiting may occur as often as several times a day. In severe cases, it may lead to dehydration and potassium loss, causing weakness and cramps.

A Cycle of Addiction

Behaviors of anorexics and bulimics are driven by the cycle of addiction. There is an emotional emptiness which in turn leads to the psychological pain of low self-esteem. The individual looks for a way to dull the pain using addictive agents (starvation or bingeing) which usually result in the need to purge or medical problems. Finally, suffering from guilt, shame, and self-hate, the individual goes back to a routine of starvation and/or bingeing and purging.

Treatment

Medical problems caused by the disorder should be diagnosed and managed first. When the medical complications are severe, an individual may be hospitalized to stabilize physical functions and monitor nutritional intake. Often, small feedings are carefully spaced because the patient cannot handle very much food at one time. In some cases, antidepressant medications are begun during the hospital stay.

Many people with eating disorders are treated on an outpatient basis. There may be counseling that includes individual and group sessions for outpatients and family, marital therapy, and specialized support for eating disorders.

For information:

National Association of Anorexia Nervosa and Associated Disorders (ANAD)
Box 7
Highland Park, IL 60035
(847) 831-3438
(847) 433-4632 (fax)
http://anad.org

Anorexia Nervosa and Related Eating Disorders (ANRED)
P.O. Box 5102
Eugene, OR 97405
(541) 344-1144
http://www.anred.com

Kahn, Ada P. *Stress A–Z: A Sourcebook for Facing Everyday Challenges.* New York: Facts On File, Inc., 1998.

eldercare   See ABSENTEEISM; DAY CARE; WORKING MOTHERS.

electricity-related injuries   Injuries from electric power lines or connections sustained while working in construction, the utility industry, telecommunications, painting, pest exterminating, and many other fields.

Basic principles of safety while working on or around electrical systems and equipment include using the right tools for the job, following procedures, consulting drawings and other documents, isolation of the equipment from energy sources, identifying the electric shock and arc flash, as well as other hazards that may be present. Circuits and conductors should be tested every time before touching them. PERSONAL PROTECTION EQUIPMENT (PPE) should be used.

The OCCUPATIONAL SAFETY AND HEALTH ADMINISTRATION (OSHA) sets forth many regulations concerning electrical safety requirements. Guidelines by OSHA as well as many industry-based organizations (such as the National Fire Protection Association) cover electrical standards for the utility and construction industries, telecommunications, power transmission and distribution, fire safety, and other related areas.

Electrical Safety Programs

Employers should develop electrical safety programs, including procedures for analyzing risks and hazards associated with each job. Attention should focus on the working environment, the condition of equipment, safe work practices, accident prevention, shock rescue procedures, lightning strikes, and preventive electrical maintenance.

Environmental factors to consider include wet or dry, indoors or outdoors, open or cramped, well-lit or dim, metal ladders in areas where overhead wires or exposed conductors are present, electrical cords over a heat source, or overloaded electrical outlets.

Conditions of equipment to consider include the age of equipment, integrity of grounding system, internal safety mechanisms, operating voltage, electrical wiring and loads incurred, and fault current available to produce arc flash.

Safe work practices include being sure that operating procedures are up to date and appropriate for the working conditions, evaluating circuit information drawings, and determining the degree and extent of hazards. Work should comply with minimum clearances when working around electrical power lines or other exposed conductors and determine approach boundaries to prevent injuries from a potential arc-flash.

Personal protection equipment (PPE) should be chosen based on potential hazards present.

Preventing Electrical Accidents

Employers and employees must focus constant attention on reducing and eliminating exposure to electrical hazards. Aspects to be watched include physical barriers around the energy source, such as fences and insulators on conductors. The work areas should be clean and dry; cluttered work areas and benches can invite accidents and injuries.

Management should assign responsibility for electrical safety at each site, have a policy for dealing with electrical safety, have training procedures, and determine the qualifications for people working on and around electrical equipment.

PREVENTING ELECTRICITY-RELATED ACCIDENTS

- Work areas should be inspected daily for hazards such as flickering lights, warm switches or receptacles, burning odors, loose connections, frayed, cracked, or broken wires.
- Choose proper cords and connectors, making sure any portable cord used to power any type of light and/or heavy-duty industrial equipment is suitable for the equipment.

- The extension cord should be at least as thick as the electrical cord for the tool.
- All testing equipment should be properly calibrated.
- Read and follow all equipment operating instructions for proper use. All equipment repairs and adjustments should be done by authorized personnel.
- Sticking switches on electrical saws should be replaced right away.
- Never operate an electric saw while wearing loose clothing, such as long, floppy sleeves.
- Follow required lock-out/tag-out procedures.
- Turn off equipment when finished with each job; disconnect energy sources; tag out the disconnected power.
- Always clean up spills on floors.

SAFETY TIPS WHILE WORKING IN ELECTRICITY-RELATED SITUATIONS

- Wear safety glasses and a hard hat when working on live circuits.
- Use electrically insulated tools and gloves.
- Look at test dates for integrity of equipment and protective clothing.
- Wear required and appropriate flame-resistant personal protective clothing.
- Protect hands by wearing appropriate safety gloves; inspect gloves for signs of wear and damage before using.
- Use ladders with nonconductive siderails.
- Follow lock-out/tag-out procedures.
- Use double-insulated power tools or ones that have ground-fault circuit interrupters protecting the circuit.
- Inspect all extension cords for wear and tear; check testing dates.
- Never drape electrical cords over heat sources.
- Do not store flammable liquids near electrical equipment, even temporarily.
- Motors with thermal protection can restart without warning; always lock out the motor before working on it.
- Do not use tin-stranded wire with solder; this promotes corrosion and limits contact area.
- If measuring voltage with respect to ground, make the ground connection first and remove it last.
- Plugs with connectors should be wired with additional slack. If there is undue strain on the cord, the grounding will be the last broken.
- Check grounding continuity on new tools and equipment before using them.

INJURIES FROM ELECTRICAL SHOCK

- Burns
- Low-voltage contact wounds
- High-voltage contact wounds from entry and exit of electrical current

- Respiratory difficulties (vaporized metal or heated air may have been inhaled)
- Infectious complications.
- Injury to bone through falls, heat necrosis (death of tissue), and muscle contractions; shoulder joint injuries and fracture of bones in the neck are common injuries caused by muscle contraction
- Injury to the heart such as ventricular fibrillation, cardiac arrest, or stoppage
- Internal and organ injuries
- Neurological (nerve) injury
- Injury to the eyes (cataracts from electrical injury have occurred up to three years after the accident)

SHOCK RESCUE PROCEDURES

According to the National Electrical Safety Foundation, certain practices should be followed immediately in response to an electrical accident.

- Call for help and follow the emergency response system as outlined in the employer's safety procedures.
- Get the approved first-aid supplies.
- Deenergize the circuit and separate the person from the energy source. Make sure you and the victim are in a safe zone, not in contact with any electrical source, away from downed or broken wires. Never grab the person or pull the person off the current with your hands; you might become part of the circuit and become injured too. Use a dry wood broom, leather belt, plastic rope, or something similar that is nonconductive, such as a wood or plastic cane with a hook on the end, to free the person from the energy source.
- Administer first aid/apply mouth to mouth resuscitation and/or CPR.
- Keep the victim lying down, warm and comfortable. Do not move the person until help comes.
- If the victim is unconscious, put him/her on side to let fluids drain.
- Make sure the victim receives professional medical attention.

FIRST AID FOR BURN VICTIMS
(ELECTRICITY-RELATED)

- Roll the person on the ground if the person's clothing is on fire.
- Cool the burn with water or saline for a few minutes. Do not remove clothing stuck to a burn.
- Remove constricting items from the victim, such as shoes, belts, and tight collars.
- Check the victim's breathing and heartbeat. If necessary, perform mouth-to-mouth resuscitation and/or CPR if necessary.

- Keep the victim warm and comfortable by covering him/her with clean, dry sheets or blankets.
- Elevate burned areas to reduce swelling.

Lightning Strikes

Each year in the United States, approximately 93 people die as a result of being struck by lightning. Outdoor workers face a high risk of suffering a fatal lightning strike. One lightning strike can injure or kill one or more people. Of those struck by lightning, 30 percent die and 74 percent have permanent disabilities. Death from a lightning strike usually occurs within one hour of injury. Most lightning strikes occur outdoors between May and September.

HOW WORKERS CAN
AVOID INJURIES FROM LIGHTNING

- Monitor weather forecasts during the thunderstorm season.
- Remind employees that lightning is present in all thunderstorms.
- Lightning often precedes rain and can strike as far as 10 miles away from the rain of a thunderstorm.
- Seek shelter immediately when thunder is heard. Avoid trees or tall objects, high ground, water, open spaces and metal objects such as tools, fences, and umbrellas.
- Remain inside a vehicle; it is safe because rubber tires are nonconductive.
- When indoors, shut off appliances and electronic devices and avoid using the telephone.
- Inspect the grounding electrode system for loose or corroded connections, which can increase the impedance of a lightning dissipation path.
- Provide surge protection at the main service panel-board to prevent line surges from traveling to equipment.

Source: Centers for Disease Control

For further information:

National Electrical Safety Foundation
1300 N. 17th Street
Suite 1847
Rosslyn, VA 22209
(703) 841-3229
www.nesf.org

See also CONSTRUCTION; FIRE SAFETY/FIRE PROTECTION; LADDERS; LOCK-OUT/TAG OUT; NATIONAL FIRE PROTECTION ASSOCIATION; PAINTERS; PLUMBERS.

electroconvulsive therapy (ECT)   A treatment that produces a convulsion by passing an electrical current through the brain; also known as electroshock therapy. Historically, this treatment was used for serious symptoms of mental illness. It is given to carefully selected patients (such as those who have DEPRESSION that is unresponsive to medications or who are suicidal) under close medical monitoring. Employees on leave of absence with severe depression may be referred for this treatment after a course of therapy with a mental health professional. Return to work can be determined by the physician in charge.

ECT has been shown to affect a variety of neurotransmitters in the brain, including norepinephrine, serotonin, and dopamine. It is also sometimes used to treat acute mania and acute schizophrenia when other treatments have failed. The number of ECT treatments needed for each person is determined according to the therapeutic response. After a course of ECT treatments, such patients usually are maintained on an antidepressant drug or lithium to reduce the risk of relapse.

The treatment can be lifesaving in people who are too medically ill to tolerate medication or who are not eating or drinking (catatonic). Side effects, including memory loss, are not uncommon. Patients must give informed consent to ECT, similar to any operative procedure.

See also MENTAL HEALTH; PSYCHIATRIST.

Kahn, Ada P., and Jan Fawcett, *Encyclopedia of Mental Health.* 2d ed. New York: Facts On File, Inc., 2000.

elevators   A necessary mode of transportation in multifloor workplaces. Elevator safety is a constant in all businesses; inspections by local authorities take place regularly. When electricity in a building must be shut off for any reason, elevators are usually unavailable for workers, and another evacuation route must be designated. Usually during fires elevators are not used, and other routes of egress must be found.

For maintenance workers, there is the hazard of working in CONFINED SPACES, often with electrical and other mechanical equipment. When working outside the elevator cab, there is a risk of falling or being crushed between moving parts of the mechanism. There is a need for adequate lighting when working in the elevator shaft and also for wearing PERSONAL PROTECTIVE EQUIPMENT (PPE).

Fear of riding in an elevator influences where an individual works or conducts business. It can be a disabling fear because it limits one's activities. Therapists treat elevator PHOBIAS with many techniques, of which the exposure therapies are the most effective. EMPLOYEE ASSISTANCE PROGRAMS may refer an individual afraid to take elevators for appropriate mental health counseling.

See also BEHAVIOR MODIFICATION; ELECTRICITY-RELATED INJURIES; EMERGENCY RESPONSE; FIRE SAFETY/FIRE PROTECTION; MENTAL HEALTH.

ELISA test   A screening test for the human immunodeficiency virus (HIV). Antibodies are found in serum that has been separated from the red blood cells. During an ELISA test this serum is placed in a tiny well containing a plastic bead coated with the proteins of HIV. Among these proteins are antigens. If there are any HIV antibodies in the serum, they will bind to the HIV antigens on the bead. An indicating substance is then added that will turn yellow if any binding has taken place. If the test is negative, and the person may have been exposed to HIV, a test again in six months is advisable. The negative result may simply mean that antibodies have not yet been produced. If the test is positive, it is repeated. If the second test is positive, the WESTERN BLOT is performed.

See also ACQUIRED IMMUNODEFICIENCY SYNDROME; HUMAN IMMUNODEFICIENCY VIRUS.

Museum of Science and Industry, Chicago.

embalmer's asthma   See WHEEZING.

emergency response   Reaction to an unforeseen situation in the workplace that threatens employees, customers, or the public. Emergencies can be human-made or naturally caused and disrupt or shut down operations, and may cause physical or environmental damage.

Emergencies and disasters can strike anywhere or any time and employees may be forced to evacuate the place of business abruptly. According to the OCCUPATIONAL SAFETY AND HEALTH ADMINISTRA-TION, workplace emergencies may include the following: floods, hurricanes, tornadoes, fires, chemical or biological weapon attacks, toxic gas releases, chemical spills, radiological accidents, explosions, civil disturbances, and workplace violence resulting in bodily harm and trauma.

Emergency Responder Respirators

In May 2002, the U.S. Centers for Disease Control and Prevention's (CDC) National Institute for Occupational Safety and Health (NIOSH) issued its first approval of respirators for occupational use by emergency responders against chemical, biological, radiological, and nuclear agents. The approved units are self-contained breathing apparatus that provide users with air from a pressurized cylinder or tank carried on the back. The approval signifies that the products are expected to protect FIREFIGHT-ERS and other responders from chemical, biological, radiological, and nuclear exposures in the line of duty. NIOSH testing criteria builds on NIOSH's existing program for certifying respirators for occupational use in traditional workplace settings such as factories, construction sites, and health care facilities. Development of the new program involved broad national support and collaboration by many agencies, organizations, and stakeholders. NIOSH is developing criteria for approving other types of respirators, such as air-purifying devices, for use by emergency responders.

See also CHEMICAL SPILLS; ELECTRICITY-RELATED INJURIES; FIRE SAFETY/FIRE PROTECTION; HAZARDOUS WASTE; NATIONAL INSTITUTE OF OCCUPATIONAL SAFETY AND HEALTH (NIOSH); NATIONAL PRIORITIES LIST; TERRORISTS; VIOLENCE.

emphysema   A chronic, obstructive pulmonary disease (COPD) that causes its victims to struggle for every breath they take. Because their lungs have lost much of their natural elasticity, people suffering from this disease cannot completely exhale the carbon dioxide that is trapped in their lungs. They fight to replace the stale air with fresh oxygen.

There is no one known cause of emphysema, but most cases are related to cigarette smoking. Other contributing factors are AIR POLLUTION and certain inhaled dusts and fumes in workplaces and other settings. The disease is not caused by a germ or a virus and it is not infectious or contagious.

Emphysema develops over time. A chronic cough and general shortness of breath are warning signs of emphysema. Sufferers do not realize they have it until the first signs of breathlessness appear, and by then delicate lung tissue may have been damaged excessively. Emphysema is a chronic illness; there is no cure.

Some people who have emphysema require use of a portable oxygen tank, making working complicated because they need to make arrangements to replenish their supplies periodically.

Living with Emphysema

Physicians can prescribe medications to relieve the feeling of breathlessness that accompanies this disease. There are also medicines that help clear mucus from the lungs and that can ward off chest infections. Also, emphysema patients can be taught by physical therapists to use their abdominal, chest, and diaphragmatic muscles to help them breathe more easily.

For information:

Chicago Lung Association
1440 West Washington Boulevard
Chicago, IL 60607
(312) 243-2000
www.lungusa.org

See also CHRONIC OBSTRUCTIVE PULMONARY DISEASE; RESPIRATORY TOXICITY; SMOKING.

Employee Assistance Programs (EAPs)   Programs designed to provide employees with help for problems they face on or off the job. Having an EAP in one's company is an important employee benefit. From the employer's point of view, anything EAPs do to improve the lives of employees helps to keep the business running successfully.

Most authors trace the origin of EAPs to the founding of Alcoholics Anonymous in 1935. In the 1960s and 1970s the scope of EAPs began to include help for such employee problems as DEPRESSION and other mental health concerns, drug abuse, divorce, and other difficulties. These programs have been expanded to include issues such as environmental stress, corporate culture, managing rapid technological change, and retraining.

How EAPs Work

There are two types of EAPs: internal and external. The majority of EAPs use independent companies that provide EAP services under a contract with the employer.

While the programs are geared to identifying employees whose personal problems may adversely affect their job performance, they also take a proactive stance in helping employees prevent problems before they occur. For example, some companies offer seminars on stress reduction, parenting, adolescents and drugs, exercise, health, and diet.

EAPs provide referrals to appropriate professional services for employees and their immediate families. Confidentiality is assured; most employees would not use an EAP if they thought their problems would be revealed.

Employers implement EAPs for a variety of reasons. One is the skyrocketing cost related to providing a medical benefits program; another is the huge cost attributed to downtime resulting from employee alcohol addiction and mental illness. A four-year study of mental health care received by employees of the McDonnell Douglas Corporation estimated that the company could save $5.1 million over three years if those employees who did not seek treatment had done so. Employees who used the EAP for chemical dependency also lost 44 percent fewer work days and filed fewer medical claims than those who did not.

Through its EAPs, Hewlett-Packard offers stress management courses to its 56,000 U.S. employees. Programs range from learning coping skills to dealing with teenage drug abuse. Additionally, Hewlett-Packard offers its employees physical activities—membership in health clubs, on-site weight rooms, basketball courts, jogging tracks, and Nautilus equipment—as a means of stress reduction and an avenue toward healthier lives. Saturn Corporation, an automobile manufacturer headquartered in Tennessee, provides one-on-one counseling by specially trained health care specialists, much of which is stress related.

Employee Assistance Professionals Association

The Employee Assistance Professionals Association (EAPA) is the world's oldest and largest membership organization for employee assistance professionals, with approximately 6,200 members in the United States and more than 30 other countries. Members include social workers, substance abuse and mental health counselors, behavioral health specialists, human resources professionals, risk management experts, and benefits specialists. The rapid pace and degree of change in the workplace underscores the importance of employee assistance programs and the concurrent need for education, training, and development of employee assistance professionals. EAPA offers education and training, professional certification, a professional journal, chapter networking, an annual conference, and acts as a resource center to help members stay current on issues affecting today's workplace. Further, EAPA protects the interests of members and the entire employee assistance professionals community through legislative and public policy efforts.

See also JOB CHANGE; JOB SECURITY; LAYOFFS.

endocrine toxicity   Adverse effects on the structure and/or functioning of the endocrine system resulting from exposure to chemical substances. The endocrine system is composed of many organs and glands that secrete hormones directly into the bloodstream; they include the pituitary, hypothalamus, thyroid, adrenals, pancreas, thymus, ovaries, and testes. Once synthesized, hormones are conveyed to a target tissue, where they function as chemical messengers that transmit information between cells. Hormone levels and interactions control normal physiological processes, maintaining the body's homeostasis. Because the endocrine system is complex, a toxicant may interfere at any of a number of points along a hormone's pathway of production, regulation, and action. Some chemicals may injure the glands that synthesize and secrete hormones, while others disrupt hormonal actions at the target organ. Compounds that are toxic to the endocrine system may cause diseases and conditions such as hypothyroidism, diabetes mellitus, hypoglycemia, reproductive disorders, and cancer.

Many toxic substances can disrupt the function of the endocrine system. For example chemicals that resemble the hormone estrogen can bind to estrogen receptors located throughout the body and either mimic the natural hormone or inhibit its actions. Exposure to such endocrine toxicants as persistent organochlorine pesticides and dioxins are being studied for their possible role in promoting hormone-induced cancers, such as breast cancer, and in lowering sperm counts and male fertility.

Specific organs and glands in the endocrine system are known to be damaged by chemical toxicants. Several chemicals and drugs can be toxic to the cells of the pancreas that produce insulin. Exposure to the rodenticide Vacor can interfere with the secretion and function of pancreatic hormones, resulting in diabetes mellitus and hyperglycemia. Polyhydroxyphenols and the drug lithium can disrupt thyroid gland function and cause hypothyroidism and goiter. Endocrine and reproductive dysfunction have been reported in men exposed to inorganic lead. Chronic exposure to lead can cause direct testicular toxicity, followed by hypothalamic or pituitary gland disturbances.

See also CHEMICAL TOXICITY.

U.S. Environmental Protection Agency Risk Assessment Forum, *Special Report on Environmental Endocrine Disruption: An Effects Assessment and Analysis,* 1997.

Energy Employees Occupational Illness Compensation Program

A program authorized by the Energy Employees Occupational Illness Compensation Program Act, which went into effect on July 31, 2001. The program delivers benefits to eligible employees and former employees of the U.S. Department of Energy, its contractors and subcontractors, or to certain survivors of such individuals, and also to certain beneficiaries of the Radiation Exposure Compensation Act.

The Department of Labor's Office of Workers' Compensation Programs is responsible for adjudicating and administering claim under the act.

Compensation of $150,000 and payment of medical expenses from the date a claim is filed is available to:

Employees of the Department of Energy, its contractors or subcontractors with radiation-related cancer if:

- The employee developed cancer after working at a facility of the Department of Energy, its contractors and subcontractors;
- The employees' cancer is determined at least as likely as not related to that employment, or
- The employee is determined to be a member of the special exposure cohort and developed one of certain listed cancers;
- Employees at facilities where they were exposed to beryllium produced or processed for the Department of Energy who developed chronic beryllium disease; and
- Employees of the Department of Energy or its contractors and subcontractors who worked at least 250 days during the mining of tunnels at underground nuclear weapons test sites in Nevada or Alaska and who developed chronic silicosis.

Compensation of $40,000 and payment of medical expenses from the date a claim is filed is available for URANIUM MINERS previously awarded benefits by the Department of Justice under Section 5 of the Radiation Exposure Compensation Act.

Employees of the Department of Energy and its contractors and subcontractors who were exposed to beryllium on the job and now have beryllium sensitivity will receive medical monitoring to check for chronic beryllium disease.

For further information:

Workers' Compensation Programs
Employment Standards Administration
Room S3524
200 Constitution Avenue, NW
Washington, DC 20210
(202) 693-0031
(202) 693-1378 (fax)

See also BERYLLIUM; SILICOSIS; SPECIAL EXPOSURE COHORT.

U.S. Department of Labor.

environment   The atmosphere in which a person works or lives. In cities throughout the United States, the Pollution Standard Index (PSI), which is a combined reading of five major pollutants—particulate matter, sulfur dioxide, carbon monoxide, ozone, and nitrogen dioxide—goes beyond acceptable standards on many days. In fact, PSI can fluctuate from as few as three to a high well over 200 in any given year. Difficulties in breathing, runny eyes, and light-headedness are just some of the symptoms caused by bad air.

Inside the workplace, environmental hazards continue to prevail. It is estimated that up to 15 percent of the population is sensitive to indoor pollutants, which may be 10 times more concentrated than those in nearby outdoor air. Some chemicals found in and around the workplace are pesticides, gas stove fumes, car exhaust, and those found in permanent press fabrics and particle board. Even water causes environmental illnesses; symptoms range from mild to disabling and are often nonspecific. Every part of the body can be affected by flu-like headaches, muscle aches, and fatigue, or more debilitating food intolerance and central nervous system problems such as memory loss, confusion, and DEPRESSION.

For information:

National Coalition Against the Misuse of Pesticides
   (NCAMP)
701 E Street
Washington, DC 20003
Suite 200
(202) 543-5450
(202) 543-4791 (fax)
www.beyondpesticides.org

National Pesticide Information Center
Oregon State University
323 Weniger Hall
Corvallis, OR 97331-6502
(800) 858-7378 (toll-free)
(541) 737-0761 (fax)
http:npic.orst.edu

National Safety Council
1121 Spring Lake Drive
Itasca, IL 60143-3201

(800) 621-7619 (toll-free)
(630) 285-1121
(630) 285-1315
http://www.nsc.org

See also AIR POLLUTION; CHEMICAL TOXICITY; DUST AND DEBRIS HEADACHES; INDOOR ENVIRONMENT; SICK BUILDING SYNDROME.

Altman, Roberta. *The Complete Book of Home Environmental Hazards.* New York: Facts On File, Inc., 1990.
Kahn, Ada P. *Stress A–Z: A Sourcebook for Facing Everyday Challenges.* New York: Facts On File, Inc., 1999.

environmental medicine   See AMERICAN COLLEGE OF OCCUPATIONAL AND ENVIRONMENTAL MEDICINE.

Environmental Protection Agency (EPA)   A U.S. governmental agency that since the 1970s has worked to protect human health and safeguard the natural environment. EPA provides leadership in environmental science, research, and education. It works closely with other federal agencies, state and local governments, and Native American tribes to develop and enforce regulations under existing environmental laws. The agency also works with industry in a wide variety of voluntary pollution prevention programs to protect workers and pursue energy conservation efforts. Each regional EPA office is responsible within its states for the execution of the agency's programs.

EPA employs 18,000 people in program offices, 10 regional offices, and 17 laboratories across the United States. EPA employees are technically trained: more than half are engineers, scientists, and environmental protection specialists. Many employees are legal, public affairs, financial, and computer specialists. The administrator of the EPA is appointed by the president of the United States.

EPA is responsible for researching and setting national standards for a variety of environmental programs and delegates to states and tribes the responsibility for issuing permits and monitoring and enforcing compliance. Where national standards are not met, EPA can issue sanctions and take other steps to assist the states and tribes in reaching the desired levels of environmental quality.

For information:

U.S. Environmental Protection Agency (EPA)
1200 Pennsylvania Avenue, NW
Washington, DC 20460
(202) 564-6953
(202) 501-1450 (fax)
www.epa.gov

environmental toxins See AGENCY FOR TOXIC SUB-STANCES AND DISEASE REGISTRY; FUNGI.

ergonomics and ergonomics regulations The science of designing the job and workplace to fit the individual, rather than forcing the individual to fit the job; job design with the worker in mind.

Ergonomics is not new. It has existed in one form or another since people began working. However, the topic of ergonomics gained national focus in the 1990s when the Occupational Safety and Health Administration (OSHA) found recordkeeping violations at a few meatpacking companies and cited them with high civil penalties. At that time, the meatpacking industry had a very high rate of repetitive stress injuries, approximately 75 times that of all other national industries.

In 2001 Labor Secretary Elaine Chao reported that work-related repetitive strain injuries and similar muscular disorders account for more than a third of all job injuries. Chao indicated the need for a solid, comprehensive approach to ergonomics and to address injuries before they occur through prevention and compliance.

Ergonomics issues arise from particular jobs including repetitiveness of chore, use of body force or posture needed to perform tasks, or aspects of the environment in which the job is done, such as poor lighting and ventilation, chair and desk height, and noise level. These can be viewed as health issues in the workplace and may be the cause of illness and injury resulting from job tasks.

Most occupational injuries and illnesses are often diagnosed as musculoskeletal disorders, while cumulative trauma disorders are reported as the fastest-growing occupational issue among the U.S. working population, according to the National Institute of Safety and Health (NIOSH).

The principal objective of an occupational ergonomic program is to identify individuals and jobs, implement medical and work interventions geared at prevention, and then evaluate the effectiveness of those interventions.

INCREASE THE SUCCESS OF ERGONOMIC INTERVENTIONS IN THE WORKPLACE

- Participatory ergonomics programs require strong in-house direction, support, and significant staff expertise in both team building and ergonomics.
- Training programs must develop both teamwork and ergonomic skills among participants.
- Team size should be kept minimal, but should include production workers engaged in the jobs studied, area supervisors, and maintenance and engineering staff who can effect proposed job improvements.
- Effective team problem-solving requires access to injury and illness information. In addition, reports on the team's objectives, progress, and accomplishments need to be circulated to the plant workforce to keep all parties informed about the program.
- Evaluation of results is an important component of a participatory ergonomic program. Such data will enable the teams to appraise their progress, provide feedback to affected or interested parties, and make suitable corrections where necessary to improve the overall effort.

Source: DHHS (NIOSH) Publication No. 95-102.

See also CARPAL TUNNEL SYNDROME; MUSICIANS' INJURIES; REPETITIVE STRESS INJURY; RIVETERS.

Brown, Stephanie. *The Hand Book: Preventing Computer Injury.* New York: Ergonomne, 1993.
Donkin, Scott W. *Sitting on the Job: How to Survive the Stresses of Sitting Down to Work—A Practical Handbook.* Boston: Houghton Mifflin Company, 1986.

ethylene dibromide (EDB) See REPRODUCTIVE TOXICITY.

ethylene glycol See ETHYLENE OXIDE.

ethylene monochloride See VINYL CHLORIDE.

ethylene oxide (EtO) A substance used as an intermediate in the production of several industrial chemicals, most notably ethylene glycol. It is also used as a fumigant in certain agricultural products and as a sterilant for medical equipment and supplies. However, EtO possesses several physical and health hazards as it is both flammable and highly reactive. Acute exposures to EtO gas may result in respiratory irritation and lung injury, headache, nausea, vomiting, diarrhea, shortness of breath, and cyanosis. Chronic exposure has been associated with cancer, reproductive effects, mutagenic changes, neurotoxicity, and sensitization.

See also CANCER; CHEMICAL TOXICITY; HAZARDOUS AND TOXIC SUBSTANCES; NEUROTOXICITY; REPRODUCTIVE TOXICITY; RESPIRATORY TOXICITY.

Occupational Safety and Health Administration, U.S. Department of Labor, March 2001.

eustress Hans Selye (1907–82), pioneer researcher in the field of stress, coined the term *eustress* to refer to "good stress." During eustress and "dis-stress" (bad stress), the body undergoes virtually the same nonspecific responses to the various positive or negative stimuli acting upon it. However, he explained, the fact that eustress causes much less damage than distress demonstrates that "how you take it" determines whether one can adapt successfully to change.

Examples of "good stress" include starting a desired new job, getting a substantial raise at work, getting married, having a planned baby, or moving to a new house. These situations, as well as others, demand adaptations on the part of the individual. Both *eustress* and *dis-stress* are part of the GENERAL ADAPTATION SYNDROME (GAS) which Selye described as being the controlling factor in how people cope with stresses in their lives.

See also COPING; DIS-STRESS; SELYE, HANS; STRESS.

Selye, Hans. *Stress without Distress*. New York: Lippincott, 1974.
———. *The Stress of Life*. Rev. ed. New York: McGraw-Hill, 1978.

excavation See CONSTRUCTION.

exercise Activities such as walking, jogging, weight lifting, using aerobic machines, skiing, swimming, cycling, or rowing. Many employees participate in daily exercise workouts, and weekends devoted to sports to combat the stress-related, physical tension in their lives at work or at home. Many workplaces have installed fitness facilities to help employees squeeze exercise into their schedules.

Exercise raises pulse rate and endorphin levels, increases the supply of blood and oxygen to muscles and vital organs, lowers blood pressure, and boosts metabolism, immune level, and energy level, in addition to relieving stress and muscle tension and improving posture.

For information:

Aerobics and Fitness Association of America
15250 Ventura Boulevard
Suite 200
Sherman Oaks, CA 91403
(800) 446-2322 (toll-free)
(877) 968-7263
(818) 788-6301 (fax)
www.afaa.com

See SELF-ESTEEM; STRESS; WORKSITE WELLNESS PROGRAMS; YOGA.

exogenous depression A type of DEPRESSION that originates outside the body. It is often reactive, caused by emotional factors, such as BURNOUT, grief, or STRESS. Exogenous depression is contrasted with endogenous depression, which researchers believe may be caused by a chemical imbalance in the body.

See also AFFECTIVE DISORDERS; DEPRESSION.

exposure assessment Identifying ways in which chemicals may reach individuals, for example, by breathing. Assessment includes estimating how much of a chemical an individual is likely to be exposed to, and estimating the number of individuals likely to be exposed.

See also CHEMICAL TOXICITY.

extractive industries Mining, quarrying, and oil and gas development (the extractive industries) are commonly thought of as dangerous work. While parts of the industry may be hazardous, the overall nonfatal injury and illness rate (6.2 nonfatal injuries and illnesses for every 100 full-time workers) is lower than the average for all industries (8.1 cases per 100 full-time workers). The incidence rate for mining is lower than for industrial sectors such as construction and manufacturing, and is comparable to that for services.

Injuries and illnesses in mining are more severe than in other industries, and fatal mining injuries occur at relatively high rates. In 1995, 156 mining workers were killed. The number of fatal accidents per 1,000 employees is the highest of all industry divisions, and more than four times the national average. Additionally, nonfatal injuries in mining tend to be more severe than those in the private sector overall. While only 31 percent of injuries and illnesses in the private sector are severe enough to result in days away from work, more than 50 percent of the mining injuries and illnesses result in days away from work. The median number of days missed is 12 for injured or ill mining workers, more than twice the average for all industries. More than a third of those injuries and illnesses are severe enough to result in more than 31 days away from work.

Within the mining division, the coal mining industries have the highest rate of nonfatal injuries, 9.1 per 100 full-time workers. The anthracite coal industry, which is concentrated in northeastern Pennsylvania, experienced 13.7 injuries or illnesses per 100 full-time workers, placing it among the 15 industries with the highest incidence rates.

Oil and gas extraction experienced a much lower incidence rate, 5.9 per 100 full-time workers, although the injury and illness rate varied dramatically by activity within the industry. The crude petroleum and natural gas industry, which includes research and administrative activities, experienced 2.3 injuries or illnesses per 100 full-time workers. The oil and gas field services industry, drilling and maintaining wells, had an injury and illness rate more than three times higher than the former.

Metals mining and quarrying experienced injury and illness rates of more than five per 100 full-time workers. Both major groups are involved principally in digging material out of open pits, so the perils associated with underground mining are largely absent. The dimension stone industry, which involves quarrying large blocks of stone, had an injury and illness rate of 9.1. This is substantially higher than the rate in industries involved in quarrying sand, gravel, clay, and other more tractable commodities.

See also MINE SAFETY AND HEALTH; SURVEY OF OCCUPATIONAL INJURIES AND ILLNESSES.

extrinsic allergic alveolitis   See HYPERSENSITIVITY PNEUMONITIS.

eye injuries/protection   An estimated 1,000 eye injuries occur in American workplaces each day, according to the U.S. Department of Labor's Occupational Safety and Health Administration (OSHA). More than $300 million per year is spent on lost production time, medical expenses, and workers' compensation due to eye injuries.

A major factor contributing to eye injuries at work is not wearing eye protection. Nearly three out of every five workers injured were not wearing eye protection at the time of the accident in a study by the Bureau of Labor Statistics (BLS). Wearing the wrong kind of eye protection for the job is related to many accidents. About 40 percent of the injured workers were wearing some form of eye protection when the accident occurred. These workers were most likely to be wearing protective eyeglasses with no side shields, though injuries to employees wearing full-cup or flat-fold side-shields occurred as well.

Flying particles are a major cause of eye injuries. The BLS survey found that almost 70 percent of accidents studied results from flying or falling objects or sparks striking the eye. Injured workers estimated that nearly three-fifths of the objects were smaller than a pinhead. Most of the particles were said to be traveling faster than a hand-thrown object when the accident occurred.

Contact with chemicals caused one-fifth of the injuries in the BLS study. Other accidents were caused by objects swinging from a fixed or attached position, such as tree limbs, ropes, chains, or tools which were pulled into the eye while the worker was using them.

Potential eye hazards exist in nearly every industry, but the BLS reported that more than 40 percent of injuries occurred among craft workers, such as mechanics, repairers, carpenters, and plumbers. More than a third of the injured workers were operatives, such as assemblers, sanders, and grinding machine operators. Laborers suffered about one-fifth of the eye injuries. Almost half the injured workers were employed in manufacturing. Slightly more than 20 percent were in construction. Those engaged in professional sports are also at high risk for eye injuries.

Common Workplace Hazards and Injuries

Common hazards include dust, concrete, and metal particles, falling or shifting debris, building materials, glass, smoke, noxious/poisonous gases, chemicals (acids, bases, fuels, solvents, lime, wet or dry cement powder), welding light and electrical arc, thermal hazards and fires, and bloodborne pathogens (hepatitis or HIV) from blood, body fluids, or human remains.

Common injuries include corneal abrasions and conjunctivitis (red eyes), concrete, metal particles, or slivers embedded in the eye, chemical splash or burn, welder's flashburn, eyeball laceration, facial contusion and black eye, bloodborne pathogen exposure from blood or other body fluids or human remains.

Steps to Reduce
Eye Injuries in the Workplace

OSHA and the states and territories operating their own job safety and health programs are working to help reduce eye injuries. Together with efforts by concerned voluntary groups, OSHA has a nationwide information campaign to improve workplace eye protection. Additionally, the National Society to Prevent Blindness has developed information and training materials for preventing eye injuries at work. Its 26 affiliates nationwide also provide consultation in developing effective eye safety programs.

TIPS FOR WORKPLACE EYE SAFETY

Have a safe work environment
Minimize hazards from falling or unstable debris.
Make sure that tools work and safety features (machine guards) are in place.
Be sure that workers, particularly volunteers, know how to use tools properly.

Keep bystanders out of the hazardous area.
Evaluate your safety hazards
Know your primary hazards.
Recognize hazards from nearby workers, large machinery, and falling/shifting debris.
Wear proper eye and face protection
Select appropriate eye protection for the hazard.
Make sure the eye protection is in good condition.
Make sure it fits properly and will stay in place.
Eye/face protection devices should not be relied upon to provide complete protection.
Prepare for eye injuries and first aid needs
Have an eye wash or sterile solutions on hand.

Protective Eyewear

Minimally, safety glasses are required at many workplaces. Safety glasses should be worn for general working conditions where there may be minor dust, chips, or flying particles. Use safety glasses with side protection such as side shields or wraparound style. Use safety glasses with antifog treatment. Use an eyewear retainer to keep the glasses tight to the face or hanging from the neck if not in use.

Goggles are better protection than safety glasses. Use goggles for higher-impact protection, greater dust, chemical splash, and welding light protection. Goggles for splash or fine dust protection should have indirect venting. Use direct vented goggles for less fogging when working with large particles. Safety goggles designed like ski goggles, with high air flow, minimize fogging while providing better particle and splash protection.

Hybrid safety glasses/goggles are safety glasses with foam or rubber around the lens. They provide better protection from dust and flying particles than conventional safety glasses with only side shields. Wraparound safety glasses that convert to goggles with a soft plastic or rubber face seal may offer better peripheral vision than conventional goggles.

For even greater face protection, a shield can be used over safety glasses/goggles. Use a face shield for highest impact, full-face protection from spraying, chipping, grinding, and critical chemical or bloodborne hazards. Face shields may be tinted or metal coated for heat and splatter protection. The curve of the face shield will direct particles or chemicals coming from the side into the eyes. Safety glasses or goggles should always be worn under a face shield.

In addition to helmets, welders should wear lenses for welding light protection marked with a "shade number" (1.5–14; 14 is the darkest). Eyes should be protected even when the helmet is lifted up. The welder, welder's helpers, and bystanders should be similarly protected.

Respirators, either full face or half mask, provide the best general dust, chemical, and smoke protection. When half-face respirators are used, the respirator must not interfere with the proper positioning of the eye protection.

Protection for Workers Wearing Prescription Eyeglasses/Contact Lenses

Workers who wear prescription glasses should wear tight-fitting goggles over normal streetwear glasses or contact lenses. Goggles should also be worn over prescription safety glasses in high dust environments. If worn alone, prescription safety glasses must have side shields. Prescription safety lenses with tempered glass or acrylic plastic lenses are not suitable for high impact. These types of safety glasses should not be used when working in debris areas unless covered by goggles or face shields. Polycarbonate lenses should be used when working in high impact areas. New safety glasses with polycarbonate lenses should be hard-coated to reduce scratching. Contact lenses may present a significant corneal abrasion risk when working in dusty areas unless tight fitting goggles or a full face respirator are worn. Full face respirators will not seal properly over streetwear glasses or safety glasses. Prescription inserts compatible with a respirator should be used. Respirators should be professionally fitted.

The National Institute for Occupational Safety and Health also recommends that workers should brush, shake, or vacuum dust and debris from hard hats, hair, forehead, or the top of the eye protection before removing the protection. Beware of rubbing eyes with dirty hands or clothing. Clean eyewear regularly.

For further information:

International Safety Equipment Association (ISEA)
1901 N. Moore Street
Suite 808
Arlington, VA 22209
(703) 525-1695
(703) 528-2148 (fax)
http://www.safetyequipment.org

American Society of Safety Engineers (ASSE)
1800 E. Oakton Street
Des Plaines, IL 60018
(847) 699-2929
(847) 768-3434 (fax)
http://asse.org

Prevent Blindness America
500 E. Remington Road
Schaumburg, IL 60173-5611
(800) 331-2020 (toll-free)
(847) 843-2020
(847) 843-8458 (fax)
http://www.preventblindness.org

See also CHEMICAL TOXICITY; PERSONAL PROTECTIVE EQUIPMENT; VIDEO DISPLAY TERMINALS.

U.S. Department of Labor, Occupational Safety and Health Administration: Program Highlights, Fact Sheet No. OSHA 92-03.

Fair Labor Standards Act (FLSA) The Fair Labor Standards Act of 1938 provides for minimum standards for both wages and overtime entitlement, and spells out administrative procedures by which covered worktime must be compensated. Included in the act are provisions related to child labor, equal pay, and door-to-door activities. The act exempts specified employees or groups of employees from the application of certain of its provisions. The FLSA affects more than 80 million full-time and part-time workers in the private sector and in federal, state, and local governments.

The U.S. Office of Personnel Management (OPM) works with Federal agencies to apply the FLSA to employees of the U.S. federal government. The OPM's regulations are published in Part 551 of Title 5, Code of Federal Regulations. Changes to the Code of Federal Regulations are published in the *Federal Register.*

See also CHILD LABOR.

falling merchandise Items from store shelves may fall and injure a worker or customer. Such injuries are also known as "big box" injuries, as many occur in warehouse-style retail establishments that sell large items in large containers. Since 1990 thousands of people have been injured and some killed by falling merchandise in retail warehouses. Fallen items range from doors, hot water heaters, and televisions to housewares and toys.

Falling merchandise incidents have the following common characteristics:

- High stacking. Safety experts say high stacking is storage of merchandise on the sales floor above eye level. A sales clerk must stretch, use a ladder or step stool, or climb on shelves to handle merchandise.

- Unsecured merchandise. Typically, stores do not use restraining safety devices such as security bars, fencing, safety ties, and shelf extenders on high shelves because of the expense involved and the employee time it might take to use them.

- Triggering events. Falling merchandise can be triggered by moving merchandise that has been stacked in an unstable manner; moving merchandise on one shelf in such a way that merchandise on an adjacent shelf falls, referred to as "push through"; stacking different size boxes on top of each other, and stacking heavy merchandise on top of lighter merchandise. Vibrations, merchandise left hanging over the lip of a shelf, and merchandise too large for a shelf can also cause the problem.

- No warning of danger. Merchandise usually falls without any warning to an unsuspecting worker or customer. Even though merchants know of the risk of falling merchandise and the potential for serious injury to workers or customers, many do not give warnings of the risks with signs, banners, or placards.

- Improper training. Often store personnel are improperly trained, or not trained at all, in stocking techniques or in recognizing and correcting the hazards of falling merchandise. Many incidents could be prevented if merchants trained employees in procedures for recognizing hazards and made sure that the merchandise is safely stacked.

See also LADDERS; SLIPS, TRIPS, and FALLS.

falls/fall protection   See CONSTRUCTION; SLIPS, TRIPS, and FALLS.

Family and Medical Leave Act of 1993 (FMLA)   A federal law, covering businesses with 50 or more employees, that mandates 12 weeks of unpaid leave for qualified employees for the birth or adoption of a child and when they or a family member have a serious health condition during a 12-month period. Employers must continue health insurance and guarantee a job on return from leave. The U.S. Department of Labor's Employment Standards Administration, Wage, and Hour Division administers and enforces the FMLA for all private, state, and local government employees, and some federal employees.

FMLA is accepted by workers and corporations because of its positive effect on retention of qualified employees.

"Serious health condition" means an illness, injury, impairment, or physical or mental condition that involves either (1) any period of incapacity or treatment connected with inpatient care in hospital, hospice, or residential medical care facilities or (2) continuing treatment by a health care provider including any period of incapacity, such as inability to work, attend school, or perform regular daily activities due to:

1. A health condition (including treatment therefor, or recovery therefrom) lasting more than three consecutive days, and any subsequent treatment or period of incapacity relating to the same condition that also includes treatment two or more times by or under the supervision of a health care provider, or one treatment by a health care provider with continuing regiment of treatment; or

2. Pregnancy or prenatal care. A visit to the health care provider is not necessary for each absence; or

3. A chronic serious health condition that continues over an extended period of time, requires periodic visits to a health care provider, and may involve occasional episodes of incapacity (such as asthma, diabetes). A visit to a health care provider is not necessary for each absence; or

4. A permanent long-term condition for which treatment may not be effective (such as Alzheimer's disease, a severe stroke, or terminal cancer). Only supervision by a health care provider is required, rather than active treatment, or

5. Any absence to receive multiple treatments for restorative surgery or for a condition that would likely result in a period of incapacity of more than three days if not treated (such as chemotherapy or radiation treatments for cancer).

Utilization of the FMLA is on the increase. According to Jane Waldfogel, writing in the *Monthly Labor Review,* "surveys indicate that family and medical leave is becoming a more important part of the experience of employers and employees. On the employer side, more establishments are offering family and medical leave policies, in many instances going beyond what is required.

The government estimates that in one year alone, from 1999 to 2000, between 4.1 million and 6.1 million workers used FMLA. There appears to be an increase in use of leave by men, particularly for the birth or adoption of a child.

Waldfogel, Jane. "Family and Medical Leave: Evidence from the 2000 Surveys." *Monthly Labor Review* September 2001. vol 124 No. 9 p. 17–23.

Kleiman Carol, "More Are Using Family Leave Act, Especially Men," *Chicago Tribune,* February 5, 2002.

U.S. Department of Labor Fact Sheet No. 028 http://www.dol.gov/dolesa/public/regs/compliance/whd/whdfs28.htm.

farmer's lung   See HYPERSENSITIVITY PNEUMONITIS; WHEEZING.

farming   The greatest workplace hazard for farmworkers is from musculoskeletal injuries, such as sprains and traumatic injuries. Farmers face hazards because of the repetitive nature of much labor-intensive farmwork; there is a great deal of bending or stooping to reach crops. Some harvesting tasks may require the worker to carry or lift heavy bags full of the harvested commodity, often while balancing on a ladder.

According to author Marc B. Schenker, one of the most serious causes of fatal injuries to farm workers is motor vehicle accidents. These often occur when workers are driving or being driven to or from fields early or late in the day on unsafe rural roads; collisions may also occur with slow-moving farm equipment such as tractors.

Large and small tractors are used on many farms; tractor attachments include tillers, carts, snow blowers, and trimmers. These tractors all have engines, use fuel, have moving parts, and carry an operator, and are often used with towed or mounted equipment. Some tractors, although small, can be overturned and cause serious injury. According to Deere and Company, a farm equipment manufacturer, the fuel used on these tractors poses a fire hazard.

Author M. L. Myers reports that children riding with adults have fallen from tractors and been crushed under the wheels or chopped by mower blades. Mowers pose two types of hazards: One is potential contact with rotating blades and the other is being struck by objects thrown from the blades. Both front-end loaders and blades are operated hydraulically; if left unattended and elevated, they are a hazard of falling on anyone under the attachment.

Farmworkers experience respiratory symptoms and disease from exposure to dust and chemicals. In dry climate farming, inorganic dust exposure may result in chronic bronchitis and dust-borne lung diseases.

Skin diseases are a common work-related health problem among farmworkers. They also experience trauma from using hand equipment such as clippers; irritants and allergens in agrochemicals; allergenic plant and animal materials, including poison ivy and poison oak, nettles, and other irritating plants; skin infections caused or worsened by heat or prolonged water contact; and sun exposure (skin cancer).

Sources of Stress

Farmers have little CONTROL over their lives; weather affects their yield, international trade dictates their prices, and government subsidies affect their income. For many families, farming is a way of life and comes with a whole set of values, standards, mores and characteristics.

Currently, farming as a vocation is also threatened by a lack of respect from the public because many farmers have to rely on government subsidies to make their livelihood. This lack of respect, added to the farmer's stress, pressure and frustration, can result in physical violence, first focused on the spouse, and then on the children. This is a major social problem, but one that cannot be really addressed because of the private, independent nature of farmers who live in relative isolation and have few options on how to change their lot.

According to an article in *Canadian Family Physician* (February 1992), farmers are disadvantaged by rural society traits, such as inability to express emotions and pride that are barriers to seeking help for their stress.

See also CHILD LABOR; DUST AND DEBRIS; FRUSTRATION; LADDERS; LUNG DISEASES; POISON IVY; STRESS; WHEEZING.

Kahn, Ada P. *Stress A–Z: A Sourcebook for Facing Everyday Challenges*. New York: Facts On File, Inc., 1998.
Myers, Melvin L. "Urban Agriculture." *Encyclopaedia of Occupational Health and Safety*. 4th ed. Vol. 3, p. 64.8. Geneva: International Labor Organization, 1998.
Schenker, Marc B. "Migrant and seasonal farmworkers." *Encyclopaedia of Occupational Health and Safety*. 4th ed. Vol. 3, p. 64.7–64.9. Geneva: International Labor Organization, 1998.

fatalities by occupation   Fatalities are highest among truck drivers followed by tractor-related farm accidents, sales occupations, and construction. However, the occupations with the largest number of fatalities are not always those with the highest risk, according to *Compensation and Working Conditions* (winter 1998). The highest risk occupations in 1997 were timber cutters and fishers.

See also CONSTRUCTION; FISHING; HIGH RISK OCCUPATIONS; LOGGING.

fatigue   See CHRONIC FATIGUE SYNDROME.

Federal Employees Compensation Act   A federal law providing workers' compensation coverage to 3 million federal and postal workers for employment-related injuries and occupational diseases. Benefits include wage replacement, payment for medical care, and where necessary, medical and vocational rehabilitation assistance in returning to work.

During fiscal year 2000, more than 176,000 new cases were created, and the program provided nearly 273,000 workers slightly more than $2 billion in benefits for work-related injuries and illnesses. Of those benefit payments, nearly $1.137 billion was for wage loss compensation, $549 million was for medical and rehabilitation services, and $107 million was for death benefit payments to surviving dependents.

See also WORKERS' COMPENSATION.

U.S. Department of Labor.

feedback   Objective information given by a supervisor, coworker, instructor, or others in a SUPPORT GROUP, to an individual who is seeking comments about his or her actions or suggestions. It is a sharing of feelings or thoughts and ideally should be given without evaluating consequences to the individual or demanding that he make a change. Negative feedback, even when given with complete objectivity, can arouse defensiveness in the individual. Positive feedback, on the other hand, enhances SELF-ESTEEM and makes the individual feel good.

See also COMMUNICATION; LISTENING.

Feldenkrais method   See BODY THERAPIES.

female reproductive health   See DANCERS; REPRODUCTIVE TOXICITY.

feng shui   A way to improve the health of a workplace is to practice a philosophy that ensures harmony and good fortune. Such is the Chinese art of geomancy, or feng shui (also fung Shuia), which involves the proper alignment of objects with geographical features. In *Hemispheres* magazine (November 1993), John Goff translates *fung shuia* as "wind and water" and defines it as "a product of a culture that honors the spirits of mountains and rivers and views the landscape as a living thing with cosmic currents."

Practiced first in Hong Kong where it influenced the design of many corporate buildings, including Citicorp International and Motorola Semiconduc-

tor's Hong Kong, Ltd., feng shui has spread to other parts of the world as well. Factors that can improve the well-being of a workplace are listed below.

USE FENG SHUI TO IMPROVE THE WELL-BEING OF A WORKPLACE

- Entryways and windows should be wide enough to allow light, which symbolizes the Sun and allows good energy to come in.
- Mirrors are particularly useful in cramped spaces and over furniture that does not face windows or doors because they reflect positive energy and deflect negative forces.
- Buildings near water are good because water is an element of wealth, insight, and motivation. Avoid building near tall buildings because they block positive energy and on cul de sacs because negative energy has no place to escape.

---

fiddler's chin   A dermatological condition seen in musicians as a result of the pressure of the chin rest against the player's neck and chin. For most musicians fiddler's chin is a source of annoyance as well as being unattractive. In many players it becomes cystic and secondarily infected, requiring draining and/or antibiotic therapy, and occasionally necessitating a rest from playing the instrument. Excision should rarely, if ever, be performed because of the inevitable continued friction at the site. The potential problems caused by a scar in the area may be worse than those posed by the original dermatitis.

See also MUSICIANS' INJURIES; PERFORMING ARTS MEDICINE.

Sataloff, Robert Thayer, Alice G. Brandfonbrener, and Richard J. Lederman. *Textbook of Performing Arts Medicine.* New York: Raven Press, 1991.

firefighters and rescue workers   Dangerous occupations that can involve deadly smoke, buildings collapsing, and heart attacks. Firefighters are often the first emergency responders at the scene of a vehicle crash, fire, flood, earthquake, or act of terrorism. About 2 million fires are reported each year in the United States, and fire departments respond to a fire every 18 seconds.

According to authors Cindy Clarke and Mark Zak, firefighters perform many duties to protect lives and minimize property destruction. Duties may include connecting hose lines to hydrants, operating pumps, or positioning ladders. They also rescue victims, administer medical aid, and salvage contents of buildings.

Clarke and Zak report that each year, on average, about 50 firefighters die from injuries on the job, accounting for about 1 percent of all fatal work injuries. In 1992–97, the total number of fatalities for firefighters was about 17 per 100,000 employed. This compares to five fatalities per 100,000 employed for all workers. Firefighters are about three times as likely to be fatally injured on the job as the average worker.

Despite efforts to reduce firefighter mortality with better protective equipment, breathing machines, and a buddy system that sends two firefighters into a burning building together, the number of deaths continues to rise. Fire and smoke are responsible for the largest proportion of deaths and for a high percentage of injuries, according to Kristin Kloberdanz, M.D., M.P.H., director of the Occupational Medicine Service at the University of Medicine and Dentistry of New Jersey.

According to Kloberdanz, the September 2001 attack on the World Trade Center saw the single highest count of firefighter deaths in the nation's history. The search also was dangerous for the firefighters sent in to replace those who had died. Every time rubble was moved, it created a vent for oxygen to feed the smoldering fires.

Other Hazards: Heart Disease and Cancer

Heart disease, either in the line of duty or years later, can develop as a result of cumulative job stress. The work is stressful because sites are often extremely hot and may be hostile. Firefighters and rescue workers wear heavy protective clothing and carry 75 to 90 pounds of equipment, including breathing apparatus. Additionally, rescue workers may find themselves in agonizing life-or-death situations, which can lead to depression or post-traumatic stress disorder (PTSD).

Firefighters and rescue workers also suffer a higher-than-normal risk of certain types of cancer, including bladder cancer and lymphoma, which experts attribute in part to the toxins that firefighters are exposed to inside burning buildings. While respirators and surplus air tanks are mandatory,

these safeguards do not prevent such toxic substances as BENZENE, ASBESTOS, and polycyclic aromatic hydrocarbons from entering the system.

Rescue workers also risk coming into contact with body fluids from victims, sprains and strains, cuts, and hearing loss, often caused by wailing sirens.

In additions to fighting building fires, firefighters are called on to control and extinguish forest fires. Some pilot aircraft to locate forest fires or use chain saws and axes to create fire trails, among other duties. Forest fires are particularly dangerous because they may increase enormously and rapidly and can surround firefighters who are trying to put them out.

See also ASBESTOS; CARBON MONOXIDE; DUST AND DEBRIS; ELECTRICITY-RELATED INJURIES; HAND AND POWER TOOLS; HEART ATTACK; HEALTH CARE WORKERS; HEPATITIS C; LADDERS; NOISE; PERSONAL PROTECTIVE EQUIPMENT; POLICE AND DETECTIVES; SLIPS, TRIPS AND FALLS.

Clarke, Cindy, and Mark J. Zak. "Fatalities to Law Enforcement Officers and Firefighters, 1992–1997." *Compensation and Working Conditions,* summer 1999, p. 3–7.
NIOSH. *Preventing Injuries and Deaths of Fire Fighters Due to Structural Collapse.* Publication No. 99-146, August 1999.
NIOSH ALERT. *Preventing Injuries and Deaths of Fire Fighters.* September 1994. DHHS (NIOSH) Publication No. 94-125.

fire safety/fire protection   Workplace fires and explosions kill 200 and injure more than 5,000 workers each year, according to the U.S. Department of Labor. In 1995 more than 75,000 workplace fires cost businesses more than $2.3 million. According to the National Safety Council, fires and burns account for 3.3 percent of all occupational fatalities. According to then Secretary of Labor Robert Reich, "Fires wreak havoc among workers and their families and destroy thousands of businesses each year, putting people out of work and severely impacting their livelihoods. The human and financial toll underscores the serious nature of workplace fires."

He continued: "There is a long and tragic history of workplace fires in this country. One of the most notable was the 1911 fire at the Triangle Shirtwaist Factory in New York City, in which nearly 150 women and young girls died because of locked fire exits and inadequate fire extinguishing systems. That tragedy helped put basic workplace safety and health considerations on the national agenda."

History repeated itself several years ago in the fire in Hamlet, North Carolina, where 25 workers died in a fire in a poultry processing plant. It appears that here, too, there were problems with fire exits and extinguishing systems.

BASIC TIPS FOR FIRE SAFETY IN THE WORKPLACE

Eliminate fire hazards
Keep workspaces free of waste paper and other combustibles, replace damaged electrical cords, and avoid overloaded circuits.

Prepare for emergencies
Make sure all smoke detectors work, know who to call in an emergency, and participate in fire drills.

Report fires and emergencies promptly
Sound the fire alarm and call the fire department.

Evacuate safely
Leave the area quickly in an emergency. Use stairs instead of the elevator, and help your coworkers.

Occupational Safety and Health Administration (OSHA) standards require employers to provide proper exits, firefighting equipment, and employee training to prevent fire deaths and injuries in the workplace. When OSHA conducts workplace inspections, it checks to see whether employers are complying with OSHA standards for fire safety.

OSHA Standards for Fire Protection and Safety

- *Fire exits.* Each workplace building must have at least two means of escape remote from each other to be used in a fire emergency. Fire doors must not be blocked or locked to prevent emergency use when employees are within the buildings. Delayed opening of fire doors is permitted when an approved alarm system is integrated into the fire door design. Exit routes from buildings must be clear and free of obstructions and properly marked with signs designating exits from the building.

- *Portable fire extinguishers.* Each workplace building must have a full complement of the proper type of fire extinguisher for the fire hazards present, excepting when the employer wishes to have employees evacuate instead of fighting small fires.

- Employees are expected or anticipated to use fire extinguishers, must be instructed on the hazards of fighting fire, how to properly operate the fire extinguisher available, and what procedures to follow in alerting others to the fire emergency.

- Only approved fire extinguishers are permitted to be used in workplaces, and they must be kept in good operating condition. Proper maintenance and inspection of this equipment is required of each employer.

- Where the employer wishes to evacuate employees instead of having them fight small fires there must be written emergency plans and employee training for proper evacuation.

EMERGENCY EVACUATION PLANNING

- Emergency action plans are required to describe the routes to use and procedures to be followed by employees. Also, procedures for accounting for all evacuated employees must be part of the plan. The written plan must be available for employee review.

- Where needed, special procedures for helping physically impaired employees must be addressed in the plan; also, the plan must include procedures for those employees who must remain behind temporarily to shut down critical plant equipment before they evacuate.

- The preferred means of alerting employees to a fire emergency must be part of the plan and an employee alarm system must be available through the workplace complex and must be used for emergency alerting for evacuation. The alarm system may be voice communication or sound signals such as bells, whistle, or horns. Employees must know the evacuation signal.

- Training of all employees in emergency action is required. Employers must review the plan with newly assigned employees so they know correct actions in an emergency and with all employees when the plan is changed.

FIRE PREVENTION PLAN

- Employers need to implement a written fire prevention plan to complement the fire evacuation plan to minimize the frequency of evacuation. Stopping unwanted fires from occurring is the most efficient way to handle them. The written plan must be available for employee review.

- Housekeeping procedures for storage and cleanup of flammable materials and flammable waste must be included in the plan. Recycling of flammable waste such as paper is encouraged. However, handling and packaging procedures must be included in the plan.

- Procedures for controlling workplace ignition sources such as smoking, welding, and burning must be addressed in the plan. Heat-producing equipment such as burners, heat exchangers, boilers, ovens, stoves, fryers, and other equipment must be properly maintained and kept clean of accumulations of flammable residues. Flammables must not be stored close to these pieces of equipment.

- All employees are to be apprised of the potential fire hazards of their job and the procedures called for in the employer's fire prevention plan. The plan shall be reviewed with all new employees when they begin their job and with all employees when the plan is changed.

FIRE SUPPRESSION SYSTEM

- Properly designed and installed fixed fire suppression systems enhance fire safety in the workplace. Automatic sprinkler systems throughout the workplace are among the most reliable firefighting means. The fire sprinkler system detects the fire, sounds an alarm and put the water where the fire and heat are located.

- Automatic fire suppression systems require proper maintenance to keep them in serviceable condition. When it is necessary to take a fire suppression system out of service while business continues, the employer must temporarily assemble a fire watch of trained employees standing by to respond quickly to any fire emergency in the normally protected area. The fire watch must interface with the employers' fire prevention plan and emergency action plan.

- Signs must be posted around areas protected by total flooding fire suppression systems which use agents that are a serious health hazards such as carbon dioxide, Halon 1211, and others. Such automatic systems must be equipped with area predischarge alarm systems to warn employees of the impending discharge of the system and allow time to evacuate the area. There must be an emergency action plan to provide for the safe evacuation of employees from within the protected area. Such plans are to be part of the overall evacuation plan for the workplace facility.

Under OSHA regulations, workers have the right to complain to OSHA about fire hazards in their workplaces. If employees request it, OSHA will keep their identities confidential to avoid the possibility of reprisals by their employers.

See also CONSTRUCTION; COMPRESSED GAS AND EQUIPMENT; FIREFIGHTERS: HAZARD COMMUNICATION; NATIONAL FIRE PROTECTION ASSOCIATION.

Adapted from Occupational Safety and Health Administration, News Release USDL: 96-423

fish cutters   See BUTCHERS AND MEAT, POULTRY, AND FISH CUTTERS.

fishing   Although commercial fishing, like many other occupations, is considerably less dangerous today than in the past, it is still the single most deadly occupation according to the Bureau of Labor Statistics CENSUS OF FATAL OCCUPATIONAL INJURIES (CFOI).

Fishers face a risk of death on the job that is 20 to 30 times greater than any other single occupation. Between 1992 and 1996 (the latest year for which data are available), between 50 and 100 fishing deaths occurred each year. This translates into 140 deaths per 100,000 workers engaged in the occupation over the period. For occupations as a whole over the same period, the fatality rate was five per 100,000.

As described by the Bureau of Labor Statistics in the article "Fishing for a Living Is Dangerous Work" (Compensation and Working Conditions, summer 1998), fishing boats often travel great distances, far from the safety of home ports. Storms in the open seas can have tremendous destructive power that can sink a typical fishing boat. Ocean storms have been known to produce waves of more than 200 feet high ("rogue waves"). Perils such as striking an underwater object or colliding with another vessel in the fog can have disastrous results.

Vessel casualties were the leading cause of fishing deaths, often involving multiple fatalities, from 1992 through 1996. Half of fishing deaths, 197, involved sinking, capsizing, collisions, explosions, and fires (see chart).

Falls from the ship or boat can result from tripping over or being caught in fishing gear, slipping on a wet or icy deck, being pulled overboard by a hook caught in clothing, or having a fishing line wrap around the legs. Falls accounted for almost one-fifth of all fishing fatalities, or 70 deaths during the 1992–96 period.

Shellfishers are more at risk of dying on the job than are finfishers. During 1992–96, shellfishing, with 160 fatalities, accounted for one-third more deaths than finfishing, with 119 fatalities. Yet the shellfishing industry employed just three-fifths as many workers as the finfishing industry.

Certified divers are often hired to assist fishers and face hazards such as poor weather conditions, murky water, unexpected underwater currents, snagged air lines, equipment malfunction, decompression problems, and dangerous marine life. Drownings accounted for one-sixth of the recorded fishing deaths between 1992 and 1996; most were diving related.

Fishers who go overboard into extremely cold water risk hypothermia and can last only six to seven minutes immersed before dying. Alaska, with one of the United States's smallest workforces, accounted for the largest number (112) of fishing deaths in 1992–96 (see chart). In Alaska, harvesting most commercial crab species takes place during the winter, when air and sea temperatures are at their lowest; high winds, snow, sleet, ice, and high seas are common and daylight hours shorter. Other cold-water states, such as Maine, Massachusetts, Oregon, and Washington, also had disproportionately high numbers of fishing deaths.

Other hazards facing the fishing industry are typical of other workplaces, such as electrocutions, being caught in winches and other machinery, homicides, and aircraft crashes.

FISHING OCCUPATION* FATALITIES BY STATE, 1992–1996

State	Number	Percent
Total	380	100
Alaska	112	29
Massachusetts	32	8
Texas	31	8
Florida	26	7
Oregon	21	6
California	21	6
Washington	20	5
Louisiana	18	5
North Carolina	18	5
Maine	17	4
Hawaii	14	4
Other**	50	13

*Includes fishers, captains, and other fishing vessel officers.
**These 50 fishing fatalities are distributed over the remaining 30 states and the District of Columbia. They also include seven fatalities occurring outside any state or territorial waters. None of these states accounted for more than five fishing fatalities.

For further information contact:

Bureau of Labor Statistics
U.S. Department of Labor
Office of Safety, Health and Working Conditions

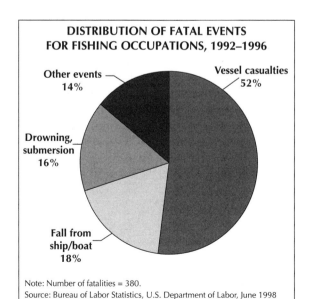

DISTRIBUTION OF FATAL EVENTS FOR FISHING OCCUPATIONS, 1992–1996

Other events 14%
Vessel casualties 52%
Drowning, submersion 16%
Fall from ship/boat 18%

Note: Number of fatalities = 380.
Source: Bureau of Labor Statistics, U.S. Department of Labor, June 1998

Postal Square Building
Room 2850
2 Massachusetts Ave NE
Washington, DC 20212-0001
(202) 691-7800
(202) 691-7797 (fax)
http://www.bls.gov

See also MACHINE ACCIDENTS.

Adapted with permission from Drudi, Dino. "Fishing for a Living is Dangerous Work," *Compensation and Working Conditions,* summer 1998, p. 3–7.

fishmeal worker's lung   See WHEEZING.

flexible work hours   Work hours that vary and may be arranged to suit the convenience of employees, such as working mothers. In her *Chicago Tribune* column, "Worklife" (June 12, 2001), writer Carol Kleiman reported on two studies that found advantages to flexible work hours. One study was by Flexible Resources, Inc., a consulting and staffing firm based in Cos Cob, Connecticut, that specialized in permanent jobs with flexible hours. The other is by Catalyst, a nonprofit agency in New York that works with businesses to advance women.

The research reported that job assignments are satisfying even though promotions are slow. Salaries are surprisingly good. Both studies included women only because they are more likely to work flexible schedules.

Both studies focused on high-ranking, well-educated, experienced professionals and did not include employees in support or administrative jobs. Lower level employees are less likely to be allowed flexible hours and more often are required to be on the job site during specific periods.

Kleiman quoted Linda Coletti, a marketing executive at a consumer product company in Stamford, Connecticut. "There's been a tremendous change in employers' attitudes since I started working flexible hours eight years ago. Some companies viewed you as a second-class citizen, but now your experience is valued."

See also WORKING MOTHERS.

Kleinman, Carol. "Price Is Right for Flexible Work Hours." *Chicago Tribune.* June 12, 2001.

fluoride   See AUTOIMMUNE DISORDERS; MUSCULOSKELETAL TOXICITY.

flutist's chin   A dermatological condition that professional flutists may encounter. This involves contact dermatitis on the lips from prolonged contact with a metal alloy mouthpiece. Acne mechanica or localized acneiform eruption of the lips can occur as a result of repetitive mechanical pressure, friction, or rubbing.

See also DERMATITIS (OCCUPATIONAL); PERFORMING ARTS MEDICINE.

food service industry   An industry that employs a wide variety of workers, from cooks, bakers, and chefs, to servers, buyers, accountants, managers, and maintenance personnel. Hazards for kitchen workers include slips, trips, and falls, back injuries from lifting heavy pots and other equipment, and cuts and burns. Skin irritations can result from having hands in water and using cleaning materials for kitchen equipment.

Protective equipment for kitchen workers includes nonslip shoes and hand protection if sharp knives are used. If working with gas, workers should know where the gas shut-off valve is and know the emergency procedure for gas leaks. To avoid electric shock, splashproof or waterproof electrical appliances should be provided and enough outlets should be available to avert the need for adapters or extension cords. To protect against fire hazards, exhaust fans and hoods should be cleaned to prevent residue buildup, rubbish should be disposed of appropriately, and workers should know where the fire extinguishers are kept and how to use them.

Hazardous cleaning materials such as oven cleaners should be labeled with information on how to use the product. The material safety data sheet (MSDS) accompanying the product should be available.

See also COOKS; DERMATITIS; HOT ENVIRONMENTS; LADDERS; MATERIAL SAFETY DATA SHEETS; PERSONAL PROTECTIVE EQUIPMENT; REPETITIVE STRESS INJURIES; SLIPS, TRIPS, AND FALLS; TEENAGE WORKERS.

Flying Physicians Association   See AEROSPACE MEDICINE.

football injuries (professional) Injuries to players can often be prevented with use of proper equipment, enforcement of rules, and the presence of health professionals at games and practices.

Clipping or hitting a player in the legs from behind can break a leg or tear knee ligaments, depending on what gives way. Grabbing the face mask can break a neck. Piling on can break a leg. Head slapping with the forearm can perforate an eardrum.

Helmets should be reconditioned and recertified frequently. Protective pads can wear down, and pants can lose their stretch so that the thigh pads slip, leaving a player vulnerable to a disabling thigh bruise.

Summer practices and warm-weather games played with a full load of equipment covering the body can lead to heat exhaustion or heat stroke. Heat exhaustion results from loss of fluids and natural body salts. Heat stroke is a medical emergency due to failure of the body's internal thermostat and is a major cause of death on the football field.

See also HOT ENVIRONMENTS; SPORTS MEDICINE.

Levy, A. M., and Fuerst, M. L. *Sports Injury Handbook.* New York: Wiley, 1993.

foot protection In any given year, there are about 120,000 job-related foot injuries, one-third of them toe injuries, according to the National Safety Council. When a job requires standing for long periods or working in potentially hazardous areas or with potentially hazardous materials, there is some risk of foot injury.

Recent Bureau of Labor Statistics research shows that injuries to feet and toes that required days away from work have been reduced significantly since 1994 when the Occupational Safety and Health Administration (OSHA) launched its first formal hazard assessment program. This program required employer personal protective equipment (PPE) programs. Foot injuries have been reduced by 21 percent, toe injuries by 39 percent, and combination foot and toe injuries by 35 percent.

If your feet are injured at work, report the injury to your supervisor promptly for necessary first aid. Then see a podiatrist if further treatment is recom-

mended. Proper foot care improves your efficiency and keeps you on the job.

Many injuries can be prevented by keeping your feet healthy and following safe work practices.

FOLLOW SAFE PRACTICES: AVOID WORKPLACE FOOT INJURIES

The following tips from the American Podiatric Medical Association can help prevent foot injuries:

- Be aware of the hazards of your job and the proper protective measures.
- Take time to do your job right. Do not take unnecessary risks.
- Be alert. Watch for hidden hazards.
- Be considerate. Watch out for other workers' safety.
- Follow the rules. Do not cut corners. Use equipment as specified.
- Concentrate on the job. Inattention can lead to accidents.
- Pace yourself. Work steadily at a comfortable speed.
- Keep your tools in place and your work area clean.

Protective Footwear Is Essential

Safety shoes and boots protect the feet, help prevent injuries to them, and reduce the severity of injuries that occur in the workplace. Only one of four victims of job-related foot injuries was wearing any type of safety shoe or boot, according to the National Safety Council. The remaining three either are unaware of the benefits of protective footwear or disregard it.

HAZARDS AND PROTECTIVE EQUIPMENT

The American Podiatric Medical Association suggests these guidelines for protective equipment against selected workplace hazards:

Falling and rolling objects, cuts and punctures
Protection: Steel-toe safety shoes; add-on devices; metatarsal guards, metal foot guards, puncture-proof inserts, shin guards.
Chemicals, solvents
Protection: Footwear with synthetic stitching, and made of rubber, vinyl, or plastic
Electric current
Protection: Shoes or boots with rubber soles and heels, and insulated steel toes
Extreme cold
Protection: Shoes or boots with moisture- or oil-resistant insulation and that can repel water (if this is a problem); insulated socks

HAZARDS AND PROTECTIVE EQUIPMENT (continued)

Extreme heat or direct flame
Protection: Overshoes or boots of fire-resistant materials
High voltage
Protection: Shoes with rubber or cork heels and soles, and no exposed metal parts
Hot surfaces
Protection: Safety shoes with wooden or other heat-resistant soles; wooden sandals; overshoes
Sanitation contamination
Protection: Special plastic booties or overshoes; paper or wood shower sandals
Slips and skids (from wet, oily shoes with wooden soles or cleated surfaces)
Protection: Nonslip rubber or neoprene soles; nonskid sandals that slip over shoes; strap-on cleats for icy surfaces
Sparking (from metal shoes parts)
Protection: Safety shoes with no metal parts and non-sparking material
Sparks, molten metal splashes
Protection: Foundry boots with elastic sides; quick-release buckles for speedy removal
Static electricity
Protection: Shoes or boots with heels and soles or cork or leather
Wetness
Protection: Lined rubber shoes or boots; rubbers or shoes of silicone-treated leather

---

Foot Injuries: Professional Athletes

In the United States, it is estimated that 15 percent of sport-related injuries affect the foot alone. In many sports, the foot absorbs tremendous shearing and leading forces, sometimes surpassing 20 times body weight. Although foot injuries can result from a variety of causes, the most common is trauma. Other causes include:

• Rapid or improper warm-up
• Overuse
• Intense workouts
• Improper footwear
• Hard playing surfaces

It is estimated that 5 percent to 10 percent of all sports related injuries involve stress fractures. Stress fractures are defined as spontaneous fractures of normal bone that result from the summation of stress, any of which by themselves would be harmless. Stress fractures of the foot were first described by Breihupt in 1855. Serving as a physi-cian in the Prussian army, Breihaupt observed fractures of the metatarsals in otherwise healthy military recruits after long marches. These became known as march fractures. Nine of the 24 members of the 1994 U.S. National World Cup Soccer Team were diagnosed with stress fractures.

Athletes returning to play after foot injury. Athletes should practice before they play, and the injury should be essentially pain free. Strength should be at least 90 percent of the unaffected limb. Mentally, athletes must feel confident that the foot injury has healed to the point where they can compete without conscious awareness of the injury. This can be assessed during practices.

See also BASEBALL INJURIES; BASKETBALL INJURIES; PERSONAL PROTECTIVE EQUIPMENT; SPORTS MEDICINE.

American Podiatric Medical Association.
9312 Old Georgetown Rd
Bethesda, MD 20814
(800) ASK APMA (toll-free)
(301) 371-9200
(301) 530-2752 (fax)
www.apna.org

Klein, John. "The Extremities of Safety: Hand and Foot Protection." *Compliance Magazine,* 9, no. 7 (July/August 2002).
National Safety Council.
Schanen, Dean E. and Timothy J. Rupp. "Athletic Foot Injuries." *Medicine Journal* 3, no. 5 (May 3, 2002).

forestry   See LOGGING.

forklift truck injuries   The forklift is a useful labor saving device with which millions of tons of materials and equipment are moved every day at the touch of a button. Industrial workplaces have come to rely on forklift trucks for their ability to lift and transport heavy loads around the plant. The power of forklifts makes them indispensable, but also dangerous. Often, when employees grow accustomed to using forklifts they stop thinking of them as a safety hazard and forget or neglect to follow important operating and maintenance procedures. When forklift injuries occur, they are usually serious due to the tremendous weight of the machines.

Forklift trucks come in various shapes and sizes:

* Industrial counterbalanced lift truck
* Industrial reach truck
* Rough terrain counterbalanced lift truck
* Telescope Materials handler
* Pedestrian-operated truck

No one should ride or operate a forklift truck except for a trained operator who is able to maintain control of the forklift and operate it smoothly when stopping, starting, lifting, and tilting.

Employees must be trained to work safely with forklifts, not just when they are hired but periodically thereafter. Refresher training for the experienced operator is just as important as first-time training for new employees, according to the Canadian Center for Occupational Health and Safety.

Forklift truck injuries can add heavy costs to the employers business. Even an incident without injury may result in costly damage to trucks, buildings, fittings, and the loads being handled.

In the United Kingdom, approximately 7,000–8,000 accidents a year involve lift trucks. Many of these are injuries where the value of life is permanently affected or fatalities occur. Approximately 20 fatalities occur per year using lift trucks. Lift truck accidents are frequently associated with lack of suitable and sufficient operator training.

formaldehyde   A chemical found in virtually all indoor workplace environments. The Occupational Safety and Health Administration (OSHA) estimates that approximately 2.1 million workers are exposed to formaldehyde. Workers most exposed include those in apparel, furniture, foundries, textile finishing, laboratories, paper mills, and plastic molding.

Formaldehyde is one of the most common chemicals in use today. As a chemical building block, its use can be traced to consumer goods through a wide spectrum of manufacturing processes. The major sources that have been reported and publicized include urea-formaldehyde foam insulation (UFFI) and particleboard or pressed wood products used in manufacturing

office furniture. It is used in consumer paper products that have been treated with UFFI resins, including grocery bags, facial tissues, and paper towels. Many cleaning agents contain formaldehyde. UFFI resins are used as stiffeners, wrinkle resisters, water repellants, fire retardants, and adhesive binders in floor coverings and carpet backings. Formaldehyde is also used as a preservative in medical laboratories and as an embalming agent in mortuaries.

Studies indicate that formaldehyde is a potential human CARCINOGEN. Airborne concentrations above 0.1 ppm (parts per million parts of air) can irritate the mucous membranes of the eyes, nose, and throat. The severity of irritation increases as concentrations increase. At 100 ppm it is immediately dangerous to life and health. Dermal contact causes various skin reactions including sensitization, which might force persons thus sensitized to find other work. The most widely reported symptoms from exposure to high levels of this chemical include irritation of the eyes and headaches. Until recently, the most serious of diseases attributed to formaldehyde exposure was ASTHMA. However, the ENVIRONMENTAL PROTECTION AGENCY (EPA) has recently conducted research that has caused formaldehyde to be strongly suspected of causing a rare type of throat cancer in long-term occupants of mobile homes.

OSHA Standard Protects Workers

To protect workers exposed to formaldehyde, the OSHA standard applies to formaldehyde gas, its solutions, and a variety of materials such as trioxane, paraformaldehyde, and resin formulations, and solids and mixtures containing formaldehyde that are sources of the substance. In addition to setting permissible exposure levels, exposure monitoring, and training, the standard requires medical surveillance and medical removal, recordkeeping, regulated areas, HAZARD COMMUNICATION, emergency procedures, primary reliance on engineering and work practices to control exposure, and maintenance and selection of PERSONAL PROTECTIVE EQUIPMENT.

The standard requires that employers conduct initial monitoring to identify all employees who are exposed to formaldehyde at or above the action level and to accurately determine the exposure of each employee so identified. If the exposure level is maintained below the action level, employers may discontinue exposure monitoring until there is a change which could affect exposure levels. The employer must also monitor employee exposure promptly upon receiving reports of formaldehyde-related signs and symptoms.

Employees who suffer significant adverse effects from formaldehyde exposure must be removed to jobs with less exposure until their condition improves. The medical removal protection benefits can continue for up to six months or until a physician determines that the employee will never be able to return to a job involving formaldehyde exposure (whichever occurs first).

Training is required at least annually for all employees exposed to formaldehyde concentrations of 0.1 ppm or greater. The training will increase employees' awareness of specific hazards in their workplace and of the control measures employed. Training also will assist successful medical surveillance and medical removal programs. These provisions are effective if employees know what signs or symptoms are related to the health effects of formaldehyde, if they know how to properly report them to the employers, and if they are periodically encouraged to do so.

Specific hazard labeling is needed for all forms of formaldehyde, including mixtures and solutions, and at certain levels, a warning that formaldehyde presents a potential cancer hazard if levels may potentially exceed 0.5 ppm.

See also AIR POLLUTION; ASSOCIATED LANDSCAPE CONTRACTORS OF AMERICA; CANCER; CHEMICAL TOXIC-ITY; INDOOR ENVIRONMENT; OCCUPATIONAL SAFETY AND HEALTH ADMINISTRATION.

fossil fuel burning   See AIR POLLUTION; CADMIUM.

foundries   See AIR POLLUTION; FORMALDEHYDE.

frostbite   See COLD ENVIRONMENTS.

frustration   Interference with an individual's impulses or desired actions by internal or external forces. Internal forces are inhibitions and mental conflict, and external forces can come from a supervisor, a coworker, instructors, friends, as well as the rules of society. Frustration results in deep feelings of discontent and tension because of unresolved problems, unfulfilled needs, or roadblocks to personal goals. Regardless of the cause, frustration is a health issue for many people in the workplace.

People who are repeatedly and constantly stressed by frustrations respond in many ways. A person who is mentally healthy usually deals with frustration in an acceptable way, sometimes with HUMOR. Others react with ANGER, HOSTILITY, AGGRESSION, OR DEPRESSION, while still others become withdrawn and passive.

See also CONTROL; COPING; GENERAL ADAPTATION SYNDROME; STRESS MANAGEMENT.

fungi   Organisms in workplace indoor air and elsewhere that can cause ALLERGIES, ASTHMA, lung diseases, and other respiratory problems and contribute to SICK BUILDING SYNDROME. The fungi that affect indoor air quality are multicellular organisms formed of microscopic branched filaments called hyphae. A visible colony of interwoven hyphae forms a mycelium, and the mycelliod fungi most commonly found indoors are called MOLDS; the terms *fungus* and *mold* are used interchangeably in this entry.

When windows in a workplace can be kept open, the kinds of fungi in indoor air normally reflect those in outdoor air. To grow and proliferate indoors, however, fungi require a suitable substrate such as wood, paper, gypsum board, or other materials that have a high cellulose content and water. Buildings where there is chronic water damage or where humidity levels are high are particularly at risk of fungal contamination.

Various aspects of fungal growth and structure have potential injurious effects on health. Certain species of fungi produce mycotoxins, natural organic compounds that initiate a toxic response in humans, including mucosal and skin irritation, immunosuppression, and systemic effects. The primary mode of human exposure to these toxic chemicals is by inhalation of spores or of material that has been contaminated by mold. Some people develop allergies, such as rhinitis and asthma, when exposed to molds. Heavy and repeated exposure to small fungal particles can also cause hypersensitivity pneumonitis in certain people.

Molds also produce various volatile organic compounds, such as alcohols and ketones. These compounds, which are responsible for the musty odor associated with the presence of molds, are irritants.

Certain species of fungi can cause infectious diseases, but this is rare, unless the exposed person is severely immunosuppressed.

Other Health Problems

Systemic effects, such as headache, fever, excessive fatigue, cognitive and neuropsychological effects, gastrointestinal symptoms, and joint pain, have also been observed in some people exposed to molds. Symptoms caused by exposure to mold should disappear once exposure ceases. It is unknown whether there is a threshold for exposure below which no health effects occur.

See also CHEMICAL TOXICITY; ENVIRONMENTAL TOXINS; SKIN AND SENSE ORGAN TOXICITY.

King, Norman, and Pierre Auger. "Indoor Air Quality, Fungi, and Health." *Canadian Family Physician,* February 2002, pp. 298–302.

furniture manufacturing An industry that includes manufacturing or refinishing of lumber, hardwood veneer and plywood, particle board, new or upholstered household furniture, wooden office furniture, lockers, office and store fixtures, milled wood products, such as doors, window frames, and the like, softwood veneer and plywood, and wooden household furniture. Furniture and wood product production may involve treating wood, painting, lacquering or staining wood, gluing wood, and stripping paint.

These industries can produce hazards in the workplace, particularly hazardous waste. If any ignitable liquids (SOLVENTS, paints, furniture stripper) are used or if wood is treated with preserving compounds, among them creosote, pentachlorophenol, arsenic, or FORMALDEHYDE, then the wastes that are generated may be hazardous.

Materials that are corrosive include acidic liquids or liquids that corrode steel at a rate greater than 0.25 inch per year. Wastes from these substances can dissolve most materials; specialized containers are necessary to resist corrosion. During handling, they tend to burn the skin.

Reactive substances, such as cyanide or sulfide compounds, may generate toxic gases under mildly acidic or alkaline conditions. Chromatic acids, perchlorates, and peroxides are common reactive substances. Wastes produced from reactive substances are hazardous as they may explode.

Other hazards come from bending and lifting heavy materials, using power tools, slips, trips, and falls, gluing, painting, and refinishing.

See also CREOSOTE; GLUERS; HAND AND POWER TOOLS; HAZARDOUS WASTE; OVERLOAD INJURIES; PAINTERS; PERSONAL PROTECTIVE EQUIPMENT; WOOD DUST; WOOD PRODUCTS INDUSTRY.

fur industry Many types of jobs relate to the production of furs. Fur pelts are obtained from fur farmers, trappers, and hunters. Steps involved in preparing furs include stripping them from the carcass, stretching and air drying them after the flesh and fatty deposits are removed, sorting them, stamping them with identifying marks, cutting them open using knives and snippers, and tanning, or soaking them in tubs or barrels for several hours to soften them, sometimes in sulfuric, hydrochloric, or other acids. Tanned pelts are treated with an oil solution, then cleaned in rotating drums to remove moisture and excess oil. Other steps may include using buffing machines and brushing and lusterizing the pelts with lacquers and resins.

Some furs are dyed at the same time as they are tanned. Many chemicals may be used in dyeing, including ammonia, ammonium chloride, formaldehyde, hydrogen peroxide, lead acetate or nitrate, oxalic acid, and others.

Hazards to workers with fur pelts include machine accidents, SLIPS, TRIPS, AND FALLS, and mishaps with hand tools. Many chemicals used in the industry may be skin irritants. These include acids, bleaching agents, and the compounds used in the dyeing process. Irritant dust may be produced when bales of pelts treated with dusting powder are unpacked or sheared. Hazardous vapors may come from degreasing solvents. Allergies may develop as a result of contact with chemicals or the dust from the furs. Good ventilation, personal respiratory protective equipment, protective clothing, rubber hand protection, foot and leg protection, and aprons should be used for protection against acids and chemicals.

Because there is much manual labor involved in moving handcarts and loading and unloading of heavy wet pelts, ergonomic injuries as well as repetitive stress injuries occur. Working in the drying rooms can produce heat stress; noise from the machines used can produce hearing impairments.

See also ALLERGIES; CHEMICAL TOXICITY; CONFINED SPACES; DUST AND DEBRIS; DERMATITIS; HOT ENVIRONMENTS; NOISE; REPETITIVE STRESS INJURIES.

Mager-Stillman, Jeanne, ed. *Encyclopaedia of Occupational Health and Safety.* Vol. 3. Geneva: International Labour Organisation, 1998, pp. 88.4–88.7.

gambling Playing a game (such as cards, slot machines, or roulette) for money or other stakes or betting on an uncertain outcome (such as a horse race or football game). Some employees participate in betting pools to gamble on sporting events. When these activities do not interfere with work, employers seem to think that the attention to a sporting event may increase morale and camaraderie among employees.

The fascination with gambling and the prospect of winning becomes an ADDICTION and a compulsion for some individuals. Employees whose gambling habits interfere with work should be referred to an EMPLOYEE ASSISTANCE PROGRAM or other counseling program.

People gamble for many reasons. Some simply enjoy the sociability of the event while others find the risk and unpredictability of the game exciting and stimulating. Some derive a sense of power and importance from winning; others may gamble out of rebellion.

A Compulsion or an Addiction

Gambling may be considered a compulsion or addiction when the gambling activity becomes the most important aspect of people's lives. Such individuals will direct all of their efforts toward obtaining money to gamble. Seeking funds to enable gambling can become a stressor. For family and friends of the addicted gamblers who may not be able to pay household bills and provide a living, it becomes a source of stress as well.

Although gambling does not involve ingesting substances, compulsive gambling has many characteristics in common with alcoholism. The National Council on Compulsive Gambling and Gamblers Anonymous has estimated that there are 6,000,000 compulsive gamblers in the United States. Typically, the compulsive gambler is a married man in his early to mid-30s, employed in a field involving money and high risks such as investment, business, or law. Usually, compulsive gamblers are outgoing, generous, and gregarious, but are prone to sudden negative mood swings. Even in serious stages of compulsive gambling, gamblers will express concern about their health, but not about their addiction to gambling and the stress caused by it.

National attention was focused on the problem of compulsive gambling in the late 1980s with the well-publicized problems of baseball star Pete Rose. Shortly afterward, a Gallup poll showed a somewhat ambivalent public attitude toward gambling. Survey results indicated that while gambling may be legal or illegal, it is nevertheless on the upsurge and extremely popular. Public sentiment ran toward increasing legalized gambling, although 61 percent of those surveyed said they thought legal gambling encouraged excessive gambling.

Historically, there have been underworld aspects surrounding gambling. Films frequently depict expensively dressed, glamorous men and women gambling in casinos in exotic locations all over the world, or seedy, down-on-their-luck characters playing cards or shooting craps and about to get raided by the police. Today, when more and more states are passing laws that allow gambling and state-run lotteries have become common, gambling has become completely accessible to people in all walks of life.

Gamblers Anonymous offers a recovery program similar to Alcoholics Anonymous. The Council on Compulsive Gambling offers a crisis intervention hot line for compulsive gamblers and their families.

For information:

Gamblers Anonymous (GA)
P.O. Box 17173
Los Angeles, CA 90017
(213) 386-8789
(213) 386-0030 (fax)
www.gamblersanonymous.org

National Council on Problem Gambling (NCPG)
208 G Street, NE
2nd Floor
Washington, DC 20002
(202) 547-9204
(202) 547-9206 (fax)
www.ncpgambling.org

See also ADDICTIONS; SELF-HELP GROUPS.

Kahn, Ada P. *Stress A–Z: A Sourcebook for Facing Everyday Challenges.* New York: Facts On File, Inc., 1998.

gardeners   Workers who may maintain grounds of a public, private, industrial, or commercial property. Gardeners dig in the soil, fertilize it, plant grass, flowers, shrubs, and trees, water lawns, flowers, and shrubs, cut the lawn, trim and edge around walks, flower beds, and walls, prune shrubs and trees, and spray lawns, shrubs, and trees with insecticides, herbicides, and fertilizers. Further tasks may include cleaning, disinfecting, repairing, and sharpening gardening tools and equipment, removing damaged leaves, branches, or twigs, raking and bagging leaves, and taking away litter and leaves.

Equipment used by gardeners includes lawn mowers, clippers, weed cutters, edging tools, shears, pruners, saws, spades, sprayers, sprinklers, spreaders, rakes, booms, shovels, trowels, knives, and other tools.

The tools with which gardeners work can cause accidents. Accidents happen as a result of worker inattention, tool slippage, or breakage, causing stabs, scratches, and amputation of fingers. There is the possibility of ejection of flying particles, such as sand and stones, during work with power mowers, causing injuries to the eyes.

A major accident hazard is falling on mud, wet soil, or grass, or tripping and falling on uneven soil or over various gardening implements. Gardeners are at risk of getting bites and stings from bees, wasps, and other insects causing pain and swelling. There is the hazard of electrocution or electric shock from contact with exposed live wires or during work with poorly insulated electrical equipment. Also, there may be acute poisoning by accidental ingestion or inhalation of pesticides or other toxic chemicals, or stabs from thorns.

Gardeners may experience excessive NOISE levels from mowers, exposure to sunlight causing heatstroke and skin melanomas, and dermatitis and other skin ailments as a result of prolonged contact with chemicals, chronic poisoning as a result of prolonged inhalation, ingestion, or absorption through the skin of chemicals containing heavy metals, such as CADMIUM, mercury, lead, and ARSENIC. They may develop allergies and dermatitis as a result of contact with plants, fungal diseases caused by fungi in the soil or on plant leaves, and parasitic diseases caused by tick, chigger, and mite bites.

Gardeners perform repetitive hand motions and may develop repetitive stress injuries, and work in nonergonomic postures, such as bending over flower beds and carrying and lifting heavy loads, and may develop back pains.

See also ALLERGIES; DERMATITIS; EYE SAFETY; GREENHOUSE AND NURSERY WORKERS; PERSONAL PROTECTION EQUIPMENT; REPETITIVE STRESS INJURIES; SLIPS, TRIPS, AND FALLS.

Stellman, Jeanne Mager, ed. *Encyclopaedia of Occupational Health and Safety.* 4th ed. Vol. 4. Geneva: International Labor Organization, 1998, pp. 103.13–103.14.

gas narcosis   See COMMERCIAL DIVING.

gas station/garage workers   See AUTO BODY REPAIR AND REFINISHING; VIOLENCE.

gastrointestinal or liver toxicity   Adverse effects on the structure and or function of the gastrointestinal (digestive) tract, liver, or gallbladder that result from exposure to chemical substances. The liver functions as a center for metabolism, processing chemicals so they can be utilized, detoxified, or excreted. While chemicals absorbed from the gastrointestinal tract are always processed by the liver, toxicants that enter the body through other routes of exposure can also reach the liver via its blood supply from the hepatic artery and the portal vein. The liver is frequently subject to injury induced by chemicals called hepatotoxins because of its role as the body's principal site of metabolism.

Necrosis, or cell death, is a common effect of acute exposure to hepatotoxic chemicals such as BERYLLIUM, phosphorus, and urethane. The necrosis can be localized in specific areas of the liver or be more widespread. The liver is usually able to recover from necrosis because of its regenerative capacity. Exposure to hepatotoxic substances can also cause fatty liver (steatosis), hepatitis, jaundice, cholestasis, chronic liver damage (cirrhosis), and cancer. Carbon tetrachloride and related chemicals, such as CHLOROFOM, are linked to steatosis, necrosis, and cirrhosis of the liver. Cancer of the liver has been associated with occupational exposures to ARSENIC, copper, and VINYL CHLORIDE.

The gastrointestinal tract is composed of the esophagus, stomach, pancreas, and small and large intestines. The gastrointestinal tract is the site of entry for chemicals that are ingested. Digestive tract exposure to toxic chemicals can cause anorexia, nausea, vomiting, abdominal cramps, and diarrhea. There are four major types of tissue response to gastrointestinal injury from toxic agents; ulceration, necrosis, inflammation, and proliferation, including cancer. Some chemicals that cause gastrointestinal injury are halogenated aromatic hydrocarbons, chlorobenzene and hexachlorobenzene, and such metals as lead, MERCURY, arsenic, and CADMIUM.

See also CHEMICAL TOXICITY; EXPOSURE ASSESSMENT.

Plaa, G. "Toxic Responses of the Liver." Chap. 10 in *Casarett and Doull's Toxicology,* edited by C. Klaasen, M. Amdur, and J. Doull. New York: Pergamon Press, 1996.
@2001 Environmental Defense. Used by permission. Scorecard is available at www.scorecard.org.

general adaptation syndrome General adaptation syndrome (GAS) refers to how the body copes with stress. Hans Selye (1907–82), an Austrian-born Canadian endocrinologist and psychologist, in his landmark book, *The Stress of Life* (1956), discussed the manifestation of stress in the whole body as it develops over time. It is through GAS that various internal organs, especially the endocrine glands and the nervous system, help individuals adjust to constant changes occurring in and around them and to "navigate a steady course toward whatever they consider a worthwhile goal."

Selye was a pioneer in an area that has continued to look at stress as a threat to wellness. The secret of health, he contended, was in successful adjustment to ever-changing conditions. Life, he said, is largely a process of adaptation to the circumstances of existence. He viewed many conditions, such as high blood pressure and some cardiovascular problems, gastric and duodenal ulcers, and certain types of allergic problems, as essentially diseases of adaptation.

Selye called his concept the general adaptation syndrome because it is produced only by agents that have a *general* effect on large portions of the body. He called it *adaptive* because it stimulates DEFENSE MECHANISMS. He used the term *syndrome* because individual manifestations are coordinated and interdependent on each other.

There are three states in GAS, Selye said. Individuals go through the stages many times each day as well as throughout life. Whatever demands are made on us, we progress through the sequence. The first is an alarm reaction, or the bodily expression of a generalized call for our defensive forces. We experience surprise and anxiety because of our inexperience in dealing with a new situation. The second stage is resistance, when we have learned to cope with the new situation efficiently. The third stage is exhaustion, or a depletion of our energy reserves, which leads to fatigue. Adaptability, Selye explained, was a finite amount of vitality (thought of as capital) with which we are born. We can draw on it throughout life, but cannot add to it.

See also COPING; DIS-STRESS; EUSTRESS, HARDINESS; SELYE, HANS; STRESS.

Selye, Hans. "The Stress of Life. New York: McGraw-Hill, 1956.
———. *Stress without Distress.* Philadelphia: J. B. Lippincott Company, 1974.

generalized anxiety disorder See ANXIETY.

genotoxicity The adverse health effect a chemical has on genes and chromosomes, primarily manifesting in gene mutations, chromosome aberrations, and changes in chromosome number. Genotoxicity may be indicative of cancer-causing chemicals.

See also CHEMICAL TOXICITY; EXPOSURE ASSESSMENT.

glass ceiling   The term *glass ceiling* refers to an invisible barrier that keeps many working women from rising to the top of their field despite good qualifications, experience, and hard work. This FRUSTRATION leads to STRESS and anxiety, and for many individuals, DEPRESSION.

There are many variations of the effects of the glass ceiling. For example, men in high-level posts may be brought from outside the organization to provide a "fresh outlook" while qualified women already in the organization are passed over. In discussions involving teamwork and negotiations, women are often kept on the periphery of the decision making process.

Teasing and harassment of women may discourage them from seeking a promotion. Women in lower-level positions are sometimes given responsible, demanding work that is not reflected in title or salary. As women attempt to progress in an organization, they may find that performance standards are higher for them than for men. Women may also be inhibited by assumptions that a feminine management style is more passive and nurturing toward fellow workers and less goal-oriented and driven than the masculine management style.

Women who do make it past the glass ceiling frequently credit the influence of a mentor, spouse, or parent. Some women avoid the glass ceiling by striking out on their own.

See also SEXUAL HARASSMENT.

glass workers/glaziers   People who install glass in windows, doors, showcases, skylights, on tabletops, or who work with glass products, including mirrors.

Work in this field involves hazards of injuries, especially cuts to hands and feet and crushing of toes caused by glass sheets and their sharp edges during cutting, moving, setting, and other handling operations. Cuts and stab wounds occur with use of chisels, knives, and glass cutting tools. Falls

from heights while setting glass in windows can result in serious trauma and even death. SLIPS, TRIPS, AND FALLS occur because of wet, slippery, and greasy floors. Eye and skin injuries occur from glass splinters. As a result of using strong reactives, such as hydrofluoric acid for etching glass and similar purposes, acute poisoning and/or chemical burns can occur.

Glass workers often work under direct sunlight and experience exposure of their eyes and skin to ultraviolet light. They often work in very cold or hot conditions and may suffer frostbite or heat stress. They may have acute musculoskeletal injuries caused by physical overexertion and awkward posture while carrying and handling bulk glass sheets. They may have cumulative trauma disorders, including CARPAL TUNNEL SYNDROME, due to repetitive work with hands and arms over a long period of time. They may have chronic poisoning or skin diseases as a result of exposure to splinters of glass containing lead, arsenic and other toxic elements. Skin conditions may result from using putties, sealants, adhesive, and SOLVENTS.

Glass cutters may have job-related stress if they fear falling from heights or fear serious accidents while cutting, handling, and setting sheets of glass.

See also STRESS.

Mager-Stillman, Jeanne, ed. *Encyclopaedia of Occupational Health and Safety.* 4th ed. Vol. 4. Geneva: International Labor Organization, 1998, p. 103.15.

Globally Harmonized System for Hazard Communication (GHS)   See HAZARD COMMUNICATION.

gloves   See HAND PROTECTION.

gluers   Workers who glue together materials such as paper, cloth, leather, wood, metal, glass, rubber, or plastic. Related occupations include adhesive workers, cementers, floor layers and wall coverers, adhesives applicators, and veneer workers. Gluers apply adhesives to surfaces or materials by spraying, dipping, or rolling, press glued materials together manually, and use clamps to bond materials together and set glue. They may trim excess material from cemented parts and may wipe surplus adhesive from seams, using a cloth or sponge. This occupation is common in many industries, including air conditioning, aircraft manufacturing and maintenance, bookbinding, car manufacturing and maintenance, floor laying and wall covering, corrugated cardboard, disposable diapers, electronics, foam mattresses, footwear, furniture, packaging, lamination, leather goods, plumbing, refrigeration, toy manufacturing and upholstering.

CHEMICAL TOXICITY HAZARDS FOR WORKERS USING GLUE

- Skin sensitization and dermatitis as a result of exposure to many solvents and other glue components, (such as epoxy resin, n-hexane, toluene, vinyl chloride)
- Vitiligo (skin depigmentation) as a result of exposure to neoprene glues
- Blistering of skin in contact with glues containing epichlorohydrin, such as epoxy glues
- Eye irritation by glues or vapors
- Asphyxia when exposed to high concentrations of n-hexane
- Irritation of the mouth, throat, and nasal cavity by toluene, trichloroethylene, or xylene; respiratory tract irritation by solvent vapors, particularly n-hexane
- Carbon monoxide poisoning from overhead hot adhesives
- Pneumoconiosis from exposure to dust or fibers of some insulating materials
- Pulmonary edema as a result of inhaling vapors
- Central nervous system effects such as headaches, dizziness, a lack of coordination as a result of inhalation of many chemicals, including toluene, xylene, trichloroethane, and trichloroethylene
- Damage to the liver by dimethylformamide, tetrahydrofuran, or vinyl chloride
- Carcinogenicty: Many glue components or solvents are considered known or possible carcinogens: chloroform, hexachloroethane, methylene chloride, benzene, and ethyl acrylate.

Source: *Encyclopaedia of Occupational Health and Safety,* 4th ed.

These workers risk injuries during work with mechanized equipment used for the mixing or application of glues; their clothing or fingers can become caught in machinery. They risk falling from ladders, dropping heavy glue containers on their toes or feet, and suffering cuts during opening of certain types of glue containers. Bursting of pressure-spraying nozzles carries a particular risk of eye damage, as does working with hot metal adhesives.

Gluers also risk splashing of irritants, allergens, and other hazardous fluids such as SOLVENTS, thinners, and liquid glues into their eyes or onto their skin. They risk electric shock or electrocution because of the use of hand-held electric tools, fires and explosions because of working near flammable solvents and other flammable materials such as paper and cardboard, wood and wood dust, and the accumulation of solvent vapors, particularly in small and inadequately ventilated places.

These workers face a high level of NOISE because of the tools they use. They may have wrist, hand, and arm problems such as tenosynovitis as a result of repetitive motion and strains and sprains caused by lifting heavy glue containers.

Gluers may experience many forms of chemical toxicity. (Some are described below.)

"Glue sniffing" to elevate mood and related intoxication and neurotoxic effects are a hazard for these workers because of their easy access to glues.

See also CARBON MONOXIDE; CARPAL TUNNEL SYNDROME; CHEMICAL TOXICITY; CONFINED SPACES; FOOT PROTECTION; ELECTRICITY-RELATED INJURIES; FIRE SAFETY/FIRE PROTECTION; GASTROINTESTINAL OR LIVER TOXICITY; HAND PROTECTION; REPETITIVE STRESS INJURIES; SKIN OR SENSE ORGAN TOXICITY.

Mager-Stellman, Jeanne, ed. *Encyclopaedia of Occupational Health and Safety.* 4th ed. Vol. 4. Geneva: International Labor Organization, 1998, pp. 103.16–103.17.

goggles, protective   See EYE INJURIES/PROTECTION.

grain handling   As defined by the U.S. Occupational Safety and Health Administration, grain handling facilities include grain elevators, feed mills, flour mills, rice mills, dust pelletizing plants, dry corn mills, soybean flaking operations, and the dry grinding operations of soycake.

There are many safety and health hazards associated with grain handling operations. Suffocation and falls are the two leading causes of deaths at grain handling facilities. Other hazards include fires, explosions, electrocutions, and injuries from improperly guarded machinery. Exposure to grain dust and associated airborne contaminants can also occur; such contaminants include molds, chemical fumigants, and gases associated with decaying and/or fermenting silage.

See also CONFINED SPACES; ELECTRICITY-RELATED INJURIES; FIRE SAFETY/FIRE PROTECTION; FUNGI (MOLDS); LOCKOUT/TAGOUT; SLIPS, TRIPS, AND FALLS.

Occupational Safety and Health Administration.

graphic arts   A field in which designers work with commercial art, visual design, and visual communication. Hazards of graphic design have changed with the advent of computer graphics, and the Internet. Now, graphic designers are concerned with potential hazards of prolonged work at a computer. Hazards from working for extended periods at a VIDEO DISPLAY TERMINAL (VDT) include eyestrain, headaches, backaches, stiff necks, sore hands and wrists, irritability, and stress. Ergonomic computer workstations, elimination of glare, and frequent work breaks enable graphic designers to work more safely.

In addition to computers, materials used by graphic arts professionals include drawing and painting materials such as markers, watercolors, oil paints, colored inks, colored pencils, dry pastels, oil pastels, dyes, acrylic paints, and gouache. Commonly used colors contain hazardous ingredients such as xylene and petroleum distillates. Pigments may contain mercury, cadmium, cobalt, and lead.

Adhesives used by graphic artists include rubber cement, spray mount, contact cement, glue sticks, and hot glue guns. Hazards include dangerous chemicals such as *n*-hexane (a neurotoxin) in some rubber cements and contact cement, airborne chemicals, and fire hazards associated with sprays adhesives and burns from hot glue guns.

SOLVENTS used by graphic artists include rubber cement, thinner, turpentine, acetone, correction fluid, and mineral spirits. Hazards include skin irritation, headaches, damage to respiratory and nervous systems, kidney and liver damage, and flammability. Aerosols used by graphic artists include fixative spray, spray markers, varnish, texture sprays, and airbrush colors. Hazards include respiratory problems, skin irritation, headaches, dizziness, and nausea from toxic chemicals such as toluene and xylene. Sprays can be flammable and they must be used away from heat or flames.

Graphic artists also use cutting tools, such as paper cutters, razor knives, and mat cutters. Precautions include careful use of equipment, keeping hands away from blades, and maintaining blades in sharp condition.

Precautions for graphic artists include working in a well-ventilated studio, wearing gloves and respirator when using oil-based materials (particularly from aerosol) and substitutions of water- and alcohol-based colors when possible. Pastels (chalks) can be hazardous when they become airborne dust. Good ventilation is essential when using any material that can be breathed into the lungs.

See also GLUERS; PRINTING PLANTS; SKIN OR SENSE ORGAN TOXICITY.

Mager-Stellman, Jeanne, ed. *Encyclopaedia of Occupational Safety and Health.* 4th ed. Vol. 3. Geneva: International Labour Organisation, 1991, pp. 96.21–96.22.

greenhouse and nursery workers   These workers are exposed to many health hazards, including skin irritants, DUST AND DEBRIS, NOISE, heat, musculoskeletal disorders (sprains and strains), pesticides, and injuries related to vehicles, machines, slips and falls, and electricity.

There is a high rate of sprain and strain injuries in nursery work, as with other agricultural activities. Authors M. M. Methner and J. A. Miles report that 38.9 percent of all reported injuries in horticultural specialties (including nurseries) were sprains and strains. Overexertion as a cause of injury was cited for 30.2 percent of reported injuries.

There are many ergonomic hazards in these occupations. For example, in a greenhouse, during propagation, the worker stands or sits at a worktable, empties a basket of plant cuttings and uses hand shears to cut them into smaller pieces. The shears are held in one hand, the plant material in the other. After each cutting, the shears are disinfected by dipping into a solution in a container at the workbench. Cutting requires very repetitive motion. Workers often report pain and numbness in the hand, wrist, and arm. After many years on the job, there is an elevated incidence of carpal tunnel syndrome.

In transporting plants from a conveyor belt to a trailer, the worker grasps containers in each hand and places them on a trailer, resulting in highly repetitive gripping and awkward postures, including shoulder, lumbar, and trunk flexion.

The pruner works with various shears to snip unwanted or dead parts off the tops and sides of plants, usually while standing or bent over. This work is associated with pain in the fingers and hand, wrist, upper extremities, and lower back.

Diseases and insects that attack plants can cause serious problems for greenhouse operators. To prevent damage, pesticides are applied to plants. With each application, the workers risk being exposed to the chemical. The two most common routes of exposure are through the skin (dermal) and through the lungs (respiratory). A less common route of exposure is by ingesting food or drinks contaminated with pesticides. Greenhouse workers who handle the chemicals or the treated plants may be poisoned if they do not follow proper safety precautions.

Methner and Miles suggest that to avoid poisoning, greenhouse and nursery workers use proper ventilation systems, use and maintain appropriate PERSONAL PROTECTIVE EQUIPMENT (PPE), such as suits, gloves, respirators, and boots, observe recommended reentry times and follow pesticide label instructions. Additionally, workers should store pesticides in a locked, well-ventilated area, post signs in areas where plants have been treated, and undergo extensive education about proper application and handling techniques. All workers who work with pesticides should be trained in appropriate disposal techniques for old pesticides and empty pesticide containers.

See also CARPAL TUNNEL SYNDROME; CHEMICAL TOXICITY; ERGONOMICS; FARMING; HAND PROTECTION; REPETITIVE STRESS INJURIES; RESPIRATORY TOXICITY; SLIPS, TRIPS, AND FALLS; STRESS.

Methner, Mark M., and John A. Miles. "Greenhouse and Nursery Operations." Mager-Stillman, Jeanne, ed. *Encyclopaedia of Occupational Health and Safety.* 4th ed. Vol. 3. Geneva: International Labor Organization, 1998, p. 64.10.

greenhouse effect   See AIR POLLUTION.

greenhouse gases   See AIR POLLUTION.

groundskeepers   See CENSUS OF FATAL OCCUPATIONAL INJURIES; GARDENERS.

grocery stores   See VIOLENCE.

guided imagery   A technique to help the individual generate vivid mental images that help reduce stress or anxiety. It creates positive mental pictures and promotes the relaxation necessary for a healing process. The individual pictures an image, such as a calm, serene lake with sailboats slowly moving along, breathes gently, and becomes more relaxed. The individual gradually learns to notice every detail of the imagined scene and how the sense of relaxation deepens with this self-talk. He or she learns, too, that this sense of calm can be created at any time by breathing and imagining the positive vision.

Some EMPLOYEE ASSISTANCE PROGRAMS encourage employees to learn this technique to cope with the pressure of the workplace. Some employer-sponsored health-promotion programs include guided imagery among their offerings.

Imagery has qualities that make it valuable in mind/body medicine and healing; it can bring about physiological changes, provide psychological insights, and enhance emotional awareness. Use of imagery, in some cases, changes the need for medication. Depending on an individual's medical condition, imagery is best used under the supervision of a physician in conjunction with holistic medicine.

Guided imagery can be used alone or together with other relaxation techniques. It is often used in conjunction with hypnosis, although the two techniques are distinct. While hypnosis serves to induce a special state of mind, imagery consists of a focused, intentional mental activity.

For information:

The Academy for Guided Imagery
P.O. Box 2070
Mill Valley, CA 94942
(800) 726-2070

See also COMPLEMENTARY THERAPIES; IMMUNE SYSTEM; RELAXATION; STRESS.

Kahn, Ada P. *Stress A–Z: A Sourcebook for Facing Everyday Challenges.* New York: Facts On File, Inc., 1998.

guilt   An emotional response to a perceived or actual failure to meet expectations of self or others. Guilt is a stressor for many people in the workplace because guilt feelings can be destructive if carried to an extreme. It can destroy people's sense of SELF-ESTEEM and feelings of capability. However, these feelings can also be constructive when the sources of guilt are understood and one learns to cope with this very common aspect of the human condition.

Some individuals, depending on differences in conscience, can steal or commit crimes against others and not feel any guilt, while others will suffer from uncomfortable guilt feelings over minor incidents. Many individuals may experience guilt feelings for not remembering the birthday of a coworker.

For some individuals, an EMPLOYEE ASSISTANCE PROGRAM or mental health counseling can help relieve some of the discomforts of guilt feelings.

See also COPING; DEPRESSION.

Kahn, Ada P. *Stress A–Z: A Sourcebook for Facing Everyday Challenges.* New York: Facts On File, Inc., 1998.

guitar players' injuries   Guitarists may encounter injuries of their fingers, hands, and wrists, as well as back discomforts if they play standing or in an awkward seated posture.

The common factor in all types of guitar playing is the position of the arms, especially the wrists. There is repetitive motion, and the need for strength of the fingers when applied against the strings and struts. Considerable dexterity is also necessary.

The use of a pick, regardless of the style of playing, tends to take a toll on the pinch muscles of the thumb and forefinger. STRESS and PERFORMANCE ANXIETY are factors that professional guitarists face regularly.

See also PERFORMING ARTS MEDICINE; REPETITIVE STRESS INJURIES; STRESS.

Sataloff, Robert Thayer, Alice G. Brandfonbrener, and Richard J. Lederman, eds. *Textbook of Performing Arts Medicine.* New York: Raven Press, 1991.

Gulf War illness   A syndrome or collection of symptoms reported by those in the armed forces who were part of Operation Desert Storm in the Persian Gulf in 1991. More than 100,000 U.S. veterans, within six to 12 months after exposure, reported a wide variety of symptoms, including skin rashes, headaches, disabling fatigue, intermittent fevers, joint and muscle pains, and short-term memory impairment.

Those who experienced Gulf War illness may have been exposed to certain chemical mixtures, possibly antinerve and nerve agents; radiological sources, primarily depleted uranium, possibly fallout from destroyed nuclear reactors; and biological sources, such as bacteria and viruses.

According to then Deputy Secretary of Defense John P. White, the Department of Defense in the late 1990s launched an aggressive health care outreach effort to evaluate the health concerns of persons with Gulf War illness symptoms. The Department of Defense allocated up to $12 million for general research on possible causes of Gulf War illnesses.

http://www.dtic.mil/armylink/news.Oct1996/a/1996102 5gulf3.html. Army News Service. "Gulf War Illness Developments." *Army Link News,* October 1996.

halogenated aromatic hydrocarbons   See IMMU-
NOTOXICITY; KIDNEY TOXICITY.

hand and power tools   Common tools used in
nearly every industry. These tools help workers
with tasks that otherwise would be difficult or
impossible to perform. However, these simple tools
can be hazardous, and have the potential for causing severe injuries when used or maintained
improperly.

Hand and power tools may include metal-cut-
ting hand tools, woodworking tools, miscellaneous
cutting tools, torsion tools, shock tools, portable
power tools, abrasive wheel tools, pneumatic
power tools, fuel-powered tools, hydraulic power
tools, and power-actuated tools. Misuse of common hand tools is a major source of injury to maintenance and construction workers. Supervisors
must ensure that every maintenance and construction worker's instruction program includes detailed
training in the proper use of hand tools.

To prevent hand and power tool accidents, the
right tool should be selected for the job. Examples
of unsafe practices include striking hardened faces
of hand tools together (such as using a carpenter's
hammer to strike another hammer, hatchet, or
metal chisel), using a file for a pry, a wrench for a
hammer, or using pliers instead of the proper
wrench.

Tools must be kept in good condition. Examples
of tools in poor condition include wrenches with
cracked work jaws, screwdrivers with broken
points or broken handles, hammers with loose
heads, dull saws, and extension cords or electric
tools with broken plugs, improper or removed
grounding lugs, or split insulation. Tools must also
be kept in a safe place; do not carry sharp tools in
pockets or leave sharp tools in toolboxes with the
cutting edges exposed.

Carrying Tools

According to guidelines from Virginia Polytechnic
Institute and State University, employees should
never carry tools in any way that might interfere
with using both hands freely while climbing a ladder or structure. A strong bag, bucket, or similar
container should be used to hoist tools from the
ground to the job. Tools should be returned in
the same manner, not brought down by hand,
carried in pockets, or dropped to the ground. Tools
should not be left where employees are moving or
walking.

Chisels, screwdrivers, and pointed tools must
never be carried in a worker's pocket. They should
be carried in a toolbox or cart, in a carrying belt
(sharp or pointed end down) like those used by
electricians and steelworkers, in a pocket tool
pouch, or in the hand, with cutting edges pointing
away from the body. Employees carrying tools on
their shoulders should be aware of clearance when
turning around and should handle tools so that
they will not strike other employees.

Personal Protective Equipment

Because workers using hand and power tools are
likely to be exposed to the hazards of flying debris,
harmful dusts or noise, they must wear appropriate
PERSONAL PROTECTIVE EQUIPMENT, advises the Occupational Safety and Health Administration.

See also ASBESTOS; BRICKLAYERS, CEMENT WORK-
ERS, AND PLASTERERS; CONFINED SPACES; CONSTRUC-
TION; ELECTRICITY-RELATED INJURIES; DUST AND
DEBRIS; ERGONOMICS; LADDERS; LOCKOUT/TAGOUT;
SAFETY; SCAFFOLDING; SLIPS, TRIPS AND FALLS; WOOD
DUST.

hand protection   Gloves may be the most common form of PERSONAL PROTECTIVE EQUIPMENT (PPE) used in the workplace. Because gloves can provide protection against a variety of hazards, including cuts, abrasions, burns, and skin contact with chemicals, it is important to select the most appropriate glove for a particular application, determine how long it can be worn, and whether it can be reused.

Workers are required to use appropriate hand protection when they are exposed to the following hazards:

- Absorption of harmful substances through the skin
- Severe cuts or lacerations
- Severe abrasions
- Punctures
- Chemical burns
- Thermal burns
- Harmful temperature extremes

Employers are required to base the selection of appropriate hand protection on the following factors:

- An evaluation of the performance characteristics of the tasks to be performed
- Conditions
- Duration of use
- The hazards and potential hazards identified

Selecting the Right Glove for the Job

Determine the performance characteristics of gloves relative to the specific hazards anticipated, including chemical hazards, cut hazards, and flame hazards. Performance hazards should be established by using standard test procedures. Employers should request documentation from manufacturers that the gloves meet the appropriate test standards for the hazards involved.

Other factors to be considered in glove selection:

- Cost effectiveness of reusing more expensive gloves versus regularly replacing cheaper ones
- Characteristics of the work performed, including a need for dexterity, duration of the work activity, frequency of use, and degree of exposure

- Toxic properties of the chemicals involved, including the ability to pass through the skin and cause systemic effects
- Ability of employees to remove gloves in a manner that prevents skin contamination. In general, any chemical resistant glove can be used for dry powders. For work with mixtures and formulated products, the gloves should be selected on the basis of the chemical component with the shortest breakthrough time, because it is possible for solvents to carry active ingredients through polymeric materials.

For further information:

National Center for Construction Education and Research (NCCER)
P.O. Box 141104
Gainesville, FL 32614-1104
(352) 334-0911
(352) 334-0932 (fax)
www.nccer.org

Adapted with permission from: Klein, John. "The Extremities of Safety: Hand and Foot Protection." *Compliance* 9, no. 7 (July/August 2002).

hangover   A disagreeable condition that occurs after consuming too much alcohol or using drugs. Sometimes sleeping medications cause hangover-like symptoms. A hangover produces physical as well as emotional symptoms that differ among individuals. Any employee appearing at work with a hangover should be referred to an EMPLOYEE ASSISTANCE PROGRAM or other appropriate counseling. Some may experience nausea, vomiting, or dizziness, while others may have HEADACHES, sleepiness, unsteadiness, blurred vision, depression, or self-pity. Many individuals may blame mixing of drinks, but drinking any one alcoholic beverage can cause a hangover.

The distinctive headache experienced as part of a hangover may be due to toxic substances that are released into the bloodstream and cause irritation of the brain membranes. Headaches may also come from the pressure of swollen blood vessels, which is an effect of alcohol. When alcohol promotes excessive urination, the resulting loss of fluid may reduce spinal fluid pressure, which has been known to bring on a headache.

Usually individuals recover from hangovers without medical assistance. Recommendations from physicians generally include aspirin or aspirin substitute, rest, and solid food as soon as possible. A cup of coffee and a meal helps most people feel better.

harassment See SEXUAL HARASSMENT.

harborworkers See FISHING; LONGSHORE AND HARBOR WORKERS' COMPREHENSIVE PROGRAM.

hardiness Term applied by Salvatore Maddi, Ph.D., a University of Chicago psychologist, to stress-buffering characteristics of people who stay healthy. People with hardiness are able to withstand significant levels of stress without becoming ill; those who are more helpless than hardy develop more illnesses, both mental and physical.

In working with executives at a major American employer, Dr. Maddi and colleagues determined three techniques that can augment hardiness as well as happiness and health.

Focusing. This technique was developed by Eugene Gendlin, an American psychologist. It is a way of recognizing signals from the body that something is wrong, such as tension in the neck or a mild headache. With stress, these conditions worsen. Maddi suggests mentally reviewing where things are not feeling just right and reviewing situations that might be stressful. Focusing increases one's sense of CONTROL over stress and enables one to make changes.

Reconstructing stressful situations. This is a technique in which you think about a recent stressful episode, such as an encounter with your superior at work, and write down three ways it might have gone better and three ways it might have gone worse. If you cannot think of what you could have done differently, focus on a person you know who deals with similar situations well and what he or she would have done. Realize that things did not go as badly as they could have. Also, realize that you can think of ways to cope better with the same situation.

Self-improvement. In this technique, you know there are some situations you cannot control or avoid, such as downsizings and layoffs. To regain your sense of control and achieve more effective COPING, choose a new task to master, such as learning a new computer skill or foreign language.

Suzanne Kobasa, a City University of New York psychologist, also used the term *hardiness* to identify and measure a style of psychological coping. Some of the characteristics people with hardiness exhibited included viewing life's demands as challenges rather than threats, responding with excitement and energy to change, and having a commitment to something they felt was meaningful, such as their work, community, or family. A third trait was a sense of being in control.

Issue of Control in Hardiness
A study reported in the *Journal of Personal and Social Psychology* (April 1995) detailed how 276 Israeli army recruits completed questionnaires on hardiness, mental health, and ways of coping at the beginning and end of a demanding four-month combat training period. Two components of hardiness, commitment and control, measured at the beginning of the training, predicted mental health at the end of the training. Commitment improved mental health by reducing the appraisal of threat. Control improved mental health by reducing appraisal of threat and by increasing the use of problem-solving and support-seeking strategies.

See also GENERAL ADAPTATION SYNDROME; LEARNED HELPLESSNESS; STRESS.

Floria, V., et al. "Does Hardiness Contribute to Mental Health During a Stressful Real-life Situation? The Roles of Appraisal and Coping." *Journal of Personal and Social Psychology* 68 (April 1995): 687–695.
Kahn, Ada P. *Stress A–Z: A Sourcebook for Coping with Everyday Challenges.* New York: Facts On File, Inc., 1998.

hatmakers See MERCURY.

"having it all" An expression that became popular during the 1980s, referring to career women who follow their chosen career, get married, and raise a family. For many, this has become a satisfying way of life, but others have experienced many frustrations. Some women feel that they are not giving adequate attention to their marriage and children, are constantly tired, and feel some guilt over having their children in day care centers.

Nevertheless, an increasing number of women opt to pursue careers. Those who are most successful say it is due to helpfulness and understanding of their spouse as well as an adequate day care situation, or deciding not to have children.

hazard communication (HazCom)   Identifying and alerting employees to dangers or hazards on the job. The goals of a hazard communication program are to ensure that employees and employers are aware of job dangers and how to protect themselves and to reduce the incidence of illness and injuries.

Generally, hazard communications programs cover chemical injuries. Chemicals pose a wide range of health hazards, such as irritation, sensitization, and carcinogenicity, and physical hazards, such as flammability, corrosion, and reactivity. The Health Communication Standard of the Occupational Safety and Health Administration is designed to ensure that information about these hazards and associated protective measures is disseminated to workers and employers. This is accomplished by requiring chemical manufacturers and importers to evaluate the hazards of the chemicals they produce or import and to provide information about them through labels on shipping containers and more detailed information sheets known as material safety data sheets (MSDSs). All employers with hazardous chemicals in their workplaces must prepare and implement a written hazard communication program, and must ensure that all containers are labeled, tagged, or marked with an appropriate hazard warning. Employees must be provided access to MSDSs and receive an effective training program for all potential exposures.

The Hazardous Chemicals Standard provided workers the right to know the hazards and identities of the chemicals to which they are exposed in their workplace. A list of the chemicals can serve as an inventory of all items for which an MSDS must be maintained. When workers have this information, they can effectively participate in their employers' protective programs and take steps to protect themselves. In addition, the standard gives employers the information they need to design and implement an effective protective program. These actions can result in a reduction of chemical sources of illnesses and injuries in the workplace.

Global Harmonization

The goal of the United States and other countries is to classify and label hazardous chemicals to promote common, consistent criteria for classifying chemicals according to their health, physical, and environmental hazards, and to develop compatible labeling and MSDSs for workers. The concept is known as the Globally Harmonized System for Hazard Communication (GHS).

See also AMERICAN INDUSTRIAL HYGIENE ASSOCIATION; CHEMICAL SENSITIVITY; CHEMICAL TOXICITY; EXPOSURE ASSESSMENT; HAZARDOUS AND TOXIC SUBSTANCES; HAZARDOUS AIR POLLUTANTS; HOSPITAL HAZARDS; MATERIALS SAFETY DATA SHEETS; NEEDLESTICK INJURIES AND PREVENTION; OCCUPATIONAL SAFETY AND HEALTH ADMINISTRATION; SOCIETY FOR CHEMICAL HAZARD COMMUNICATION; SOLVENTS; SPILL EXPOSURE.

Occupational Safety and Health Administration

Hazardous Air Pollutants (HAPs)   Chemicals that cause serious health and environmental effects. Health effects include CANCER, birth defects, nervous system problems, and death due to massive accidental releases such as occurred at the Union Carbide pesticide plant in Bhopal, India. Hazardous air pollutants are released by sources such as chemical plants, dry cleaners, printing plants, and motor vehicles.

See also AIR POLLUTION; CHEMICAL TOXICITY; CLEAN AIR ACT OF 1990; EXPOSURE ASSESSMENT; HAZARD COMMUNICATION; HAZARDOUS AND TOXIC SUBSTANCES; NEUROTOXICITY; PARTICULATE MATTER.

hazardous and toxic substances   According to the Occupational Safety and Health Administration (OSHA), U.S. Department of Labor, hazardous and toxic substances are chemicals present in the workplace which are capable of causing harm. In this definition, the term *chemicals* includes dusts, mixtures, and common materials such as paints, fuels, and solvents. OSHA currently regulates exposure to approximately 400 substances. The OSHA Chemical Sampling Information file contains listings for approximately 1,500 substances; the Chemical Substances Inventory of the Environmental Protection Agency lists information on more than 62,000 chemicals or chemical substances. Some libraries maintain files of material safety data sheets for more than 100,000 substances.

OSHA provides guidelines related to chemicals for workers and employers as well as for physicians, industrial hygienists, and other occupational safety and health professionals who may need such information to conduct effective occupational safety and health programs.

See also CHEMICAL TOXICITY; DUST AND DEBRIS; ENVIRONMENTAL PROTECTION AGENCY; HAZARDOUS WASTE; HAZARD COMMUNICATION; MATERIAL SAFETY DATA SHEETS; OCCUPATIONAL SAFETY AND HEALTH ADMINISTRATION; REPRODUCTIVE TOXICITY; SOLVENTS.

hazardous materials, transporting   See BROWNFIELDS.

hazardous waste   Dangerous unused materials from nuclear generators. Hazardous waste management standards vary, depending on the viewpoints of those who are generators, transporters, owners or operators of treatment, storage, or disposal facilities.

Generators, those who create hazardous waste, must determine whether their generated material is a solid waste or a hazardous waste. There are two methods to make determination of hazardous waste. The substance may be a "listed" waste, one of hundreds of substances that the Environmental Protection Agency (EPA) has placed on a list of hazardous waste, or the substance may be a "characteristic" waste, one that exhibits any of four hazardous waste characteristics: corrosivity, ignitability, reactivity, or toxicity.

Generators must comply with some or all of the rules of the federal Resource Conservation and Recovery Act (RCRA) depending upon whether they are large-quantity generators, small-quantity generators, or conditionally exempt small-quantity generators. Some states have stricter generator classifications systems than the federal.

Hazardous materials transporters must obtain an identification number from the EPA, comply with manifest and recordkeeping requirements, ensure that the shipment has appropriate labels, markings, and placards, and respond properly to releases of hazardous waste during transport. Additionally, hazardous waste transporters are subject to various Department of Transportation regulations.

Universal waste is a general term the EPA uses to describe certain widely generated hazardous wastes, such as certain batteries, pesticides, and thermostats.

See also ENVIRONMENTAL PROTECTION AGENCY; HAZARD COMMUNICATION; HAZARDOUS AND TOXIC SUBSTANCES.

HAZCOM training   See HAZARD COMMUNICATION; HAZARDOUS WASTE.

headaches   Pains in the head from the outer linings of the brain and from the scalp and its blood vessels and muscles; headaches occur due to tension in or stretching of these structures. Headaches are a workplace concern because of their discomfort and unpredictability. They may be caused by a reaction to stressful situations with coworkers or supervisors as well as to overindulgence in alcohol, extreme fatigue, and certain infections.

Headaches are fairly common in DEPRESSION and sleep disorders, as well as those suffering from BOREDOM. The National Headache Foundation estimates that more than 80 million Americans develop headaches each year that are serious enough to warrant treatment by a physician.

Types of Headaches

Tension or muscle contraction headaches, caused by tightening in the muscles of the face, neck, and scalp, may result from stress or poor posture; they may last for days or weeks and can cause variable degrees of discomfort. About 90 percent of all headaches are classified as tension headaches.

Cluster headaches is a term that refers to the characteristic grouping in a series of attacks; the pain is generally very intense and is almost always one-sided (during a series, the pain remains on the same side). In a new series, it can occur on the opposite side. Cluster headaches are not associated with the gastrointestinal disturbances or sensitivity to light that typically accompany other vascular headaches, such as migraine.

Temporomandibular joint (TMJ) headaches cause a dull ache in and around the ear that gets worse when one chews, talks, or yawns. Sufferers may hear a clicking sound on opening the mouth and feel soreness in the jaw muscles. Stress, a poor bite, or grinding of the teeth may bring on the headache.

Caffeine headaches occur in some individuals who drink too much CAFFEINE in coffee, tea, and soft drinks. Some people can relieve their symptoms by eliminating drinks containing caffeine from their diet. Others, however, who drink large quantities of the liquids and stop abruptly, may suffer caffeine withdrawal symptoms, including headaches, irritability, depression, and sometimes nausea; relief may occur with ingestion of a caffeinated beverage.

Migraine Headaches

Migraine or vascular headaches are characterized by the throbbing sensation that occurs when blood vessels in the head dilate or swell. Migraine is often a debilitating condition that occurs in periodic attacks, with each attack lasting from four to 72 hours. Symptoms may include intense pain, often associated with nausea, vomiting, appetite loss, and an unusual sensitivity to light and/or sound. Migraines generally start on either side of the head and usually remain one-sided. Of 23 million American migraine sufferers, 60 percent are women. Men and women between the ages of 35 and 45 years of age seem to suffer most from migraine headaches. More than three-fourths of migraine sufferers come from families in which other members have the same disorder.

Common migraine headaches start unexpectedly, while classic migraine is usually preceded by a warning symptom known as an aura, which occurs five to 30 minutes prior to the headache. Typically, the aura includes hallucinations of jagged light or color, speech impairment, perception of strange odors, confusion, and tingling or numbness in the face or limbs.

Migraine Headaches: A Toll on Productivity

Because migraine headaches usually recur, sufferers become concerned that an attack will happen at work or before an important appointment. Migraine headaches often begin during a period of time filled with anxieties, such as around the time of a job performance review, or around the time of a personal source of stress, such as divorce or illness in the family.

Migraine headaches, which often occur in members of the same family, may result from a predisposing genetic biochemical abnormality. Also, personality traits may play a role in determining who gets migraines. Although there is no typical personality associated with these headaches, some migraine sufferers have characteristics of compulsivity and PERFECTION.

Common Migraine Triggers

In a susceptible person, the migraine trigger might be something seen, smelled, heard, eaten, or experienced; it may be one particular trigger or a combination of factors.

Approximately 20 percent of all migraine sufferers have sensitivity to a specific food or foods. Knowing that certain foods may trigger migraines is an additional source of stress. Many individuals find that certain foods (such as cheese, chocolate, and red wine) containing a substance known as tyramine trigger migraine attacks. Sodium nitrite, a preservative used in ham, hot dogs, and many other sausages, is a trigger for some people. Although some migraine researchers have recommended that all migraine sufferers avoid these foods, only about 30 percent of people who have migraine headaches experience this reaction to some foods. Not eating or missing meals can cause low blood sugar levels, which are also a migraine trigger.

Identifying and avoiding the triggers that cause headaches is one of the most significant management techniques for controlling headache frequency and stress.

COMMON MIGRAINE TRIGGERS

- Dietary habits (See detailed listing following).
- Environmental factors, such as weather, bright lights, glare, or noise.

- Emotional factors, such as depression, anxiety, resentment, or fatigue.
- Motion sickness, lack of sleep or too much sleep, eyestrain, and a fall or head injury.
- Hormonal triggers, such as menstrual cycle, oral contraceptives, or estrogen supplements.
- Medications, such as overuse of over-the-counter pain relievers and some prescription medications.

DIETARY FACTORS:
POSSIBLE MIGRAINE ATTACK TRIGGERS

- Caffeinated foods and drinks: coffee, tea, chocolate, cocoa, colas/soft drinks
- Alcohol: especially red wine, vermouth, champagne, beer
- Dairy products: aged cheeses, sour cream, whole milk, buttermilk, yogurt, and ice cream
- Breads: sourdough, fresh yeast, and some types of cereals
- Vegetables: some types of beans (broad, Italian, lima, lentil, fava, soy), sauerkraut, onions, peas
- Snacks: nuts, peanuts, peanut butter, pickles, seeds, sesame
- Meats: organ meats, salted meats, dried meats, cured meats, smoked fish, meats with nitrites (such as hot dogs, sausages, lunch meat)
- Fruits: most citrus fruits, bananas, avocados, figs, raisins, papaya, passion fruit, red plums, raspberries, plantains, pineapples
- Monosodium glutamate (MSG): a flavor enhancer often used in restaurants and also in seasoned salt, instant foods, canned soup, frozen dinners, pizza, potato chips
- Soups: particularly those containing MSG; soups made from bouillon cubes
- Desserts: chocolate, licorice, molasses, cakes/cookies made with yeast
- Seasonings and flavorings such as soy sauce, some spices, garlic powder, onion powder, salt, meat tenderizers, marinades
- Hunger: missing meals, fasting, dieting

Therapies for Headaches

Treatments for headaches include nonpharmacological treatments, such as BIOFEEDBACK, MEDITATION, and RELAXATION techniques, as well as prescription medications. In the mid-1990s, a medication called sumatriptan succinate became available in tablet form. A highly selective serotonin receptor-agonist for the treatment of migraine with or without aura, it is not indicated for cluster headaches.

For migraine or vascular headaches, medication is targeted toward altering responses of the vascular system to stress, hormonal changes, noise, and other stimuli. Such medications affect the dilation reaction of the blood vessels. Ergot, a naturally occurring substance that constricts blood vessels and reduces the dilation of arteries, has historically been a popular medication. Ergot may be given by inhalation, injection, orally, or rectally. Some people find that if they take the ergot medication early enough in prepain stages of an attack they can abort their headaches or at least reduce their intensity.

Some vascular headaches are helped with prophylactic (preventive) measures. The drug of choice for prevention of migraine in carefully selected patients is propranolol. Propranolol is a vasoconstrictor that can be taken daily for as long as six months. This drug may slow down the vascular changes that occur during the migraine attack; it is frequently prescribed for some individuals who have headaches more than once each week. Propranolol has an advantage over ergot medications in that rebound headaches are not brought on by discontinuance of propranolol.

Medication for muscle contraction headaches is directed toward relieving muscular activity and spasm. Analgesics (pain relievers) commonly used are aspirin, dextropropoxyphene, and ethoheptazine. Injection with anesthetics and corticosteroids may be helpful.

For treating cluster headaches, choice of medications depends on the frequency and severity of headaches, as well as response to previous treatments. Some drugs used include ergotamine, methysergide, cyproheptadine, lithium, and steroids, as well as oxygen inhalation and histamine desensitization. These treatments should only be used under the careful guidance of a physician who is familiar with their use.

In depressed individuals, some antidepressant drugs may provide relief from headaches including migraine; examples are the monoamine oxidase inhibitors (MAOIs), such as phenelzine sulfate.

Complementary Therapies

A wide variety of COMPLEMENTARY THERAPIES may be helpful for headache sufferers. Some individuals experience relief with their use and without medication, while others use them in conjunction with medication. Alternative therapies should be discussed with the attending physician. Although some people can relieve their headache pain with alternative therapies, for others these therapies act as an adjunct or complement to pharmacological therapy, making the sufferer more receptive to medical treatment.

Biofeedback involves teaching a person to control certain body functions through thought and willpower with feedback from an electronic device.

Meditation (also known as transcendental meditation), is a technique of inward contemplation that helps some people relieve anxieties and in turn relieve some headaches, by relaxation. During meditation, the mind and other organs in the body slow down, heart rate decreases, breathing becomes slower, and muscle tensions diminish.

Acupuncture has been successfully used to treat some headache sufferers. Acupuncture probably works because the needle insertions somehow stimulate the body to secrete endorphins, naturally occurring hormonelike substances that kill pain. Acupressure involves pressing acupuncture points with hands, and can be done by a professional as well as a trained layperson.

For information:

American Headache Society (AHS)
19 Mantua Road
Mount Royal, NJ 08061
(856) 423-0043
(856) 423-0082 (fax)
http://www.ashnet.org

National Headache Foundation
428 West St. James Place
2nd Floor
Chicago, IL 60614
(888) NHF-5552 (toll-free)
(773) 388-6399
(773) 525-7357 (fax)

See also GUIDED IMAGERY; HANGOVER; HYPNOSIS.

Diamond, Seymour. *The Hormone Headache: New Ways to Prevent, Manage, and Treat Migraines and Other Headaches.* New York: Macmillan, 1995.

Inlander, Charles B., and Porter Shimer. *Headaches: 47 Ways to Stop the Pain.* New York: Walker and Company, 1995.

Maas, Paula, and Deborah Mitchell. *The Natural Health Guide to Headache Relief: The Definitive Handbook of Natural Remedies for Treating Every Kind of Headache Pain.* New York: Pocket Books, 1997.

head protection See PERSONAL PROTECTIVE EQUIPMENT.

health care workers Employees who work in health care settings, such as hospitals, nursing homes, or laboratories. There are approximately 6 million persons working in more than 6,000 U.S. hospitals and nearly 1 million workers providing care in a variety of community health settings, including patient homes, where available control measures are more limited than in the hospital setting.

Female nurse's aides and licensed practical nurses are approximately two and a half times more likely to experience a work-related low-back disorder than all other female workers. Workplace assaults, such work organization issues as inadequate staff, poor indoor air quality, and exposure to infectious agents and drug-resistant infections such as tuberculosis pose challenges to many health care workers.

Many health care workers are at a higher risk of occupational exposure to a number of airborne and bloodborne infectious diseases relative to the general population. For example, urban health care workers have a rate of seropositivity on tuberculin skin tests approximately eight times that of the U.S. population. There are hospital-based outbreaks of multidrug resistant tuberculosis (TB), with 17 documented cases among workers. In prevaccine surveys, the annual incidence of hepatitis B virus (HBV) among physicians and dentists was five to 10 times higher than among blood donors. The Centers for Disease Control estimated that in 1994 there were approximately 1,100 occupationally acquired HBV infections in health care workers in the United States, causing 250 to 1,000 cases of clinical acute hepatitis and 50 hospitalizations.

Although the incidence of occupational hepatitis C virus infection among health care workers is unknown, occupational exposure accounts for approximately 2 percent of all cases of hepatitis C. Dentists, particularly oral surgeons, have been found to have a significantly higher seropositivity rate than blood donors.

As of December 1996, the Centers for Disease Control reported 163 United States health care workers with documented or possible occupational transmission of human immunodeficiency virus (HIV) as a consequence of the approximately 800,000 needlestick injuries that occur each year.

According to authors Jane Lipscomb and Lina Rosenstock, the first case of occupational transmission of HIV infection to a health care worker, documented in 1984, raised fear among health care workers and their families. As a consequence, advances in occupational health and infection control practices occurred. The passage of the Occupational Safety and Health Administration's Bloodborne Pathogens Standard in 1991 provided important protection for healthcare workers at risk of HIV, HBV, and other bloodborne infections. Additionally, the Centers for Disease Control advised recommendation of chemoprophylaxis (protection against chemicals) for exposed workers after occupational exposures associated with high risk for transmission of HIV.

Historical Perspective

Although the practice of occupational health dates back to the late 1800s, and national professional societies in occupational medicine and nursing were established in 1916 and 1942 respectively, health care workers did not become a focus of study and prevention strategies until much later. As recently as the 1950s, there was no consensus regarding the occupational risk of exposure. A number of factors may have caused this lack of consensus, including fear that young people would avoid nursing careers if they knew the risks involved. When TB declined significantly in the general public but remained elevated in the medical profession, TB was recognized as an occupational hazard.

Latex Allergies

Increased use of examination and surgical gloves by health care and other exposed workers has increased the incidence of latex allergy. Lipscomb and Rosenstock estimate the prevalence of latex allergy between 7 and 10 percent, with atopic workers at even greater risk.

Future of Health Care Workers' Safety

Primary prevention should be the focus of the future. Nonhazardous substances can be substituted for hazardous ones, workers can be isolated from hazardous exposure, engineering controls such as local and dilution ventilation can be in place, administrative controls can cover work practices, and PERSONAL PROTECTIVE EQUIPMENT can be used.

Several psychosocial and organizational factors may correlate with hazards, such as risk-taking personality profiles or perceived conflict of interest between providing optimal patient care and protecting oneself from exposure.

Adequate staffing and appropriate staff mix to meet the increasing acuity of hospitalized patients may have a relationship with work-related injuries among nurses, according to a study by the Institute of Medicine.

The National Institute of Occupational Safety and Health (NIOSH) is focusing on the challenges facing health care workers through the National Occupational Research Agenda (NORA), developed to guide occupational safety and health research. NIOSH collaborates with 500 organizations and individuals (including infection control professionals and front-line health care workers) who provided input into the agenda. Priorities include infectious diseases, allergic and irritant dermatitis, asthma and chronic obstructive pulmonary disease, low back disorders, indoor exposures, and organization of work.

See also BACK INJURIES; BLOODBORNE PATHOGENS; CHEMICAL TOXICITY; CONFINED SPACES; FORMALDEHYDE; FUNGI; HEPATITIS C; HUMAN IMMUNODEFICIENCY VIRUS; INDOOR ENVIRONMENT; NEEDLESTICK PROTECTION; NOISE; SHIFT WORK; SLIPS, TRIPS, AND FALLS; REPETITIVE STRESS INJURIES; STRESS; TUBERCULOSIS; VIOLENCE.

Lipscomb, Jane, and Lina Rosenstock. "Healthcare Workers: Protecting Those Who Protect Our Health." *Infection Control and Hospital Epidemiology* 18, no. 6 (June 1997).

health insurance   Insurance protection that provides payment of benefits for covered sicknesses or injuries. This may include short- and long-term disability, dental, medical and vision care, and in some cases, accidental death coverage as well as other specific benefits. While health insurance was once considered a fringe benefit, it is now a common expectation of employees.

Health insurance began as indemnity insurance, with programs in which the insured worker was reimbursed or the provider was paid for covered expenses after services were rendered.

Today, health insurance may mean coverage by one of many forms of managed care, including HEALTH MAINTENANCE ORGANIZATIONS, preferred provider organizations, or other types of prepaid plans. Many employers provide health insurance for their retirees as well as current employees.

See also MANAGED CARE.

health maintenance organizations (HMOs)   Health insurance plans offered to many employed persons, sometimes as an alternative to a form of indemnity insurance, that offer prepaid, comprehensive health coverage for both hospital and physician services. The HMO provides, offers, or arranges for coverage of designated health services needed by plan members for a fixed, prepaid premium. The HMO is paid monthly premiums or capitated rates by the payers, which include employers, insurance companies, government agencies, and other groups.

The HMO must meet specifications of the federal HMO Act of 1973 as well as meet rules and regulations of each state. Under the federal HMO Act, an entity must have three characteristics to call itself an HMO: it must be an organized system for providing health care or otherwise assuring health care delivery in a geographic area, it must have an agreed-upon set of basic and supplemental health maintenance and treatment services, and it must serve a voluntary enrolled group of people. The four most prevalent models of HMOs are the group model, individual practice association, network model, and staff model. Many HMOs are hybrids of two or more of these types.

An HMO contracts with health care providers, such as physicians, hospitals, and other health professionals. Members of the HMO are required to use participating or approved providers for all health services and generally all services must be approved by the HMO through its utilization review program. Members enroll for a specified period of time, usually one year, and in most instances, have an option to move in or out of an HMO annually if their employer offers more than one option of health insurance.

There has been controversy over whether HMOs use "gatekeepers" to reduce the number of health care services members use. However, many persons are satisfied with the services of their HMOs. Employees often re-enroll during open enrollment periods each year.

In some parts of the country, HMOs also cover persons covered by Medicare.

See also HEALTH INSURANCE; MANAGED CARE.

health promotion   The science and art of helping people change their lifestyle to move toward a state of optimal health. According to the *American Journal of Health Promotion,* optimal health is defined as a balance of physical, emotional, social, spiritual, and intellectual health. Lifestyle change can be facilitated through a combination of efforts to enhance awareness, change behavior, and create environments that support good health practices. Of the three, supportive environments will probably have the greatest impact in producing lasting change.

Efforts of the *American Journal of Health Promotion* have included formation of the Health Promotion Research Foundation, providing advice to national health promotion organizations, creating a grassroots effort to build health promotion into the national agenda, and participating in international health promotion efforts.

Many WORKSITE WELLNESS PROGRAMS are based on recommendations for goals set by the journal. A survey reported in 2002 by Hewitt Associates, a global human resources consulting firm, indicated that 93 percent of U.S. companies offer some level of health promotion, up from 89 percent in 1996. Survey findings indicated that 72 percent of employers offer education or training such as counseling for lifestyle habits, 42 percent of businesses have financial incentive and disincentive initiatives, giving gifts or cash to employees who participate in health appraisals or screenings. An example of a disincentive is charging employees more for insurance if they smoke. Further, 75 percent of companies used health screenings to detect high blood pressure or cholesterol or screen for breast cancer and other types of cancer.

For further information:

American Journal of Health Promotion
6689 Orchard Lake Road
#322 West Bloomfield, MI 48322-3409
(248) 682-0707
inquiries@HealthPromotionJournal.com

See also WELLNESS COUNCILS OF AMERICA.

Health Research Group (HRG) A division of Public Citizen (a nongovernmental organization), HRG works for protection against unsafe workplaces, foods, drugs, and medical devices and advocates for greater consumer control over personal health decisions. A monthly health letter and a monthly letter on prescription drugs are available.

For information:

Health Research Group (HRG)
1600 20th Street, NW
Washington, DC 20009
(202) 588-1000
(202) 588-7796 (fax)
www.citizen.org/hrg

Public Citizen
1600 20th Street, NW
Washington, DC 20009
(202) 588-1000
(202) 588-7798 (fax)
www.citizen.org

health risk assessment See WORKSITE WELLNESS PROGRAMS.

hearing loss See also BROWNFIELDS; DISABILITIES; MUSICIANS' INJURIES; NOISE.

heart attack Known medically as myocardial infarction, a heart attack is sudden death of part of the heart muscle, characterized in most cases by severe, unremitting chest pain. Contributory factors to a heart attack include STRESS, high blood pressure and TYPE A PERSONALITY.

When a heart attack starts, the individual may be short of breath, restless, feel nauseated, vomit, or lose consciousness. *It is crucial to respond immediately to a suspected heart attack.* In mild cases, pain and other symptoms are very slight or do not develop at all, in which case the attack is known as a "silent heart attack." Such an episode may be discovered only by subsequent tests.

Fear of having a heart attack is a common source of stress, because many signs of anxieties and PHOBIAS (including hyperventilation, palpitations, and faintness) mimic some of the signs of a heart attack. Such fears are not unfounded; heart attack is the leading cause of death for both men and women in the United States. Every year, 1.5 million Americans have a heart attack; one-third of them die as a result. However, treatment of heart attacks with clot-dissolving drugs, for example, has helped reduce the death rate dramatically.

Once the coronary artery gets blocked by a clot, a heart attack can occur quite suddenly. Within minutes of a heart attack, the heart muscle begins to change. Deprived of oxygen, the affected portion of the heart muscle deteriorates and dies; surrounding tissue may also be damaged. The longer the artery remains blocked, the greater the damage and possibility of death. According to the American Heart Association, about 60 percent of all heart attack deaths occur within the first hour. Fear, unfamiliarity with the symptoms, and denial are some of the reasons why people delay getting help. Many deaths from heart attack can be prevented with proper and prompt treatment.

Symptoms of a Heart Attack

If these warning signs occur, individuals should get help immediately.

HEART ATTACK WARNING SYMPTOMS

- A crushing chest pressure or pain in the center of the chest that lasts more than a few minutes or goes away and comes back. The discomfort may be felt as a burning sensation that can be mistaken for severe heartburn.
- Chest pain that spreads to the shoulders and arms or the left or both sides, as well as to the neck or back
- Nausea, vomiting, sweating, cold sweats, shortness of breath, palpitations, light-headedness, or faintness
- A sensation of impending doom

Symptoms may be mild, or severe, or even completely absent. Often, older individuals have the fewest or mildest symptoms of heart attack. Few people have all the classic signs. The sooner a person receives appropriate medical treatment, the greater the chances of surviving a heart attack and avoiding permanent damage to the heart. Some potent new drugs that can prevent the death of the heart muscle work only if they are given within the first few hours after the heart attack.

WHAT TO DO IF A HEART ATTACK IS SUSPECTED

Coworkers or employers can assist immensely if they know what to do in response to the emergency, including cardiopulmonary resuscitation (CPR) procedures. Also:

- Do not spend time trying to reach a physician. Have someone call the local emergency number (911 in many urban areas) or an ambulance service. Tell the dispatcher heart attack is suspected.
- If getting to a hospital is faster by car, have someone drive the person there instead of waiting for an ambulance.
- Ask to be taken to an area hospital equipped with 24-hour emergency cardiac care.

If you are the victim:

- Try to stay calm. Lie down, propped up with pillows. Agitation can increase the likelihood of abnormal, life-threatening heart rhythms.
- Have someone call your personal physician.

Concerns After a Heart Attack

Individuals who have suffered a heart attack have an increased risk of suffering another one in the following few years. They live with anxiety about this probability. Many such individuals benefit from psychological counseling. The chances of surviving for many years can be improved by attention to lifestyle changes, including more RELAXATION, increased exercise, better diet, reduction of OBESITY, and cessation of SMOKING. An individual who has had a heart attack should have regular check-ups by a physician. Support and exercise groups can be helpful.

For information:

American Heart Association
7320 Greenville Avenue
Dallas, TX 75231-4596
(214) 373-6300
(800) 242 USA1 (toll free)
(214) 373-6300
(214) 987-4334 (fax)
www.americanheart.org

National Heart, Lung and Blood Institute
9000 Rockville Pike
Bethesda, MD 20891-2486
(301) 496-5166
(301) 402-0818 (fax)
www.nhlbi.nih.gov

See also ANXIETY; BIOFEEDBACK; MEDITATION.

heat illness/heat stress   See HOT ENVIRONMENTS.

heel spur   See FOOT PROTECTION.

help lines   See HOT LINES; SELF-HELP GROUPS; SUPPORT GROUPS.

Henry's law   See COMMERCIAL DIVING.

"HEPA" filters   See ASBESTOS.

hepatoxins   See GASTROINTESTINAL OR LIVER TOXICITY.

hepatitis C   A liver disease caused by the hepatitis C virus (HCV), which enters the liver cells. In about 15 percent of cases, hepatitis C infection is acute, meaning it is cleared spontaneously by the body and there are no long-term consequences.

Unfortunately, in the majority of cases (85 percent) the infection becomes chronic and slowly damages the liver over many years. Over time, these damages can lead to cirrhosis (or scarring) of the liver, end-stage liver disease, and liver cancer.

Hepatitis C is spread through exposure to HCV-infected blood, which may occur through needle-stick injuries, contaminated tattooing or body piercing equipment, transfusions with HCV-infected blood, contaminated hemodialysis equipment, and in other ways. Workers at risk of acquiring hepatitis C in the workplace are those who are exposed to human blood or blood products and needlestick injuries. Transmission in the workplace is possible if skin is punctured by a contaminated sharp, or broken skin or mucous membrane is splashed with blood or bloody fluid. The risk of hepatitis can be reduced by implementing infection control guidelines specific to each workplace. Universal precautions usually include preventing exposure to semen, vaginal secretions, synovial cerebrospinal fluid, pleural fluid, peritoneal fluid, and amniotic fluid.

According to the blood-borne pathogens standard issued by the Occupational Safety and Health Administration in 1991, employers must provide nurses and other employees who have contact with blood or other infectious materials with free hepatitis-B vaccine, gloves, gowns, goggles, face masks, and other necessary protective equipment, immediate medical evaluation and follow-up if exposed, confidential treatment, and protection of medical records. Additionally, employers must make sure that universal precautions are practiced institution-wide, and that employees know which materials are potentially infectious, provide puncture- and leak-proof containers for sharps disposal, remove hazards whenever possible by changing the design of the workplace, and train employees during orientation and annually about hazards and prevention.

The prevalence of hepatitis C is higher among veterans than in the general population, particularly among Vietnam War veterans. Of 325,000 veterans tested for HCV from 1998 through 2000 as part of a national screening program, 30 percent, or 65,000, were found to be HCV positive.

The rate of hepatitis C infection is higher in the prison population than in the general population, with estimates ranging form 28 percent to 67 percent. This is probably due to the fact that injection drug use is more common among those who are in prison. About 80 percent of the nation's estimated 1.7 million drug injection users have been through the prison system, according to the Schering Corporation, a pharmaceutical firm.

About one-third of people with HIV, primarily those who acquired HIV through injection drug use or through a blood transfusion, are also infected with the hepatitis C virus.

Hepatitis A and Hepatitis B

Hepatitis A (once called infectious hepatitis) is thought to be spread by a virus from an infected person's feces directly or indirectly contaminating food, drinking water, or someone else's fingers. Food handlers can transmit the virus, so appropriate handwashing is essential.

Hepatitis B (once referred to as serum hepatitis) is mainly sexually transmitted or spread by mechanisms in which an infected person's blood is inoculated into someone else, for example, by needle sharing among drug abusers, razor sharing, or ear piercing.

The non-A, non-B hepatitis virus is the cause of most transfusion-associated hepatitis cases. Vaccines are available against viral hepatitis (type B). Vaccines are generally offered or recommended only to those who are at high risk of infection, such as health care workers and drug addicts.

For further information:

American Nurses Association
600 Maryland Avenue SW
Suite Washington, DC 100W
(800) 274-4ANA (toll-free) or (800) 274-4262 (toll-free)
(202) 651-7000 (fax)
www.nursingworld.org

See also HAND PROTECTION; HEALTH CARE WORKERS; HOSPITAL HAZARDS; NEEDLESTICK INJURIES AND PREVENTION; PERSONAL PROTECTIVE EQUIPMENT.

herbicides   Materials used as weed control for commercial vegetable crops. Effects from exposure to herbicides and pesticides can be acute or chronic. The potential for poisoning can be reduced by careful storage and handling. These materials should be kept in a separate room or building used only for storage purposes, and should be dry and ventilated.

Herbicides have the same mode of entry into the human body as other pesticides: through the skin, by swallowing, and by breathing. Paraquat, for example, is highly toxic orally and can be fatal. The arsenicals, such as MSMA and DSMA, can be fatal if swallowed. According to J. Tredaway Ducar, University of Florida, Cooperative Extension Service, Institute of Food and Agricultural Sciences, herbicides are not as toxic to humans as insecticides, rodenticides, and nematicides, because plants have different sites of action than humans or animals. However, some may accumulate in the body and be fatal when a certain concentration is reached.

Workers who may be most affected by herbicides include forestry, greenhouse, and nursery employees. Requirements for protection include use of PERSONAL PROTECTIVE EQUIPMENT (PPE), observing restricted-entry intervals (REIs), and notifying workers about areas where applications are taking place or where REIs are in effect. There should be a decontamination facility, worker training, monitoring of handlers, cleaning, inspection, and maintenance of PPE. Appropriate training must be provided for noncertified pesticide handlers.

For further information:

J. Tredaway Ducar
Assistant Professor
Agronomy Department
Cooperative Extension Service
Institute of Food and Agricultural Sciences
University of Florida
Gainesville, FL 32611
P.O. Box 110500
(352) 392-1811 ext. 201
(352) 392-1840 (fax)
http://www.agronomy.ifas.ufl.edu

See also AGENT ORANGE; FARMING; GULF WAR SYNDROME.

high-risk occupations High-risk occupations may be defined as occupations that carry the greatest number of fatalities and nonfatal injuries. Work-related injuries and fatalities result from multiple causes and occur in many occupational and industrial settings. Various organizations keep track of these statistics and statistics may vary from one database to another.

According to the National Occupational Research Agenda (NORA), a health service research organization, between 1980 and 1992, more than 77,000 workers died as a result of work-related injuries. In four industries—mining, construction, transportation, and agriculture—occupational-injury fatality rates were notably and consistently higher than all other industries. Motor vehicle-related deaths in the transportation sector, machine-related deaths in agriculture, electrocutions and fatal falls in construction, homicide in retail trade and public administration, and deaths due to falling objects in mining and logging were significant because of particularly high rates of death from injury.

NORA also reported that the workplaces with the highest number of serious nonfatal injuries included eating and drinking establishments, hospitals, and grocery stores. Workers facing higher risks of serious nonfatal injuries were concentrated in the manufacturing sector and include workers in shipbuilding, wooden building and mobile home manufacture, foundries, sawmills, and meatpacking plants.

According to the U.S. Department of Labor's Bureau of Labor Statistics (BLS), outdoor occupations have exhibited the highest rates of fatal injuries. Fishers and loggers posted unusually high rates of fatal work injuries, rates 25–30 times higher than the national figure of about five deadly injuries per 100,000 workers.

In addition to fishing and timber cutting, nine other outdoor occupations exceeded the national fatality rate by a wide margin. These other occupations included airplane pilots, structural metalworkers, taxicab drivers, electrical installers and repairers, farm operators, managers and supervisors, construction laborers, truck drivers, driver–sales workers, and farmworkers.

According to the BLS, manufacturing activities commonly result in some of the highest rates of nonfatal injuries and illnesses resulting in workdays lost.

According to the National Institute for Occupational Safety and Health (NIOSH) *Chartbook, 2000,* by occupational group the highest rates of fatal injuries occurred among transportation and agricultural workers, forestry, and fishing workers.

Research Recommended on High-Risk Occupations

The National Occupational Research Agenda (NORA) of NIOSH advises research on high risk occupations. High-risk groups targeted by NORA include construction workers, loggers, miners, farmers, farmworkers, adolescents, and older workers. Multiple factors and risks contribute to traumatic injuries, including characteristics of workers, workplace/process design, work organization, economics, and other factors. Priorities are deaths caused by motor vehicles, machines, violence, and falls, as well as traumatic injuries caused by falls and contact with machines, equipment and tools.

For further information:

Office of Safety, Health, and Working Conditions
Census of Fatal Occupational Injuries
Bureau of Labor Statistics
2 Massachusetts Avenue NE
Washington, DC 20212-0001
Phone: (202) 606-6175

See BUTCHERS AND MEAT, POULTRY, AND FISH CUTTERS; FATALITIES BY OCCUPATION; FIREFIGHTERS AND RESCUE WORKERS; FISHING; LOGGERS; MINE SAFETY AND HEALTH; SLIPS, TRIPS, AND FALLS; TOXICOLOGY REPORTS AND FATAL INJURIES.

Bureau of Labor Statistics, U.S. Department of Labor, Census of Fatal Occupational Injuries—1993.

hockey injuries (professional)   In hockey, cuts and bruises, pulls and strains, separations and dislocations are common. There are dangerous areas of the rink, such as posts, which players may hit. Players are constantly twisting and turning, stressing the upper thigh, abdomen, and pelvic areas. They are balanced on a thin metal blade. The combination of strength and balance leads to a number of groin, abdominal, and back pulls and strains.

The hockey puck, a small projectile traveling up to 100 miles an hour, may result in contusions and broken bones, especially of the foot and lower leg.

See also SLIPS, TRIPS, AND FALLS; SPORTS MEDICINE.

home care industry   Many workers are involved in the home care industry, including physicians, nurses, case managers, health care aides, therapy specialists, social workers, laboratory technicians, nutritionists, and transportation providers.

Demand for health care services continues to increase as there are more early discharges from hospitals, increasing outpatient surgeries, and technical advances and pharmaceutical developments that have lengthened the survival of chronically ill patients. Some home care patients have AIDS, are on dialysis or ventilators, receive chemotherapy, or suffer from mental illness and physical disabilities. Health care workers manage intravenous therapy, tracheostomy care, and wound irrigations, in addition to managing the risks inherent in home environments.

Potential hazards to home care workers include potential violence from clients or others, exposure to communicable diseases, ergonomic issues such as lifting the patient, physical conditions (poor lighting, broken stairs), hazardous chemicals, environmental tobacco smoke, and oxygen equipment.

Hazards can be controlled, reduced, or eliminated, according to "Health and Safety in the Home Care Environment," a publication of the Health Care Health and Safety Association of Ontario. Here are some tips:

- Modify the environment; for example, use lifting devices
- Use policies and procedures determined by employers (for example, training in specific work practices)
- Practice good hygiene (such as handwashing, proper body mechanics)
- Use personal protective equipment (such as gloves, eye protection)

See also ERGONOMICS AND ERGONOMICS REGULATIONS; EYE INJURIES/PROTECTION; HAND PROTECTION; HEALTH CARE WORKERS; NEEDLESTICK INJURIES AND PREVENTION; PERSONAL PROTECTIVE EQUIPMENT; SLIPS, TRIPS, AND FALLS.

homicide in the workplace   See AGGRESSION; VIOLENCE.

hospital hazards According to the Occupational Safety and Health Administration, workers in hospitals face potential hazards that are biological, chemical, psychological, physical, environmental, mechanical, and biomechanical. The following chart indicates examples.

See also BLOODBORNE PATHOGENS; CHEMICAL TOXICITY; CONFINED SPACES; HEALTH CARE WORKERS; FORMALDEHYDE; FUNGI; HEPATITIS C; HUMAN IMMUNODEFICIENCY VIRUS; INDOOR ENVIRONMENT; NEEDLESTICK PROTECTION; NOISE; SHIFT WORK; SLIPS, TRIPS, AND FALLS; REPETITIVE MOTION INJURIES; STRESS; TUBERCULOSIS; VIOLENCE.

hostility A persistent attitude of deep resentment and intense ANGER. It may be the result of stressful workplace situations or from personal sources of STRESS for the individual. The hostile person may have an urge to retaliate against a person or situation. During some situations of intense FRUSTRATION, deprivation, or discrimination, feelings of hostility may be a normal reaction. However, hostile attitudes also may occur during ANXIETY attacks, in obsessive-compulsive disorder, or DEPRESSION. Some people who have antisocial personalities frequently have hostile attitudes.

At best, hostile people are simply grouchy. At worst, they are consumed by hatred. Hostile people may have tense-looking faces and bodies. They are easily excitable. They seem to have a chip on their shoulders and bitterness toward the world. They

HOSPITAL HAZARDS

Categories of Potential Hazards Found in Hospitals

Hazard Category	Definition	Examples found in the hospital
Biological	Infectious/biological agents, such as bacteria, viruses, fungi, or parasites, that may be transmitted by contact with infected patients or contaminated body secretions/fluids	Human immunodeficiency virus (HIV), vancomycin resistant enterococcus (VRE), methicillin resistant staphylococcus aureus (MRSA) hepatitis B virus, hepatitis C virus, tuberculosis
Chemical	Various forms of chemicals that are potentially toxic or irritating to the body system, including medications, solutions, and gases	Ethylene oxide, formaldehyde, glutaraldehyde, waste anesthetic gases, hazardous drugs such as cytotoxic agents, pentamidine ribavirin
Psychological	Factors and situations encountered or associated with one's job or work environment that create or potentiate stress, emotional strain, and/or other interpersonal problems	Stress, workplace violence, shift work, inadequate staffing, heavy workload, increased patient acuity
Physical	Agents within the work environment that can cause tissue trauma	Radiation, lasers, noise, electricity, extreme temperatures, workplace violence
Environmental, Mechanical/ Biomechanical	Factors encountered in the work environment that cause or potentiate accidents, injuries, strain, or discomfort	Tripping hazards, unsafe/unguarded equipment, air quality, slippery floors, confined spaces, cluttered or obstructed work areas/ passageways, forceful exertions, awkward postures, localized contact stresses, vibration, temperature extremes, repetitive/ prolonged motions or activities, lifting and moving patients

Source: Occupational Safety and Health Administration November 2001

may be sarcastic and moody and respond aggressively when challenged.

For many individuals, hostilities in the workplace can be worked out through better COMMUNICATION skills, BEHAVIOR THERAPY, use of MEDITATION and RELAXATION, and psychotherapy.

See also AGGRESSION; BODY LANGUAGE; COMPLEMENTARY THERAPIES; PSYCHOTHERAPIES; TYPE A PERSONALITY.

Kahn, Ada P. *Stress A–Z: The Sourcebook for Facing Everyday Challenges.* New York: Facts On File, Inc., 1998.

hot environments   Workers in foundries, laundries, construction projects, canneries, bakeries, and many other places often face hot conditions that pose hazards to safety and health. Environmental factors that affect the worker's discomfort in a hot work area include temperature, humidity, radiant heat (such as from the sun or a furnace), and air velocity. The person's age, weight, fitness, medical condition, and acclimatization to heat are also factors.

The body reacts to high external temperature by circulating blood to the skin, which increases skin temperature and allows the body to give off excess heat through the skin. However, if muscles are being used for physical labor, less blood is available to flow to the skin and release the heat. The body sweats to maintain a stable internal body temperature in hot situations. However, sweating is effective only if the humidity level is low enough to permit evaporation and if the fluids and salts lost are adequately replaced.

According to the Safety and Health Department of the International Brotherhood of Teamsters (IBT), the body stores excess heat if it cannot dispose of it. When this happens, the body's core temperature rises and the heart rate increases. As the body continues to store heat, the individual begins to lose concentration and has difficulty focusing on a task, may become irritable or sick, and loses the desire to drink, possibly resulting in fainting and death if the person is not removed from the heat stress.

According to the IBT, most heat related problems can be prevented by following some basic precautions. For example, new employees and workers returning from an absence of two weeks or more should have a five-day period of acclimatization, beginning with 50 percent of the normal workload and time exposure the first day and gradually building up to 100 percent on the fifth day. Engineering controls, general ventilation, and spot cooling by exhaust ventilation at points of high heat production may be helpful. Shielding is required as protection from radiant heat sources.

Employee education is vital so that workers are aware of the need to replace fluids and salt lost through sweat and can recognize dehydration, exhaustion, fainting, heat cramps, salt deficiency, heat exhaustion, and heat stroke.

Heat Stroke

In hot environments, heat stroke is the most serious health problem for workers. It is caused by the failure of the body's internal mechanism to regulate its core temperature. Signs include mental confusion, delirium, loss of consciousness, convulsions, or coma. While awaiting medical help, the victim must be removed to a cool area and his or her clothing soaked with cool water and fanned vigorously to increase cooling. Prompt first aid can prevent permanent injury to the brain and other vital organs.

Heat Exhaustion

Heat exhaustion results from loss of fluid through sweating when a worker has not consumed enough fluids, taken in enough salt, or both. Symptoms of heat exhaustion (although the victim is still sweating) include extreme weakness or fatigue, giddiness, nausea, or headache. The skin is clammy and moist and the body temperature normal or slightly higher. The victim should rest in a cool place and drink an electrolyte solution to quickly restore potassium, calcium, and magnesium salts.

Heat Cramps

Painful spasms of the muscles occur when workers drink large quantities of water but do not replace their bodies' loss of salt. Tired muscles are usually the ones most susceptible to cramps. Cramps may occur during or after working hours and may be relieved by taking liquids by mouth or saline solutions intravenously for quicker relief, if medically advised.

Fainting (Heat Syncope)

Workers unacclimatized to a hot environment and standing still may faint. Victims usually recover quickly after a brief period of lying down. Moving around, rather than standing still, will usually reduce the possibility of fainting, according to the IBT.

Heat Rash

Heat rash, also known as prickly heat, may occur in hot and humid environments where sweat is not easily removed from the surface of the skin by evaporation. If extensive or complicated by infection, heat rash can be very uncomfortable and result in temporary disability. Resting in a cool place and allowing the skin to dry can prevent it.

See also COOKS; CONFINED SPACES; CONSTRUCTION.

Safety and Health Department, International Brotherhood of Teamsters.

hot lines Hot lines are telephone lines maintained by trained personnel to provide crisis intervention service or information on a given topic. Throughout the United States, hot lines cover many concerns related to workplace issues, stress, and mental health. In many cases, the numbers for information and help are toll free and usually operate on a 24-hour basis. Most city telephone directories list of some of the available hot lines.

See also MENTAL HEALTH; SELF-HELP GROUPS; STRESS; SUPPORT GROUPS.

housemaid's knee See BURSITIS.

human immunodeficiency virus (HIV) The HIV virus is considered responsible for causing the infection that leads to acquired immunodeficiency syndrome (AIDS), which continues in epidemic proportions in the United States and elsewhere in the world in the early 2000s.

How the Virus Is Transmitted

The virus is usually transmitted by direct exchange of body fluids, such as blood or semen, or by using contaminated needles. Many individuals are anxious about contracting the virus through eating in restaurants in which infected individuals may work or working in a place with an infected individual. In most cases, these anxieties are unfounded, as the virus does not survive outside the body, according to research reports.

Individuals who suspect their partners of high-risk sexual contacts, such as homosexual men or prostitutes, should seek medical advice about screening for and preventing transmission of the HIV virus. Use of condoms during sexual intercourse is promoted as a way to prevent the transmission.

Concerns About Getting HIV from a Health Care Professional

Some people fear contracting the HIV virus when having blood drawn or dental and medical procedures done. According to an article in *Health* (September 1992), the person who draws the blood presents virtually no risk. To infect a person, a health professional who is HIV positive would have to get stuck with the needle and in turn stick that person with the contaminated needle. There is little likelihood of this happening. In the case of dental hygienists who manipulate sharp instruments inside a person's mouth, they would have to injure themselves and bleed into exposed tissue in that person's mouth.

The article says that stress can be reduced by being sure that health care professionals take universal precautions. Look over the doctor's or dentist's office. Equipment and instruments should look clean. Personnel should wash their hands before and after procedures, and should wear gloves, masks, and eye guards during procedures in which body fluids might splatter. Protective gear should be changed or discarded between patients. Needles and other sharp objects should be disposed of in secure containers. Anything that goes in your mouth or inside your body should arrive in sterile packaging, be disinfected or be sterilized by autoclave or dry heat.

For information:

CAIN (Computerized AIDS Information Network)
1213 North Highland Avenue
P.O. Box 38777
Hollywood, CA 90038
(213) 464-7400 ext. 450

National AIDS Hotline
(800) 243-7889 (TTY/TDD)
English Hotline: (800) 342-AIDS
Spanish Hotline: (800) 344-SIDA
International Hotline: (301) 217-0023
(800) 342-2437

CDC National Prevention Information Network
   (NPIN)
P.O. Box 6003
Rockville, MD 20849-6003
(800) 243-7012 (toll-free)
(800) 458-5231
(301) 562-1050 (fax)
www.cdcnpin.org

   See also ACQUIRED IMMUNODEFICIENCY SYNDROME;
AIDSINFO; ELISA TEST; WESTERN BLOT.

Japenga, Ann. "The Secret." *Health,* September 1992.
Kahn, Ada P., and Linda Hughey Holt. *Midlife Health: Every Woman's Guide to Feeling Good.* New York: Avon Books, 1989.

humor   A positive emotion that usually provides a helpful release of boredom and stress for many people in the workplace. Humor is healthy because it may actually ease pain and may help the respiratory system by exercising the lungs. Laughter, the expression of humor, may influence the immune system by stimulating production of certain hormones that help to lift the mood.

   Humor is a universal language and thus has universal appeal. The basis for much humor is that we are prepared for one thing and something else happens. Although we are startled, we know there is no danger, and we release our surprise in laughter. Thus a story with an unexpected ending, or a game of peek-a-boo for an infant, can seem humorous and elicit a laughter response.

   Shared humor relieves anxiety in stressful group situations, such as when deadlines approach. In work situations, a humorous approach can help one face sources of stress and daily disappointments. Esther Blumenfeld and Lynne Alpern, in their book *Humor at Work,* outline some characteristics of stress-reducing humor, which can be used in the workplace as well as in other settings. However, the authors warn against misusing humor, which can actually lead to stress.

   Humor may relieve stressful workplace situations by reducing tension. Joking about universal human frustrations and faults encourages people to relax and laugh. Those who delight in poking fun at themselves can build rapport with others. This can create a supportive atmosphere of fun and caring, allowing workers to note the positive aspects of human relationships.

HARMFUL WORKPLACE HUMOR: SITUATIONS TO AVOID

- Poking fun at other people's individual shortcomings.
- Reflecting anger.
- Offending with inappropriate use of sexual references or profanity.
- Dividing a group by put-downs.
- Using a stereotype to denigrate a person or group.
- Creating a cruel, abusive, and offensive atmosphere.

Historical Overview of Humor in the Workplace

Ancient scholars understood the role of humor. The Book of Proverbs says: "A merry heart doeth good like a medicine." Conversely, many individuals who suffer from depression lose their sense of humor and few things make them smile or laugh. Studies in the late 20th century suggested that an ability to enjoy humor and to laugh affects mental as well as physical health. Norman Cousins's book *Anatomy of an Illness* (1977), stimulated interest in use of humor in recovery from both mental and physical illness. While fighting ankylosing spondylitis, he checked out of the hospital and spent weeks watching Marx Brothers movies and other comedies. He believed that the positive feelings aroused by humor and laughter helped him recover. Increasingly, hospitals and health care practitioners are bringing humor programs into their compendia of therapies.

   For information:

International Laughter Society
16000 Glen Una Drive
Los Gatos, CA 95030
(408) 354-3456

   See also LAUGHTER.

Blumenfeld, Esther, and Lynne Alpern. *Humor at Work.* Atlanta, Ga.: Peachtree Publishers, Ltd., 1994.

Fry, William F., and Waleed A. Salameh, eds. *Handbook of Humor and Psychotherapy.* Sarasota, Fla.: Professional Resources Exchange, 1987.

hydrofluoric acid/hydrofluoric acid toxicity See GLASS WORKERS/GLAZIERS; SKIN AND SENSE ORGAN TOXICITY.

hydrogen sulfide See SKIN AND SENSE ORGAN TOXICITY.

hypersensitivity pneumonitis (HP) An inflammation of the lungs caused by repeated inhalation of a foreign substance, such as an organic dust, a fungus, or a mold. The immune system of the body reacts to these substances, called antigens, by forming antibodies, molecules that attack the invading antigen and try to destroy it. The combination of antigen and antibody produces acute inflammation, or pneumonitis (a hypersensitivity reaction), which later can develop into chronic lung disease that impairs the ability of the lungs to take oxygen from the air and eliminate carbon dioxide.

Hypersensitivity pneumonitis is sometimes called allergic alveolitis. *Allergic* refers to the antigen-antibody reaction, and *alveolitis* means an inflammation of the alveoli, tiny air sacs in the lungs where oxygen and carbon dioxide are exchanged.

Typical changes occur in the lungs of persons who have HP. In the acute stage, there are large numbers of inflammatory cells throughout the lungs and the air sacs may be filled by a thick fluid mixed with these cells. In the subacute stage, disease extends into the small breathing tubes, or bronchioles, and the inflammatory cells collect into tiny granules called granulomas. Finally, in the chronic stage, the previously inflamed parts of the lungs become scarred and unable to function, as in pulmonary fibrosis.

Farmer's lung is a type of HP that is caused by antigens from tiny microorganisms living on moldy hay. After a time, very little of the allergenic material is needed to set off a reaction in the lungs.

Bird fancier's lung is a form of external allergic alveolitis caused by the inhalation of avian proteins present in droppings and feathers of certain birds, particularly pigeons and caged birds. As in farmer's lung, there is an acute and a chronic form.

Malt workers' lung is caused by inhalation of malt dust.

illiteracy   The inability to read or write. It interferes with the ability to obtain employment. People who are unable to read or write or who do one or both poorly may develop techniques to hide or compensate for their lack. Embarrassment may keep them from seeking help. For children, the illiteracy of a parent can also be a source of embarrassment and cause them a great deal of stress.

Illiteracy is a fairly common problem in the United States. Estimates are that 75 percent of unemployed Americans are illiterate. In the early 1990s, the New York Telephone Company had to give 60,000 people an entry-level exam in order to hire 3,000 employees. Some major corporations have had to use graphics on assembly lines to compensate for workers' inability to read simple phrases. As jobs have become increasingly technical and the economy has shifted from an industrial to a service base, more jobs will require skills that include reading and writing ability.

A study of emergency room and clinic patients at two public hospitals reported that a high proportion of them are unable to read and understand basic written medical instructions, according to an article in the *Journal of the American Medical Association* (December 5, 1995). The study raises the question of whether the estimated 40 million to 44 million adults in the United States who are functionally illiterate and another 50 million adults who are only marginally literate are leaving doctors' offices and hospitals without understanding the next steps to take to ensure their good health.

The authors commented that patients with limited literacy skills who have difficulty reading informed consent forms present a troubling ethical issue: "The ethical obligation of physicians to explain the risks and benefits of any procedure or treatment is fundamental to the physician-patient relationship. Patients unable to understand informed consent forms cannot intelligently participate in their own care."

Learning disabilities account for some illiteracy; however, there is not always agreement among educators to what extent. There is a growing movement in American education to reduce illiteracy by treating reading and writing as learning disabilities at an early stage in schooling.

At the end of the 20th century, many community organizations took on illiteracy as a project. Volunteers work with people who need help reading and writing with good results.

immune system   A collection of cells and proteins that works to protect the body from potentially harmful, infectious microorganisms such as bacteria, viruses, and fungi. The immune system also plays a role in the control of cancer and is responsible for the phenomena of allergy, hypersensitivity, and rejection problems when organs or tissues are transplanted.

See also ALLERGIES; CANCER; FUNGI; HYPERSENSITIVITY PNEUMONITIS; HUMAN IMMUNODEFICIENCY VIRUS; IMMUNOTOXICITY.

immunotoxicity   Adverse effects on the functioning of the immune system resulting from exposure to chemical substances. Altered immune function may lead to increased incidence or severity of infectious diseases or cancer, since the immune system's ability to respond adequately to invading agents is suppressed. Identifying immunotoxicants is difficult because chemicals can cause a wide variety of complicated effects on immune function. A number of environmental and industrial chemicals can adversely affect the immune system. Exposure to ASBESTOS, BENZENE, and halogenated aromatic hydrocarbons such as POLYBROMINATED BIPHENYLS (PBBs), POLYCHLORINATED BIPHENYLS (PCBs), and dioxin can lead to immunosuppression. Toxic agents can also cause autoimmune diseases, in which healthy tissue is attacked by an immune system that fails to differentiate self-antigens from foreign antigens. For example, the pesticide dieldrin induces an autoimmune response against red blood cells, resulting in hemolytic anemia.

Allergens are compounds that stimulate the immune system and can cause hypersensitivity reactions or allergies. Many chemicals induce allergic reactions producing a variety of symptoms, such as asthma, rhinitis, and anaphylaxis. The industrial chemical toluene diisocyante (TDI) and metals such as nickel and BERYLLIUM are examples of allergenic agents.

See also ALLERGIES; CHEMICAL TOXICITY.

Dean, J., M. Murray, and E. Ward. "Toxic Responses of the Immune System." Chap. 9 in *Casarett and Doull's Toxicology,* edited by C. Klaassen, M. Amdur, and J. Doull. New York: Pergamon Press, 1996.
Luster, M. I. "Immunotoxicology: Clinical Consequences." *Toxicology and Industrial Health* 12, no. 3 (1996): 533–535.
Environmental Defense
www.scorecard.org/health-effects

incinerators   See WASTE INDUSTRY.

indecision   See DECISION MAKING.

indoor environment (indoor air quality)   The quality of the indoor environment can affect the health of workers in a building. According to World Health Organization estimates, 30 percent of office buildings worldwide may have significant problems, with 10 percent to 30 percent of occupants experiencing health effects perceived to be related to indoor air quality.

While the proportion of the estimated 20 million to 30 million United States workers who experience serious health problems is small, the large aggregate numbers make the associated economic costs high. These are estimated at tens of billions of dollars per year, including the costs of health care and ABSENTEEISM, reduced worker productivity, building investigations, and building improvements. These costs do not include the enormous costs of closure or renovation of many buildings each year in attempts to solve these problems. Furthermore, the office and indoor job sectors continue to expand along with the proportion of modern, energy-efficient buildings in which these health problems tend to occur.

By 1988, the NATIONAL INSTITUTE FOR OCCUPATIONAL SAFETY AND HEALTH (NIOSH) found that more than 20 percent of its calls were about indoor air quality. Of the more than 500 investigations done by NIOSH, more than 50 percent had a primary problem of inadequate ventilation. The next most common findings were inside contamination (15 percent), outside contamination (10 percent), and building materials themselves (4 percent.)

Ventilation in some workplaces may have deteriorated because of energy conservation following the oil crisis in the 1970s. The need to conserve energy led to reduced ventilation. Buildings were sealed to exclude hot summer air and cold winter air. Computers and other office technologies led to more heat output, chemical hazards, and job stress.

Nearly 70 percent of U.S. workers, or approximately 89 million persons, are employed in nonindustrial, nonagricultural indoor work environments. Some indoor environmental conditions have been associated with increased risks of nonspecific symptoms, respiratory disease, and impaired performance. Some health-related complaints associated with poor air quality are similar to those of flu or colds: HEADACHES, sinus problems, congestion, dizziness, nausea, fatigue, and irritation of the eyes, nose, or throat. The indoor environment is usually not the suspected cause of occupant symptoms unless the symptoms are shared by a number of workers.

Indoor air quality is good when it is free of odors and dust, not too still or too drafty, and is a comfortable temperature and humidity. Factors associated with possible complaints about indoor air quality include new furnishings, renovation, poor air circulation, and persistent moisture.

Possible sources of contamination in office buildings and manufacturing plants include tobacco smoke, dust, poor maintenance of heating, ventilation, and air-conditioning (HVAC) systems, cleaning supplies, pesticides, building materials, furnishings, and cosmetics. They cause indoor air quality problems when concentrations are excessive. Dusty surfaces, stagnant water, and damp materials provide an environment for microbial growth. When mold spores and other microbial particles become airborne, some building occupants may experience allergic reactions. One potential but extremely rare infection known as Legionnaire's disease is caused by *Legionella* bacteria.

Disease transmission by inhalation or airborne infectious aerosols may be influenced by factors affecting indoor concentrations of infectious agents, transport pathways between individuals, viability of infectious agents, or susceptibility of individuals.

Contaminants. Contaminants may come from inside or outside the building. Indoor sources of contaminants include cigarette smoke, renovation and remodeling materials, dirt, deteriorating lining in the ventilation system, cleaning compounds, correction fluids, copy machines, laser printers, and pesticides. Outdoor sources include car exhaust, pollen, and industrial emissions from nearby buildings.

Ventilation. Fresh air should be brought to all occupied spaces to remove contaminants that occur in normal use. An evaluation includes determination of the quantity and quality of fresh air. It should address how well the distribution system is functioning. The air system must be balanced and assure good mixing. Fresh air intakes should be evaluated. Outside air should enter the system freely, not impeded by louvers. If air comes in, it should be fresh, not potentially contaminated by nearby industrial discharge, such as a loading dock where trucks idle.

In some cases, measurements of carbon dioxide and total airborne hydrocarbons are taken to help determine the adequacy of the ventilation. If the air circulation is poor and the fresh air insufficient, carbon dioxide, which is produced primarily from people breathing, builds up. While carbon dioxide is not itself hazardous, it is used as a marker of a lack of fresh air and good ventilation.

Carbon dioxide (CO_2). The Occupational Safety and Health Association (OSHA) standard for indus-

trial environments is based on the potential toxic effects of CO_2. The OSHA standard for carbon dioxide is 5,000 parts per million (ppm), but it is recognized that when indoor levels rise above 700–800 ppm, building occupants report discomfort. Carbon dioxide is often the only useful measure taken and can provide valuable information if done properly.

Odors. Our sense of smell can be an important qualitative measurement device. For example, if vehicle exhaust enters the building, carbon dioxide as well as carbon monoxide levels will increase. Vehicle exhaust is accompanied by an odor that people are quick to recognize and complain about. Smoking contributes to both carbon dioxide and total hydrocarbon level in the air.

Volatile hydrocarbons. A test of ventilation adequacy can pick up traces of cleaning chemicals, perfumes, exhaust, paints, art materials, cigarette smoke, carpet glues, and so on. As with carbon dioxide, OSHA standards for industrial environments for many of these same hydrocarbons found in trace levels in office air are much higher than those considered acceptable for ambient air quality. There are no national standards for indoor air quality, although some agencies such as the California Air Resources Board are considering promulgating such measures.

Particulates. Airborne dust particles are a common problem in offices and other workplaces. Potential sources of particulates in the air include old or dirty carpeting, paper dust, chalk, and outside dirt that gets tracked in. If ventilation filters are overloaded or breached, or some part of the insulation of the ductwork deteriorates, the ventilation system itself can become a source of contamination. Construction dust may get into the ventilation system. Systems designed with an open return plenum are particularly susceptible.

If filters are changed regularly and the system is intact and functions well, routine cleaning of the ductwork should not be necessary. Evidence of draft around the air suppliers on the ceiling indicate an excess of room dirt that is caught there by static electricity caused by the flow of air. It is not due to dirt in the ductwork itself.

Bioaerosols. Levels of airborne mold or bacteria or their by-products are sometimes measured. The most common measurement is of viable airborne mold levels, the spores that will grow in an agar petri dish. Mold is always present in indoor as well as outdoor air and varies seasonally and from place to place. A visual inspection for evidence of water damage, a history of leaks, or chronic dampness is often more useful than measurement in determining the potential for mold.

For comfort, good temperature control and relative humidity levels between 30 and 50 percent are recommended. Levels below 30 percent indicate air that may be dry enough to irritate mucous membranes. Air that is too humid, with relative humidity higher than 60 percent, may cause moisture to form and mold to grow.

Authors M. J. Mendell et al, in an article in the *American Journal of Public Health,* summarized indoor environment factors:

- Rate and effectiveness of outdoor air ventilation, which dilutes concentrations of indoor aerosols

- Rate and efficiency of air filtration

- Disinfection, as by ultraviolet light, which may deactivate infectious organisms

- Rate of air recirculation, which influences transport between regions of the building

- Density of occupancy, use of private workspaces, or use of barriers between occupants, which influence the effective distance between individuals

- Temperature and humidity of air, which affect the period of viability of infectious aerosols and human susceptibility

- Indoor toxic or fungal exposures, which may alter human susceptibility to infection

Building-related Asthma and Allergic Disease

According to Mendell et al, about 18 million indoor workers have ALLERGIES, and about 5 million (most with allergies) have ASTHMA. Asthma is increasing globally in much of the developed world, and part of this increase may be related to indoor environmental quality. Studies conducted in schools and residences have indicated that moisture and mold problems (also common in nonindustrial workplaces) are related to lower-respiratory-tract symptoms associated with asthma. Serious allergic diseases such as hypersensitivity pneumonitis and asthma have been documented among office workers. Causes have included microbiological exposures resulting from water leaks, contaminated ventilation system components, and other building inadequacies.

Exposures to allergens such as dust mites, cockroaches, rodents, and pollen, as well as exposure to tobacco smoke has been associated with allergy and asthma in residential studies. These same exposures occur in the nonindustrial work environment; however, their magnitude and effects are not yet determined.

Barriers to Improving Indoor Workplace Environment

Social and economic forces influence whether available health-related information is put into action. Decisions affecting indoor environmental quality are made primarily by building professionals, including architects and engineers, and owners. These decisions occur during design, construction, operation, maintenance, and renovation, and in the course of activities related to sales, rental, and use.

According to Mendell et al, some of the barriers that may obstruct consideration of indoor environment quality include:

- Limited information, guidelines, and standards on the relation of indoor environmental quality to health

- Lack of necessary products and services for measuring or controlling indoor environmental quality

- Lack of documentation of the costs versus benefits of specific health-protective building practices

- Decision making habits based on lowest first costs

Incentives to Increase Healthful Features in Buildings

Mendell et al suggest that the following incentives may increase implementation of healthful features and practices in indoor workplace environments:

- Codes, regulations, and laws (local, state, or federal) based on science, professional consensus, or both

- Nonregulatory government actions, such as tax incentives, subsidies, demonstration projects, guidelines, and education

- Guidelines from professional consensus groups or other sources establishing a standard of care

- Financial section incentives

- Avoidance of liability

- Scientific data documenting that improving indoor environmental quality can diminish adverse effects among building occupants

- Educational or informational activities for building professionals and occupants

Need for Research on Indoor Work Environments

According to Mendell et al, indoor nonindustrial work environments were designated a priority research area through the nationwide process that created the National Occupational Research Agenda (NORA). A multidisciplinary research team used member consensus and quantitative estimates, with extensive external review, to develop a specific research agenda. They identified 21 priority areas in which new research could most effectively reduce work-related illnesses, injuries, and deaths in the coming decade. The team outlined the following priority research topics: building-influenced communicable respiratory infections, building-related asthma/allergic diseases, and nonspecific building-related symptoms; indoor environmental science; and methods for increasing implementation of healthful building practices. Available data suggest that improving building environments may result in health benefits for more than 15 million of the 89 million U.S. indoor workers, with estimated economic benefit of $5 billion to $75 billion annually. Research on these topics, requiring new collaborations and resources, offers enormous potential health and economic returns.

Although there are limitations in available scientific documentation, some guidance and standards are available on health-protective building practices. According to Mendell et al, many current building codes, standards, and guidelines, although intended to be health protective, are based primarily on practical experience within the building sector or on non-health-related criteria such as perceived acceptability of air (that is, immediate perception of odor or irritants), and these codes are not always sufficiently health protective. Additional scientific research is needed to provide health bases for standards and practices and to develop knowledge of indoor environmental and building science to implement these practices while considering cost and energy efficiency.

Further, Mendell et al suggest that the availability of information on health-protective building practices and of adequate building science and technology does not in itself guarantee implementation in buildings for the benefit of occupants. A complex set of institutional and economic barriers and incentives affects decisions on design, operation, and maintenance of buildings. Even with recognized potentially fatal building-related illnesses such as Legionnaires' disease, implementation of available prevention strategies is not universal. Current building costs generally regulate only the design and construction of buildings. Few U.S. legal standards, excepting ordinances in several states, mandate that occupied buildings provide healthful indoor air quality, comfortable thermal conditions, or even some minimum amount of outside air. Mendell et al recommend that nonregulatory incentives now determine most postconstruction decisions on building environments.

Mendell and coauthors (the NORA Indoor Environment Team) included expertise from fields of engineering, architecture, occupational medicine, epidemiology, industrial hygiene, physiology, and chemistry. They formulated priorities for research on health in indoor work environments. They suggest that these priorities will require new collaborations and resources. Implementation of this research agenda will provide knowledge on which employers and unions, building owners and managers, financial institutions, professional associations, and government can base policies.

Table 1 provides estimates (as available) of the total adverse health effects produced by U.S. indoor work environments and of the proportions of adverse effects preventable by improving these environments. The estimated potential annual reductions in adverse health effects include 5 million to 7 million communicable respiratory infec-

Improving the Health of Workers in Indoor Environments: Priority Research Needs for a National Occupational Research Agenda

TABLE 1. ESTIMATED HEALTH IMPACTS OF CONTAMINANTS IN INDOOR WORK ENVIRONMENTS IN THE UNITED STATES, AND POTENTIAL BENEFITS OF IMPROVED ENVIRONMENTS (ALL STATISTICS FOR 1996 UNLESS NOTED)

Contaminant-Related Health Effect	Number of Workers with Health Effect due to Work or Non-work Exposures (of 89 million total indoor workers in United States)	Health Impacts		Estimated Potential Annual Reduction in Health Effect Among Indoor Workers with Improved Work Environments [%] and number
		Severity	Frequency (duration)	
Communicable respiratory infections—building-influenced, occupant sources (e.g., influenza, common cold, tuberculosis	Influenza and common cold: 52 million cases; tuberculosis not in health-care or prison settings: unknown	Usually moderate, fewer than 70,000 hospital-izations and unquantified fatalities	~0.58 cases of common cold and influenza per year among working age population; (duration varies, days to months)	[Estimated 10% to 14%] 5 million–7 million cases (estimate has substantial uncertainty)
Asthma, hypersensi-tivity pneumonitis, and allergic disease	Asthma: 4.7 million, allergies: 18 million	Allergies—mild to severe; asthma—mild to fatal	Asthma and allergies: many to all days per year (duration of both usually chronic)	[Estimated 6% to 15%] asthma episodes among 0.3–0.7 million cases; allergy episodes among 1 million–3 million cases (estimates have substantial uncertainty)
Nonspecific building-related symptoms (acute effects of indoor exposures or conditions, including so-called sick building syndrome)	35 million–60 million workers with one or more weekly building-related symptoms (effects from work exposures only)	Usually mild to moderate	Often while at work (chronic with chronic exposure)	[Estimated 20% to 50%]; 8 million–30 million cases (estimate has substantial uncertainty)
Respiratory infections—building sources (Legionnaires' disease, Pontiac fever, and fungal infections)	2,700–6,000 estimated cases per year of Legionnaires' disease, unknown number of Pontiac fever and fungal infection cases	Legionnaires' disease: often severe, 5% to 15% of documented cases are fatal; Pontiac fever: moderate; fungal infections: can be severe or life threatening	Legionnaires' disease and Pontiac fever: usually once per lifetime (duration varies); fungal infections: varies	[Unknown, probably fairly high (e.g., >50%)]; Legion-naires' disease: 1,400–3,000 cases, including>70 deaths; Pontiac fever, fungal infections: unknown

(continues)

TABLE 1. ESTIMATED HEALTH IMPACTS OF CONTAMINANTS IN INDOOR WORK ENVIRONMENTS IN THE UNITED STATES, AND POTENTIAL BENEFITS OF IMPROVED ENVIRONMENTS (ALL STATISTICS FOR 1996 UNLESS NOTED) *(continued)*

| Contaminant-Related Health Effect | Number of Workers with Health Effect due to Work or Non-work Exposures (of 89 million total indoor workers in United States) | Health Impacts | | Estimated Potential Annual Reduction in Health Effect Among Indoor Workers with Improved Work Environments [%] and number |
		Severity	Frequency (duration)	
Health effects of environmental tobacco smoke	Among 10 million–30 million exposed—acute irritation, respiratory effects, reproductive effects: unknown; cardiovascular effects: 2,000–11,000 deaths; lung cancer; 100–600 cases. (effects from work exposures only)	Acute irritation—mild to moderate; respiratory and reproductive effects—moderate to severe; cardiovascular effects—severe to fatal; lung cancer—fatal	Acute irritation—with exposure; respiratory effects—chronic; cardiovascular effects and cancer—chronic, often fatal	[100%] 2,000–11,000 cardiovascular disease deaths; 100–600 lung cancer cases including 90–530 deaths

TABLE 2. ESTIMATED ANNUAL ECONOMIC IMPACTS OF CONTAMINANT-RELATED HEALTH EFFECTS IN INDOOR WORK ENVIRONMENTS IN THE UNITED STATES, AND POTENTIAL BENEFITS OF IMPROVED ENVIRONMENTS (ALL STATISTICS FOR 1996 UNLESS NOTED)

Contaminant-Related Health Effect	Annual Economic Impacts		Estimated Economic Consequence for Indoor Workforce due to Work or Non-work Exposures	Estimated Economic Benefits Possible with Improved Indoor Work Environments
	Health Care Costs of Effects due to Work or Non-work Exposures	Costs from Absence due to Illness and from Other Performance Losses due to Work or Nonwork Exposures		
Communicable respiratory infections—building-influenced; occupant sources (e.g., influenza, common cold, tuberculosis)	$10 billion in health care costs	$19 billion in absence from work $3 billion from reduced performance at work	$32 billion	$3 billion–$4 billion (estimate has substantial uncertainty)
Asthma, hypersensitivity pneumonitis, and allergic disease, building-related	asthma, $2.6–2.8 billion; allergic rhinitis, $580 million, other, not estimated	Asthma, $340 million; allergic rhinitis, $377 million; other, not estimated	$3.9 billion–4.1 billion	$200 million to $600 million (estimate has substantial uncertainty)
Nonspecific building-related symptoms (acute effects of indoor exposures or conditions, including so-called sick building syndrome)	Unknown (effects from work exposures only)	$20 billion–70 billion (effects from work exposures only)	$20 billion–70 billion (effects from work exposures only)	$4 billion–70 billion (estimate has substantial uncertainty)
Respiratory infections—building sources (Legionnaires' disease, Pontiac fever, and fungal infections)	Legionnaires' disease: $26 million–40 million in health care costs; Pontiac fever: minimal health care costs; Fungal infections: unknown costs	Legionnaires' disease: $5 million–8 million in absence from work; Pontiac fever: unknown absence costs 1 week/case; fungal infections: unknown costs	Greater than $30 million–50 million	Tens of millions of dollars
Health effects of environmental tobacco smoke	$30 million–140 million in health care costs for cardiovascular disease and lung cancer (effects from work exposures only)	(costs of absence from work and other performance losses not estimated)	$30 million–140 million (costs of absence from work and other performance losses not estimated; effects from work exposures only)	$30 million–140 million (costs of absence from work and other performance losses not estimated)

tions, a 6 percent to 15 percent reduction in exacerbation of asthma among the 4.7 million indoor workers with asthma, and a 20 percent to 50 percent reduction in nonspecific building-related symptoms.

Table 2 provides estimates of the adverse economic consequences of contaminant-related health effects in indoor work environments and of the potential economic benefits from improved indoor work environments. The most uncertain estimate, according to Mendell et al, is that for productivity losses from building-related symptoms. The estimates in Table 2 indicate that the combined annual costs of these adverse health effects range from $50 to $100 billion, with about 5 billion to 75 billion potentially preventable.

For further information:

Mark J. Mendell, Ph.D., M.P.H.
Lawrence Berkeley National Laboratory
1 Cyclotron Road
MS90–3058
Berkeley, CA 94720
mjmendell@lbl.gov

American Industrial Hygiene Association
2700 Prosperity Avenue
Suite 250
Fairfax, VA 22031
(703) 849-8888
(703) 207-3561 (fax)
infonet@aiha.org

National Institute of Occupational Safety and Health
Division of Surveillance, Hazard Evaluations and Field Studies
4676 Columbia Parkway
R-16
Cincinnati, OH 45226
(513) 841-4445
(513) 841-4486 (fax)

See also AIR POLLUTION; ALLERGIES; ASTHMA; DUST; FUNGI; MOLD; RESPIRATORY TOXICITY; SICK BUILDING SYNDROME; SMOKING.

Mendell, Mark J., William J. Fisk, Kathleen Kreiss, et al. "Improving the Health of Workers in Indoor Envi-

ronments: Priority Research Needs for National Occupational Research Agenda." *American Journal of Public Health* 92, no. 9 (September 2002): 1430–1440.
Yale Medical School, Department of Internal Medicine.

industrial hygiene   A profession in which occupational health, safety, and environmental professionals are concerned primarily with the control of environmental health hazards that arise out of the workplace or the community. Industrial hygienists are scientists and engineers committed to keeping workers, their families, and the community healthy and safe. They play a vital role in ensuring that federal, state, and local laws and regulations are followed in the work environment.

ISSUES INDUSTRIAL HYGIENISTS FACE

- Emergency response planning
- Ergonomics/cumulative trauma disorders
- Exposure and risk assessment strategies
- Indoor environmental quality
- Workplace environmental exposure levels
- Noise hazards
- Practice standards and guidelines
- Respiratory protection
- Risk assessment
- Sampling and laboratory analysis

Source: American Industrial Hygiene Association

WHAT INDUSTRIAL HYGIENISTS DO

- Investigate and examine the workplace for hazards and potential dangers
- Make recommendations for improving safety of workers and the surrounding community
- Conduct scientific research to provide data on possible harmful conditions in the workplace
- Develop techniques to anticipate and control potentially dangerous situations in the workplace and the community
- Train and educate the community about job-related risks
- Advise government officials and participate in the development of regulations to ensure the health and safety of workers and their families
- Ensure that workers are properly following health and safety procedures

Source: American Industrial Hygiene Association

The American Industrial Hygiene Association, founded in 1939, with more than 12,000 members, is one of the largest international associations serving the needs of occupational and environmental health professionals practicing industrial hygiene in industry, government, labor, academia, and independent organizations.

For information:

American Industrial Hygiene Association
2700 Prosperity Avenue
Suite 150
Fairfax, VA 22031
(703) 849-8888
(703) 207-3561 (fax)
http://www.aiha.org

See also ERGONOMICS AND ERGONOMIC REGULATIONS; NOISE; INDOOR ENVIRONMENT; REPETITIVE STRESS INJURIES.

infection control   See HEALTH CARE WORKERS; NEEDLESTICK INJURIES AND PREVENTION; PERSONAL PROTECTIVE EQUIPMENT.

instrumental musical injuries   See MUSICIAN'S INJURIES; PERFORMING ARTS MEDICINE.

international air pollution   Canada and Mexico, neighbors of the United States, share the air at international borders. Pollution moves across the borders and can be serious. The CLEAN AIR ACT OF 1990 includes provisions for cooperative efforts to reduce pollution that originates in one country and affects another.

See also AIR POLLUTION; INTERSTATE AIR POLLUTION.

International Brotherhood of Teamsters (IBT)
One of the largest labor unions in the world, with 1.4 million members, formed in 1903. The union represents a diverse group of workers, ranging from airline pilots to zookeepers. One out of every 10 union members in the United States is a Teamster.

Objectives of this international union include securing improved wages, hours, working conditions, and other economic advantages through organization, negotiations, and collective bargaining.

Further, objectives include providing educational advancement and training for employees, members, and officers, promoting the principle of free collective bargaining, and advancing the rights of workers, farmers, and consumers. The union communicates workers' needs to employers and politicians, protect workers' health and safety, and work to keep jobs in North America.

The IBT supports local unions with:

- Advice and assistance from safety and health experienced organizers, negotiators, safety and health professionals, researchers, attorneys, auditors, and communications specialists
- Coordination of national contract negotiations, political action, and organizing
- Training and educational programs for Teamsters officers, business agents, stewards, and members

For further information:

International Brotherhood of Teamsters
25 Louisiana Avenue, NW
Washington, DC 20001
(202) 624-6800
(202) 624-8102 (fax)
www.teamster.org

See also AMERICAN FEDERATION OF LABOR-CONGRESS OF INDUSTRIAL ORGANIZATIONS.

International Ladies' Garment Workers Union (ILGWU)   A U.S.-based labor organization formed in 1900 by the amalgamation of several local unions. At that time, attempts by workers to organize were hampered by clashes between anarchists and socialists. In the early years, many members were sympathetic to various radical movements.

In the 1940s, under the leadership of David Dubinsky, the ILGWU developed into one of the nation's most powerful and progressive unions, with a wide range of member benefits, including loans and technical assistance. Dubinsky retired in 1966. In 1967 the Dubinsky Foundation was established, with the purpose of making grants to causes and institutions in line with ILGWU objectives. From 1968 to the early 1990s, the union lost more than 300,000 workers through diminished U.S. employment as a result of low-cost imports and the transfer of factories overseas.

In 1995 the 125,000-member ILGWU merged with the 175,000-member Amalgamated Clothing and Textile Workers' Union to form UNITE!, the Union of Needletrades, Industrial and Textile Employees.

International Occupational Hygiene Association
(IOHA) An international organization that conducts a wide range of activities intended to promote and develop occupational hygiene worldwide. From its creation in 1987, the IOHA has grown to more than 20 member organizations, representing more than 20,000 occupational hygienists worldwide. Member organizations in the United States include the American Conference of Governmental Industrial Hygienists and the American Industrial Hygiene Association.

The IOHA provides an international voice of the occupational hygiene profession through its recognition as a nongovernmental organization (NGO) by the International Labour Organization and the World Health Organization. IOHA also cooperates with the work of other international organizations such as the International Commission on Occupational Health.

As an association of organizations, overall objectives are to promote and develop occupational hygiene throughout the world, to promote the exchange of occupational hygiene information among organizations and individuals, to encourage the further development of occupational hygiene at a professional level, and to maintain and promote a high standard of ethical practice in occupational hygiene.

For further information:

IOHA Secretariat
Suite 2, Georgian House
Great Northern Road
Derby
DE1 1LT
United Kingdom
Email: admin@ioha.com

See also AMERICAN CONFERENCE OF GOVERNMENTAL INDUSTRIAL HYGIENISTS; AMERICAN INDUSTRIAL HYGIENE ASSOCIATION.

International Labour Organisation (ILO) A specialized agency of the United Nations involving national delegations of government, employers, and worker representatives. The purposes of the ILO include promoting voluntary cooperation of nations to improve labor conditions, raising living standards, and fostering economic and social stability throughout the world. The ILO sets standards covering all aspects of working life, including human rights, through adoption of recommendations and conventions.

The ILO was established in 1919 by the Treaty of Versailles as an affiliated agency of the League of Nations and became the first affiliated specialized agency of the United Nations in 1946.

The ILO holds its annual International Labour Conference in Geneva, Switzerland, usually in June with approximately 2,500 attendees. There is a U.S. branch of the ILO in Washington, D.C., which has a library that includes materials on labor, child labor, women, occupational safety, and health.

For information:

International Labour Organisation
4, route des Morillons
CH-1211 Geneva 22
Switzerland
41 22 7996111
41 22 79888685 (fax)
http://www.ilo.org

International Labour Organisation–U.S.
1828 L Street, NW
Suite 600
Washington, DC 20036
(202) 653-7652
(202) 653-7687 (fax)
http://www.us.ilo.org

International Safety Equipment Association
(ISEA) A trade association in the United States for companies that manufacture safety equipment. Member companies design and manufacture cloth-

ing and equipment used in factories, construction sites, hospitals and clinics, farms, schools, and laboratories. Included in the association are products for head, eye and face, respiratory, hearing, hand and foot protection, environmental monitoring instruments, safety warning signs and symbols, emergency eyewash and showers, first aid kits, clean room garments, and safety apparel.

The common goal of ISEA member companies is protecting the health and safety of people exposed to hazardous and potentially harmful environments.

For information:

International Safety Equipment Association (ISEA)
1901 N. Moore Street
Suite 808
Arlington, VA 22209
(703) 525-1695
(703) 528-2148 (fax)
www.safetyequipment.org

See also CONSTRUCTION; PERSONAL PROTECTIVE EQUIPMENT.

interstate air pollution   In many areas, two or more states share the same air. These states are in the same air basin, defined by geography and wind patterns. Often, air pollution moves out of the state in which it is produced into another state. Some pollutants, such as the power plant combustion products that cause acid rain, may travel over several states before affecting health, environment, and property. The CLEAN AIR ACT OF 1990 includes many provisions, such as interstate compacts, to help states work together to protect the air they share. Reducing interstate air pollution is very important since many Americans live and work in areas where more than one state is part of a single metropolitan area.

See also AIR POLLUTION.

International Union of Bricklayers and Allied Craftworkers (BAC)   A service organization formed in 1865 which became an international union in 1881 and was given its current name in 1975. BAC was one of the first unions to support the eight-hour workday which took effect nationally in 1901. By the 1950s, BAC's membership included bricklayers, stone and marble masons, cement masons, plasterers, tilers, terrazo and mosaic workers, cleaners, and caulkers.

Objectives of the BAC include promoting or establishing programs to meet the health care, retirement, unemployment, and other needs of BAC members and their families, advancing the skills, efficiency, and working knowledge of BAC members through apprentice and training programs, maintaining relationships with other labor organizations, and raising public awareness of the need to improve the lives of workers across the world.

For information:

International Union of Bricklayers and Allied
   Craftworkers
1776 I Street, NW
Washington, DC 20006
(202) 783-3788
www.bacweb.org

See also CONSTRUCTION.

interstitial lung diseases   See ASBESTOS; BERYLLIUM; HYPERSENSITIVITY PNEUMONITIS; SILICOSIS.

irritant contact dermatitis   (ICD)
See DERMATITIS.

isocyanates   Chemicals known to cause asthma.
See also ASTHMA.

janitors, custodians, maintenance workers
Those who keep office buildings, hospitals, stores, apartment buildings, hotels, and other buildings clean and in good condition. Some only do cleaning, while others may fix leaky faucets, empty trash cans, do painting and carpentry, replenish bathroom supplies, mow lawns, and maintain heating and air conditioning equipment. They may mop floors, clean bathrooms, vacuum carpets, dust furniture, make minor repairs, and exterminate insects and rodents.

In hospitals they may also wash bed frames and disinfect and sterilize equipment and supplies. In hotels, maintenance people may also deliver irons, ironing boards, and rollaway beds to guest rooms.

Janitors use varied equipment, tools, and cleaning materials. They usually work inside heated, well-lighted buildings. However, they sometimes work outdoors, sweeping walkways, mowing lawns, or shoveling snow. Working with machines can be noisy, and they may encounter toxic substances while cleaning bathrooms, trash rooms, or exterminating pests. Janitors may suffer cuts, bruises, and burns from machines, hand tools, and chemicals. They spend most of their time on their feet, sometimes lifting or pushing heavy furniture or equipment. Many tasks, such as sweeping, require bending, stooping, and stretching, resulting in back injuries and sprains. Scrubbing and other tasks result in repetitive motion injuries. Janitors and cleaners use cleaning and other chemicals, which may cause irritation and other problems in the eyes, nose, throat, and skin.

Because most office buildings are cleaned while they are empty, many janitors and maintenance people work evening hours. Some, however, such as school and hospital custodians, may work in the daytime. Some janitors are assigned to shifts to cover the 24-hour period. Part-time cleaners usually work in the evenings and on weekends. Many are also victims of violence, partially due to working nights and being alone in isolated places.

According to recent workers' compensation data from the state of Washington, six out of every 100 janitors have lost-time injuries every year. Eye irritation or burns accounted for 40 percent of these injuries, skin irritation or burns, 36 percent, and chemical fumes, 12 percent.

See also BOREDOM; CHEMICAL TOXICITY; COLD ENVIRONMENTS; ELECTRICITY-RELATED INJURIES; FOOT PROTECTION; FUNGI (MOLD); GARDENERS; HAND PROTECTION; HOSPITAL HAZARDS; HOT ENVIRONMENTS; NOISE; PEST CONTROL WORKERS; REPETITIVE STRESS INJURIES; SHIFT WORK; SKIN OR SENSE ORGAN TOXICITY; SLIPS, TRIPS, AND FALLS; VIOLENCE.

Bureau of Labor Statistics.

jewelry stores   See VIOLENCE.

job change   Making the transition to a new position. Regardless of whether the change involves continuing to work for the same company or for a new one, it can be stressful for many people. There are pros and cons in both situations. Coming from the outside means the individual does not have to worry about dealing with coworkers or friends. However, without a mentor or friend in a new company, the worker has no one to rely on or to explain corporate policies and politics. Starting out fresh also means not knowing what others are good at, who are the hard workers, and who goofs off.

Promotion, whether from within or without, can also significantly raise stress levels because it raises fear of incompetence and fear of failure. Usually these fears subside once the new position is mastered and evidence of success becomes visible.

See also DOWNSIZING; JOB SECURITY; LAYOFFS; NETWORKING.

Snyder, Don J. *The Cliff Walk: A Memoir of a Job Lost and a Life Found*. Boston: Little, Brown, 1997.

job security   Lack of job security is a major cause of instability and stress for workers throughout the world. This was not so 30 to 40 years ago. Then, many employers had implicit or explicit long-term employment contracts with their workers, contracts that emphasized management's commitment to minimize the need for LAYOFFS. Wages and job benefits usually increased over the years, and it was not unusual for the company to pay the total cost of employees' health care and charge minimally for family coverage. This job security led workers to expect to remain in their jobs for many years and it was not unusual for workers to devote their entire working lives to one company, perhaps retiring with the traditional gold watch and the company pension.

During the later 1990s, DOWNSIZING, layoffs, MERGERS, and other organizational changes have greatly altered job security. Employers are no longer sharing their wealth; raises and employee benefits have been scaled back. Full-time jobs are harder to find. According to *Money* magazine (September 1995) since 1991, a staggering 1 million out of the 7.5 million jobs created in the United States has been a temporary position.

To cope with dwindling job security, in addition to the option of operating their own business, suggestions in *Money* include that workers consider themselves free agents or skilled artisans; set new professional goals, look for new jobs while still employed, build portable skills, set up a network made up of five to 10 trusted colleagues, clients, former bosses, and other professionals who know the worker's track record and opportunities available in his/her field, create an escape hatch (options, lateral moves, further education), and be ready to accept change.

See also DOWNSIZING; JOB CHANGE; LAYOFFS; MENTAL HEALTH; MERGERS; NETWORKING.

Alderman, Lesley. "Here's How You Can Work on Job Security." *Money,* September 1995.

jumper's knee   See BASKETBALL INJURIES (PROFESSIONAL).

Kabat-Zinn, Jon Jon Kabat-Zinn, Ph.D., is a professor of medicine and founder and Director of the Stress Reduction Clinic at the University of Massachusetts Medical Center in Worcester. He is the author of numerous books, including *Mindfulness Meditation in Everyday Life, Meditation for Daily Living,* and *Full Catastrophe Living: Using the Wisdom of Your Body and Mind to Face Stress, Pain and Illness.*

Dr. Kabat-Zinn is a proponent of mindfulness meditation, a more than 2,000-year-old Buddhist method of living fully in the present. This is an approach that offers a unique way to cope with stress and illness. Mindfulness meditation can help induce deep states of relaxation and, at times, directly improve physical symptoms. Other forms of meditation involve focusing on a sound or the sensation of breath leaving and entering the body. Anything else that comes up in the mind during meditation is seen as a distraction to be disregarded. Mindfulness, on the other hand, is "insight" meditation, encouraging the meditator to note any thoughts as they occur and observe them nonjudgmentally, moment by moment, as events occur in one's awareness. This practice of observing thoughts, feelings, and sensations can help one become calmer and have a broader perspective on one's life. It involves a significant commitment to oneself; it is a way of life.

In his writings, Kabat-Zinn explains how to live in the moment by taking up such techniques as "nondoing," trust, and concentration. He shows readers meditation postures and ways to meditate, including visualizing mountains and lakes, and concentrating on walking or standing.

Like many mind/body techniques, mindfulness has just begun to be explored scientifically. Typically, the training program for mindfulness meditation is eight weeks long. Controlled studies are investigating whether mindfulness meditation can influence the healing process and help in treating many diseases.

For further information:

Stress Reduction Clinic
University of Massachusetts Medical Center
55 Lake Avenue North
Worcester, MA 01655
(508) 856-1616

See also COMPLEMENTARY THERAPIES; MEDITATION; RELAXATION.

Kabat-Zinn, Jon. *Full Catastrophe Living: Using the Wisdom of Your Body and Mind to Face Stress, Pain and Illness.* New York: Delacorte, 1991.
———. *Wherever You Go, There You Are: Mindfulness Meditation in Everyday Life.* New York: Hyperion, 1993.
Kahn, Ada P., and Jan Fawcett. *Encyclopedia of Mental Health.* 2d ed. New York: Facts On File, Inc., 2001.

karoshi A Japanese term meaning "death from overwork," synonymous with *stress* in Japan. C. Frank Lawlis, Ph.D., wrote in *Alternative Therapies* magazine (July 1995), "People [in Japan] are literally dying at their workstations. It appears that their entire physiological system collapses or shuts down."

Lawlis draws from a 1989 study by Chiyoda Fire and Marine Insurance, Ltd., one of the top insurance carriers in Japan, covering more than 100,000 Japanese corporations. Chiyoda conducted a major study on health problems that Japanese people are likely to encounter. One important conclusion of the study was that in 40 percent of the health problems, stress played a major role.

As a result, Chiyoda established N.C. Wellness, a company that developed programs integrating Oriental medicine into a health promotion program for employees and citizens incorporating transpersonal psychology—chosen because of its close alignment with mental fitness—in its teaching.

Buildings housing the programs were constructed to focus on tranquil space and function. At the same time, they were designed as places where "interference from everyday affairs is barred" and where the environment to practice the mind-body and awareness elements of balance is enjoyable and protective.

The first prototype center was opened in Kichjoji, Musashino-shi, Tokyo, in June 1994. The core program offered at this site incorporated five "directions": self-management, self-promotion, self-discovery/purpose of life, fun and pleasure, and interpersonal skills and community.

See also ACCULTURATION.

keyboard instrument players' injuries (professional)   Injuries sustained while playing pianos, organs, claviers, harpsichords, synthesizers, and other keyboard instruments. Playing keyboard instruments combines movements of the fingers, arms, and torso. The number of musculoskeletal injuries in pianists is directly related to the number of repetitive activities of the fingers. Also, using fingers repeatedly fatigues and stresses many tissues. Overuse syndrome results just as it does in industry among riveters and welders.

Posture is a factor in producing injuries, as a sitting position is required both for practice and performance in keyboard playing. Those who do attempt to play standing for any length of time may develop problems with hands and wrists due to the hyperextended wrist position. Benches can present problems, particularly for organists of small stature or who have disproportionately short arms. Some benches are adjustable, but if they are not, they may induce discomfort in the players. Some keyboardists sit too high or too low. Many keyboardists develop back fatigue. Distance from the keyboard is another factor. Many people sit too close, and if they keep raising their shoulders when they play, discomfort may result. The neck is also a frequent location of pain and tension among pianists, as it is in other musicians and occupational groups.

Recent injuries are specific to people who play electronic keyboards. While these lighter-action keyboards may seem easier to play, they are actually harder, because many players have a tendency to press harder than they would on a naturally-weighted keyboard to overcompensate for the lack of resistance.

If keyboardists' injuries are untreated, injuries can cause permanent damage. Professionals have been known to stop performing, both temporarily and permanently, because of injuries.

See also CARPAL TUNNEL SYNDROME; PERFORMING ARTS MEDICINE; REPETITIVE STRESS INJURIES.

Sataloff, Robert Thayer, Alice G. Brandfonbrener, and Richard J. Lederman, eds. *Textbook of Performing Arts Medicine.* New York: Raven Press, 1991.

Mark, Thomas. *What Every Pianist Needs to Know About the Body.* Chicago: GIA Publications, 2003.

kidney toxicity   Adverse effects on the kidney, ureter, or bladder that result from exposure to chemical substances. Toxic injury to the kidney is known to occur as a result of occupational, accidental, or therapeutic exposure to certain chemicals. Renal toxicants include halogenated hydrocarbons, such as carbon tetrachloride and trichloroethylene, and the heavy metals CADMIUM and lead.

The kidney is the major excretory organ in the body, and it also performs nonexcretory functions, such as regulating blood pressure and blood volume. Since the kidneys receive approximately 25 percent of cardiac output, any chemical in systemic circulation is delivered to them in relatively high amounts. This makes the kidney unusually susceptible to the toxic effects of chemicals. Some nephrotoxic agents cause acute injury to the kidney, while others produce chronic changes that can lead to renal failure or cancer. The consequences of renal failure can result in permanent damage that requires dialysis or kidney transplantation.

See also CHEMICAL TOXICITY.

Hook, J., and W. Hewitt. "Toxic Responses of the Kidney." Chap. 11 in *Casarett and Doull's Toxicology,* edited by C. Klaasen, M. Amdur, and J. Doull. New York: Pergamon Press, 1996.

kinesics The study of communication as expressed through facial expression and other body movements. Theories and techniques of studying this type of nonverbal communication were developed by Ray L. Birdwhistell (1918–94), who found that certain gestures and expressions were typically masculine or feminine and also related to regional and national groups. BODY LANGUAGE also changes with mood, health, age, and degree of tension or relaxation. Birdwhistell developed his theories with the use of photography and developed a notation system of symbols called kinegraphs to describe gestures and expressions. Understanding nonverbal communication is important in job interviews and reviews.

Birdwhistell, Ray L. *Kinesics and Context.* Philadelphia: University of Pennsylvania Press, 1970.

L

laboratory workers People who work in a laboratory may perform tests or research according to prescribed standards to determine chemical and physical characteristics or composition of solid, liquid, or gaseous materials for purposes such as quality control. Laboratory workers are employed in industries including chemical, petroleum and petrochemical, food, rubber, polymer, metallurgical and metal finishing, and paper, and in universities, schools, research institutes, hospitals and medical clinics, public and private testing, inspection and quality assurance laboratories.

Laboratory workers may handle a wide variety of materials and equipment, including disposable glass and plastic equipment, securing devices, automatic dispensing equipment, filters, pumps, gas-, liquid- and solid-sampling instruments, particle-counting instruments, heating, cooling, and temperature-measure equipment.

JOB HAZARDS FACING LABORATORY WORKERS

- Slips, trips, and falls on wet floors
- Cuts and stabs from sharp edges and broken glass
- Fires and explosions from uncontrolled chemical reactions
- Falls of heavy objects from overhead storage shelves
- Electrocution and electric shock
- Burns and scalds from flames, hot surfaces, hot gases and liquids
- Chemical burns from corrosive fluids
- Flying particles from bursting centrifuges and autoclaves
- Acute poisoning from a wide variety of poisonous gases, liquids, and solids used as starting materials or released in chemical reactions
- Damage to eyes from laser beams, splashes of chemicals, corrosive gases, and flying particles
- "Freeze burn" or frostbite from skin contact with cold surfaces or liquefied gases

---

- Exposure to a wide variety of chemical substances
- Exposure to many biological agents through inhalation, ingestion, skin, eye contact, accidental injection, or laboratory animal bites
- Eyestrain from work with optical and electron microscopes, computer terminals, and work in dark or semi-dark rooms
- Musculoskeletal problems from routine work in a fixed position
- Hand stress from repetitive manual operations

See also ANIMAL HANDLERS; CHEMICAL TOXICITY; EYE INJURIES/PROTECTION; HEALTH CARE WORKERS; FIRE SAFETY/FIRE PROTECTION; HOSPITAL HAZARDS; NEEDLESTICK INJURIES; PERSONAL PROTECTION EQUIPMENT; REPETITIVE STRESS INJURIES.

Mager-Stillman, Jeanne, ed. *Encyclopaedia of Occupational Health and Safety.* 4th ed. Vol. 4. Geneva: International Labour Organisation, 1998, pp. 103.20–103.21.

laborers See CENSUS OF FATAL OCCUPATIONAL INJURIES.

labor unions See AMERICAN FEDERATION OF LABOR-CONGRESS OF INDUSTRIAL ORGANIZATIONS; INTERNATIONAL BROTHERHOOD OF TEAMSTERS.

ladder Occupations that involve use of ladders include construction, plumbing, heating and air conditioning, electrical work, and roofing. According to the American Academy of Orthopedics, more than 500,000 people a year in the United States are treated for ladder-related injuries. About 300 people die from ladder-related injuries annually. Estimated annual cost of ladder-related injuries is $11 billion, including work loss, medical, legal, liability, and pain and suffering expenses.

ENCOURAGE SAFETY: CHOOSE THE RIGHT LADDER

- Ladder style: Step or extension. Both may be needed for a job. A stepladder can be used indoors and outdoors but are usually shorter than standard ladders. Use an extension ladder primarily outdoors where extra height is required. An extension ladder can be used indoors where high ceilings are hard to reach.
- Size of ladder: For stepladders, the height of the ladder plus four feet equals the total reach. For example, a four-foot ladder can be used to reach an eight-foot ceiling. Use a six-foot ladder to reach a 10-foot ceiling, and so on. For an extension ladder, the base and upper sections must overlap. Thus a 20-foot extension ladder is only good for about 17 feet. The ladder must travel above the roofline two to three feet so that it can be used for balance as one climbs onto the roof.
- Duty rating: Ladders are sold by duty rating, which means the weight a ladder is rated to carry. The more weight it will hold, the stronger it must be.
- Construction material: Choices are wood, aluminum, and fiberglass.
- Wood ladders are solid and sturdy. However, they are heavy and therefore cumbersome and somewhat difficult to transport. Wood must be maintained to prevent cracking, splitting, and rotting. Wood is economical and does not conduct electricity when clean and dry. When doing electrical work, choose a fiberglass ladder.
- Ladders made from high-strength aluminum are lightweight, but salt air or chemicals can corrode and weaken an aluminum ladder. Aluminum ladders conduct electricity.
- Fiberglass ladders are lighter than wood but heavier than aluminum. They are not subject to rot, do not bend easily, and do not conduct electricity.

See also CONFINED SPACES; CONSTRUCTION; ELECTRICITY-RELATED INJURIES; SLIPS, TRIPS, AND FALLS.

lasers Devices that produce coherent, intense, directional beams of light of a single wavelength. Advanced technology enables increasing use of lasers in the workplace. Lasers can be hazardous if safe work systems and appropriate controls are not established and followed.

Repeated exposure to relatively low-powered lasers, or from a single exposure to medium-powered lasers, may cause long-term damage to sight or minor damage to the skin. Exposure to high-level lasers may cause depigmentation, severe burns, and possible damage to underlying organs. High-powered lasers may cause fire hazards.

Lasers may produce hazards from airborne contaminants released during laser use, collateral radiation, high voltage electricity, cryogenic coolants and flying particles during laser cutting or welding.

Lasers are used for cutting and welding, and scientific lasers are used in a wide range of applications. Medical lasers are used on eyes and for microsurgery, neurosurgery, and dermatology. Lasers are also used in many other ways, including optical fibers and for display and entertainment, instrumentation, and security systems.

To prevent injuries, hazards and risks must be assessed before lasers are used. Suitability of the laser type should be considered, as well as the capability of the laser to injure people, the environment in which the laser is used, and operator training.

Where there is a risk to health and safety from laser use, employers should consider eliminating laser use, substitution with a safer alternative, isolating the laser (a closed laser operation should be used where practical), engineering controls, including interlocks, workplace layout, shielding materials and warning signs, administration and procedural controls to assure that exposure limits are not exceeded, and use of PERSONAL PROTECTIVE EQUIPMENT.

At all times, workers should avoid looking into a laser beam or a laser reflection. Lasers should be used in a controlled area with emphasis on controlling the path of the laser beam. Only authorized personnel should operate lasers.

Protective eyewear specifically designed for protection against non-ionizing radiation lasers and laser systems may include goggles, face shields, spectacles, or prescription eyewear using special filter materials or reflective coatings.

Lasers used in presentations as remote pointing devices for slides, overheads, and computer projections can also be hazardous to a worker's health if used improperly. The penlike laser pointer, which produces a fine beam, can be hazardous to the unprotected eyes of the individuals who look directly at the laser beam.

See also DERMATITIS; EYE INJURIES/PROTECTION.

latex allergy See ALLERGIES; HEALTH CARE WORK-ERS; HOSPITAL HAZARDS.

laughter An individual's response, such as a smile, chuckle, or explosive sound, to something that inspires joy or scorn. The ability to laugh, and its companion, a sense of HUMOR, can provide psychological relief from stress, ANXIETY, and HOSTIL-ITY in the workplace. Laughter helps individuals deal with stressful situations at work or in social situations.

Laughter may be a defense against personal feelings of self-consciousness or embarrassment. An ability to laugh at oneself can be an important coping mechanism against these stresses. However, many people find it difficult to poke fun at themselves and to acknowledge that they have made a mistake. Individuals suffering from DEPRESSION often lose their ability to laugh and see no humor in their lives or the world around them.

The Curative Powers of Laughter

Maintaining a sense of humor can help most people stay healthy. It causes the body to have a physiological response, and the immune system benefits. For example, when one laughs, various muscles tense, then relax, which can result in toning. Breathing gets faster, allowing the body to take in more oxygen and to get rid of more carbon dioxide. Heart and pulse rate and blood pressure also increase, promoting more vigorous circulation, and an increase in the brain's chemical transmitters aids mental alertness.

Research shows that laughter, like exercise, can stimulate the brain to secrete endorphins. Endorphins increase one's sense of physical and mental well-being and, to some extent, relieve pain.

The curative power of laughter is not a 20th-century discovery. The *Book of Proverbs* says: "A merry heart doeth good like a medicine." Norman Cousins (1915–90), former editor of the *Saturday Review* and later a member of the faculty of the medical school at the University of California at Los Angeles, used the curative power of laughter to help himself recover from a degenerative disease of the body's connective tissue. Following is an excerpt from Cousins's book *Anatomy of an Illness* (1979), in which he described the benefits of laughter:

> I made the joyous discovery that ten minutes of genuine belly laughter had an anesthetic effect and would give me at least two hours of pain-free sleep. . . . Exactly what happens inside the human mind and body as the result of humor is difficult to say. But the evidence that it works has stimulated the speculations not just of physicians but of philosophers and scholars over the centuries.

Cousins checked out of the hospital and spent weeks watching Marx Brothers movies and other comedies. He attributed his recovery to the positive feelings that laughter aroused in him.

Research in Laughter

In an article titled "Laughter" in *American Scientist,* University of Maryland psychologist Robert R. Provine attempted to shed some light on laughter as a stereotyped, species-specific form of COMMUNI-CATION. Among other things, Provine's research provides a novel approach to the mechanisms and evolution of vocal production, speech perception, and social behavior.

The laugh tracks of television situation comedies—attempts to stimulate contagious laughter in viewers—and the difficulty of extinguishing "laugh jags," fits of nearly uncontrollable laughter, are familiar phenomena. "Rather than dismissing contagious laughter as a behavioral curiosity," Provine suggests, we should recognize it and other laugh-related phenomena as clues to broader and deeper issues.

For information:

International Laughter Society
16000 Glen Una Drive
Los Gatos, CA 95030
(408) 354-3456

See also HUMOR.

Peter, Laurence J. *The Laughter Prescription: The Tools of Humor and How to Use Them.* New York: Ballantine Books, 1982.
Provine, Robert R. "Laughter." *American Scientist* 84, no. 1 (January–February 1996).
Roach, Mary. "Can You Laugh Your Stress Away?" *Health,* September 1996.

law enforcement officers   See POLICE; VIOLENCE.

laws about workplace safety   Laws regarding workplace safety and health establish regulations designed to eliminate personal injuries and illnesses from occurring in the workplace. The laws consist primarily of federal and state statutes. Federal laws and regulations preempt state laws where they overlap or contradict each other.

The major statute protecting the health and safety of workers is the Occupational and Safety Health Act. Congress enacted this legislation under its constitutional grant of authority to regulate interstate commerce. OSHA requires the secretary of labor to promulgate regulations and safety and health standards to protect employees and their families. Every private employer who engages in interstate commerce is subject to the regulations promulgated under OSHA.

As explained by the Legal Information Institute of Cornell Law School, in order to aid the secretary of labor in promulgating regulations and enforcing them, the act established the National Advisory Committee on Occupational Safety and Health. The secretary of labor may authorize inspections of workplaces to ensure that regulations are followed, examine conditions about which complaints have been filed, and determine what regulations are needed. If an employer is violating a safety or health regulation, a citation is issued.

The act establishes the Occupational Safety and Health Review Commission to review citation orders of the secretary of labor. The commission's decision is also subject to judicial review. The secretary of labor may impose fines of varying amounts according to the type of violation and length of noncompliance with the citation. The secretary of labor may also seek an injunction to restrain conditions or practices that pose an immediate threat to employees. The act also established the National Institute of Occupational Safety and Health, which, under the secretary of health and welfare, conducts research on workplace health and safety and recommends regulations to the secretary of labor. Federal agencies must establish their own safety and health regulations. The regulations that have been promulgated under the act are extensive and fill five volumes of the Code of Federal Regulations.

Under the act, states are not allowed without permission of the secretary of labor to promulgate any laws that regulate an area directly covered by these regulations. They may, however, regulate in areas not governed by federal regulations. If they wish to regulate areas covered by the act, they must submit a plan for federal approval. The number of state regulations varies. California is an example of a state that has chosen to adopt many of its own regulations in place of those promulgated under the act.

See also OCCUPATIONAL AND SAFETY HEALTH ADMINISTRATION.

layoffs   Reductions in workforce have become very common. In the early 2000s, more than ever, there seems to be no job security, and the big organization that took care of its workers is a thing of the past.

During the recession of the 1980s, job reduction was blamed on national or international business conditions. At the end of the 20th century, more and more companies reduced their workforces in attempts, they claim, to save money after MERGERS or acquisition or realize productivity gains.

Layoffs also result from plant closings, work slowdowns, or corporate "downsizings." Being laid off is different from being fired, though the individual will probably feel the same stress. When workers are fired, it may be because their performance is lacking; when layoffs occur, performance is rarely cited.

Typically, there are five emotional stages that follow a termination and they are not unlike those felt at the time of any major loss:

Stage One: Denial. *It must be some mistake, this can't be happening* to *me.*

Stage Two: Self-Blame. *I must have done something wrong. How did I screw up?*

Stage Three: Anger. *Why did management do this to me?*

Stage Four: Depression. *It's not worth getting out of bed in the morning.*

Stage Five: Acceptance. *What happened may be all for the best.*

On virtually every indicator of mental and physical health, layoffs have a negative impact. People who lose their jobs are often anxious, depressed, unhappy, and generally dissatisfied with their lives. They have reduced self-esteem, are short-tempered, and are fatalistic and pessimistic about the future. Thus, job loss is clearly hard on one's health and it is important to get control over one's life and one's stress after a job loss.

See also DOWNSIZING; JOB SECURITY.

lead poisoning　See CARDIOVASCULAR OR BLOOD TOXICITY; KIDNEY TOXICITY; NEUROTOXICITY; SKIN OR SENSE ORGAN TOXICITY.

learned helplessness　According to Martin E. P. Seligman (b. 1942), an American psychologist, *learned helplessness* refers to a feeling of helplessness and stifling of motivation brought about by exposure to aversive events over which people have no CONTROL. Such situations lead to feelings of powerlessness, BOREDOM, and DEPRESSION, and the worker becomes passive and nonassertive.

In experiments, Seligman and Steven Maier, another psychologist, exposed animals to pathologic amounts of psychological stressors. Those stressors included loss of control and predictability within certain contexts, a loss of outlets for FRUSTRATION, a loss of sources of support, and a perception of life worsening. The animals had trouble coping with many varied tasks, such as competing with other animals for food or avoiding social AGGRESSION. Such animals have a motivational problem; they are helpless because they do not even attempt to cope with a new situation.

The condition that the animals experienced was a condition very similar to depression in humans. Later on, Seligman coined the term *learned optimism* to refer to the opposite behavior, in which an individual does not give up but persists toward a goal.

See also COPING; GENERAL ADAPTATION SYNDROME; LEARNED OPTIMISM.

Seligman, Martin E. P. *Learned Optimism.* New York: Alfred A. Knopf, 1991.

learned optimism　A term coined by Martin E. P. Seligman in his book *Learned Optimism* (1991) describing attitudes and behaviors people exhibit when they face the stress of failures and disappointments that inevitably are a part of experiences in the workplace as well as in personal life. According to Seligman, individuals learn in childhood to explain setbacks to themselves. Some are able to say and believe: "It was just circumstances; it's going away quickly, and there is much more in life." Scientific evidence has shown that this optimism is vitally important in overcoming defeat, promoting achievement, and maintaining or improving health. He documents the effects of optimism on the quality of life.

In his book, Seligman shows how to stop automatically assuming guilt, how to get out of the habit of seeing the direst possible implications in every setback, and how to be optimistic.

The opposite is *learned helplessness,* a term Seligman coined earlier, which relates to an attitude of hopelessness about the future and future activities.

See also COPING; GENERAL ADAPTATION SYNDROME; LEARNED HELPLESSNESS.

Seligman, Martin E. P. *Learned Optimism.* New York: Alfred A. Knopf, 1991.

leather tanning　See TANNING.

leukemia　See BENZENE; CARDIOVASCULAR OR BLOOD TOXICITY; CHEMICAL TOXICITY.

life change events　See GENERALIZED ADAPTATION SYNDROME; LIFE CHANGE SELF-RATING SCALE; SELYE, HANS.

life change self-rating scale　The original life change self-rating scale was developed as a predictor of illness based on stressful life events by authors Holmes and Rahe and presented at the Royal Society of Medicine in 1968. In many variations, this type of rating scale has been used to help individuals determine their composite stress level within the last year.

To take this test, mark any of the changes listed below that have occurred in your life in the past

12 months. Your total score indicates the amount of stress you have been subjected to in the one-year period. Your score may be useful in predicting your chances of suffering illness in the next two years due to physiological effects of serious stressors.

LIFE CHANGE SELF-RATING SCALE

Event	Value
Death of spouse	100
Divorce	73
Marital separation	65
Death of close family member	63
Personal injury or illness	53
Marriage	50
Fired from work	47
Marital reconciliation	45
Retirement	45
Change in family member's health	44
Pregnancy	40
Sex difficulties	39
Addition to family	39
Business readjustment	39
Change in financial status	38
Death of close friend	37
Change to different line of work	36
Foreclosure of mortgage or loan	30
Change in work responsibilities	29
Son or daughter leaving home	29
Trouble with in-laws	29
Outstanding personal achievement	28
Spouse begins or stops work	26
Starting or finishing school	26
Change in living conditions	25
Trouble with boss	23
Change in residence or school	20
Change in recreational habits	19
Change in church or social activities	19
Change in sleeping habits	16
Change in eating habits	15
Vacation	13
Christmas season	12
Minor violation of the law	11
Your total score:	

What Your Score Means

A total score of less than 150 may mean you have only a 27 percent chance of becoming ill in the next year. If your score is between 150 and 300, you have a 51 percent chance of encountering poor health. If your score is more than 300, you are facing 80 percent odds that you will become ill. As the score increases, so do the odds that the problem will be serious. To avoid these consequences, attention to RELAXATION and STRESS relief can help.

Adapted from Holmes and Rahe, Life Change Measurements as a Predictor of Illness, proceedings, Royal Society of Medicine, 1968.

lifting   See OVERLOAD INJURIES.

lightning strikes   See ELECTRICITY-RELATED INJURIES.

limousine drivers   See CHAUFFEURS.

liquid oxygen   See AEROSPACE MEDICINE.

liquor stores   See VIOLENCE.

listening   Hearing with thoughtful attention is a skill necessary for good COMMUNICATION between individuals in the workplace. It is an active process in which one gives complete attention to what others are saying and how they are saying it. According to Deborah Tannen, author of *Talking from 9 to 5: How Women's and Men's Conversational Styles Affect Who Gets Heard, Who Gets Credit, and What Gets Done at Work,* "Listening taps two important areas, gathering information and developing relationships." Active listening can reduce the stress of communication not only in business but personal life as well.

By using nonverbal gestures such as a nod of the head or a smile, active listeners can convey concern and reinforce or encourage the other's verbalizations. Listeners contribute by asking good questions, providing FEEDBACK on what they hear, and seeking consensus or pointing out differences of opinion within a group. On the other hand, people feel listened to when more than just their ideas get heard; they feel valued, and they will contribute a lot more to the conversation.

BETTER LISTENING SKILLS FOR THE WORKPLACE

- Focus on the speaker; use eye contact. Keep interruptions, such as phone calls and other conversations, down to a minimum.
- It helps to question the speaker. You can gently guide a conversation, show that you are interested in what he/she is saying, and what you might want to learn.
- Don't judge the person speaking, concentrate on the information he/she is presenting.

See also BODY LANGUAGE.

Kahn, Ada P. *Stress A–Z: A Sourcebook for Facing Everyday Challenges.* New York: Facts On File, Inc., 2000.

Nichols, Michael P. *The Lost Art of Listening.* New York: Doubleday, 1995.

Tannen, Deborah. *Talking from 9 to 5: How Women's and Men's Conversational Styles Affect Who Gets Heard, Who Gets Credit, and What Gets Done at Work.* New York: William Morrow, 1994.

lithium See BIPOLAR DISORDER; DEPRESSION.

liver toxicity See GASTROINTESTINAL OR LIVER TOXICITY.

lockout/tagout Programs designed to prevent accidental startup of machines or equipment and to prevent releasing stored energy during maintenance or servicing. Every year workers are maimed, injured, and killed in accidents because they failed to disconnect the power source of machinery they are working on or because a fellow worker restarted the equipment, not knowing anyone was in danger. The procedures for securing power sources and alerting all persons that power is to not be restored are spelled out in the Occupational Safety and Health Administration (OSHA) standard called lockout/tagout (LO/TO). Equipment is isolated from energy sources through use of specific procedures that involve applying locks and/or tags as direct controls.

OSHA requirements for lockout/tagout apply to all servicing and maintenance of equipment where accidental startup or unexpected release of energy can occur. Departments involved in these activities are responsible for developing and implementing a lockout/tagout program.

Employers should develop a written program that establishes general lockout/tagout procedures, including the sequence of steps to follow for all lockouts. The program should include where specific lockout procedures are to be used, where tagout alone is permitted, and what types of locks and tags can be used. Workers should receive general and specific training. Lockout/tagout requirements do not apply to work on cord- and plug-connected equipment.

See also CONSTRUCTION; ELECTRICITY-RELATED INJURIES; OCCUPATIONAL HEALTH AND SAFETY ADMINISTRATION; RIVETERS; WELDING.

Office of Environment, Health and Safety
317 University Hall
#1150
University of California
Berkeley, CA 94720-1150
(510) 642-3073 or (510) 642-3073
http://www.ehs.berkeley.edu

logging According to the Bureau of Labor Statistics Census of Fatal Occupational Injuries (CFOI), logging was the second most dangerous occupation (behind fishing) during 1992–96. With more than 128 deaths per 100,000 workers, logging surpassed fishing as the most dangerous occupation in 1997. Loggers comprise .5 percent of the total workforce in America, yet they account for nearly 2 percent of all fatalities.

Each year, between 100 and 150 loggers lose their lives, and many more suffer nonfatal injuries. Loggers face a risk of fatal work injury approximately 27 times greater than the average for all occupations.

The tools and equipment used in logging, such as chain saws and logging machines, pose hazards wherever they are used. As loggers use their tools and equipment, they are dealing with massive weights and irresistible momentum of falling, rolling, and sliding trees and logs. Logging occupations are physically demanding, involving lifting, climbing, and other strenuous activities in remote locations, frequently far from medical services. Additionally, because the work is performed outdoors, loggers often face adverse weather conditions, irregular terrain, and pests such as mosquitoes, blackflies, and deerflies.

Trees themselves are a menace to loggers. Of the 772 fatal injuries to loggers in 1992–97, 70 percent resulted directly from contact with trees and logs. Some 60 percent of logging fatalities occurred as a result of being struck by falling objects, almost all of which were trees and logs. Various types of non-roadway vehicular accidents, including those caused by tractors and skidders, accounted for 7 percent of fatalities; loggers crushed or struck by rolling logs accounted for 5 percent; and falls from trees, 2 percent.

STATES WITH THE LARGEST NUMBER OF LOGGING FATALITIES, 1992–97

State	Fatalities[1]		Percent of Logging Workforce
	NUMBER	PERCENT	
All States[2]	772	100	100
North Carolina	55	7.1	2.9
Mississippi	51	6.6	3.3
Kentucky	45	5.8	3.7
Virginia	42	5.4	2.8
Washington	41	5.3	9.7
Alabama	37	4.8	6.0
Pennsylvania	33	4.3	3.3
Oregon	32	4.2	7.0
West Virginia	31	4.0	2.0
Montana	29	3.8	2.0
Texas	29	3.8	4.5
Tennessee	27	3.5	5.3
Georgia	25	3.2	5.0
California	24	3.1	2.4
South Carolina	23	3.0	1.3

1 Includes supervisors.
2 Not all states had logging fatalities between 1992 and 1997.
Source: *Compensation and Working Conditions,* Winter 1998.

FATAL OCCUPATIONAL INJURIES TO LOGGERS BY YEAR, 1992–97

Year	Logging Occupations					
	Total		Supervisors, Forestry and Logging		Timber Cutting and Logging	
	NUMBER	RATE	NUMBER	RATE	NUMBER	RATE
1992–97	772	128.3	76	81.7	696	136.8
1992	146	162.2	13	108.3	133	170.5
1993	135	121.8	11	64.7	124	133.3
1994	131	123.6	19	95.0	112	130.2
1995	110	100.0	12	92.3	98	101.0
1996	129	139.2	10	62.5	119	157.3
1997	121	128.7	11	73.3	110	140.7

1 The rate represents the number of fatal occupational injuries per 100,000 employed workers and was calculated as follows: $(N/W) \times 100,000$ where
N = the number of fatal work injuries to workers 16 years of age and older.
W = the number of employed workers 16 years of age and older.
100,000 = number of workers.
Employment figures are annual average estimates of employed civilians 16 years of age and older from the Current Population Survey (CPS), 1992–97
Source: U.S. Department of Labor, Bureau of Labor Statistics, in cooperation with state and federal agencies, Census of Fatal Occupational Injuries, 1992–97.

Nonfatal injuries. Logging injuries that do not result in a fatality but require time away from work to recuperate most often occur to the torso and the lower extremities. In 1996, the most recent year for which data are available, there were an estimated 2,136 cases involving time away from work. However, this statistic does not account for the self-employed, government workers, or workers in agricultural establishments with fewer than 11 employees.

MOST REPORTED INJURIES FOR TIMBER CUTTERS (LOGGERS)

Nature of Injury	Number of Cases	Percent of Total Cases
Total, 1996	2,136	100
Sprains, strains	713	33
Fractures	359	17
Bruises	305	14
Cuts, punctures	209	10
Bodily pain	87	4
All other	463	22

Lost time from work. Between 1992 and 1996, more than 30 percent of the logging injury cases resulted in 31 or more lost workdays and almost 17 in 1996. (See chart following.)

TREND IN NONFATAL INJURIES AMONG LOGGERS

Year	Number of Injuries
1992	4,537
1993	4,522
1994	3,479
1995	2,779
1996	2,136

For further information:

Division of Safety Research
National Institute for Occupational Safety and Health
1095 Willowdale Road
Morgantown, WV 26505-2588

(304) 285-5894 or (800)-35-NIOSH
www.cdc.gov/niosh

See also CENSUS OF FATAL OCCUPATIONAL INJURIES.

Sygnatur, Eric F. "Logging is Perilous Work," *Compensation and Working Conditions,* Winter 1998, pp. 3–9.

Longshore and Harbor Workers' Compensation Program A U.S. government program that provides more than $670 million in monetary, medical, and vocational rehabilitation benefits in more than 72,000 cases annually for maritime workers and various other classes of private industry employees disabled or killed by employment injuries or occupational diseases.

According to the U.S. Department of Labor, the program also maintains more than $2 billion in securities to ensure the continuing provision of benefits for these injured workers in cases of

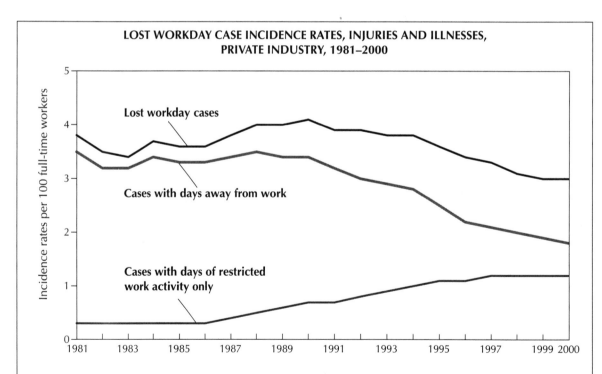

LOST WORKDAY CASE INCIDENCE RATES, INJURIES AND ILLNESSES, PRIVATE INDUSTRY, 1981–2000

Note: The incidence rate for lost workday cases declined steadily from 4.1 cases per 100 full-time workers in 1990 to 3.0 cases per 100 full-time workers in 2000. Rates for the two types of lost workday cases moved in opposite directions during that period.

Source: Bureau of Labor Statistics, U.S. Department of Labor, December 2001

employer insolvency. Claimants depend upon timely receipt of these benefits to provide food, housing, and minimal standards of living for themselves and their families.

Several other statutes extend the provisions of the act to cover other classes of private industry workers, including those engaged in the extraction of natural resources of the outer continental shelf, employees on U.S. defense bases, and those working under contract with the U.S. government for defense or public work projects outside the continental United States.

During fiscal year 2000, more than $670 million in compensation and medical benefits was paid in approximately 72,000 cases covered under these compensation acts.

U.S. Department of Labor.

longshoremen   See COMMERCIAL DIVING.

lost workdays   Days on which, because of occupational injury or illness, the employee was away from work or limited to restricted work activity. Days away from work are those days on which the employee would have worked but could not. Days of restricted work activity are those days on which the employee was assigned to a temporary job, or worked at a permanent job less than full time, or worked at a permanent job but could not perform all duties normally connected with it. The number of lost workdays (consecutive or not) does not include the day of injury or onset of illness or any days on which the employee would not have worked even though able to work.

National Safety Council.

lumber   See LOGGING.

lung cancer   The leading cancer killer in both men and women. In the United States in 2000, there were an estimated 164,100 new cases of lung cancer and an estimated 156,900 deaths from lung cancer.

A leading cause of cancer is on-the-job exposure to cancer-causing substances or carcinogens. ASBESTOS is a well-known work-related substance that can cause lung cancer. Many other substances, including URANIUM, ARSENIC, and certain petroleum products also can cause cancer. Many jobs involve exposure to these and other carcinogens, including working with certain types of insulation, working in coke ovens, and repairing brakes. When exposure to job-related carcinogens is combined with SMOKING, the risk of getting lung cancer is sharply increased.

Lung cancer takes many years to develop. Changes in the lung can begin almost as soon as a person is exposed to cancer-causing substances. Soon after exposure begins, a few abnormal cells may appear in the lining of the bronchi (the main breathing tubes). If a person continues to be exposed to the cancer-causing substance, more abnormal cells will appear. These cells may be then become cancerous and form a tumor.

Types of Lung Cancer

There are two main types of lung cancer: non-small-cell lung cancer and small-cell lung cancer. Non-small-cell lung cancer is much more common. It usually spreads to different parts of the body more slowly than small-cell lung cancer. Squamous-cell carcinoma, adenocarcinoma, and large-cell carcinoma are three types of non-small-cell lung cancer. Small-cell lung cancer also called oat-cell cancer, and accounts for about 20 percent of all lung cancers.

Causes of Lung Cancer

Radon is considered to be the second leading cause of lung cancer in the U.S. today. Radon gas can come up through the soil under a building and enter through gaps and cracks in the foundation or insulation, as well as through pipes, drains, walls or other openings. Radon causes between 15,000 and 22,000 lung cancer deaths each year in the U.S. Estimates are that 12 percent of all lung cancer deaths are linked to radon. Radon has been found in every state. Because radon cannot be seen or smelled, the only way to detect it is to measure radon levels. Exposure to radon in the workplace in combination with cigarette smoking greatly increases the risk of lung cancer. For smokers, exposure to radon at work is an even greater health risk.

For further information:

American Lung Association
1740 Broadway
New York, NY 100 19-4374
(800) LUNG USA (toll-free)
(212) 315-8700
(212) 315-8872 (fax)
www.lungusa.org

See also CHEMICAL TOXICITY; ENVIRONMENTAL PROTECTION AGENCY; FARMER'S LUNG; MESOTHELIOMA; RADON.

lung diseases, occupational   See ASTHMA; CHRONIC OBSTRUCTIVE PULMONARY DISEASE; EMPHYSEMA.

machine accidents Getting caught or hit by moving machine parts. Machine accidents are a major cause of on-the-job injuries.

When working around any machine that rotates, slides, or presses, one should use extreme caution. Never wear loose fitting clothing or jewelry that could get caught in the machine. Use safeguards, shields, and appropriate lock-out procedures. One should not work on a machine unless specifically trained to do so.

See also DEATHS IN THE WORKPLACE; LOCKOUT/TAGOUT.

male reproductive health See REPRODUCTIVE TOXICITY.

malt fever See BREWING.

malt workers' lung See HYPERSENSITIVITY PNEUMONITIS.

managed care A term covering many varieties of health insurance, including health maintenance organizations (HMOs) and preferred provider organizations (PPOs). The premise on which HMOs are based is that insurance companies provide specified services for a prepaid fee to an enrolled population. In many cases, employers and employees share the costs for coverage of employees and their families. HMOs and other forms of managed care are also available to retirees as a supplement to Medicare. Enrollment in managed care plans rose significantly after 1973 when a federal law paved the way for insurance companies to finance and deliver health care. In 1996 about 60 percent of Americans were enrolled in some sort of managed care health plan, up from 36 percent in 1992. The increase was due in large part to employers shifting their workers away from the traditional, and considerably more expensive, "fee-for service" health insurance plans.

Critics of HMOs claim that HMOs limit the patient's choice of doctors, while proponents claim HMOs deliver better, more closely monitored care. Some managed care plans have physicians as their employees, while other plans compensate physicians on a "capitation" basis, or the number of patients which they serve.

As health care costs spiraled upward, health plans became the subject of criticism for enacting limits on what managed care would cover. In most cases, managed care plans limit the number of mental health visits for which a patient may be covered annually.

In the early 2000s HMOs have been touted for bringing affordable health coverage to a wide range of consumers, as well as criticized for cutting costs by limiting treatment options and patient choice. Doctors and patients increasingly are seeking new ways to regulate the managed care industry by giving patients new rights, including the ability to sue their health plans. Controversy continues over how to protect patients without further driving up already expensive health care costs.

See also HEALTH INSURANCE.

manic-depressive illness See AFFECTIVE DISORDERS; BIPOLAR DISORDER.

manufacturing Manufacturing accounted for three-fifths of all newly reported occupational illnesses for private industry in 1999. Within the manufacturing industry, the rate for cases with days of restricted work activity decreased in 1999, but the rate for cases with days away from work

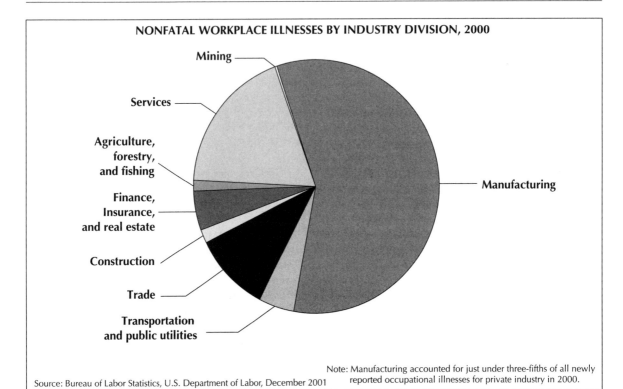

NONFATAL WORKPLACE ILLNESSES BY INDUSTRY DIVISION, 2000

Mining

Services

Agriculture, forestry, and fishing

Finance, Insurance, and real estate

Construction

Trade

Transportation and public utilities

Manufacturing

Source: Bureau of Labor Statistics, U.S. Department of Labor, December 2001

Note: Manufacturing accounted for just under three-fifths of all newly reported occupational illnesses for private industry in 2000.

remained about the same as the previous three years. Lost workday cases have declined since 1995. (See charts.)

See also CENSUS OF FATAL OCCUPATIONAL INJURIES; LOST WORKDAYS; NONFATAL OCCUPATIONAL INJURIES.

maritime workers See FISHING; LONGSHORE AND HARBOR WORKERS' COMPENSATION PROGRAM.

masonry See BRICKLAYERS, CEMENT WORKERS, AND PLASTERERS; CONSTRUCTION; LADDERS; SCAFFOLDING.

massage therapy A form of body therapy in which the practitioner applies manual techniques such as kneading, stroking, and manipulation of the soft tissues of the body, the skin, muscles, tendons, and ligaments with the intention of positively affecting the mental health and physical well-being of the client. Many employers bring a

massage therapist to their worksite to help employees relieve STRESS and body aches caused by workplace tension and anxieties such as burnout and frustration.

A professional massage increases blood flow and relaxes muscles. Massage therapy can provide soothing RELAXATION or deeper therapy for specific physical problems. It can aid in recovery from pulled muscles or sprained ligaments. Massage therapy can also ease the discomforts of back pain and exhaustion, as well as the pains of certain repetitive stress injuries related to on-the-job activities.

According to the American Massage Therapy Association, once the massage is underway, many beneficial reactions are set in motion. Massage therapy can hasten the elimination of waste and toxic debris stored in muscles, increase the interchange of substances between the blood and tissue cells, and stimulate the relaxation response within the nervous system. Responses to massage therapy can help to strengthen the immune system, improve posture, increase joint flexibility and range of motion, and reduce blood pressure.

Types of Massage

The most universally understood Western form of massage is Swedish, also called Esalen. It consists of many types of strokes: gliding the hand across the skin, kneading, lifting, squeezing, and grasping the muscles, gentle pushing, friction, vibration, jostling and rocking, and percussion (hacking, chopping, and rapid pounding).

Oriental massage, sometimes referred to as SHI-ATSU or acupressure, involves pressing at certain points along invisible energy meridians that practitioners claim run through the body; the practitioner looks for tight spots, knots, or anything that interferes with the flow of energy.

Deep tissue massage uses slow strokes and deep finger pressure to combat aching muscles, such as a stiff neck or bad back. Sports massage is a combination of stretching and Swedish or deep-tissue massage performed before or after strenuous exercise.

REFLEXOLOGY, the massage of the hands, feet and ears, is based on the belief that specific areas govern all parts of the body. For example, the tips of the toes correspond to the head, while the inside arch of the foot reflects the spine. The theory is that by stimulating the nerve endings of the different organs in the body, changes can be affected.

Choosing a Massage Therapist

According to the American Massage Therapy Association (AMTA), a qualified massage therapist should have a solid foundation in physiology and be knowledgeable about the inner workings of the body. Therapists from an accredited school have usually completed 500 hours of training, including classes in anatomy, first aid, and cardiopulmonary resuscitation.

The AMTA, founded in 1943, is the largest and oldest national organization representing the profession. Membership in the AMTA is limited to those who have demonstrated a level of expertise through testing and/or education. All AMTA therapists must agree to abide by the AMTA code of ethics. AMTA membership increased from less than 5,000 in 1986 to approximately 46,400 in 2003.

Patricia Deer, a certified massage therapist and owner of Energy Breaks in Chicago, says that a good neck and shoulder massage may contribute toward better mental performance as well as relief of stress. One study reported that people who received 15-minute seated massages during their workday showed brain-wave patterns consistent with greater alertness. Those people were also able to complete arithmetic problems twice as fast and with half the errors as they did before the massage. "Employers are increasingly recognizing the benefits of 'mini tune-ups' for people who sit at desks or computers much of the day," says Deer.

For information:

American Massage Therapy Association
800 Davis Street
Suite 100
Evanston, IL 60201
(847) 864-0123
(847) 864-1178 (fax)
http://www.amtamass.org

See also COMPLEMENTARY THERAPIES; BODY THERAPIES; MIND-BODY CONNECTIONS.

Kahn, Ada P., and Jan Fawcett. *Encyclopedia of Mental Health.* New York: Facts On File, Inc., 2001.

Shulman, Karen R. and Gwen E. Jones. "The effectiveness of massage therapy intervention on reducing anxiety in the workplace." *Journal of Applied Behavioral Science.* 1996. June; Vol 32 (2): 160–173.

material safety data sheets (MSDS)   A product safety information sheet prepared by manufacturers and marketers of products containing toxic chemicals. These sheets can be obtained by requesting them from the manufacturer. MSDSs should be posted in workplaces where toxic chemicals are used.

See also CHEMICAL TOXICITY.

Personick, Martin E., and Katherine Taylor-Shirley. "Profiles in Safety and Health: Occupational Hazards of Meatpacking." *Monthly Labor Review.* January 1989.

Schlosser, Eric. "The Chain Never Stops." *Mother Jones,* July/August 2001.

Bureau of Labor Statistics. U.S. Department of Labor. *Occupational Outlook Handbook, 2000–2001,* March 2000.

meatpacking See BUTCHERS AND MEAT, POULTRY, AND FISH CUTTERS.

meditation A learned technique to relieve stress and improve mental health involving deep RELAXATION brought on by focusing attention on a particular sound or image and breathing deeply. Thoughts are directed away from work, family, relationships, and the environment. During meditation, the heart rate, blood pressure, and oxygen-consumption rate decreases, temperature of the extremities rises, and muscles relax. Many EMPLOYEE ASSISTANCE PROGRAMS and health promotion programs at workplaces encourage employees to learn techniques of meditation.

Meditation also has been shown to reduce a number of medical symptoms and improve health-related attitudes and behaviors. For example, people with chronic obstructive pulmonary disease (COPD) who practiced meditation reduced the frequency and severity of episodes of shortness of breath and visits to emergency rooms. People with heart disease, hypertension, cancer, diabetes, and chronic pain have reported having more self-confidence, more CONTROL in their lives, and are better able to manage stress after mastering the meditation technique. Meditation has been used successfully by individuals who have PANIC ATTACKS AND PANIC DISORDER.

Meditation may bring out increased efficiency by eliminating unnecessary expenditures of energy. Individuals who practice meditation sometimes report a beneficial surge of energy marked by increased physical stamina, increased productivity on the job, the end of writer's or artist's "block," or the release of previously unsuspected creative potential.

Learning to Meditate

The basics include sitting in a quiet room with eyes closed and breathing deeply and rhythmically with attention focused on the breath. Also, there may be a focus on either a special word or "mantra," such as "peace," that is repeated over and over again, or steadily watching an object such as a candle flame for 20 minutes one or more times daily.

Meditation relies on the close links between mind and body. During meditation the alpha brain waves indicate that the body is relaxed and free from physical tension and mental strain. BIOFEEDBACK monitoring has indicated that meditation encourages the brain to produce an evenly balanced pattern of alpha and theta brain wave rhythms. This means that the body is relaxed and the mind calm yet alert. The "relaxation response" sets in, which is the opposite of the physical tension that results from stress.

Individuals who meditate frequently report that they are more aware of their own opinions after beginning meditation. They are not as easily influenced by others as they were previously and can arrive at decisions more quickly and easily. They may become more self-assertive and more able to stand up for their own rights effectively. Additionally, researchers have shown that the meditating person may become less irritable in his or her interpersonal relationships within a relatively short period of time after beginning meditation.

Types of Meditation

Modern meditation techniques are derived from spiritual practices in Eastern cultures dating back more than 2,000 years. Traditionally, the benefits of the techniques have been defined as spiritual, and meditation has constituted a part of many religious practices. In the latter part of the 20th century, however, simple forms of meditation were used for stress management with excellent results. Contributing to the rising interest is the fact that these meditation techniques are related to biofeedback (which also emphasizes a delicately attuned awareness of inner processes) and to muscle relaxation and visualization techniques used in BEHAVIOR THERAPY.

There are two basic types of meditation: concentration and insight. Concentration types, such as transcendental meditation, often use a sound or silently repeated phrase to focus attention and screen out extraneous thoughts or stimuli. Insight-oriented meditation, such as mindfulness meditation, accepts thoughts and feelings that arise from moment to moment as objects of attention. The goal of mindfulness is an increased awareness of what is happening in the mind and body right now. Recognition and acceptance of present reality provides the basis for changes of attitudes and conditions.

MEDITATION MAY BENEFIT EMPLOYEES WITH PROBLEMS SUCH AS THE FOLLOWING

- Tension or anxiety
- Chronic fatigue
- Insomnia and hypersomnia
- Abuse of alcohol or tobacco
- Excessive self-blame
- Chronic subacute depression
- Irritability, low tolerance for frustration
- Strong tendencies to submissiveness
- Difficulties with self-assertion
- Prolonged bereavement reactions

See also BENSON, HERBERT; COMPLEMENTARY THERAPIES; GUIDED IMAGERY; STRESS; TRANSCENDENTAL MEDITATION.

Benson, Herbert. *The Relaxation Response.* New York: Morrow, 1975.
Chopra, Deepak. *Creating Health: How to Wake Up the Body's Intelligence.* Boston: Houghton Mifflin, 1991.
Kabat-Zinn, Jon. *Full Catastrophe Living: Using the Wisdom of Your Body and Mind to Face Stress, Pain and Illness.* New York: Delacorte, 1991.
———. *Wherever You Go, There You Are: Mindfulness Meditation in Everyday Life.* New York: Hyperion, 1993.
Kerman, D. Ariel. *The H.A.R.T. Program: Lower Your Blood Pressure without Drugs.* New York: HarperCollins, 1992.
Mahesh Yogi, Maharishi. *Science of Being and Art of Living: Transcendental Meditation.* New York: Meridian, 1995.

melancholia   See DEPRESSION.

mental health   An individual's ability to negotiate the daily challenges and social interactions of life, without experiencing undue emotional or behavioral incapacity; mental health is more than just the absence of mental disorders. Mental health can be affected by many factors, ranging from exogenous stresses that are difficult to manage to biological defects or organic disease that impair brain function

Good mental health includes a balance between mind, body, and spirit. Physical illness influences mental health, and both affect the human spirit. Increasingly, health professionals acknowledge these important links and look at the individual with a total perspective.

The workplace affects the mental health of most people in varying degrees and for varied reasons. Some people are stressed because they have too much work, while others are stressed because they are bored. Interactions with coworkers and supervisors can lead to stress. Additional sources of stress include environmental factors, such as noise, poor lighting, or lack of fresh air, as well as the FRUSTRATION of being underpaid and overworked.

Contemporary technology-related stressors at the workplace range from back strain due to sitting at a computer terminal, to repetitive stress syndrome (carpal tunnel syndrome) from use of computers, to standing on a manufacturing assembly line.

Each occupation carries with it particular stresses, many of which are hidden by the employees. For example, secretaries may resent doing the same chores over and over. Data processors may be bored with their work. Physicians may find regulations imposed on them by managed care companies and insurance companies stressful. Accountants find the tax preparation season particularly stressful, while air controllers are under constant pressure every minute at work. Lawyers must meet the demands of their clients as well as the superiors in their law firms.

The issue of CONTROL is an important one in determining level of workplace anxiety. Those who feel they have more control over their situations, such as flexibility with work schedules or ability to set their own deadlines, may experience less stress than those who have no sense of control. PERSONAL SPACE is another issue. Workers who feel they have no privacy may feel more stressed than those who have offices or spaces with doors.

People with fairly controllable jobs include computer programmers, writers, artists, appliance repairpersons, and truck drivers. While these jobs can be very demanding, the minute-to-minute pace may be relatively unhurried. Certain employees may have slow-paced jobs with uncontrollable factors. These include janitors, security guards, and bus drivers. Employees with fast-paced and controllable professions include some physicians in private practice, business executives, and city administrators. People in fast-paced and uncontrollable professions include waiters, cashiers, firefighters, and nurses.

Job mismatches can lead to mental health concerns. For some individuals, leaving the job is the solution. However, for many, that solution is not practical. Most people cannot walk way from their professions or businesses. The more realistic solution is coping better with current pressures.

Tips for Better Mental Health in the Workplace

Some of the challenges to mental health in the workplace can be eased by taking certain actions. Listen carefully when someone is speaking to you instead of planning your response as they are speaking. Careful listening can help prevent misunderstandings which might make you angry. Additionally, ask for feedback, which is another person's perception of what you are doing or saying. Feedback is not judgmental. Speak with your coworkers or superiors at the appropriate place and time. Do not initiate a difficult conversation without appropriate privacy. Finally, always ask for a clear statement of performance expectations. Confront a superior with questions about job role and expected outcomes.

In the 2000s, many workers face the additional stress of possible and actual downsizing, during which many employees are laid off. Some take early retirement and others find new jobs.

See also ANXIETY; AUTONOMY; BOREDOM; COPING; DEPRESSION; DOWNSIZING; EMPLOYEE ASSISTANCE PROGRAMS; ERGONOMICS; LISTENING; MEDITATION; PHOBIAS; RELAXATION; STRESS; WORKSITE WELLNESS PROGRAMS; YOGA.

Adams, Scott. *The Dilbert Principle: A Cubicle's-Eye View of Bosses, Meetings, Management Fads, and Other Workplace Afflictions.* New York: HarperBusiness, 1997.

Field, Tiffany, Olga Quintino, et al. "Job Stress Reduction Therapies." *Alternative Therapies* 3, no. 4 (July 1997).

Kahn, Ada P. *Stress A–Z: The Sourcebook for Facing Everyday Challenges.* New York: Facts On File, Inc., 2000.

Murphy, Lawrence R. "Stress Management in Work Settings: A Critical Review of the Health Effects." *American Journal of Health Promotion* 11, no. 2 (November/December 1996): 112–135.

Peterson, Michael. "Work, Corporate Culture, and Stress: Implications for Worksite Health Promotion." *American Journal of Health Behavior* 21, no. 4 (1997): 243–252.

Rosch, Paul J. "Measuring Job Stress: Some Comments on Potential Pitfalls." *American Journal of Health Promotion* 11, no. 6 (July-August 1997): 400–401.

Zeitlin, Lawrence R. "Organizational downsizing and stress related illness." *International Journal of Stress Management* 2, no. 4 (October 1995): 207–219.

mentor   An older, more experienced and higher-ranking individual in an organization or business who promotes the career of a younger, lower-ranking person with assistance and advice. Mentors serve as role models and teachers and have been shown to be a key element in the rise to success for many individuals in businesses. Although they are not necessarily close friends of their protégés, friendships may develop. They serve to make the protégé comfortable in the field or corporate structure. A mentor may also use his or her influence directly to promote the protégé's career. For this reason, mentors are rarely in a direct line of authority over the protégé because of the problems of jealousy and resentment from colleagues. The mentor offers support to the protégé in terms of professional decisions or crisis.

Most mentor relationships grow somewhat spontaneously out of work situations and usually start with requests for advice or help. Frequently neither side is precisely aware when the relationship started. A mentor is usually drawn to a younger employee because of his or her talent, ambition, and interest in the field of origination. Although the benefits to the protégé are obvious, there are also definite benefits to the mentor, most obviously a sense of generosity and satisfaction. A mentor may also be at a point in his or her career when she or he has reached the pinnacle but feels the need for further accomplishment. In acquiring a protégé, a mentor also gains support for his or her ideas or programs within the organizations. She may also accumulate information from the lower-ranking person about problems or other matters within the organization that could not be acquired through more formal methods.

Mentor relationships may also benefit the organization. For example, protégés are integrated into the organization in a way that enhances formal training and are groomed for higher positions. Relationships with mentors provide for longevity and lower employee turnover and promote communication and understanding among the different levels in an organization.

With all of their benefits, there are also problems inherent in the mentor-protégé relationship. For example, a male-female relationship may turn into a romance or at least give the appearance of doing so. Even without this element, the relationship may promote envy or charges of favoritism. A mentor-protégé relationship is inherently temporary, since the object of the protégé is advancement in the organization, but one of the two may hang on and become dependent on the relationship in a destructive way. The protégé may also experience difficulties if the relationship is interrupted because the mentor is transferred or becomes ill or unable to function for some other reason. Either side may also fall in the corporate opinion if one makes a blunder or performs poorly.

Kahn, Ada P., and Jan Fawcett. *Encyclopedia of Mental Health.* 2d ed. New York: Facts On File, Inc., 2001.

mercury A naturally occurring element that is present throughout the environment. Human activity releases some mercury into the air, water, and soil. According to the U.S. Environmental Protection Agency's (EPA) 1997 report, coal-fired power plants are the biggest source of mercury emissions to the air, followed by municipal waste combustors, medical waste incinerators, and hazardous waste combustors. Mercury concentrations in air are usually low and of little direct concern.

Inhalation of mercury vapor in workplaces is a common cause of mercury poisoning that may result in shortness of breath, alter brain function, and in severe cases, cause impairment of vision and a type of irreversible dementia. Mercury encephalopathy is a type of brain damage that can occur.

The expression "mad as a hatter" arose because many hat makers often suffered from mental confusion, slurred speech, and tremors as a result of inhaling poisonous mercury-laden vapors when making felt hats.

The EPA has taken a number of actions to reduce mercury pollution, including issuing stringent regulations for industries that significantly contribute to mercury pollution. These actions, once fully implemented, will reduce nationwide mercury emissions caused by human activities by about 50 percent below 1990 levels.

U.S. industrial demand for mercury dropped 75 percent from 1988 to 1997. The drop is attributed to federal bans in mercury additives in paint and pesticides; industry efforts to reduce mercury in batteries; increasing state regulation of mercury emissions and mercury in products; state-mandated recycling programs; and voluntary actions by industry.

For further information:

Environmental Health Clearinghouse
2605 Meridian Parkway
Suite 115
Durham, NC 27113
(800) 643-4794
(919) 361-9408 (fax)
http://infoventures.com/e-hlth

See also REPRODUCTIVE TOXICITY.

mergers The transformation of two or more corporations into one organization for reasons of growth, economy of scale, diversification, or vertical integration. They were increasingly common in the late 1990s and the early 2000s.

In their book *The Human Side of Mergers and Acquisitions,* A. F. Buono and J. L. Bowditch state, "Mergers and acquisitions can sufficiently transform the organizational structures, systems, processes; in one or both of the firms people often feel stressed, disoriented, frustrated, confused, and even frightened."

Emotions felt by employees during mergers may arise in stages and can be conflicting. These emotions range from shock, disbelief, ANGER, and hopelessness to excitement and high expectations for the future. When the merger is completed, employees move slowly toward acceptance, often experiencing a period of mourning and grief. When a proposed merger does not go through, it usually means that either company is seeking change and some time down the road the change will occur. This outlook compounds the stress for employees, particularly at the management level where job redundancy is likely.

An analysis of layoff announcements in the summer months of 1995 by the outplacement firm of Challenger, Gray, and Christmas showed that one out of three jobs cut was the result of mergers.

Such job cuts could be attributed to corporate restructuring and plant and office closings.

Staff reductions that occur due to mergers may create less dissatisfaction and bitterness when they are handled with sensitivity and concern. Where possible, staff redundancies can be managed through attrition, early RETIREMENT, and attractive severance packages. When involuntary termination is necessary, decisions should be made objectively and supported by outplacement assistance and related job search services.

Most of those who lose their jobs through mergers may have little financial loss, as they are usually white-collar employees who are given generous severance packages. However, they often experience the stress of having to rethink their careers and perhaps relocate to obtain new employment.

See also DOWNSIZING, LAYOFFS; MENTAL HEALTH.

Buono, Anthony F., and James L. Bowditch. *The Human Side of Mergers and Acquisitions: Managing Collisions Between People Cultures and Organizations*. San Francisco: Jossey-Bass, 1989.
Kahn, Ada P. *Stress A–Z: A Sourcebook for Facing Everyday Challenges*. New York: Facts On File, Inc., 1998.

mesothelioma   Pleural mesothelioma is a cancer in the sac lining of the chest, covering areas around the lungs and inside the ribs. The only known cause of this disease is exposure to ASBESTOS. In many cases, the exposure occurred 20 or more years before symptoms are noticed. Many shipbuilders and construction workers have developed this disease. Treatment for mesothelioma has improved significantly in recent years, particularly when it is diagnosed early. There is ongoing research, and trials of pharmaceutical protocols are underway.

Pleural mesothelioma occurs in 70 percent of cases of mesothelioma. The other type is peritoneal mesothelioma.

Most insulation materials used before the mid-1970s contained asbestos. Many other construction materials also contained asbestos, including:

Insulation on pipes
Fireproofing spray insulation
Boiler insulation

Insulating cements, plasters, and joint compounds that came in powder form and created dust before being completely mixed with water
Fire brick and gunite used for internal insulation of furnaces, boilers, and other vessels
Roof, floor, and ceiling tiles
Transite siding
Automotive brakes and clutches

Many employees worked with asbestos, including the following:

Insulators who installed asbestos insulation
Shipyard and navy personnel
Boilermakers
Plumbers, pipe fitters, and steamfitters, particularly those who worked on ships
Plasterers working with fireproofing spray on steel beams
Electricians, mechanics, bricklayers, carpenters, and other building trades workers
Steelworkers
Refinery and other industrial workers

See also ASBESTOS; LUNG CANCER; OCCUPATIONAL LUNG DISEASES.

metal mining   See EXTRACTIVE INDUSTRIES.

metal smoldering   See CADMIUM.

methyl mercury   See NEUROTOXICITY.

migrant workers   Employees who travel to find seasonal work and live transiently near their workplace, usually some type of farming or crop growing. Migrant workers face the occupational health hazards of farming as well as the health and safety hazards of poverty and migrancy. In the United States, there are an estimated 5 million migrant and seasonal farmworkers, although precise numbers are difficult to determine.

In the United States, migrant agricultural workers are predominantly young Hispanic males, although farmworkers also include whites, blacks, Southeast Asians, and other ethnic groups.

Migrant workers must deal with substandard working conditions and few benefits. Less than one-fourth have health insurance. The general health status of migrant workers is related to their working conditions and low income. In many places, they have little access to medical care, nutrition, sanitation, housing, and education. Crowded living conditions may also contribute to the increased risk of acute infectious illnesses. Farmworkers see physicians less frequently than non-farm working populations. For many, preventive services such as immunizations, dental care, and vision care are inadequate.

Many workers lack access to basic sanitary facilities at the worksite. Studies have shown the contribution of infectious diseases to deaths and illnesses in this population. Many migrant workers have tuberculosis, as well as other chronic diseases including those related to the cardiovascular and respiratory systems. Traumatic injuries contribute to a high death rate, similar to the numbers from this cause among farmers.

Author Michael Schenker reports that the health status of children of migratory workers is a concern because of the impact of lack of preventive health services. Children are exposed to the hazards of farmwork at an early age, both by doing farmwork and living in the farming environment. Children under five years of age are most at risk of unintentional injury from farm hazards such as machinery and animals. Over 10 years of age, many children work, particularly during labor shortages such as seasonal harvests. Exposure to agrochemicals is a particular problem, as children may be unable to read warnings on chemical containers and may not be aware of recent field application of chemicals. Farmworkers are at increased risk of illness from pesticides while working in the fields. Exposures most commonly occur from direct contact with the spray of application equipment, from prolonged contact with recently sprayed foliage or from drift of pesticide applied by aircraft or other spray equipment.

See also CHILD LABOR; FARMING; PESTICIDES.

Schenker, Marc B. "Migrant and Seasonal Farmworkers." *Encyclopaedia of Occupational Health and Safety.* 4th ed. Geneva: International Labor Organization, 1998.

military injuries   See AGENT ORANGE; GULF WAR SYNDROME.

mill worker's asthma   See ASTHMA; WHEEZING.

mind/body connections   Links among the brain and other organ systems. Research studies have demonstrated that psychological as well as physical stress affects health. Increasingly, workplaces are recognizing that BEHAVIOR THERAPY and COMPLEMENTARY THERAPIES such as GUIDED IMAGERY, RELAXATION, BIOFEEDBACK, and HYPNOSIS are useful adjuncts in the comprehensive care of many employees, many of whom have mental health concerns.

Mind/body medicine involves many treatments and approaches ranging from meditation and relaxation training to social support groups designed to engage the mind in improving physical and emotional well-being. Some EMPLOYEE ASSISTANCE PROGRAMS include lectures and classes in mind-body connections.

According to Herbert Benson, M.D., author of *The Relaxation Response,* "Too often in the practice of modern medicine, the mind and body are considered to be separate and distinct, which is not in our best interests. Because of specialization, patients are no longer treated as whole persons. Instead, we are separated into groups of organs and specific symptoms are not considered in context."

In *The Mind/Body Effect,* Dr. Benson emphasized the need for practicing behavioral medicine, which incorporates the principles of medicine, physiology, psychiatry, and psychology. Patients are viewed in their entirety with the realization that what happens in their mind has direct bearing on the state of their physical health. He makes it clear that psychological factors often induce physical ailments. He suggests that in extreme cases, fear and a sense of hopelessness can even induce death.

Many conditions have been found to respond to such techniques when they are used alone or in combination with standard medical and surgical treatments. These include high blood pressure, coronary artery disease, cancer, chronic pain, TEM-

POROMANDIBULAR JOINT SYNDROME, HEADACHES, and irritable bowel syndrome.

ADVANTAGES OF TEACHING MIND/BODY TECHNIQUES IN THE WORKPLACE

- Can be used along with standard medical practices
- Financial cost of procedures is low
- Physical and emotional risk is minimal; potential benefit is great
- Many can be taught by paraprofessionals
- No high-tech interventions
- May improve quality of life by reducing pain and symptoms for people with chronic diseases
- May help control or reverse certain underlying disease processes
- May help prevent disease from developing

See also MEDITATION; SOCIAL SUPPORT SYSTEM; SUPPORT GROUPS; WORKSITE WELLNESS PROGRAMS.

Benson, Herbert. *The Relaxation Response.* New York: Avon Books, 1975.
———. *Beyond the Relaxation Response.* New York: Berkeley Press, 1985.
———. *The Mind/Body Effect: How Behavioral Medicine Can Show You the Way to Better Health.* New York: Simon and Schuster, 1979.
Borysenko, Joan. *Minding the Body, Mending the Mind.* New York: Bantam, 1988.
Kerns, Lawrence L. "A Clinician's Guide to Mind-Body Treatments." *Chicago Medicine* 97, no. 22 (November 21, 1994).

mindfulness meditation See COMPLEMENTARY THERAPIES; KABAT-ZINN, JON; MEDITATION; MIND/BODY CONNECTIONS.

mine safety and health Mining the Earth, underground and on the surface, for coal, ore, and stone remains one of the most dangerous industries in the United States, according to the NATIONAL INSTITUTE FOR OCCUPATIONAL SAFETY AND HEALTH (NIOSH). Unpredictable geological conditions, confined workspaces, poor visibility, and the use of large, powerful equipment are hazards in mining. Coal and metal miners who suffer injuries tend to lose twice as many days of work as workers in other industries.

Metal and nonmetal mining includes production of metals such as gold and copper, nonmetals such as salt and phosphate, and production of stone, sand, and gravel. These mining techniques and conditions are diverse and differ substantially from those in the coal sector.

Approximately 400,000 miners are employed in more than 11,000 surface and underground mines in the United States. Each year, an estimated 2,000 miners die from lung diseases caused by exposure to coal mine DUST AND DEBRIS. The Federal Black Lung Program paid more than $18 billion to beneficiaries in the 1980s.

NIOSH reports that mining has the highest rate of fatal injuries of all U.S. industries. More than 80 miners die from fatal work injuries each year. However, the MINE SAFETY AND HEALTH ADMINISTRATION reports that total mining fatalities reached the lowest level in history in 2001. In 1993, according to NIOSH, one in eight underground coal miners was injured on the job, nearly twice the average of U.S. industries.

The chart compares the rate of traumatic occupational fatalities for mining and all industries between 1983 and 1992, and indicates the dramatically higher number of mining fatalities.

Preventing Diseases among Miners

Silicosis, an often fatal lung disease, is caused by inhaling fine particles of silica. Each year, thousands of coal workers are afflicted with silicosis, even though prevention information is readily available. To reduce silicosis among miners, NIOSH disseminated information to inspectors, miners, and employers throughout the surface mining industry describing steps to prevent silicosis. Further, NIOSH has produced a video for the surface mining community and provides technical assistance to establish a program providing health screening and follow-up care for surface miners in Pennsylvania.

To reduce the health risks of underground and surface coal miners and to prevent pneumoconiosis (BLACK LUNG DISEASE), NIOSH describes methods of monitoring worker exposures, procedures for medical screening and surveillance of miners, and the use of PERSONAL PROTECTIVE EQUIPMENT. Further, NIOSH recommends an exposure limit for respirable coal mine dust to protect miners from respiratory diseases.

DISTRIBUTION OF DAYS LOST BY ACCIDENTS: SURFACE OPERATIONS, 1996–2000

Category	Percentage
Handling materials	34
Slip or fall	27
Machinery	14
Powered haulage	15
Hand tools	9
All others	7

Source: Mine Safety and Health Administration

DISTRIBUTION OF FATALITIES BY ACCIDENTS: UNDERGROUND MINING, 1996–2000

Category	Percentage
Fall of ground	48
Powered haulage	23
Machinery	10
Electrical	3
Falling, rolling, or sliding rock or material	3
Hand tools	3
Slip or fall	3
Hoisting	3
All other	4

Source: Mine Safety and Health Administration

LOST TIME INJURIES BY ACCIDENTS: SURFACE OPERATIONS, 1996–2000

Category	Percentage
Handling materials	34
Slips and falls	27
Hand tools	11
Machinery	11
Powered haulage	10
All others	7

Source: Mine Safety and Health Administration

LOST TIME INJURIES BY ACCIDENTS: UNDERGROUND MINING, 1996–2000

Category	Percentage
Handling materials	33
Fall of ground	16
Slip or fall	15
Powered haulage	12
Machinery	11
Hand tools	7
Stepping, kneeling on object	2
All others	4

Source: Mine Safety and Health Administration

History of Mine Safety

The history of mine safety in the United States goes back to 1891 when Congress passed the first federal statute governing mine safety. The 1891 law was relatively modest legislation that applied only to mines in U.S. territories, and among other things, established minimum ventilation requirements at underground coal mines and prohibited operators from employing children under 12 years of age.

In 1910, following a decade during which the number of coal mine fatalities exceeded 2,000, Congress established the Bureau of Mines as a new agency in the Department of the Interior. The bureau was charged with the responsibility to conduct research and to reduce accidents in the coal mining industry, but was given no inspection authority until 1941, when Congress empowered federal inspectors to enter mines. In 1947 Congress authorized the formation of the first code of federal regulations for mine safety.

The Federal Coal Mine Safety Act of 1952 provided for annual inspections in certain underground coal mines, and gave the bureau limited enforcement authority, including power to issue violation notices and imminent danger withdrawal orders. The 1952 act also authorized the assessment of civil penalties against mine operators for noncompliance with withdrawal orders or for refusing to give inspectors access to mine property, although no provision was made for monetary penalties for noncompliance with the safety provisions. In 1966 Congress extended coverage of the 1952 Coal Act to all underground coal mines.

The first federal statute directly regulating noncoal mines did not appear until the passage of the Federal Metal and Nonmetallic Mine Safety Act of 1966, which provided for the promulgation of standards, many of which were advisory, and for inspections and investigations; however, its enforcement authority was minimal.

The Federal Coal Mine Health and Safety Act of 1969, generally referred to as the Coal Act, was more comprehensive and more stringent than any previous federal legislation governing the mining industry. The Coal Act included surface as well as underground coal mines within its scope, required two annual inspections of every surface coal mine and four at every underground coal mine, and dramatically increased federal enforcement powers in coal mines. The Coal Act also required monetary penalties for all violations and established criminal penalties for knowing and willful violations. The safety standards for all coal mines were strengthened, and health standards were adopted. The Coal Act included specific procedures for the development of improved mandatory health and safety standards, and provided compensation for miners who were totally and permanently disabled by the progressive respiratory disease known as pneumoconiosis, or black lung disease.

In 1973, the Secretary of the Interior, through administrative action, created the Mining Enforcement and Safety Administration (MESA) as a departmental agency separate from the Bureau of Mines. MESA assumed the safety and health enforcement functions formerly carried out by the bureau to avoid any appearance of conflict of interest between the enforcement of mine safety and health standards and the bureau's responsibilities for mineral resource development.

In 1977 Congress passed the Federal Mine Safety and Health Act (Mine Act), the legislation which currently governs MSHA's activities. The Mine Act amended the 1969 Coal Act in many ways, and consolidated all federal health and safety regulations of the mining industry, coal as well as noncoal mining, under a single statutory system. The Mine Act strengthened and expanded the rights of miners, and enhanced protection of miners from retaliation for exercising such rights.

Mining fatalities dropped sharply under the Mine Act, from 272 in 1977 to 86 in 2000. The Mine Act also transferred responsibility for carrying out its mandates from the Department of the Interior to the Department of Labor, and named the new agency the Mine Safety and Health Administration (MSHA). Additionally, the Mine Act established the independent Federal Mine Safety and Health Review Commission to provide for independent review of the majority of MSHA's enforcement actions.

See also CONFINED SPACES; SILICOSIS; VIBRATION WHITE FINGER.

Mine Safety and Health Administration (MSHA)
The mission of the MSHA is to administer the provisions of the Federal Mine Safety and Health Act of 1977 (Mine Act) and to enforce compliance with mandatory safety and health standards as a means to eliminate fatal accidents; to reduce the frequency and severity of nonfatal accidents; to minimize health hazards; and to promote improved safety and health conditions in the nation's mines. MSHA carried out the mandates of the Mine Act at all mining and mineral processing operations in the United States, regardless of size, number of employees, commodity mined, or methods of extraction.

See also EXTRACTIVE INDUSTRIES; MINE SAFETY AND HEALTH.

monitoring   Measurement of air pollution is referred to as monitoring. The ENVIRONMENTAL PROTECTION AGENCY (EPA) and state and local agencies measure the types and amounts of pollutants in community air. The CLEAN AIR ACT OF 1990 requires certain large polluters to perform enhanced monitoring to provide an accurate picture of their pollutant releases. Enhanced monitoring programs may include keeping records on materials used by the source, periodic inspections, and installation of continuous emission monitoring systems (CEMS). Continuous emission monitoring systems measure how much pollution is being released into the air.

See AIR POLLUTION.

mood disorders   According to the fourth edition of the American Psychiatric Association's *Diagnostic and Statistical Manual of Mental Disorders,* mood disorders have a disturbance in mood as the predominant feature. Mood episodes include major depressive episode, manic episode, mixed episode, and hypomanic episode. Mood disorders include major depressive disorder, dysthmic disorder, and bipolar disorder. Supervisors who suspect a mood disorder in an employee should talk with the employee and make a referral to an EMPLOYEE ASSISTANCE PROGRAM or appropriate therapist.

See also AFFECTIVE DISORDERS; BIPOLAR DISORDER; DEPRESSION.

American Psychiatric Association. *Diagnostic and Statistical Manual of Mental Disorders.* 4th ed. Washington, D.C.: American Psychiatric Association, 1994.

Fawcett, Jan, Bernard Golden, and Nancy Rosenfeld. *New Hope for People with Bipolar Disorder.* Roseville, Calif.: Prima Publishing, 2000.

motor vehicle injuries/deaths According to a report issued by the National Institute for Occupational Safety and Health (NIOSH) in 1998, workers are more likely to die from traffic-related motor vehicle crashes than from any other hazard on the job, including workplace violence and machine-related injuries.

According to the NIOSH report, three workers are killed every day, more than 1,000 each year, while driving, riding in, or working around motor vehicles in traffic. Highest risks are in the trucking service and CONSTRUCTION industries. By occupation, the largest number of vehicle deaths occurs among truck drivers.

NIOSH found that workers fatally injured in vehicle crashes were mostly male (93 percent); most were age 25–54 (70 percent); most were drivers (76 percent) as opposed to pedestrians or vehicle passengers; and most were not using any type of safety restraint (62 percent).

TRAFFIC-RELATED MOTOR VEHICLE CRASHES: INDUSTRIES WITH THE HIGHEST AVERAGE ANNUAL RATES OF DEATH PER 100,000 WORKERS

Trucking	12.1
Petroleum products	5.2
Agriculture crop production	4.2

TRAFFIC-RELATED MOTOR VEHICLE CRASHES: OCCUPATIONS WITH THE HIGHEST ANNUAL AVERAGE FATALITY RATES PER 100,000 WORKERS

Truck drivers	12.2
Garbage collectors	11.5
Sheriffs/bailiffs	7.1
Farmworker supervisors	5.2
Surveying and mapping technicians	5.1

NIOSH recommends that businesses identify appropriate measures for preventing traffic-related death and injury among employees. Effective steps may include:

- Establishing and enforcing a written policy requiring drivers and passengers always to use seat belts.
- Providing a seat belt for the driver and each passenger in each employer-provided vehicle, and limiting the number of passengers to the number of seat belts
- Conducting driver's license background checks on prospective drivers before they are hired
- Ensuring that drivers comply with designated speed limits and prohibiting workers from driving on the job when they are fatigued
- Ensuring that employees in construction and maintenance zones wear high-visibility clothing and use appropriate barriers and traffic control
- Equipping new vehicles with appropriate occupant protection such as seat belts, and wherever feasible and appropriate, with other safety features, such as antilock brakes.

See also CONSTRUCTION; FARMING; LOGGING; POLICE; VIOLENCE; WASTE INDUSTRY.

multiple chemical sensitivity syndrome (MCS syndrome) Belief that one's symptoms are caused by a very low-level exposure to chemicals in the environment. The term *chemical* is used to refer broadly to many natural and artificial chemical agents, some of which have several chemical constituents. According to M. K. Magill and Anthony Suruda, MCS syndrome has led to controversies among clinicians, researchers, patients, lawyers, legislators, and regulatory agencies.

People with MCS syndrome say severe symptoms interfere with daily work and life. They often report that they had no symptoms before a single large exposure, which is then followed by exacerbation of symptoms in response to previously tolerated low-level exposures. Symptoms generally occur as central nervous symptoms, respiratory and mucosal irritation, or gastrointestinal problems. Commonly reported symptoms, according to Magill and Suruda, include fatigue, difficulty concentrating, depressed mood, memory loss, weakness, dizziness, headaches, heat intolerance, and arthralgias.

Individuals exposed to pesticides have been reported to have more severe symptoms than those exposed to chemicals during a building remodeling, say Magill and Suruda.

EXAMPLES OF EXPOSURES PRECIPITATING SYMPTOMS OF MULTIPLE CHEMICAL SENSITIVITY

Aerosol air freshener
Asphalt pavement
Cigar and cigarette smoke
Diesel exhaust, diesel fuel
Dry cleaning fluid
Floor cleaner
Furniture polish
Garage fumes
Gasoline exhaust
Insecticide repellent
Insecticide spray
Marking pens
Oil-based paint
Paint thinner
Public restroom deodorizers
Tar fumes from roof or road
Tile cleaners
Varnish, shellac, lacquer

Excerpted from Lax, M. B., and P. I. Henneberger. "Patients with Multiple Chemical Sensitivities in an Occupational Health Clinic: Presentation and Follow-up." *Archives of Environmental Health* 50 (1995): 425–431.

To manage MCS syndrome, Magill and Suruda advise establishing a respectful and empathetic physician-patient relationship. Goals should be to maximize rehabilitation, control (not cure) symptoms, and treat concomitant psychiatric and physical illness. They recommend encouraging activity as tolerated, desensitization to symptom-producing situations, relaxation exercise, and avoiding unproven therapies, isolation, and social withdrawal.

See also AIR POLLUTION; ASPHALT FUMES; CHEMICAL SENSITIVITY; CHEMICAL TOXICITY; DIESEL EXHAUST; DRY CLEANING; ENVIRONMENT; RELAXATION; SICK BUILDING SYNDROME; STRESS.

Magill, Michael K., and Anthony Suruda. "Multiple Chemical Sensitivity Syndrome." *American Family Physician*, September 1, 1998.

municipal waste and incinerator facilities   See CADMIUM.

musculoskeletal disorders   See CONSTRUCTION; OVERLOAD; MUSCULOSKELETAL TOXICITY; VIDEO DISPLAY TERMINALS.

musculoskeletal toxicity   Adverse effects on the structure and/or functioning of the muscles, bones, and joints that result from exposure to chemical substances. Although injuries arising from repetitive motion or cumulative trauma are among the most common causes of musculoskeletal disorders, chemical hazards can also play a role in musculoskeletal disease. Exposure to toxic substances such as COAL DUST and CADMIUM has been shown to cause adverse changes to the musculoskeletal system. The bone disorders arthritis, fluorosis, and osteomalacia are among the musculoskeletal diseases that can be induced by occupational or environmental toxicants.

Rheumatoid arthritis is an autoimmune disease of the connective tissue characterized by joint inflammation and pain. It is often chronic and progressive, leading to deformities and disability. An increased incidence of rheumatoid arthritis has been associated with prolonged exposure to silica and coal dust. Occupational exposure to fluoride can cause the skeletal disorder fluorosis, in which fluoride rather than calcium is deposited in bone. Symptoms of fluorosis include aches, pains, changes in the teeth, and increased density of bone and soft tissue. Osteomalacia, a painful degenerative disease involving the gradual softening and bending of bones, is caused by exposure to the toxicant cadmium.

See also AUTOIMMUNE DISORDERS.

Morse, L. H. "Unusual Occupational Rheumatologic and Musculoskeletal Disorders." *Occupational Medicine* 7, no. 3 (1992): 423–432.
Steenland, D., and D. Goldsmith. "Silica Exposure and Autoimmune Diseases." *American Journal of Industrial Medicine* 28, no. 5 (1995): 603–608.

musician's injuries/illnesses   Injuries or illnesses sustained while practicing or performing. Environmental concerns about musicians' workplaces include social, economic, and health issues. For some, social life outside of their musical circles is difficult to maintain because of their work hours, usually evenings and weekends. Some need to supplement incomes with second jobs, creating fatigue and sleep deprivation. Others may have nutritional insufficiencies because of irregular mealtimes.

In addition to the technical aspects of playing a musical instrument, factors relating to illness and injury include the number of rehearsals and quantity of repertoire, acoustic properties of the environment, its temperature, seating and lighting conditions, and the space provided per player. Pit orchestras are commonly regarded as among the highest risk because of the limited space, the sound properties, and the often poor lighting. According to authors Sataloff, Brandfonbrener, and Lederman, musicians who play outdoors risk insect bites, falling stage parts, and excessive cold and heat.

Musicians who spend time in recording studios may find these sessions very stressful; players may also experience STRESS and PERFORMANCE ANXIETY before performances.

Players of different instruments experience different maladies. Keyboard artists experience repetitive use of their hands. String instrumentalists experience injuries related to instrument size, string caliber and tension, bow grip, and additional factors. String instrumentalists frequently report head, neck, and shoulder discomforts. String players also experience dermatological problems such as "practice points" and FIDDLER'S CHIN. Some players have variably sensitive spots on their necks. Some players have a similar area where the clavicle is rubbed by the instrument. Occasionally players have a contact allergy to the resin used on the bow hairs to enhance contact with the strings. Calluses on fingers may pose another annoyance for string players. Some violinists and violists develop TEMPOROMANDIBULAR JOINT (TMJ) problems as a result of displacing the left side of the jaw against the chin rest, thus stressing the right TMJ.

Faulty posture of all instrumental players can result in back strain and other neuromuscular discomforts. Carrying a heavy instrument, such as a cello or French horn, can lead to musculoskeletal discomforts and back strain.

Playing of wind instruments can be impaired if the player has ASTHMA, because a significant bronchospasm is a major impediment. Some players use an inhaled bronchodilator prior to playing. Brass players encounter musculoskeletal hazards, primarily involving the facial musculature, or the embouchure. Lip problems are particularly common among brass instrumentalists. External problems relate to the pressure of the mouthpiece against the lips and the position of the lips relative to the mouthpiece. Mouthpieces come in a variety of metals; many players are allergic to the nickel used in mouthpieces.

Because of frequent tuning of the many strings, harpists may encounter problems with the right wrist and hand, as well as repetition stress injuries because of the turning motions of operating the tuning key. Percussion players (tympanists) may experience injuries because of repetitive actions of the hands, wrists, arms, and shoulders, and vibrations from a variety of drumhead surfaces.

Vision is a concern for all musicians, as they must be able to read music directly in front of them as well as watch the conductor (or, in a chamber group, watch other players). Many use specially prescribed glasses; pianists generally use a lens that is just for reading music. Conductors who use a score may have special vision requirements.

Research on Musicians' Injuries

The most comprehensive study done on musicians' injuries was undertaken for the International Conference of Symphony and Opera Musicians (ICSOM) in 1986 by Fishbein et al. From a population of more than 4,000 representing 48 American orchestras, 2,212 responses were received. Of these, 76 percent indicated having had a medical problem severe enough to affect performance. The majority of these problems were painful musculoskeletal syndromes, most frequent among string players (78 percent). Of nonstring musicians, 75 percent also had a severe medical problem. In a 1986 study involving eight orchestras in Australia, the United States and England, researchers found a 64 percent occurrence of overuse syndrome, which when the least severe of these was subtracted, amounted to 42 percent with a more significant level of symptoms.

Researchers have found a slightly higher incidence of injuries among female musicians than male musicians. Research still goes on, but speculations for the reasons of the gender differences include playing techniques, repetitious actions, stress, hand size, and joint condition.

Lifestyles of some musicians, particularly popular or rock musicians, may differ from classical musicians. Some may use drugs and alcohol, possibly leading to ADDICTIONS and alcoholism. In all musicians, smoking can lead to the deterioration of pulmonary function and reduced resistance to infection.

See also BELTING; CLARINETIST'S CHEILITIS; CONDUCTORS (MUSICAL); GUITAR PLAYERS' INJURIES; HEARING LOSS; KEYBOARD INSTRUMENT PLAYERS' INJURIES; PERFECTION; PERFORMING ARTS MEDICINE; PERFORMING ARTS MEDICINE ASSOCIATION; REPETITIVE STRESS INJURIES; WIND INSTRUMENT PLAYERS' INJURIES.

Fishbein, M., et al. "Medical Problems among ICSOM Musicians." *Medical Problems of Performing Artists* 3 (1988): 1–14.

Fry, H. J. H. "Incidence of Overuse Syndrome in the Symphony Orchestra." *Medical Problems of Performing Artists* 1 (1986): 51–55.

Sataloff, R. T., A. G. Brandfonbrener, and R. J. Lederman. *Textbook of Performing Arts Medicine.* New York: Raven Press, 1991.

music in the workplace   Music is a basic social and cultural activity of humankind, involving sounds produced by the voice or instruments. Music is often used to reduce stress and help people relax. Music is often played in the workplace as background to the sounds of people moving about, talking, and machines clattering. Often, employees in their own workspaces choose the type of music that most reflects their interests and helps them relieve stress and stay relaxed.

Historical Background: Music and Healing

Using music as a stress reliever is not a new concept. In Greek mythology, Apollo was god of both music and medicine. His son Aesculapius became god of medicine and cured mental diseases with song and music. Plato, the Greek philosopher, believed that music influenced a person's emotions and character. According to the Bible, David's harp playing relieved King Saul's melancholy (DEPRESSION).

Music and Stress Reduction

Music may be effective in reducing stress in the workplace because it addresses the whole person concurrently and simultaneously on physical, affective, cognitive, and social levels. Music usually has few if any side effects, relative ease of administration, and increasing therapeutic promise as indicated by studies in many fields.

Researchers have looked at the influences of music in managing stress in many anxiety-provoking situations. One example is test taking; anxiety levels appear to rise in the absence of music, while they are held constant with music. Music may have more effect on highly anxious subjects. Stimulating music may increase worry and emotionality; more sedative music decreases these feelings.

PHYSICAL EFFECTS OF MUSIC IN THE WORKPLACE

- Heart rate acceleration is correlated with loudness, tempo, and musical complexity; heart rate deceleration is correlated with resolution of musical conflict, decreasing loudness, and slowing tempo.
- Stimulating music increases heart rate; sedative music decreases heart rate.
- Rock music leads to heart deceleration.
- Tachycardia (fast heartbeat) is associated with driving rhythms and increasing dynamics; bradycardia (slow heartbeat) is associated with changes in rhythm, texture, and dynamics.
- Sedative music significantly increases finger temperature.
- Blood pressure is affected by listening to music, but the type of music that affects these changes is unknown; music is effective in reducing blood pressure in essential hypertensives.
- Music that is enjoyed increases respiration.
- Music decreases stomach acid production.
- Popular music produces more electroencephalograph (EEG) changes than classical music, particularly in middle-aged subjects. Popular music causes a decrease in blood flow to the brain in young adults; classical music promotes brain blood flow enhancement in middle-aged subjects.

Surgeons and Music

A study reported in the *Journal of the American Medical Association* offered data to support the belief of many surgeons that music calms them and aids their performances. Researchers at State University of New York, Buffalo, devised a controlled laboratory experiment in which 50 male surgeons, age 31–61—all of whom reported that they typically listen to music during surgery—performed a complex math task under three separate conditions: while listening to music of their own choosing, while listening to music selected by the researchers, and with no music.

Changes in skin conductance, pulse rate, and blood pressure, all responses associated with stress, were dramatically lower with the physicians' music, somewhat lower with the researchers' music, and highest with no music at all. Music also appeared to improve speed and accuracy. Researchers selected Pachelbel's *Canon in D*, an orchestral piece often used in commercially prepared stress reduction tapes. Participants' selections covered a range of musical styles including a range of classical, jazz, and Irish folk. Category of music, regardless of tempo or instrumentation, seemed to have no significant impact on results, as long as the music was of the surgeon's own choosing.

Researchers pointed out that since all participants were already enthusiastic believers in the benefits of music and eager to participate in this study, they did not speculate about the effects on surgeons who customarily choose not to listen during surgery.

See also COMPLEMENTARY THERAPIES; STRESS MANAGEMENT.

Aldridge, David. "The Music of the Body: Music Therapy in Medical Settings." *ADVANCES, The Journal of Mind-Body Health* 9, no. 1 (winter 1993).

Allen, I., and J. Blascovich. "Effects of Music on Cardiovascular Reactivity among Surgeons." *Journal of the American Medical Association* (1994): 882–884.

Crowley, Susan L. "The Amazing Power of Music." *Bulletin*, American Association of Retired Persons, February 1992.

Kahn, Ada P. *Stress A–Z: A Sourcebook for Coping with Everyday Challenges*. New York: Facts On File, Inc., 1998.

naphthalene   A colorless-to-brown solid with a mothball-like or tarlike odor. It is insoluble in water but soluble in benzene, alcohol, ether, and acetone. The principal health effects of naphthalene are hemolytic anemia (damage to red blood cells) and local respiratory tract irritation (nose and throat). Naphthalene is readily absorbed by inhalation, ingestion, and contact with the skin.

The main use of naphthalene is in manufacturing phthalic anhydride, a chemical intermediate with a wide range of uses, such as dyes and pesticides. It is also used in the manufacture of naphthalene sulphonic acids which in turn are used in the manufacture of plasticizers for concrete, in the manufacture of an ingredient for plasterboard, as dispersants in synthetic and natural rubbers, and in tanning agents for the leather industries. Naphthalene is used in the manufacture of mothballs and has limited use in theatrical pyrotechnics. It is also present in creosote, which is used for pressure impregnation of timber and for timber treatment by immersion, spraying, or brushing. Tar containing naphthalene is used in some specialty paints and waterproof membranes.

See also RESPIRATORY TOXICITY; SKIN AND SENSE ORGAN TOXICITY; TANNING.

NASA   See ASSOCIATED LANDSCAPE CONTRACTORS OF AMERICA.

National Center for Research in Vocational Education (NCRVE)   Funded by the Office of Vocational and Adult Education of the U.S. Department of Education, NCRVE ceased operation on December 31, 1999. NCRVE played a key role in developing a new concept of workforce development. The center's mission was to strengthen school-based and work-based learning to prepare all individuals for lasting and rewarding employment, further education, and lifelong learning. The NATIONAL RESEARCH AND DISSEMINATION CENTERS FOR CAREER AND TECHNICAL EDUCATION now furthers this effort.

National Consumers League (NCL)   Founded in 1899, the National Consumers League is the nation's pioneer consumer group working to bring consumer power to bear on workplace and marketplace issues. NCL worked for child labor provisions in the Fair Labor Standards Act (passed in 1938) and more recently has helped organize the Child Labor Coalition (CLC), which is committed to ending child labor exploitation in the United States and abroad.

For information:

National Consumers League
1701 K Street, NW
#1200
Washington, DC 20006
(202) 835-3323
(202) 835-0747 (fax)
www.nclnet.org

See also CHILD LABOR; CHILD LABOR COALITION; FAIR LABOR STANDARDS ACT.

National Depressive and Manic-Depressive Association (NDMDA)   A national association that recognizes the biochemical nature of bipolar and unipolar affective disorders and the disruptive psychological impact of the illnesses on patients and families. Its purpose is to provide personal support and direct service to persons with major DEPRESSION or manic-depression and their families, to educate the public concerning the nature and management of these disorders, and assist patients suffering with depression and manic-depression in gaining access to effective care.

Membership in the group not only provides information and support, but a source of self-esteem and dignity for those suffering from depressive disorders and their families. Many employed persons are referred to the NDMDA through EMPLOYEE ASSISTANCE PROGRAMS.

In addition to the service aspect of local chapters, the national organization fights the stigma associated with mental illness, promotes funding for research to improve diagnosis and treatment, and lobbies for adequate insurance coverage for the treatment of these disorders. There are chapters throughout the United States and Canada.

For information contact:

NDMDA
730 North Franklin Street
Suite 501
Chicago, IL 60610
(800) 826-3632 (toll-free)
(312) 642-7243 (fax)
http://www.ndmda.org

See BIPOLAR DISORDER.

National Fire Protection Association (NFPA) An international nonprofit membership organization founded in 1896 with more than 75,000 members representing nearly 100 nations. NFPA serves as the world's leading advocate of fire prevention and is an authoritative source on public safety.

NFPA's activities extend from development of codes and standards to prevention education and professional training. The NFPA has developed many codes related to fire protection that have been accredited by the AMERICAN NATIONAL STANDARDS INSTITUTE (ANSI).

For further information:

National Fire Protection Association
1 Batterymarch Park
Quincy, MA 02269-9101
(617) 770-3000
(617) 770-0700 (fax)
www.nfpa.org

See also FIRE PROTECTION/FIRE SAFETY.

National Foundation for Depressive Illness A group of lay and professional people organized to advance private and public education about DEPRESSION and its treatment. There is a toll-free telephone number which gives a recorded message concerning symptoms of depression and offering to send a list of local referrals and literature. Many employees are referred to the foundation through EMPLOYEE ASSISTANCE PROGRAMS.

For information contact:

National Foundation for Depressive Illness
P.O. Box 2257
New York, NY 10116
(800) 239-1265 (toll-free)
(212) 268-4260
(212) 268-4434 (fax)
http://www.depression.org

See also MENTAL HEALTH.

National Institute for Occupational Safety and Health (NIOSH) Established by the Occupational Safety and Health Act of 1970, NIOSH is part of the Centers for Disease Control and Prevention (CDC) and is the federal institute responsible for conducting research and making recommendations for the prevention of work-related illnesses and injuries. Special concerns of NIOSH include: occupational health, industrial hygiene, toxicology and hazards of industrial materials and conditions; chemical engineering, nursing, medicinal, and physiological aspects of occupational health hazards; prevention and treatment of injurious effects on health; poisonous gases, vapors, mist, and dust; radiation; heat and humidity; noise; and effects of pesticides.

For further information:

National Institute for Occupational Safety and Health
Centers for Disease Control and Prevention
Public Health Services
U.S. Department of Health and Human Services
Robert A. Taft Laboratories
4676 Columbia Parkway
Cincinnati, OH 45226
(800) 356-4674
(513) 533-8573 (fax)
http://www.cdc.gov/niosh

National Institute of Mental Health (NIMH) A
U.S. government agency that supports and conducts research concerning prevention, diagnosis, and treatment of mental illnesses. Studies benefit individuals with mental health problems, those at risk of developing problems, and concerned employers, families, and friends. NIMH is part of the Alcohol, Drug Abuse, and Mental Health Administration, a component of the U.S. Department of Health and Human Services.

For information contact:

National Institute of Mental Health
6001 Executive Boulevard
Room 8184
MSC 9663
Bethesda, MD 20892-9663
(800) 421-4211 (toll-free)
(301) 443-4513
(301) 443-4279 (fax)
http://www.nimh.nih.gov

National Institute on Drug Abuse A part of the
U.S. Alcohol, Drug Abuse, and Mental Health Administration (ADAMHA), its function is to provide leadership, policies, and goals for governmental work in preventing, controlling, and treating narcotic addiction and drug abuse, and in rehabilitating affected individuals through referrals from employers and physicians.

For further information contact:

National Institute on Drug Abuse
National Institutes of Health
6001 Executive Boulevard
Room 5213
Bethesda, MD 20892-9561
(301) 443-1124
http://www.nida.nih.gov

See also MENTAL HEALTH.

National Mental Health Association A volunteer
nongovernmental organization for the prevention of mental illness and promotion of mental health, with more than 650 chapters nationwide. Goals of the organization include protecting the rights of people with mental health problems, educating the public about MENTAL HEALTH and promoting research concerning all aspects of mental health. EMPLOYEE ASSISTANCE PROGRAMS often make referrals to chapters and utilize the association's educational materials.

For information contact:

National Mental Health Association
1021 Prince Street
Alexandria, VA 22314-2971
(800) 969-6642
(703) 684-7722
(703) 684-5968 (fax)
http://www.nmha.org

National Priorities List (NPL) A listing by the
ENVIRONMENTAL PROTECTION AGENCY of sites that have undergone preliminary assessment and inspection to determine which locations pose an immediate threat because of toxic materials to persons working or living nearby.

National Safety Council The leading advocate in
the United States for safety and health. Founded in 1913 and chartered by the U.S. Congress in 1953, the mission of the council is "to educate and influence society to adopt safety, health and environmental policies, practices and procedures that prevent and mitigate human suffering and economic losses arising from preventable causes."

The council is a nonprofit, nongovernmental, international public service organization. According to the council, unintentional injuries are the fifth leading cause of death in this country and the leading cause of death for Americans under 45 years old. The council believes that such incidents are not just random occurrences, but instead result from multiple conditions involving the interactions of machines and environments with people as they live, work, and play. The council defines "accidents" as unplanned, unwanted, and nearly always preventable events.

As a nongovernmental organization, the National Safety Council has no authority to legislate or regulate. It can, however, influence public opinion, attitudes, and behavior. The council serves as an objective and impartial intermediary by bringing safety and health professionals representing industry and labor together with government and public-interest representatives to form national coalitions on key safety, health, and environmental issues.

Compilation of Injury Data

National Safety Council statisticians have created a comprehensive system for tracking and compiling injury and illness data, including annual publication of *Injury Facts,* an authoritative compendium of safety and health statistics. Council researchers also produce the *Journal of Safety Research,* an interdisciplinary scientific quarterly. The Council's Environmental Health Center, based in Washington, D.C., is a leading provider of credible and timely information and community-based programs on environmental and public health issues.

For further information:

National Safety Council
1121 Spring Lake Drive
Itasca, IL 60143-3201
(630) 285-1121
(800) 621-7619 (toll-free)
(630) 285-1315 (fax)
www.nsc.org

National Toxicology Program (NTP) A program of toxicological testing for those substances most frequently found at sites on the NATIONAL PRIORITIES LIST of the Environmental Protection Agency, and which also have the greatest potential for workplace exposure.

See also ENVIRONMENTAL PROTECTION AGENCY.

National Transportation Safety Board (NTSB)
An independent federal agency charged by Congress with investigating every civil aviation accident in the United States and significant accidents in the other modes of transportation, including railroad, highway, marine, and pipeline, and issuing safety recommendations aimed at preventing future accidents. The NTSB also works with states, community groups, and others to promote passage of safety legislation consistent with their recommendations.

For information:

National Transportation Safety Board
490 L'Enfant Plaza, SW
Washington, DC 20594
(202) 314-6000
www.ntsb.gov

natural gas industry See EXTRACTIVE INDUSTRIES.

needlestick injuries (NSIs) and prevention
According to the Occupational Safety and Health Administration (OSHA), approximately 5.6 million workers in the health care industry and related occupations are at risk of occupational exposure to bloodborne pathogens, including human immunodeficiency virus (HIV), hepatitis B virus (HBV), hepatitis C virus (HBV), and others.

According to a report by OSHA in March 1999, an estimated 600,000 to 800,000 needlestick injuries and other percutaneous (though the skin) injuries occur annually among health care workers. Nurses sustain the majority of these injuries and as many as one-third of all sharps injuries have been reported to be related to the disposal process. The Centers for Disease Control estimates that 62 to 88 percent of sharps injuries can potentially be prevented by the use of safer medical devices. Needlestick injuries and other sharps-related injuries that result in occupational bloodborne pathogens exposure, continue to be an important public health as well as workplace concern.

Congress passed the Needlestick Safety and Prevention Act in November 2000 directing OSHA to revise its bloodborne pathogens standard to describe in greater detail its requirements for employers to identify and make use of effective and safer medical devices. Since then, OSHA has been educating employers, health care workers, and the general public on OSHA's revision to the bloodborne pathogens standard.

The revision will help reduce needlestick injuries among health care workers and others who handle medical sharps. According to Secretary of Labor Elaine Chao, "Prevention is the best medicine. By revising this standard, OSHA is giving employers a stronger tool to help reduce serious injuries and illnesses caused by needles and sharps."

New provisions of the standard require employers to maintain sharps injury logs and involve non-managerial employees in selecting safer medical devices. Enforcement of these provisions began in July 2001. "Safe needles protect workers from deadly injuries," said R. Davis Layne, Acting OSHA Administrator.

Bloodborne Pathogens Standards

The Needlestick Safety and Prevention Act directs specific revisions to the standard, including clarifying the requirement for employers to select safer needle devices as they become available and involving employees in identifying and choosing the devices.

OSHA's standard revision specifies the types of controls, such as safer medical devices in the health care setting. Below are definitions of terms included in the revision:

Sharps with engineered sharps injury protections includes non-needle sharps or needle devices used for withdrawing fluids or administering medications or other fluids that contain built-in safety features, or mechanisms that effectively reduce the risk of an exposure incident.

Needleless systems are devices that do not use needles for the collection or withdrawal of body fluids, or for the administration of medication or fluids.

Engineering controls include all control measures that isolate or remove a bloodborne pathogen hazard from the workplace. The revision now specifies that "self-sheathing needles" and "safer medical devices, such as sharps with engineered sharps injury protections and needleless systems" are engineering controls.

Employers must review their exposure control plans annually to reflect changes in technology that will help eliminate or reduce exposure to bloodborne pathogens. That review must include documentation of the employer's consideration and implementation of appropriate commercially available and effective safer devices.

Employers must solicit input from nonmanagerial health care workers regarding the identification, evaluation, and selection of effective engineering controls, including safe medical devices. Examples of nonmanagerial workers include those in different departments of the facility, such as geriatric, pediatric, nuclear medicine, and others.

Employers with 11 or more employees, who are required to keep records by current recordkeeping standards, must maintain a sharps injury log. The log must be maintained in such a way as to assure employee privacy and will contain, at minimum, the type and brand of device involved in the incident, if known, and the location and description of the incident.

See also HEPATITIS C; HEALTH CARE WORKERS; HUMAN IMMUNODEFICIENCY VIRUS.

nervous breakdown   A nonmedical term referring to any one of several mental health disorders in an acute phase. The term is used when an individual loses control of his or her emotions and is no longer able to control behavior. Popularly, the term is applied to severe anxieties as well as more severe psychoses, but a better term might be "emotional breakdown."

The individual may be unable to work or concentrate, unable to sleep, will have little interest in eating, may cry frequently, become fearful, and may become severely depressed. Physical symptoms may include fast heartbeat, dizziness, headaches, fainting, and sweating palms. These symptoms interfere with activities of daily living as well as work.

Many employed persons experience some of these symptoms for brief periods of time. It is when they last for a long time that they produce a breakdown.

Avoiding an emotional breakdown can be best accomplished by developing an ability to share one's feelings and emotions with another person. Just talking to another person helps many people get their life situations in a better focus before their emotional system goes on overload and breaks down. Many breakdowns occur at times of transition and change, such as job change, layoffs, middle age, marriage, divorce, and parenthood. At times of transition a person is more insecure, with good reason, and hence more vulnerable to emotional swings.

See also ANXIETY DISORDERS; DEPRESSION; MENTAL HEALTH; STRESS.

networking   Using individual contacts to gain important information, employment, power, or some type of financial advantage. The contacts used in networking are generally mutually advantageous to all parties and may be arrived at informally, even socially. Networking involves an exchange of favors and usually breaks down if an individual is always on the receiving or giving end. An example of networking in action is when someone gets a job or information about a job possibility through relatives, friends, friends of friends, or teachers, rather than registering with an employment agency or contacting employers listed in help wanted ads.

Networks may be created by certain similarities of their members' goals. For example, women's networks have coalesced in fields such as business and politics to counteract the hold of the perceived or actual "old boy network" of men on such institutions. Networking has been used in sales techniques, to market creative work and ideas, and to advance social programs.

Individuals who are not social minglers have more trouble networking than those who are joiners and have large circles of friends and acquaintances, both business and social. Being a successful "networker" involves extroverted personality traits such as meeting new people easily and a willingness to become involved in a cause or activity or a group.

Boe, Anne, and Bettie B. Youngs. *Is Your "Net" Working?: A Complete Guide to Building Contacts and Career Visibility.* New York: Wiley, 1989.
Steinem, Gloria. *Outrageous Acts and Everyday Rebellions.* New York: New American Library, 1983.

neurotoxicity   Adverse effects on the structure or functioning of the central and/or peripheral nervous system resulting from exposure to chemical substances. Neurotoxicants can cause changes that lead to generalized damage to nerve cells (neuronopathy), injury to axons (axonopathy), or destruction of the myelin sheath (myelinopathy). It is well established that exposure to certain agricultural and industrial chemicals can damage the nervous system, resulting in neurological and behavioral dysfunction.

Exposure to chemical agents can trigger a wide range of adverse effects on the nervous system. Neurotoxic substances can alter the propagation of nerve impulses or the activity of neurotransmitters and can disrupt the maintenance of the myelin sheath or the synthesis of protein. As a result, neurotoxicological assessments require the administration of a battery of functional and observational tests. Neurotoxicity is most commonly measured by neurological tests that assess cognitive, sensory, and motor function.

Symptoms of neurotoxicity include muscle weakness, loss of sensation and motor control, tremors, alterations in cognition, and impaired functioning of the autonomic nervous system.

Central Nervous System and Neurotoxicity

The central nervous system (CNS) is composed of the brain and spinal cord. It is responsible for the higher functions of the nervous system (conditioned reflexes, learning, memory, judgment, and other functions of the mind). Chemicals toxic to the CNS can induce confusion, fatigue, irritability, and other behavioral changes. Methyl mercury and lead are known CNS toxicants. Exposure to these metals can also cause degenerative diseases of the brain (encephalopathy).

Peripheral Nervous System and Neurotoxicity

The peripheral nervous system (PNS) includes all the nerves not in the brain or spinal cord. These nerves carry sensory information and motor impulses. Damage to the nerve fibers of the PNS can disrupt communication between the CNS and the rest of the body. The organic solvents carbon disulfide, n-hexane, and trichloroethylene can harm the PNS, resulting in weakness in the lower limbs, prickling or tingling in the limbs (paresthesia), and loss of coordination.

See also CHEMICAL TOXICITY.

Needleman, H. L. Behavioral Toxicology. *Environmental Health Perspectives* 103 (Supplement 6) (1995): 77–79.
@2001 Environmental Defense used by permission. Scorecard is available at www.scorecard.org

neurotransmitters   See DEPRESSION.

new hires   See SAFETY.

n-hexane   See NEUROTOXICITY.

nickel   See IMMUNOTOXICANTS; SKIN OR SENSE ORGAN TOXICITY.

nicotine dependence Nicotine in tobacco is responsible for dependence on tobacco. Nicotine in tobacco smoke passes into the bloodstream after it is inhaled; in chewing tobacco, the nicotine is absorbed through the lining of the mouth. In habitual smokers, nicotine increases the heart rate, narrows blood vessels, raises blood pressure, stimulates the central nervous system, reduces fatigue, increases alertness, and improves concentration. Regular smoking results in tolerance, and a higher intake is required to bring about the desired effects. Many employers offer cessation programs at the workplace to encourage employees to stop smoking.

See also ADDICTIONS; SMOKING.

NIOSH See NATIONAL INSTITUTE FOR OCCUPATIONAL SAFETY AND HEALTH.

NIOSH Pocket Guide to Chemical Hazards A source of general industrial hygiene information for workers, employers, and occupational health professionals. The *Pocket Guide* presents key information and data in abbreviated tabular form for 677 chemicals or substance groupings, among them manganese compounds, tellurium compounds, inorganic tin compounds, and so on, that are found in the work environment.

The industrial hygiene information in the *Pocket Guide* should help users recognize and control occupational chemical hazards. The chemicals or substances contained include all substances for which the National Institute for Occupational Safety and Health (NIOSH) has recommended exposure limits (RELS) and those with permissible exposure limits (PELs) as found in the Occupational Safety and Health Administration (OSHA) General Industry Air Contaminants Standard.

The *Pocket Guide* lists the toxicologically important routes of entry for each substance and whether contact with the skin or eyes is potentially hazardous as well as potential symptoms of exposure, and organs affected by exposure to each substance. It also presents a summary of recommended personal protection practices for each toxic substance. These recommendations supplement general work practices (such as avoiding eating, drinking, or smoking where chemicals are

used). Recommendations include immediate care for injuries, for skin, clothing removal, changing of clothing, eyewash fountains and/or quick drench facilities, first aid, and respirator use.

For information:

National Institute for Occupational Safety and
  Health
Centers for Disease Control and Prevention
4676 Columbia Parkway
Cincinnati, OH 45226
(800) 356-4674
(513) 533-8573 (fax)
www.cdc.gov/niosh/npg

See also NATIONAL INSTITUTE FOR OCCUPATIONAL SAFETY AND HEALTH; OCCUPATIONAL SAFETY AND HEALTH ADMINISTRATION; PERMISSIBLE EXPOSURE LIMITS; RECOMMENDED EXPOSURE LIMITS.

National Institute for Occupational Safety and Health.

nitrogen dioxide See COMBUSTION POLLUTANTS.

nitrogen oxide See RESPIRATORY TOXICITY.

nitrogen tetroxide See AEROSPACE MEDICINE.

nitrous oxide Compressed gases such as nitrous oxide are often used to obtain the cold temperatures needed for cryosurgery. Cryosurgical instruments that use compressed gas are designed to allow the gas to expand through a valve inside the metal tip of the cryosurgical probe, causing the tip to reach extremely low temperatures. If the exhaust gas from the probe is improperly vented, nitrous oxide concentrations in the air can reach several thousand parts per million (ppm) during a cryosurgical procedure, according to the National Institute of Occupational Safety and Health (NIOSH). Depending on the room ventilation, levels may remain elevated for long periods following the procedure. NIOSH recommends that exposures should be minimized to prevent short-term behavioral and long-term reproductive health effects that can be caused by nitrous oxide.

As gas is under considerable pressure, the discharge end of the tubing can be exhausted directly outdoors. This can be accomplished by placing the end of the hose out of a window or attached to a pipe placed through a wall or ceiling to the outdoors. Care should be taken to assure that the discharge location is not an area where people are normally present or in close proximity to an outside air intake or window where the nitrous oxide could reenter the building.

Even with proper ventilation systems, leaks can occur that can cause high levels of nitrous oxide in the work area. The equipment manufacturer should be consulted to determine what routine maintenance is necessary for the particular cryogenic unit. NIOSH recommends that periodic leak testing of all fittings and connections be conducted to minimize this source of exposure.

See also DENTISTRY; HEALTH CARE WORKERS.

National Institute of Occupational Safety and Health.

noise   A workplace health issue because of its psychological as well as physiological effects. It can be wanted, unwanted, or distracting. The volume or frequency of the noise can be stressful as well as physically debilitating. Certain forms of noise, such as loud music, may simply annoy some workers, while others feel more productive when listening to certain types of music.

Workers in certain occupations are more prone to injuries from noise. These include rock musicians, machine shop workers, and lumber mill employees. As chronic noise levels approach 85 decibels, significant potential for permanent hearing loss increases. Usually, hearing loss occurs only on specific frequency levels, depending on the amount of the exposure. It may be difficult for a worker to become aware of a hearing loss until it evolves significantly. The federal government

NONFATAL OCCUPATIONAL ILLNESSES BY CATEGORY OF ILLNESS, PRIVATE INDUSTRY, 1996–2000

Category	Number (000)					Percent of Total Illness Cases				
	1996	1997	1998	1999	2000	1996	1997	1998	1999	2000
Total illness cases	439.0	429.8	391.9	372.3	362.5	100	100	100	100	100
Skin diseases or disorders	58.1	57.9	53.1	44.6	41.8	13	13	14	12	12
Dust diseases of the lungs	3.5	2.9	2.1	2.2	1.7	1	1	1	1	(2)
Respiratory conditions due to toxic agents	21.7	20.3	17.5	16.5	14.7	5	5	4	4	4
Poisoning	4.8	5.1	4.0	4.4	3.3	1	1	1	1	1
Disorders due to physical agents	16.8	16.6	16.6	15.1	13.9	4	4	4	4	4
Disorders associated with repeated trauma	281.1	276.6	253.3	246.7	241.8	64	64	65	66	67
All other occupational illnesses	53.0	50.4	45.4	42.9	45.1	12	12	12	12	12

Category	Incident Rate				
	1996	1997	1998	1999	2000
Total illness cases	52.2	49.8	44.2	41.2	39.4
Skin diseases or disorders	6.9	6.7	6.0	4.9	4.6
Dust diseases of the lungs	.4	.3	.2	.2	.2
Respiratory conditions due to toxic agents	2.6	2.4	2.0	1.8	1.6
Poisoning	.6	.6	.5	.5	.4
Disorders due to physical agents	2.0	1.9	1.9	1.7	1.5
Disorders associated with repeated trauma	33.5	32.0	28.5	27.3	26.3
All other occupational illnesses	6.3	5.8	5.1	4.7	4.9

Source: Bureau of Labor Statistics, U.S. Department of Labor December 2001

mandates that workers exposed to high levels of noise wear protective ear equipment.

See also BROWNFIELDS.

Girdano, Daniel A., George S. Everly, Jr., and Dorothy E. Dusek. *Controlling Stress and Tension: A Holistic Approach.* Englewood Cliffs, N.J.: Prentice Hall, 1990.

noise-induced hearing loss   See NOISE.

nonfatal occupational injuries   Of the 5.7 million nonfatal injuries and illnesses reported in private industry for 1999, 5.3 million were injuries. The remainder of these (372,000) cases were work-related illnesses. Sixty-six percent (246,700 cases) of the workplace illnesses were disorders associated with repeated trauma, such as carpal tunnel syndrome, according to the Bureau of Labor Statistics, U.S. Department of Labor (DOL).

In private industry, nine industries (including eating and drinking places, hospitals, nursing and personal care facilities, grocery stores, and department stores) each with at least 100,000 injuries, accounted for about 1.6 million injuries, or 30 percent of the 5.3 million total, according to the DOL.

The DOL reported that rates for nonfatal workplace injury and illness incidence rates per 100 full-time workers declined from 1995 to 1999 in all industry divisions. The DOL ranked nonfatal workplace injuries and illnesses for agriculture, forestry, and fishing, mining, construction, manufacturing, transportation and public utilities, trade, finance, insurance, and real estate and services.

In private industry, nonfatal occupational illnesses categorized by the DOL for the period 1996–2000 included skin diseases or disorders, dust diseases of the lungs, respiratory conditions due to toxic agents, poisoning, disorders due to physical

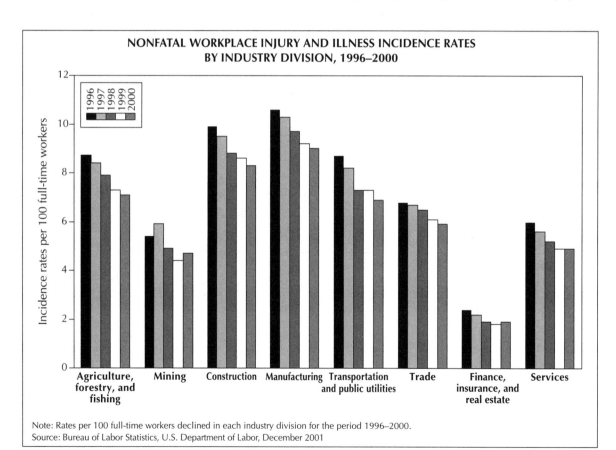

NONFATAL WORKPLACE INJURY AND ILLNESS INCIDENCE RATES BY INDUSTRY DIVISION, 1996–2000

Incidence rates per 100 full-time workers

1996
1997
1998
1999
2000

Agriculture, forestry, and fishing   Mining   Construction   Manufacturing   Transportation and public utilities   Trade   Finance, insurance, and real estate   Services

Note: Rates per 100 full-time workers declined in each industry division for the period 1996–2000.
Source: Bureau of Labor Statistics, U.S. Department of Labor, December 2001

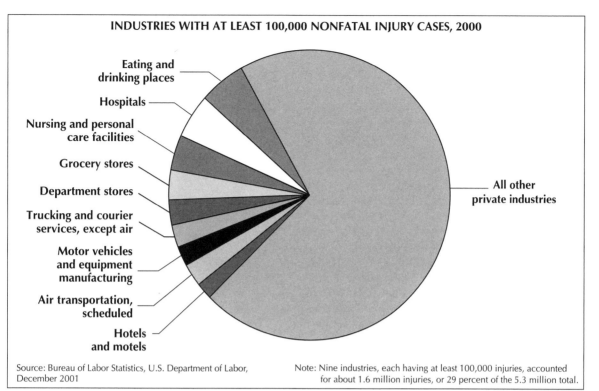

INDUSTRIES WITH AT LEAST 100,000 NONFATAL INJURY CASES, 2000

Eating and drinking places

Hospitals

Nursing and personal care facilities

Grocery stores

Department stores

Trucking and courier services, except air

Motor vehicles and equipment manufacturing

Air transportation, scheduled

Hotels and motels

All other private industries

Source: Bureau of Labor Statistics, U.S. Department of Labor, December 2001

Note: Nine industries, each having at least 100,000 injuries, accounted for about 1.6 million injuries, or 29 percent of the 5.3 million total.

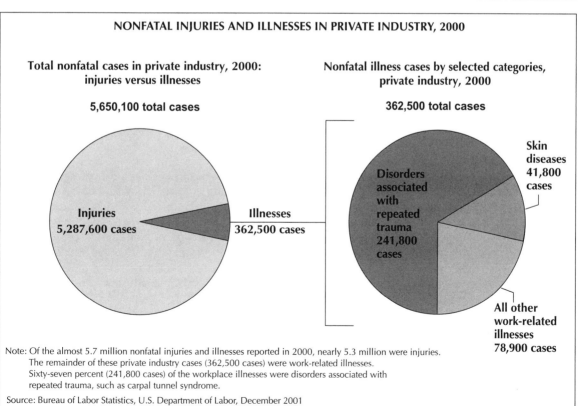

NONFATAL INJURIES AND ILLNESSES IN PRIVATE INDUSTRY, 2000

Total nonfatal cases in private industry, 2000: injuries versus illnesses

5,650,100 total cases

Injuries 5,287,600 cases

Illnesses 362,500 cases

Nonfatal illness cases by selected categories, private industry, 2000

362,500 total cases

Disorders associated with repeated trauma 241,800 cases

Skin diseases 41,800 cases

All other work-related illnesses 78,900 cases

Note: Of the almost 5.7 million nonfatal injuries and illnesses reported in 2000, nearly 5.3 million were injuries. The remainder of these private industry cases (362,500 cases) were work-related illnesses. Sixty-seven percent (241,800 cases) of the workplace illnesses were disorders associated with repeated trauma, such as carpal tunnel syndrome.

Source: Bureau of Labor Statistics, U.S. Department of Labor, December 2001

agents, disorders associated with repeated trauma, and other occupational illnesses. (See charts.)

See also FATALITIES BY OCCUPATION.

nonverbal communication   See BODY LANGUAGE; COMMUNICATION.

nuclear weapons workers   Employees involved in production of nuclear weapons. Since World War II, hundreds of thousands of men and women have worked toward building U.S. nuclear defense. Thousands of Americans developed disabling or fatal illnesses as a result of exposure to BERYLLIUM, ionizing radiation, and other hazards unique to nuclear weapons production and testing. Often these workers were neither adequately protected from, nor informed of, the occupational hazards to which they were exposed.

In October 2000 the United States enacted the Energy Employees Occupational Illness Compensation Program Act, a complex law providing health care and compensation for nuclear weapons workers. This law sets out responsibilities to compensate workers. The Departments of Labor, Health and Human Services, and Energy are responsible for developing and implementing actions to compensate these workers and their families in a manner that is compassionate, fair, and timely.

Historical Background

According to Arjun Makhijani in the *Bulletin of Atomic Scientists,* while the government was building nuclear warheads in the 1950s, there was denial that some 600,000 nuclear workers had been put at risk of radiation exposure. When workers sought compensation, the government and its contractors fought them. Nuclear weapons contractors signed agreements that completely excused them from any liability, even in cases of gross negligence. However, in April 2000, then-Energy Secretary Bill Richardson acknowledged that nuclear weapons workers as a group had been put at risk by exposure to radiation and other toxic substances.

Many workers were exposed to fallout as a result of participation in atmosphere testing programs. Tests were conducted in 1946 at Bikini atoll, and underwater using a plutonium bomb. The explosion threw 1 million tons of intensely radioactive

spray into the air, leaving plutonium "hot spots" over a wide area. However, radiological teams monitoring the tests did not have the ability to make accurate measurements in the field. Unfortunately, food was washed with contaminated water, radioactive materials were deposited in nearly every ship's evaporator pipes that provided water for drinking, cooking, and bathing, and surfaces such as wooden decks absorbed the radioactivity.

In 1990 the first law acknowledging possible radiation-related harm was passed. Called the Radiation Exposure Compensation Act (RECA), the law provided health care and compensation for people who had lived downwind from the Nevada Test Site and for uranium miners, the first nuclear workers to be compensated by Congress. The Atomic Energy Commission, the predecessor to the Energy Department, was aware that high levels of radon gas, as well as toxic dust suspended in poorly ventilated uranium mines, would cause lung cancer and other diseases. "Instead of improving conditions in the mines, the government chose to monitor the miners," said Makhijani.

The 1990 legislation created a list of cancers for which atomic workers might seek compensation. Included were:

Various types of leukemia
Multiple myeloma
Non-Hodgkin's lymphoma
Primary cancer of the breast (in women)
Esophagus, stomach, small intestine, pancreas, bile
   duct, gall bladder and liver

In 1999 the *Washington Post* revealed that uranium processed at the Paducah enrichment plant in Kentucky was contaminated with plutonium, and the government admitted that it had put workers at risk. The presence of plutonium, even in trace amounts, increases the dangers to workers. Plutonium is about 100,000 times more radioactive than natural uranium. Officially, plutonium contamination in uranium was supposed to be 20 parts per billion. That limit was often exceeded at Paducah. According to Makhijani, investigation of other uranium enrichment plants at Oak Ridge, Tennessee, and Portsmouth, Ohio, showed similar problems.

These uranium enrichment plant workers did not have the protections provided to plutonium workers, who used gloveboxes when processing materials. At uranium enrichment facilities, radioactive dust is carried off by ventilation systems installed in hoods. This difference is the technical basis for the place carved out in the new compensation law for those who worked at the three uranium enrichment sites, known as the "special exposure cohort."

According to Makhijani, workers at the three enrichment plants and at the Amchitka test site in Alaska who developed cancer will be compensated without having to prove that they were exposed. The plutonium exposures at the enrichment plants and the apparent loss of exposure data at Amchitka were used to justify including workers from these four sites in the cohort. However, workers at other sites have to prove that their exposures were large enough that their cancers were "at least as likely as not" caused by their exposure to radiation. This requirement will leave out many people whose cancers were caused by workplace exposures. Complicating their cases is the fact that radiation records were incomplete and it is thus impossible to calculate radiation doses confidently.

More groups of victims may be added to the legislation in the future. These could include the families of workers who may have been exposed to radioactivity brought home in cars or on clothes, and those living near weapons plants whose environment was often contaminated with radiation and other toxic substances.

Fire Protection at Nuclear Power Plants

The Nuclear Regulatory Commission requires fire protection programs at U.S. commercial nuclear power plants to guard against the probability of occurrence and consequences of fire. The fire protection program is designed to reasonably ensure that a fire will not prevent safe shutdown functions from performing and will not significantly increase the radioactive releases to the environment.

See also CANCER; FIRE SAFETY/FIRE PROTECTION; NATIONAL FIRE PROTECTION ASSOCIATION; PERSONAL PROTECTION EQUIPMENT.

U.S. Nuclear Regulatory Commission
11555 Rockville Pike
MSO16C1
Rockville, MD 20852

(301) 415-1759
(301) 415-1757 (fax)
http://www.nrc.gov/reactors/operating

Makhijani, Arjun. "The Burden of Proof." *Bulletin of the Atomic Scientists* 57, no. 4 (July 2001): 49.
Clinton, Bill. "Providing Compensation to America's Nuclear Weapons Workers." *Weekly Compilation of Presidential Documents* 36, no. 49 (December 11, 2000): 3025.

nurses See BACK INJURIES/BACK PAIN; HEALTH CARE WORKERS; NEEDLESTICK INJURIES AND PREVENTION.

nursing home workers Major sources of injuries and illnesses in nursing home workers include resident handling, slips, trips, and falls, contact with objects and equipment, assaults and violent acts, and exposure to harmful substances. Bureau of Labor Statistics data indicate that nursing aides, orderlies, and attendants account for 70 percent of nursing home injuries that result in days away from work. Female employees have more injuries that result in lost workdays than male employees.

Workers in nursing homes may include registered nurses, licensed practical nurses, other health aides, maids, cooks, janitors, and laundry workers. In 1996 the Occupational Safety and Health Administration unveiled an outreach and enforcement initiative to protect workers in nursing homes and personal care facilities that emphasized helping employers reduce injuries and illnesses through effective safety and health programs. The initiative also addressed potential nursing home hazards, including back injuries, slips and falls, workplace violence, and risks from bloodborne pathogens and tuberculosis.

Many nursing home workers face hazards similar to those faced by workers in hospitals and in the home care industry.

See also BACK INJURIES, BACK PAIN; BLOODBORNE PATHOGENS; HEALTH CARE WORKERS; HOME CARE INDUSTRY; NEEDLESTICK INJURIES AND PREVENTION; SLIPS, TRIPS, AND FALLS; TUBERCULOSIS; VIOLENCE.

nursing mothers In 2000 at least 20 states had legislation protecting mothers who breast-feed. The number of states with legislation addressing nursing mothers in the workplace nearly doubled that year. An example is the state of Illinois, which in 2001 regulated that employers must accommodate nursing mothers. Under the Illinois Nursing Mothers in the Workplace Act, an employer must provide unpaid break time for mothers who need to express breast milk for an infant.

The law applies to employers who have more than five workers other than immediate family. The break time must, if possible, run concurrently with break time already provided to the employee. An employer is exempt, however, if it would unduly disrupt an employer's operations.

An employer must also make reasonable efforts to provide a room or other location near the work area other than a toilet stall to allow the mother privacy. The law represents a good compromise for workers and employers, said Kim Clarke Maisch, state director of the National Federation of Independent Business, which has about 21,000 mostly small-business members in Illinois.

In 2002 the Hawaii legislature passed an amendment to its fair employment practices law stating that no employer can prohibit an employee from expressing breast milk during any meal period or other break period required to be provided by the employer by law or by a collective bargaining agreement.

In 1998 other states, such as California, Florida, and Texas, had enacted laws regarding nursing mothers. A California law simply urges all employers to support and encourage working mothers who want to continue breast-feeding. Both the Texas Breast Feeding Rights and Policies Law and the Florida Public Health Law encourage breast-feeding in the workplace by allowing businesses that develop a policy supporting worksite breast-feeding to use the designation "mother-friendly" or "baby-friendly" in their promotional materials.

President Clinton signed a law making breast-feeding legal on all federal property where a woman and her child have a right to be. Under the law, it is illegal to ask a woman who is nursing her infant child to move from federal property.

Many major corporations have already included mother-friendly programs in their employee benefits packages. These companies have been prompted by studies citing the decreased rate of ABSENTEEISM of mothers who continue to breast-feed after returning to the job and the lower medical bills of nursing mothers and their children.

Some companies report that accommodating mothers has been excellent for their bottom line, estimating a return of up to 400 percent of funds invested in lactation programs. While the issue of mothers breast-feeding in the workplace is largely left to the discretion of individual employers, facilitating a lactation program may be in employers' own good interest.

Help for Nursing Mothers

The La Leche League, an international organization devoted to assisting women with breast-feeding, advises women who have an employment problem to educate the employer on how breast-feeding will benefit the company. Cite illnesses for which breast-feeding reduces the risk and discuss practical solutions that can work. Some mothers may benefit from discussing the issue ahead of time with their employer, and others may decide it is better to say nothing and just pump when they return to work. Breast-feeding mothers should decide where they can express milk in privacy, as well as how much time is needed to express. If it takes more than 15 minutes, or if the separations because of work affect the milk supply, assistance may be needed. If it appears that a breast-feeding woman might get fired or need to sue her employer, an attorney should be consulted. Time frames apply to these lawsuits.

For further information:

La Leche League International (LLLI)
P.O. Box 4079
Schaumburg, IL 60168-4079
(847) 519-7730
(800) LA-LECHE (toll-free)
(847) 519-0035 (fax)
www.lalecheleague.org

See also WORKING MOTHERS.

Cohen, Rona, and Marsha B. Mrtek. "The Impact of Two Corporate Lactation Programs on the Incidence and Duration of Breastfeeding by Employed Mothers." *American Journal of Health Promotion* 8, no. 6 (July/August 1994).

Cohen, Rona, Marsha B. Mrtek, and Robert G. Mrtek. "Comparison of Maternal Absenteeism and Infant Illness Rates among Breastfeeding and Formula-feeding Women in Two Corporations." *American Journal of Health Promotion* 10, no. 2 (November/December 1995).

nutrition   Good mental and physical health in the workplace, as in all aspects of life, depends on good nutrition. The body and mind need many nutrients to function optimally. Nutrition is affected by emotional, biological, cognitive, and sociocultural factors. Many employers offer nutrition education programs as part of their health promotion activities.

Alcoholism and substance abuse can suppress the appetite, leading to a decrease in food intake. Additionally, excessive alcohol intake impairs liver and pancreatic functioning and often results in gastric inflammation. Nutrients taken in by the alcohol abuser may be malabsorbed; vitamin B complex, magnesium, zinc, folic acid, and vitamin K are just a few examples.

Severe ANXIETY, STRESS, and overwork can interfere with an individual's ability to meet optimal nutrition. For example, severe anxiety increases the release of epinephrine and norepinephrine. These hormones shunt blood from the digestive organs to the muscles, heart, and brain. Also, during stress, the body prepares itself for fight or flight. The body's response to stress is to fuel itself for this response, and the body increases its release of glucocorticoids as well as growth hormone. Glucocorticoids increase glucose production, while growth hormone decreases the effectiveness of insulin in glucose metabolism. Decreased blood flow, along with the increased glucose production, creates a state of anorexia in which the individual has a decreased intake of essential nutrients.

The cultural emphasis on thinness has led many to poor nutritional habits in an effort to lose weight; hence, poor body image may interfere with proper nutritional intake.

See also EATING DISORDERS; HEALTH PROMOTION; WORKSITE WELLNESS PROGRAMS.

obesity   Obesity—an excess of body fat—is a national public health concern and a concern of many workplace health promotion programs.

While the words *obese* and *overweight* are often used synonymously, they are actually different. An obese person is defined as being 20 percent or more above ideal body weight. Scientists use a scale called the body mass index (BMI) to measure obesity. BMI is computed by multiplying weight in pounds by 700 and dividing the result by the square of height in inches. *Overweight* refers to an excess of total fat, bone, muscle, and water. Obesity is a source of STRESS and ANXIETY for many of the one-third of all Americans who are obese, and many are fast realizing that crash diets alone will not solve their problem. Obesity can affect a person's SELF-ESTEEM, mental well-being, and productivity at work. It can lead to social withdrawal and have debilitating effects on the body.

The public image of obesity is changing; once obesity was simply considered the look of a moral failing of laziness or gluttony. However, recent breakthroughs in the genetics of obesity and drugs under development to fight obesity are contributing to a view, long shared by researchers and many overweight Americans, that obesity is a long-term disease.

Although obesity occurs when the calories absorbed by the body exceed those that are being used, obese people do not necessarily eat more than those who are not. It is thought that obese people have a lower metabolic rate, which is the amount of energy needed to maintain the body's functions.

Since children of obese parents are much more likely to be obese than children of thin parents, genetics may play a role in obesity. However, psychologist Kelly D. Brownell, director of the Yale Center for Eating and Weight Disorders, has said that "genetics may cause obesity to occur, but our environment makes it happen." By *environment* he means "a world in which we are inundated with media images of thinness that few of us could attain; filled with labor-saving devices that keep us physically inactive; and full of cheap, seductive food that is rich and fat in calories."

Researchers agree that a healthy diet and exercise can fight obesity. A reducing diet should provide the obese adult 500 to 1,000 calories fewer than his or her energy requirements. Regular exercise, that burns extra calories, particularly aerobic exercise, is considered a must. Increasing physical activity not only controls weight, but protects against many illnesses, including diabetes, heart disease, and cancer.

See also EATING DISORDERS; HEALTH PROMOTION; NUTRITION; WORKSITE WELLNESS.

American Society of Bariatric Physicians (ASBP)
5453 East Evans Place
Denver, CO 80222-5234
(303) 770-2526
(303) 779-4834 (fax)
www.asbp.org

Merz, Beverly, ed. "Obesity Drugs Redux." *Harvard Women's Health Watch* 4, no. 6 (February 1997).
For information:

occupational contact dermatitis   See DERMATITIS.

occupational health   See OCCUPATIONAL MEDICINE; WORKPLACE WELLNESS PROGRAMS.

occupational illness   Any abnormal condition or disorder, other than one resulting from an occupational injury, caused by exposure to environmental factors associated with employment. According to the Bureau of Labor Statistics' *Record-keeping Guidelines for Occupational Injuries and Illnesses* (1986) the term includes acute and chronic illnesses or diseases which may be caused by inhalation, absorption, ingestion, or direct contact.

occupational injury   Any injury, such as a cut, fracture, sprain, or amputation, that results from a work accident or from exposure involving a single incident in the work environment.

See also OCCUPATIONAL ILLNESS.

occupational lung disease   The number one work-related illness in the United States based on the frequency, severity, and preventability of diseases. According to the American Lung Association, these diseases are usually caused by extended exposure to irritating or toxic substances that may cause acute or chronic respiratory ailments, although severe single exposures can cause chronic lung disease as well.

Although occupational lung diseases are not often curable, they are always preventable. Improving ventilation, wearing protective equipment, changing work procedures, and educating workers are the key factors for prevention.

Smoking can act synergistically to increase the severity of these diseases. Smokers who are exposed to carcinogens such as asbestos and radiation greatly increase their chances of getting lung cancer and other lung diseases.

Occupational lung cancer is attributable to inhalation of carcinogens in the workplace such as asbestos, coal, and petroleum-related carbon compounds. In 1998 approximately 17,315 lung cancer deaths were attributable to inhalation of these carcinogens in the workplace.

Byssinosis (BROWN LUNG DISEASE) is a chronic condition involving obstruction of the small airways, severely impairing lung function. It is caused by dusts from hemp, flax, and cotton processing. Between 1979 and 1996 byssinosis caused 120 deaths; an estimated 35,000 current and former textile workers have been disabled.

Coal workers' pneumoconiosis, also known as BLACK LUNG DISEASE, is caused by the inhalation of coal dust. An estimated 4.5 percent of coal miners are affected; about 0.2 percent have scarring on the lungs, the most severe form of the disease. Between 1979 and 1996, 14,156 deaths were attributed to black lung disease, according to the American Lung Association.

SILICOSIS results from exposure to free crystalline silica in mines, foundries, blasting operations, and stone, clay, and glass manufacturing. Silicosis substantially raises the risk of other types of lung disease, particularly tuberculosis. Between 1979 and 1996, 2,694 deaths were attributed to silicosis. Each year, silicosis is listed as the cause of death on death certificates of 300 people, a rate that has been stable since the mid-1980s. About 1.6 million workers are believed to have been exposed to silica dust, and almost 60,000 are expected to suffer from some degree of silicosis.

Occupational ASTHMA occurs when a worker is exposed to substances such as dusts, vapors, gases, or fumes that trigger an asthma attack. Occupational asthma represents an estimated 15 percent of the cases of adult asthma.

Hypersensitivity pneumonitis is caused by the inhalation of fungus spores from moldy hay, bird droppings, or other organic dusts. Repeated exposure causes the air sacs of the lungs to become inflamed; parts of the lungs may then develop fibrous scar tissue and cease to function normally in breathing.

See also ALLERGY; ASBESTOS; LUNG CANCER; SMOKING.

American Lung Association
1740 Broadway
New York, NY 10019
(800) 586-4872 or (800) LUNG-USA
(212) 315-8872 (fax)
www.lungusa.org

occupational medicine   A field of medicine dedicated to promoting the health of workers through preventive medicine, clinical care, research, and education. Occupational medicine encompasses pre-employment physicals, return-to-work examinations, health screenings, nutrition and fitness education, drug testing, and immunization programs, as well as worksite wellness programs and safety and ergonomic programs at the workplace.

The American College of Occupational and Environmental Medicine (ACOEM), founded in 1916, is the largest U.S. medical society in this field. ACOEM members treat job-related diseases, identify and resolve workplace hazards, institute rehabilitation methods, and provide care. ACOEM publishes the monthly *Journal of Occupational and Environmental Medicine* as well as several newsletters and position papers.

The American Academy of Physician Assistants in Occupational Medicine (AAPAOM) is an educational organization representing physician assistants whose common interest is caring for working persons and preventing workplace illness and injury.

The Office of Occupational Medicine (OOM), part of the Occupational Safety and Health Administration (OSHA), is staffed by board-certified occupational medicine physicians and others, including a nurse and a toxicologist. The OOM provides medical, toxicological, and epidemiological support to OSHA field offices and interacts with other federal agencies regarding health and workplace issues. For example, the OOM has provided support on a number of respiratory protection issues, the hazard of silicosis, tuberculosis in the workplace, and support for protection against bloodborne pathogens through the standard-setting process.

For information:

American College of Occupational and Environmental Medicine
1114 N. Arlington Heights Road
Arlington Heights, IL 60004
(847) 818-1800
(847) 818-9266 (fax)
http://www.acoem.org

American Academy of Physician Assistants in Occupational Medicine
950 North Washington Street
Alexandria, VA 22314-1552
(800) 596-439
www.aapa.org

See also ERGONOMICS; INDUSTRIAL HYGIENE; WORKSITE WELLNESS PROGRAMS.

Occupational Safety and Health Administration (OSHA)

OSHA was created in 1971 with the mission of ensuring safe and healthful workplaces in America. Since 1971 workplace fatalities have been cut in half and occupational injury and illness rates have declined 40 percent. At the same time, U.S. employment has doubled from 56 million workers at 3.5 worksites to 111 million workers at 7 million sites.

In fiscal year 2002 OSHA's staff numbered 2,316, including 1,123 inspectors; the agency's budget was $443 million. Sharing the responsibility for oversight of workplace safety and health are 26 states that run their own OSHA programs with 3,105 employees, including 1,378 inspectors.

Under the George W. Bush administration, OSHA focused on four strategies: leadership, strong, fair, and effective enforcement, outreach, education, and compliance assistance, and voluntary partnerships. OSHA's Strategic Partnership Program targets areas of construction, shipbuilding, food processing, logging, and nursing homes and includes partnerships that zero in on specific hazards.

Occupational Safety and Health Act of 1970

This federal law was passed to assure safe and healthful working conditions for working Americans. The act authorizes enforcement of standards developed under the act, assists and encourages states in efforts to assure safe and healthful working conditions, and provides for research information, education, and training in the field of occupational safety and health.

The purposes of the act are many. It:

- Encourages employers and employees in their efforts to reduce the number of occupational safety and health hazards at workplaces and stimulates employers and employees to institute new and to perfect existing programs for providing safe and healthful working conditions.

- Provides that employers and employees have separate but interdependent responsibilities and rights with respect to achieving safe and healthful working conditions.

- Authorizes the secretary of labor to set mandatory occupational safety and health standards applicable to businesses affecting interstate commerce, and by creating an Occupational Safety and Health Review Commission, to carry out adjudicatory functions under the act.

- Provides for research in the field of occupational safety and health, including the psychological factors involved, and develops innovative methods, techniques, and approaches for dealing with occupational safety and health concerns.

- Explores ways to discover latent diseases, establishing causal connections between diseases and work in environmental conditions, and conducts other research relating to health problems, in recognition of the fact that occupational health standards present problems often different from those involved in occupational safety.

- Provides medical criteria that will assure in a practical way that no employee will suffer diminished health, functional capacity, or life expectancy as a result of work experience.

- Provides for training programs to increase the number and competence of personnel engaged in the field of occupational safety and health.

- Provides for development and promulgation of occupational safety and health standards.

- Provides an effective enforcement program, which includes a prohibition against giving advance notice of any inspection and actions for any individual violating this prohibition.

- Encourages states to assume the fullest responsibility for administration and enforcement of their occupational safety and health laws by providing grants to states to assist in identifying needs and responsibilities in areas of occupational safety and health, to develop plans in accordance with the provisions of this act, to improve the administration and enforcement of state occupational safety and health laws, and to conduct associated experimental and demonstration projects.

- Provides for appropriate reporting procedures with respect to occupational safety and health, which will help achieve the objectives of this act and accurately describe the nature of the occupational safety and health problem.

- Encourages joint labor-management efforts to reduce injuries and disease arising out of employment.

Filing OSHA Complaints

OSHA deals with complaints based on two questions: Who filed it? (For example, a complaint by an employee who gives a name is given greater consideration than a complaint from an anonymous employee.) What does the complaint allege? (A complaint about a condition that could kill someone is given greater consideration than a complaint about a record-keeping violation.)

All workplaces in the United States are under the jurisdiction of an area office. Complaints should be filed with the area office that has jurisdiction over the location of your workplace. Whether you file your complaint in writing or by telephone, you can give OSHA your name or register the complaint anonymously. However, OSHA gives less priority to complaints made anonymously. If you give OSHA your name, you can request that OSHA not disclose your name to your employer. OSHA is required to protect your identity; however, on some occasions employers learn the identity of a complainant even though OSHA was instructed to protect his or her identity.

You will be asked to answer many questions, including a description of the hazard that you think exists and the number of employees exposed to or threatened by each hazard. If you have photographs or accident reports involving the hazard, include those. Specify the particular building or worksite where the alleged violation is taking place. Draw a map if that will help. If your employer or another government agency already knows about the hazard involved in your complaint, tell OSHA as specifically as possible.

Some complaints result in an investigation and others result in an inspection. Inspections often take place if the complaint, signed by a current employee or employee representative, reports a hazard that is a violation of the law with "reasonable particularity," if there is a physical hazard from which illnesses or injuries have occurred, or if there is an "imminent danger" which might harm employees if it is not corrected immediately.

Inspections may follow a complaint about a business that has been cited by OSHA for an egregious violation within the past three years.

For further information:

Occupational Safety and Health Administration
U.S. Department of Labor
200 Constitution Avenue, NW
Washington, DC 20210
(800) 321-OSHA (Fatalities or life-threatening emergencies only)
(202) 693-2106 (fax)
http://www.osha.gov

odors See INDOOR ENVIRONMENT.

ohashiatsu A form of therapy useful for relief of stress that is based on the same system of Oriental medicine as acupuncture. The practice may be included in some WORKSITE WELLNESS PROGRAMS. Ohashiatsu addresses the body's "energy meridians" and points along those meridians called *tsubos*. Instead of using needles, however, the practitioner of ohashiatsu uses hands, elbows, and sometimes even knees as tools. The goal is for the patient to achieve a feeling of deep RELAXATION, harmony, and peace.

Ohashiatsu adds psychological and spiritual dimensions to traditional SHIATSU by incorporating Zen philosophy, movement, and MEDITATION to balance the energy of body, mind, and spirit.

See also COMPLEMENTARY THERAPIES; MIND-BODY CONNECTIONS.

oil acne and chloracne See DERMATITIS.

oil and gas well drilling and servicing See EXTRACTIVE INDUSTRIES.

opportunistic infections See ACQUIRED IMMUNODEFICIENCY SYNDROME (AIDS).

overload See BACK INJURIES, BACK PAIN; CONSTRUCTION; ERGONOMICS AND ERGONOMICS REGULATIONS; PHYSICAL LOAD/PHYSICAL OVERLOAD.

overwork See *KAROSHI.*

ozone See CARDIOVASCULAR OR BLOOD TOXICITY; RESPIRATORY TOXICITY.

painters (commercial) Workers who apply paint to surfaces and prepare walls, metal, wood, or other surfaces for painting. Because of their work, many accident hazards are present. Painters erect SCAFFOLDING and set up LADDERS for work above ground level. They remove fixtures (such as pictures, nails, and electric-switch covers), remove old paint using paint remover, scrapers, wire brushes, or blowtorches. They fill holes, cracks, and joints with caulk, putty, plastic, or other fillers. They smooth surfaces using sandpaper, steel wool, and/or brushes. They wash and treat surfaces with cleaning materials. They apply coats of paint, varnish, stain, enamel, or lacquer to surfaces using brushes, spray guns, rollers, or electrostatic equipment. Some cut stencils and brush or spray decorations and lettering on surfaces.

Because of the nature of their work and their awkward body postures when painting (particularly ceilings), neck and shoulder pains, sprains and strains of the upper limbs, and musculoskeletal disorders are common. Many experience knee pain and injuries to the cartilage of the knee joints, as well as cardiorespiratory strains when using respiratory-protection equipment. Painters of small articles experience eyestrain.

Reports have indicated that painters may be at increased risk of cancer of the lungs, bladder, stomach, kidneys, esophagus and the large intestines, and leukemia, when using paint containing BENZENE, mental impairment as a result of exposure to SOLVENTS, endocrine disorders, chronic bronchitis and respiratory obstructive diseases, mixed-dust pneumoconiosis, renal failure, and chronic eye damage as a result of long-term solvent exposure.

There is also a risk in the mechanical or chemical stripping or burning of old paints. Use of pigments containing lead, ARSENIC, or MERCURY in modern paints is now restricted and may be prohibited by law except for some specialized applications.

ACCIDENT HAZARDS FOR PAINTERS

- Falls from heights (such as ladders and platforms)
- Slips and falls on slippery floors
- Electrocution or electric shock from faulty electrical equipment or through contact of metallic ladders with electric lines
- Injection of paint into skin on fingers and hands while working with high-pressure airless spraying equipment
- Wood splinters in the skin when preparing wood surfaces for painting
- Eye injuries from high-pressure paint jets or sanding or from solvent drops splashed into the eyes
- Cuts, stabs, or abrasions in fingers and hands during surface preparation
- Fire and explosions of flammable paint solvents
- Asphyxiation in confined spaces due to deficiency of oxygen and the presence of solvent vapors
- Fire and explosions of flammable paint solvents when working in confined spaces with poor ventilation
- Skin abrasions from ladder rungs
- Clothes catching fire when covered with paints or oil
- Paint-splashing accidents from burst piping or when trying to unclog spray nozzles
- Noise from spray guns
- Exposure to cold, rain, snow, and winds in winter, or to heat in summer
- Poisoning by lead in primers and by other metal components of paints (mercury and arsenic compounds)

See also CANCER; CONFINED SPACES; ELECTRICITY-RELATED INJURIES; ERGONOMICS; EYE PROTECTION; FIRE PROTECTION; HAND PROTECTION; SLIPS, TRIPS, AND FALLS.

"Painter (non-art)" in *Encyclopaedia of Occupational Health and Safety.* 4th ed. Vol. 2. Geneva: International Labor Organization, 1998, pp. 103.23–103.24.

panic attacks and panic disorder   A panic attack is a short period (five to 10 minutes) of sudden, intense fear or discomfort, usually for no rational apparent reason. The feeling may cause extreme stress in the affected individual because it is usually accompanied by a fear of dying, a sense of imminent danger or impending doom, and an urge to escape. EMPLOYEE ASSISTANCE PROGRAMS offer referrals to appropriate sources for counseling.

Panic attacks are considered one of several ANXIETY DISORDERS.

The word *panic* is derived from Pan, whom Greeks worshipped as their god of flocks, herds, pastures, and fields. Pan loved to scare people and make eerie noises to frighten passersby. The fright he aroused was known as "panic."

How Panic Attacks Are Diagnosed

Organic factors as the cause of the disturbance should be ruled out. The panic incident must include at least four or more of the characteristic symptoms, which are a sense of breathing difficulty, palpitations or rapid heartbeat, sweating, trembling, shaking, feelings of smothering or choking, chest pains, nausea or abdominal distress, dizziness or lightheadedness, and chills or hot flushes.

Hyperventilation (fast, shallow breathing) worsens the symptoms and leads to a pins-and-needles sensation and to a feeling of derealization or depersonalization. These symptoms are usually the result of underlying emotional conflicts such as fear of being trapped or loss of emotional support.

According to the fourth edition of the *Diagnostic and Statistical Manual of Mental Disorders* (1994), typically, the first attack occurs in individuals in the late teens. Initially, attacks are unexpected and do not occur immediately before or on exposure to a stressful situation, as do simple PHOBIAS or social phobias. Later in the course of the disorder, certain situations may be identified with a panic attack, such as crossing a bridge or being on an escalator. Once a panic attack has occurred in a particular setting, the individual may become fearful that it will happen again and tend to avoid that situation. If the panic attacks happen in the workplace or on the way to work, the employee may tend toward frequent absenteeism.

What Is Panic Disorder?

When panic attacks recur frequently and disrupt an individual's life, the condition is known as panic disorder. Sufferers (1 percent to 2 percent of the population) may have attacks ranging from two or three a day to two to four times a week. This type of disorder tends to fluctuate and worsens when the individual comes under stress. Panic disorder usually begins during periods of choices, transitions, separation, and added responsibilities. There is often a family history of panic disorder.

In diagnosing panic disorder, the essential feature is the presence of recurrent, unexpected panic attacks followed by at least one month of persistent concern about having another panic attack, worry about the possible implications or consequence of the attacks, or a significant behavioral change related to the attacks.

Personality Characteristics and Panic Disorder

Personality characteristics of those who have panic disorder vary considerably. However, H. Michael Zal, a clinical professor of psychiatry at the Philadelphia College of Osteopathic Medicine, has observed some common factors. Persons with panic disorder or agoraphobia have demonstrated personality traits of dependency, avoidance, low SELF-ESTEEM, and interpersonal sensitivity. One attribute common to panic-prone people may include placing a great value on CONTROL. Any loss or threatened loss of control, particularly changes in their lifestyles, causes them to feel anxious and stressed. According to Dr. Zal, panic-prone people overvalue their independence and feel great discomfort in acknowledging their dependency needs. They are often reluctant to accept help and prefer helping others. As perfectionists and compulsive individuals, they have high expectations of themselves and others.

It is difficult to estimate how many men suffer from panic disorder because men may attempt to mask their symptoms by drinking alcohol. This type of self-medication can develop into a secondary problem. Many men go to family physicians, see multiple specialists, or end up in emergency rooms, thinking they have physical disorders. They complain of lower gastrointestinal problems, which are sometimes a symptom of panic disorder. When the panic disorder is treated, these gastrointestinal symptoms disappear.

Getting Help for Employees Who Have Panic Disorder

Often a combination of therapies is specifically chosen for each individual. Treatment begins with education about the illness and encouragement to reenter situations that the person has come to avoid. Treatment may involve cognitive therapy (changing how one thinks and deals with feelings of anxiety), BEHAVIOR THERAPY (changing how one acts in response to certain situations and using desensitization techniques to gradually become exposed to avoided situations), or medical treatment.

Three-quarters of patients who take drugs need long-term drug therapy, while another 25 percent will not be helped regardless of how long they take drugs. Overall, a quarter of the patients who do take drugs are helped permanently and will not have to continue them.

Employers, coworkers, and family members can help in recognizing panic disorders by being alert to the individual's level of anxiety. Because symptoms can be hidden, repeated avoidance of situations is often the best clue. Others can give the sufferer support and be good listeners. Instead of enabling the person to avoid a situation, others can help him or her make a small step forward by finding something positive in that effort.

See also AGORAPHOBIA; MENTAL HEALTH; NATIONAL MENTAL HEALTH ASSOCIATION; SOCIAL PHOBIA.

American Psychiatric Association. *Diagnostic and Statistical Manual.* 4th ed. Washington, D.C.: American Psychiatric Association, 1994.
Kahn, Ada P. "Family Members Can Help Sufferers Cope with Attacks." *Chicago Tribune,* June 23, 1991.
Kahn, Ada P. "Panic Attacks." *Chicago Tribune,* June 23, 1991.
Zal, H. Michael. *Panic Disorder: The Great Pretender.* New York: Insight Books, Plenum Press, 1990.

paper and pulp See PULP, PAPER, AND PAPERBOARD MILLS.

papermill worker's disease See ALLERGIES; SNEEZING.

parasites See ALLERGIES; COMMERCIAL DIVING; PLUMBERS.

particulate matter (PM-10) An air pollutant including dust, soot and other tiny bits of solid materials that are released into and move around in the air. Particulates are produced by many sources, including burning of diesel fuels by trucks and buses, incineration of garbage, mixing and application of fertilizers and pesticides, road construction, industrial processes such as steel making, mining operations, agricultural burning (field and slash burning), and operation of fireplaces and woodstoves. Particulate pollution can cause eye, nose, and throat irritation and other health problems for nearby workers.

See also AIR POLLUTION; AIR QUALITY CONTROLS; CHEMICAL TOXICITY; CLEAN AIR ACT OF 1990; HAZARDOUS AIR POLLUTANTS.

particulates See AIR POLLUTION; INDOOR ENVIRONMENT.

peer group A group whose members are of equal standing with each other: people who are of the same age or educational level, or who have the same job or profession. Peer group relationships are important throughout life. Working people who seek new friends and acceptance in a group are looking for peer relationships.

Peers are crucial to psychological development of the individual throughout life. Throughout school years, young people rely on their peers as important sources of information and may use peers as standards by which to measure themselves. Many look to their peers as models of behavior and for social reinforcement as often as they look to their own families.

For adults, the increasing mobility that often cuts them off from family and long-time friends has made the development of peer relationships in the workplace and other social and community activities extremely important.

Peer Pressure

Peer pressure is the influence of the peer group on the individual. It begins in adolescence, because teenagers want to belong to a group. Teenagers react to the physical changes they are going through, as well as their changing responsibilities and experiences by close bonding with those in their own age group. Young people in the workplace may form their own group for lunchtime and social outings.

Peer pressure is subtle in the ways it affects adults. It may be caused by advertising or it may be human nature that among peers there will always be leaders who have the power to influence.

See also MENTOR; SELF-ESTEEM.

pentachlorophenol poisoning (PCP poisoning)
A chlorinated hydrocarbon insecticide and fungicide. It is primarily used in sawmills to protect timber from fungal rot and wood-boring insects, as an industrial wood preservative for utility poles, cross arms, fence posts, and similar structures. It is registered for use by the U.S. Environmental Protection Agency (EPA) as an insecticide (termicide), fungicide, herbicide, mulluscide, algicide, disinfectant, and as an ingredient in antifouling paint.

Workers with potentially high exposure to PCP are those involved in wood preservation, lumber mill workers, carpenters, loading-dock workers, and pesticide applicators.

PCP is readily absorbed into the skin, the lungs, and the gastrointestinal lining. Internally, in large doses, PCP is toxic to the liver, kidney, and nervous system. In certain concentrations, PCP is irritating to mucous membranes and skin. Contact dermatitis is common among workers in contact with PCP. In a study of employees involved in the manufacture of PCP, CHLORACNE was found in 7 percent, and the risk was significantly higher among employees with documented skin contact compared to employees without skin contact.

Short-term exposure to pentachlorophenol can lead to poisoning that is rapidly fatal. Even small amounts passing through the skin can cause sweating, high fever, breathing trouble, chest and abdominal pain, and death. Brief exposure can damage the liver, kidney, skin, blood, lungs, nervous system, and gastrointestinal tract. Contact can irritate the eyes, nose, and throat.

The Occupational Safety and Health Administration has established PERMISSIBLE EXPOSURE LIMITS for the skin for pentachlorophenol.

perchloroethylene   See DRY CLEANING.

perfection   The state of being expert, proficient, flawless, without fault or defect. Although this is an unrealistic goal, a drive toward the impossible and unattainable is something for which many people in the workplace strive. Perfectionists are very achievement oriented. They are unable to select what is important and have the mistaken idea that perfectionism equals quality.

The perfectionist faces stresses and frustration with failure of any kind, imagined, real, large, or small. The obsession with perfection ultimately results in fragmentation of self, loss of efficiency, sleep deprivation, less time for exercise, rest, and quiet meals, increased use of alcohol and drugs, and, ultimately, exhaustion. The perfectionist ideal leaves out the important fact that people are only human and have limitations of body, mind, and spirit.

Many people believe the myth that overachieving will bring recognition. Today's society measures individuals in terms of productivity and accomplishment. However, there is a delicate balance between the amount of work the human body and mind can do and the amount of time required for rest and regeneration. That balance point differs for each person and is affected by feelings of stress, emotional overload, illness, and fatigue.

Overcoming Perfectionism

People who are plagued by the need to be perfect and the stresses that are incurred should realize their own limitations and reevaluate personal priorities. They must decide what is important and what is not and set realistic deadlines, short- and long-term goals, and choose values that matter.

CONQUER PERFECTIONISM IN THE WORKPLACE

- Look for sources of satisfaction in simple pleasures.
- Pursue special outside interests such as painting, music, gardening, reading, handicrafts, etc.
- Take better care of yourself with improved diet, rest, and exercise.
- Concentrate on the process of achieving a goal instead of the goal itself.
- Establish friendships outside work and family.
- Set personal priorities at work and for oneself and stay with them.
- Find time to be alone and become better acquainted with yourself.

See also MENTAL HEALTH; PERSONALITY; SELF-ESTEEM; STRESS.

Kahn, Ada P. *Stress A–Z: A Sourcebook for Facing Everyday Challenges.* New York: Facts On File, Inc., 1998.
Riess, Dorothy Young. "The Perils of Perfection." *Better Health Newsletter,* March 1989.

performance anxiety Many people experience extreme stress over any kind of performance because they fear FAILURE, CRITICISM, or not measuring up to real or imaginary standards. This is known as performance anxiety. Issues of SELF-ESTEEM are involved. Time and energy spent in thinking about fears may interfere with concentration, preparation, and performance. Performance anxiety may result from the prospect of giving a speech before coworkers or having a review with a supervisor.

For some individuals, performance anxiety may cause loss of sleep, indigestion, dizziness, or even faintness. However, if properly directed, the nervous energy generated by stress before a performance can become an advantage. When focused on the best possible outcome, for example that there will be a standing ovation, the individual will be challenged to do a good job.

Coping with Performance Anxiety

Many individuals use MEDITATION and deep breathing exercises to reduce stress before performances. Others carry a good luck charm to reduce anxieties with a placebo-like effect. Some follow certain rituals before every performance: establishing a routine for getting dressed, avoiding certain foods or beverages (caffeine and alcohol particularly) or taking a walk. For severe cases of performance anxiety, physicians may prescribe medication; however, medications may have side effects.

See also MENTAL HEALTH; PUBLIC SPEAKING; SOCIAL PHOBIA; STRESS.

performance review A review that is sometimes held separately from the salary review; an annual or biennial management evaluation of how well an employee is doing the job. The evaluations, held face-to-face, may be a source of stress for both the managers and the employees. According to Dr. Susan E. Brodt, assistant professor of business administration at Duke University, "The process (of job evaluations) often is so stressful because most companies do not do them correctly." Brodt researched how 100 firms do employee reviews and concluded that they may be a waste of time because the important topics such as salary, goals, and objectives are often not discussed. Brodt added that appraisals "generally are conducted too late to change performance, often long after problems occur. They are anxiety-filled and people tend to avoid sensitive subjects." Finally and tragically, Brodt continues, they can lead to misunderstandings in which talented employees are fired or forced to leave the company.

Chris B. Bardwell, a Chicago-based human resource consultant, argues in favor of performance reviews "because employees need to know areas in which they should improve and also areas where they are having success."

However, it has been reported that when layoffs occur, employees often feel that performance evaluations are either not used at all or are purposely downgraded to justify terminations. One study on termination showed that 75 percent of the survey respondents had recently received "excellent" or "outstanding" reviews and were still let go. Performance reviews are often seen as political tools, inflated to assure maximum merit raises and deflated to speed up the termination procedure, depending on corporate circumstances.

See also JOB SECURITY; LAYOFFS; MERGERS.

performing arts medicine A multidisciplinary branch of health care focusing on performing artists that encompasses prevention of injuries as well as treatment of practice and performance-linked injuries.

Medical literature on the occupational problems of musicians goes back at least to the early 18th century. In a treatise titled *Diseases of Workers,* Bernardino Ramazzini described the fatigue and malfunction of the right hand and arm associated with excessive writing. This could be translated into the current concept of writer's cramp or REPETITIVE STRESS INJURIES; a similar effect can happen to a player of a musical instrument. In the 19th century, a textbook of neurology described a case of a pianist whose thumb involuntarily curled into the palm of the hand while playing.

Although health hazards in the arts have been recognized for hundreds of years, the medical specialty evolved in the late 1970s and early 1980s. Arts medicine has advanced medical care, heightened awareness of health hazards, and improved artistic training and practice and performance techniques. In the 1980s several groups organized to promote exchange of information and discussion between arts groups and health care providers. These include the International Arts Medicine Association, the International Society for Music in Medicine, and the PERFORMING ARTS MEDICINE ASSOCIATION (PAMA). Advancements in the field have led to development of numerous facilities that provide care specifically for performing artists throughout the United States, Canada, Australia, and Europe.

There are many challenges in arts medicine. Performance artists are subject to all human ills and frailties. However, because of the nature of the demands in musical, dance, and theater performance, physical condition requirements are different than those in the general population. Seemingly small irritations or minor pains can threaten the career of a performer.

Traditional medical training does not provide necessary background in areas of performing arts medicine or sports medicine. Thus the development of these fields has come from an understanding and interaction among physicians, performers, or athletes, as well as members of other health care disciplines.

To successfully treat performing arts injuries, the medical community must recognize the significance of both the ailment as well as the psychological significance that performers attach to their problems. Psychological components play a vital role in successful therapy, according to Brian A. Roberts in his article "Musicians and Medicine: A View of Arts Medicine in Canada." Physicians need to realize the significance of complaints. For example, for a singer or actor a sore throat can cancel an important and lucrative performance. For wind instrument players, recovery from such common conditions as Bell's palsy can result in what looks asymptomatic to a physician on visual diagnosis, but the player still cannot play properly because he or she cannot yet form an embouchure. Such trivial matters as small cold sores (herpes simplex) can be totally debilitating for a brass instrument player, says Roberts.

Hearing loss may be an occupational hazard for musicians. This happens not only to rock musicians, but also to players in symphony orchestras. Hearing loss is a problem because of musicians' extreme dependence on this sense; also, their work and environment places them in jeopardy. In the case of popular musicians, including guitarists, the acutely and highly amplified sound system is hazardous.

Rock musicians can help prevent hearing loss by standing behind or beside, rather than in front of their amplifiers. Instrumentalists sitting in front of the brass section constantly have loud sounds in their ears. Certain instruments, such as violins, may cause hearing loss in the performers who play them. There is a cumulative risk to the hearing of the left ears of violinists and violists due to the proximity of that ear to the sound, both airborne and vibratory, through the instrument.

Harpists have the logistical problem of transporting their instrument. Frequent tuning of the many strings of a harp as well as repetitive turning motions of operating the tuning key may cause problems of the right wrist and hand. Although the instrument is tipped back into its playing position, the intent is to have it balanced without actually resting any weight against the right shoulder. When this balance is not achieved, a number of subsequent muscular problems, primarily with the right shoulder and upper arm, may occur. The position of the harpist in relation to the instrument can also present a problem depending on the size of the musician. The sitting height of the musician should be determined by what is comfortable rather than by the height of the bench, which may come with the harp.

Other complex issues are associated with arts medicine. These include the diverse physical and metabolic health issues associated with dancers, pneumonia in bagpipers, and shoulder and elbow disorders in symphony orchestra conductors.

Overuse Syndrome and Pain

Overuse (or abuse) is a common factor in performance injuries. A synonym for *overuse* is *repetitive stress injury.* It may be the most common hazard faced by professional musicians (as well as professional athletes). It is literally a breakdown of the small muscles in the hand, and overstrain of the joint at the base of the thumb where there is highly geared leverage, and also of the wrist joint. Overuse occurs when these structures are stressed beyond their tolerance, and in some ways, are like athletes' injuries.

Overuse injury may be brought about by excessive, undisciplined, or sporadic practice. This applies to keyboardists, wind instrumentalists, string players, and percussionists. Danger signs are usually pain in the hand and wrist but may also be in the shoulder or elbow. While there may be some aching in the small muscles of the hand and other parts of the upper arm after a long practice session, the pain of repetitive stress injury is more intense and persists after practice ceases.

It is difficult to eliminate problems of overuse by altering simple motions involved in the process of making music. While it is possible to improve the ergonomic conditions involved in playing music to some degree, it is difficult for a performer to change what is tied to their perception of artistic necessity and instrumental technique from which a particular tone or expression is derived.

Many players of musical instruments develop localized pain. Common complaints include cymbalist's shoulder, flutist's forearm, and guitarist's nipple. Brass players may develop problems in their lips, jaws, tongue, and teeth. Changes in tooth alignment, which may follow dental procedures, present special and potentially disabling problems for wind players for whom embouchure is critical. Arts medicine specialists in dentistry treat such problems. Wind instrument players may develop pharyngoceles or laryngoceles, appearing as large "air bags" in the neck that protrude as they play. They sometimes interfere with performance and require treatment, says Sataloff.

Temporomandibular joint (TMJ) problems are encountered commonly in violinists and violists as a result of displacing the left side of the jaw against the chin rest, thus also stressing the right TMJ. According to authors Robert Sataloff, Alice Brandfonbrener, and Richard Lederman, the approach to treatment is generally dual: a technical approach by reducing the pressure and the displacement of the instrument against the jaw, and a dental approach through the use of a splinting device and exercise.

Lower back pain is a problem for many instrumentalists, particularly pianists and other keyboardists who sit on benches without back support during long hours of practice. Musicians, particularly violinists and violists, often develop neck and back problems. Skin abrasions and even cysts occur under the left side of the jaw at the contact point of the instrument in many string players. Dermatological problems also occur in flutists.

In his article "Occupational Maladies of Musicians: Their Cause and Prevention," in the *International Journal of Music Education,* Hunter J. H. Fry offered suggestions for musicians to lower their risk of being disabled:

- Segmentalize practice. Practice twice a day instead of practicing for one long session.

- Do not practice too long without a break. The length of the break can vary, but 25 or 30 minutes of practice should be followed by a small break.

- When facing auditions or examinations, increase the practice load gradually instead of suddenly; do not have some days without any practice at all.

- If during practice there is aching in the hands, elbows, or shoulders, rest for at least an hour until it subsides. If pain recurs or persists, it should be reported, despite the fact that an audition is coming.

- If an exercise causes pain, stop it immediately and discuss it with a coach later on.

Respiratory Dysfunction: A Threat to Singers and Wind Instrumentalists

Respiratory dysfunction can impair the technique of a singer or wind instrumentalist by causing lip dysfunction and other problems. Trumpeters, trombonists, flutists, oboists, and clarinetists have common complaints, including fatigue during playing, lip and throat pain, loss of upper range, and

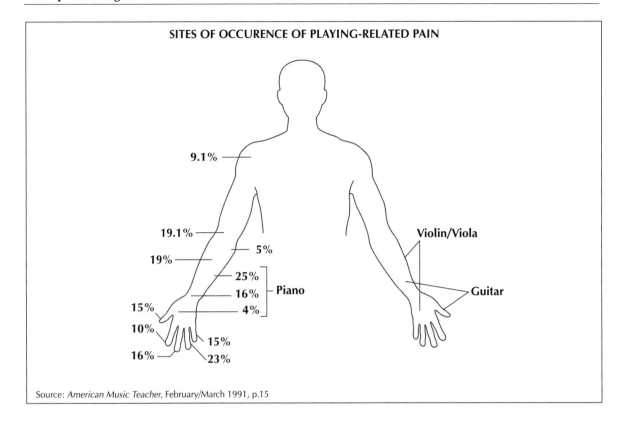

SITES OF OCCURENCE OF PLAYING-RELATED PAIN

9.1%

19.1%

19%

5%

25%
16%   Piano
4%

15%

10%

16%

15%

23%

Violin/Viola

Guitar

Source: *American Music Teacher*, February/March 1991, p.15

inability to sustain long notes. Consistent control of the airstream is necessary for woodwind or brass performance, as well as for singers.

According to Robert Sataloff in his article "Arts Medicine: An Overview" in *American Music Teacher,* respiratory disease is an important cause of technical dysfunction in singers and instrumentalists, as well as in other performers who strain inappropriate muscles in the neck, face, and lips to compensate for deficient support by impaired breathing. The most common obstructive airway disease is ASTHMA. Appropriate treatment of asthma in performers is important because successful maintenance therapy can enable them to continue their chosen careers.

Fry in 1984 reported that most wind players believed that cigarette smoking was deleterious to wind playing. Those who had previously smoked but who had quit noticed a gratifying improvement in breath control. Medical evidence has indicated the destructive effect of smoking on lung tissue over a period of time causing emphysema.

Hand Injuries

Hand medicine may be the most advanced specialty of arts medicine. Pianists, violinists, harpists, and other instrumentalists have hand injuries that are successfully treated by a multidisciplinary team. Such a team may include a hand surgeon, physical therapist, radiologist, and music coaches, teachers, and trainers. The team should observe the musician playing the instrument, because many problems may be caused by subtle habits.

Incomplete control over the hands at the keyboard or on the strings is a symptom of overuse. This may come from excessive, ineffective practicing with unbalanced muscle development, possibly resulting in nearly crippling problems that could end an instrumentalist's career. Chronic pain is also a common symptom. Other common symptoms among musicians are pain, tightening, weakness, stiffness, fatigue, pins and needles, swelling, temperature change, and redness. Such problems result in loss of control and decreased facility, endurance, speed or strength, and tension. Many musicians with these problems stop playing, alter their practice or change their fingering, technique, or repertoire. Some have related problems in their forearms, elbows, upper arms, or shoulders.

Hand problems also affect clarinetists who develop pain in the right thumb from the weight of the instrument and position used to hold it. Oboists have the same problem. Double bass players may have lower back discomfort. Cellists may have postural problems and often respond to a seating adjustment. Percussionists may suffer tissue damage from the elbow downwards, showing damage mainly in the muscle origins from the elbows, extensor muscles from the forearm and the muscles of the hand, ligaments of the wrist and base of thumb. Many instrumentalists experience repetitive stress injuries.

Voice Medicine

Through the National Association of Teachers of Singing, *The Journal of Singing*, *The Journal of Voice*, the Voice Foundation's annual symposium, and many other sources, singing teachers have become familiar with recent advances in caring for professional singers and professional voice users. In the mid-1800s singing teacher Manuel Garcia invented indirect mirror laryngoscopy through which physicians began examining the vocal folds routinely, thus improving the care of voice disorders. However, voice medicine did not develop as an accepted subspecialty of otolaryngology until the 1980s. Speech-language pathologists have continued to develop new skills to address subtle voice problems of singers and actors.

In voice, one of the most difficult techniques to correct is the *Knödel*, which is translated literally as "dumpling". With this technique, the singer pushes the larynx down with the back of the tongue. This technique is used by singers to accommodate, however incorrectly, the instinctive need to sing with a lowered larynx. While singing with the lower laryngeal position is a correct technique, getting it this way by depressing the back of the tongue down onto the voice box is not an acceptable way of doing it. With health-threatening techniques that impinge on sound, the therapist is hampered by the apparent artistic needs of the patient.

Voice medicine is based on an understanding of the anatomy and physiology of the voice. Consequently, laryngologists caring for voice patients take histories to investigate all physical functions. Voice problems may include hoarseness, loss of control, decreased vocal endurance, pitch inaccuracies, loss of agility, a "wobble," pain while speaking or singing, and others. In professional performers, such problems are often physical in origin. Mild endocrine disorders, gastroesophageal reflux, early neurologic dysfunction, alterations in balance or posture following a sprained ankle, and many other seemingly unrelated problems may be responsible for a voice complaint and may disable a voice professional.

Professional voice users include not only singers and actors, but also clergy, politicians, teachers, sales personnel, telephone operators, and anyone else whose ability to function in the workplace suffers if vocal quality, volume, or endurance are impaired. Physical examination of voice professionals includes not only a complete ear, nose, and throat examination and examination of cranial nerves, but also special factors. For example, a singer or actor should be examined while singing or reciting a part of a role. This examination should include a singing or speaking passage demonstrating the complaint, if possible.

Mental Health Aspects

Performance artists experience STRESS regularly. They face demands for PERFECTION, public scrutiny, and constant competition. In a survey of more than 2000 professional musicians performing in 48 member orchestras of the International Conference of Symphony and Opera Musicians (ICSOM), stage fright was the most frequent complaint. It was mentioned by 24 percent of respondents as a health problem with 16 percent reporting it as a severe health problem. While stage fright is a universal phenomenon, most successful performers have evolved methods of coping with or compensating for it. There are both psychological and somatic components to stage fright. Apprehension, irritability, and fear of making a mistake or having a memory slip are some of the psychological symptoms associated with performance anxiety, according to Richard Lederman in his article in *American Music Teacher*. Performers have devised methods to deal with these symptoms, such as exercise, yoga, meditation, or deep breathing. Some have turned to drugs, including alcohol, tranquilizers, and sedatives. Some have been successful with these measures, but there is a great potential for abuse and harm. Use of beta-blockers, such as a propranolol, has been much debated, according to Lederman. However, these drugs block some of the physical manifestations of performance anxiety that are most detrimental to performance, including tremor, rapid heart rate, and sweaty palms.

There is considerable strain on the performer and the performer's family, who may accompany the performer on an extensive tour. Most problems of successful performers are usually kept under control. However, some situations are very trying and marital strife or divorce can result.

When stress is unmanageable or interferes with the performer's artistic ability or life, intervention by a mental health professional may be useful to help the performer regain sufficient control over his or her life, permitting continuation of a career.

Depression is another psychological problem of performers. Issues include postperformance letdown, and depression facing a performer in decline or approaching termination of a career.

See also BELTING; CONDUCTORS MUSICAL; GUITAR PLAYERS' INJURIES; MENTAL HEALTH; MUSICIANS' INJURIES; THEATER (ACTOR) INJURIES.

Fry, Hunter J. H. "Occupational Maladies of Musicians: Their Cause and Prevention." *International Journal of Music Education* 2 (1984): 59–63.

Lederman, Richard. "An Overview of Performing Arts Medicine." *American Music Teacher,* February/March 1991, pp. 12–17.

Roberts, Brian A. "Musicians and Medicine: A View of Arts Medicine in Canada." *Canadian Music Educator* 36, no. 4 (1995): pp. 3–8.

Sataloff, Robert. "Arts Medicine: An Overview." *American Music Teacher* 50, no. 2 (October/November 2000): 33–38.

Sataloff, Robert Thayer, Alice G. Brandfonbrener, and Richard J. Lederman, eds. *Textbook of Performing Arts Medicine.* New York: Raven Press, 1991.

Wolfe, Mary L. "Correlates of Adaptive and Maladaptive Musical Performance Anxiety." *Medical Problems of Performing Artists* 4, no. 1 (March 1989): 49–56.

Performing Arts Medicine Association (PAMA)

A nonprofit organization for physicians and other professionals involved in treatment and/or research in the field of performing arts medicine. Organized in 1989, the PAMA is dedicated to improving health care for performing artists by developing educational programs and promoting communication of health-related information among physicians, performers, managers, and teachers in the performing arts. Additionally, the PAMA fosters research on the causes and prevention of injuries and health problems common in the performing arts.

The quarterly journal of the PAMA, *Medical Problems of Performing Artists,* provides a forum for medical issues relating to musicians and dancers.

For information:

Performing Arts Medicine Association (PAMA)
c/o Mary Fletcher
P.O. Box 61228
Denver, CO 80206
artsmed@aol.com

peripheral nervous system   See NEUROTOXICITY.

permanent disability or permanent impairment
Any degree of permanent nonfatal injury. It includes any injury that results in the loss, or complete loss of use, of any part of the body, or any permanent impairment of functions of the body or a part thereof.

See also NATIONAL SAFETY COUNCIL.

permissible exposure limits (PELS)   Regulatory limits on the amount or concentration of a substance in the air. The U.S. Department of Labor's Occupational Safety and Health Administration (OSHA) sets PELS to protect workers against the health effects of exposure to hazardous substances. PELS may also contain a skin designation.

PELS for nearly 500 hazardous chemicals were established in 1971, when OSHA was created, and are based on research conducted primarily in the 1950s and 1960s. Since then, new information became available indicating that in most cases these early exposure limits are outdated and do not adequately protect workers. OSHA has given priority to establishing an ongoing and cyclical rule-making process to update PELS and to add new ones as needs arise. OSHA has proposed new PELS for a limited number of hazardous substances and continues to address this priority issue.

Many of the chemical substances assigned a permissible exposure limit by OSHA are used in industrial settings. Potential health effects of exposure to these chemicals vary widely. Both chronic and acute effects on virtually every bodily system have been reported, including sensory irritation, sensitization, metabolic disturbances, cardiovascular, neurological, respiratory, liver, and kidney disease, reproductive effects, and cancer.

The National Institute for Occupational Safety and Health (NIOSH) has the statutory responsibility for establishing recommended exposure levels for workers. NIOSH has identified recommended exposure levels (RELS) for 667 hazardous substances. The American Conference of Government Industrial Hygienists (ACGIH) has developed hundreds of exposure limits that are more protective than OSHA's. Many U.S. companies use the current ACGIH levels or other internal and more protective limits.

Occupational Safety and Health Administration.

peroxides   Chemical substances, including hydrogen peroxide. Peroxides and hydroperoxides are highly reactive and may be extremely shock-sensitive explosives. Peroxides can form readily in certain organic materials, particularly ethers. Simply moving or just screwing the cap off a bottle that is contaminated with peroxides can lead to an explosion, injury, and/or death.

Persons most at risk for these injuries include chemists and laboratory workers. Workers who may be exposed to peroxides should read their MATERIALS SAFETY DATA SHEET and be watchful for peroxide-formers.

personality   The sum of all of the individual's behavioral and emotional tendencies. Personality develops from the interaction of many complex factors, including heredity and environment. Many theorists hold that genetics is more important than environment, while others take the opposite view.

Personality characteristics may be predictors of how well an individual does his or her job or integrates with others in the workplace. According to studies by psychologist Suzanne O. Kobasa and associates at the University of Chicago, survivors, or people with "hardiness," share three specific personality traits that appear to afford them a high degree of stress resistance: they are committed to what they do, they feel in CONTROL of their lives, and they see change as a challenge rather than a threat.

Personality Tests

Personality tests are questionnaires designed to determine the suitability of an individual for a particular field of work or job assignment, determine various traits, and at times, assist in psychological research. These tests measure many aspects of an individual's personality, such as how easily they are disturbed by sources of stress at work, how they might interact with coworkers, and their degree of extroversion or introversion.

In some individuals, negative personality traits and patterns are severe enough to interfere with effective work. Personality disorders involve behaviors or traits that affect recent and long-term functioning. Patterns of perceiving and thinking are usually not limited to isolated episodes, but are deeply ingrained, inflexible, maladaptive, and severe enough to cause mental stress or anxieties, or interfere with interpersonal relationships and normal functioning on the job.

See also HARDINESS; HOSTILITY; MENTAL HEALTH; STRESS; TYPE A PERSONALITY; TYPE B PERSONALITY; TYPE C PERSONALITY.

personal protective equipment (PPE)   All clothing and other work accessories designed to create a barrier against workplace hazards. Example include safety goggles, eye and face protectors, blast shields, hard hats, hearing protectors, gloves, respirators, aprons, and work boots.

The U.S. Occupational Safety and Health Administration (OSHA) sets many PPE regulations, including regulations for those who work with chemicals. Some of the important OSHA PPE regulations for chemical workers include requirements that employers perform a written hazard assessment, select appropriate PPE to protect workers, and maintain a written record indicating that all such employees have been properly trained before performing any job task requiring PPE. Training must include knowing when PPE is necessary, what PPE is necessary, how to properly put on, remove, adjust, and wear PPE, limitations of the PPE, and the proper care, maintenance, useful life, and disposal of the PPE.

OSHA requires that MATERIAL SAFETY DATA SHEETS (MSDS) list information about appropriate PPE for each substance. Not all PPE is appropriate at all times. For example, some gloves will do little to protect from certain chemicals. Also, an organic vapor cartridge respirator will be useless as protection from an atmosphere deficient in oxygen.

In addition to using PPE appropriately, workers need to understand that every piece of PPE has limitations. For example, gloves may develop small holes and respirator cartridges generally do not indicate when they need replacement. Even appropriate PPE does not provide a 100 percent guarantee of safety.

PPE should not be used as a substitute for engineering, work practice, and/or administrative controls to prevent exposure to hazardous chemicals.

See also EYE INJURIES/PROTECTION; FOOT PROTECTION; HAND PROTECTION; OCCUPATIONAL SAFETY AND HEALTH ADMINISTRATION; RESPIRATORS.

personal space   The invisible zone of privacy that people unconsciously maintain. Although personal space is something rarely noticed, when it is invaded people may feel stressed and become anxious, irritated, and even hostile. Workplace cubicles that are too close together can be a source of stress for some workers.

Anthropologists have reported that people follow established rules regarding how far apart they stand, depending largely on their relationship to each other. For example, friends, spouses, lovers, parents, and children tend to stand inside a "zone of intimacy," or within arm's reach, while a personal zone of about four feet is comfortable for conversation with coworkers and others in the workplace.

The size needed for personal space depends on many variables, including the individual's cultural background, gender, and the nature of the occasion. Individuals from north European or British ancestry usually want about a square yard of space for conversation in uncrowded situations. However, people from more tropical climates choose a smaller personal area and are more likely to reach out and touch the occupant of another space. In Mediterranean and South American societies, social conversations include much eye contact, touching, and smiling, typically while standing at a distance of about a foot. In the United States, however, people usually stand about 18 inches apart for a social conversation; while they will shake hands, they tend to talk at arm's length.

Understanding cultural and gender differences in interpretations of personal space is becoming more important as intercultural trade and business transactions escalate. The interpretation of personal space leaves much room for misinterpretation. Consultants have developed businesses interpreting for people of all nationalities the meaning and use of personal space to relieve the possibilities for occurrences of stressful situations. It is possible that a culture's use of space is evidence of a reliance on one sense over another. For example, Middle Easterners get much of their information through their senses of smell and touch, which require a close approach, while Americans rely primarily on visual information, backing up in order to see an intelligible picture.

See also CROWDING; MENTAL HEALTH, STRESS.

Davis, Lisa. "Where Do We Stand?" *In Health,* September/October 1990.

Padus, Emrika, ed. *The Complete Guide to Your Emotions and Your Health.* Rev. ed. Emmaus, Pa.: Rodale Press, 1994.

pest control workers   Pest control workers face many health hazards. While traveling in cars or trucks, they are at risk of accidents due to long drives with heavily loaded vehicles, often towing trailers and mechanical spraying equipment, sometimes on bad roads and during inclement weather conditions. Those who fly in light aircraft or helicopters are at risk of aircraft crashes, exposure to pesticides carried in the cockpit on their clothes and footwear, or accidentally while flying through a cloud of sprayed pesticides (drift cloud) and as a result of leakage from containers. Workers on the ground involved in aerial pesticide applications face the risk of being struck by aircraft during take-off landing, taxiing, or low-altitude flights. They are also exposed to pesticides as a result of pesticide-loaded aircraft crashes and leakages.

On the ground, workers may suffer SLIPS, TRIPS, AND FALLS, especially when carrying containers and other heavy loads. Foot injuries occur when stepping on sharp discarded objects while spraying in fields. Other hazards include bursting of overpressurized spraying containers, resulting in pesticide splashes that may hit the worker, the risk of hernia as a result of strenuous movements when lifting and loading heavy loads and acute poisoning when applying pesticides while not wearing protective masks. Between rails of a railroad, workers are at risk of being hit by a train. Workers are at risk of being infected by diseases transmitted by fleas or other insects during extermination work.

Pesticide workers face many hazards of CHEMICAL TOXICITY. They may have various skin effects, such as itching, erythema, blistering, photosensitization as a result of exposure to vapors, spray and gaseous forms of pesticides, particularly through direct skin contact. They may suffer chloracne and porphyria-cutanatarda as a result of contact with chlorinated pesticides. Additionally, they may experience various eye irritations as a result of exposure to certain chemicals, mouth and throat irritation, and various pulmonary diseases, including lung edema, pneumonitis, asthmatic reactions, and pneumoconiosis from pesticide dusting. Gastrointestinal effects may include abdominal pains, cramps, diarrhea, nausea, vertigo, and headaches. Nervous system effects may include neurotoxicity, neuropathy, effects on cognitive functions, ANXIETY, and insomnia. Disorders of the endocrine and reproductive system may include infertility, spon-

taneous abortion, stillbirth, sterility, congenital defects, and perinatal death. There may be effects on blood and the circulatory system, especially due to chlorinated hydrocarbons as pesticides. Pesticide workers may also have musculoskeletal and soft tissue problems and carcinogenic effects. They may develop backaches due to vibrations, inadequate vehicle suspension, uncomfortable seats, and wet and humid working conditions.

Pesticide workers face STRESS resulting from the fears of potential overexposure to pesticides and of failing periodic health check-ups.

Firefighters engaged in extinguishing pesticide-involved fires may experience skin burns as a result of excessive exposure of unprotected skin to pesticides, electric shocks caused by contact with defective electromechanical equipment, electric hazards while exterminating pests around power lines, skin and eye irritations, chest tightness, nausea, limb numbness, and asphyxia.

See also CHLORACNE; DERMATITIS; ELECTRICITY-RELATED INJURIES; FIREFIGHTERS; HAZARDOUS AIR POLLUTANTS; HAZARDOUS AND TOXIC SUBSTANCES; INDOOR ENVIRONMENT; MUSCULOSKELETAL TOXICITY; REPRODUCTIVE TOXICITY; SKIN AND SENSE ORGAN TOXICITY; STRESS MANAGEMENT.

Mager-Stillman, Jeanne, ed. *Encyclopaedia of Occupational Health and Safety.* 4th ed. Vol. 4. Geneva: International Labor Organization, 1998, p. 103.25–103.26.

pesticides   See HERBICIDES; PEST CONTROL WORKERS.

phobias   Irrational, intense fears of objects or situations and a strong desire to avoid those objects or situations. Most people have minor fears, experiencing some anxiety when unable to avoid contacts with bugs or bees, for example. However, when a fear interferes with working or social functioning, causes significant distress, and is out of proportion to any real or apparent danger, it is considered a phobia. A phobia may become apparent to a supervisor when an employee refuses to make a speech before a sales force, fly in an airplane for business, drive over a bridge to see a customer, or engage in activities considered routine for most employees.

People who have phobias cannot explain or understand their fears. Nor can they voluntarily control their anxiety response and their need to avoid the dreaded stimulus or situation.

Phobic reactions that occur when the phobic stimulus appears include:

- Persistent and irrational panic, dread, horror, or terror
- Rapid heartbeat, shortness of breath, trembling, and overwhelming desire to flee the situation
- Avoidance of the situation

Phobias are classified by the American Psychiatric Association in the fourth edition of the *Diagnostic and Statistical Manual of Mental Disorders* as the most common form of ANXIETY DISORDERS. People of all ages, at all income levels, and in all geographic locations suffer from phobias. Between 5.1 percent and 12.5 percent of Americans suffer from phobias. Broken down by age and gender, phobias are the most common mental health concern among women in all age groups and the second most common illness among men over age 25.

Types of Phobias

Phobias cannot be neatly classified because fear of almost any situation can occur and may be associated with any other psychological symptoms. However, in a general way, phobias can be classified as:

Specific phobias (also known as simple phobias). Specific phobias are characterized by a persistent, irrational fear of and compelling desire to avoid specific situations or objects. The number of specific phobias is endless, as individuals can be phobic about almost any object or situation.

Commonly recognized specific phobias relate to particular animals (dogs, rats, mice, birds, spiders, or snakes); enclosed spaces (claustrophobia), such as being in an elevator or sitting in the middle of a theater row; darkness; heights; or thunderstorms. Some specific phobias have to do with transportation, such as driving across bridges, riding in trains, or flying in airplanes.

Phobias related to the sight of blood or injury are unique types of specific phobias. Unlike other specific phobias, which cause increased pulse and other physiological signs of arousal, blood and injury phobias produce lower pulse and blood pressure and bring on fainting spells.

A person who has a specific phobia experiences stressful physiological symptoms and behavior typical of many phobic disorders. However, because these fears are so specific, individuals can usually manage to avoid contact with the object of their phobia. On the other hand, individuals who fear common situations, such as riding in elevators or going over bridges, may not easily avoid these stressful stimuli.

How simple phobias start is not well understood. Researchers differ in their explanations; some report that direct conditioning, for example, a traumatic event, is an important factor, while others say that indirect learning experiences or exposure to negative instructions and vicarious experiences are also influential. Opinions vary regarding family influences on specific fears. While some experts say that the majority of simple phobics come from families in which no other member of the family shares the same fear, some studies have found relatively strong associations between the fears of mothers and children. Many simple phobics are dependent or anxious individuals, and their family backgrounds may have contributed to these characteristics. Individuals who have simple phobias may not recall the origin of their fear.

Specific phobias can begin at any age. However, certain phobias are more common among certain age groups. For example, infants often fear loud noises and strangers. A fear of animals, prevalent in children between the ages of nine to 11, stays with many girls after age 11 but disappears in most boys. Fear of aging occurs most commonly in people over age 50.

Social phobia. Social phobia involves fear of being scrutinized by others. People with social phobias may fear making mistakes, being criticized, and making a fool of themselves. They also may fear eating or making a speech in public, using public toilets, writing in public, and making complaints. Because of the fear of interacting with the opposite sex, strangers, or aggressive individuals, social phobics are stressed in social or business situations such as parties, meetings, and interviews. Some individuals will participate in the activity only when they cannot be seen, for example, swimming in the dark. Social phobias develop over many months or years, but sometimes a precipitating event can be determined.

Social phobics have ongoing problems with excessive stress, generalized anxiety, dependence, and depression. Sweating, fainting, blushing, and vomiting may all be symptoms of social phobia.

Usually social phobias begin in a range from 15 to 30 years of age. They tend to persist throughout adulthood, unlike specific or simple phobias, which tend to diminish as the individual enters young adulthood. Many social phobics have traits that interfere with social and marital adjustment.

Some social phobics attribute their fears to direct conditioning, some to vicarious factors, and some to instructional and informational factors; direct negative learning experience may play an important role. Development of social phobias may be influenced somewhat by parental behavior. For example, parents who have few friends and are socially anxious in the presence of others may influence their children to react in similar ways. Also, the presence of anxiety in children is often associated with criticism and verbal punishment.

Agoraphobia. Agoraphobia may be the most stressful and serious of the phobias. Agoraphobics are afraid to leave a safe place such as their home or be apart from a safe person such as a spouse or close relative. Such separations cause intense anxiety and panic. A small percentage of agoraphobics remain house bound, sometimes for many years.

Symptoms of agoraphobia include a wide range of avoidance behaviors, including a fear of entering public places or open spaces, traveling, social interaction, and even being alone. Agoraphobics often have physiological symptoms such as palpitations, lightness in the head, weakness, atypical chest pain, and difficulty in breathing. Some agoraphobics have panic attacks. Agoraphobics express fears of losing CONTROL, going insane, embarrassing themselves, and dying.

Phobias of internal stimuli. These are fears that develop without reason, such as fear of dying from an illness such as cancer, heart disease, or venereal disease, for which there are no physical symptoms.

Some of these fears, which occur in both sexes, may be regarded as an extreme form of hypochondria. Often characteristic of depressive illnesses, these phobias often improve when the depression improves.

Obsessive phobias. Examples of obsessive phobias are fear of harming people or babies, fear of swearing, or fear of contamination, which leads to obsessive hand washing and cleaning. Such phobias usually occur along with other obsessive-compulsive symptoms.

Treatment of Phobias

Qualified psychiatrists, psychologists, social workers, and other mental health professionals treat phobias with many forms of therapy, ranging from BEHAVIOR THERAPY to psychoanalysis. Many people are helped with BIOFEEDBACK, RELAXATION, GUIDED IMAGERY, and MEDITATION.

Sometimes antianxiety drugs and a variety of other medications can help people face their phobic situations and overcome them. Pharmacological treatment for phobias varies with individuals and should be undertaken only with supervision by a physician or mental health professional.

See also COMPLEMENTARY THERAPIES; MENTAL HEALTH; PANIC ATTACKS AND PANIC DISORDER; PERFORMANCE ANXIETY; PSYCHOTHERAPIES; PUBLIC SPEAKING; SOCIAL PHOBIA; STRESS.

American Psychiatric Association. *Diagnostic and Statistical Manual of Mental Disorders.* 4th ed. Washington, D.C.: American Psychiatric Association, 1994.

Bourne, Edmund J. *The Anxiety and Phobia Workbook.* Oakland, Calif.: New Harbinger Publications, 1995.

Kahn, Ada P., and Jan Fawcett. *The Encyclopedia of Mental Health.* 2d ed. New York: Facts On File, Inc., 2001.

Monroe, Judy. *Phobias: Everything You Wanted to Know, But Were Afraid to Ask.* Springfield, N.J.: Enslow Publishers, 1996.

phosgene   See CHEMICAL TOXICITY; SOLDERING.

phosphorus   See GASTROINTESTINAL OR LIVER TOXICITY.

photo-allergic and photo-irritant contact dermatitis (PACD and PICD)   See DERMATITIS.

photosensitization Heightened reactivity of the skin to sunlight, usually due to the action of certain drugs or to exposure of certain chemicals.

See also SKIN OR SENSE ORGAN TOXICITY.

physical load (physical overload) Lifting too much, or lifting improperly, while straining, over-reaching, bending, or twisting. Physical overload is a leading cause of work-related injuries. To avoid physical overload, learn and use proper lifting techniques. Never bend or twist while lifting or carrying, and whenever possible, use mechanical help.

Occupations that may carry the highest physical workloads include manual forest work, operation of portable machines such as chainsaws, and operation of machines that require heavy lifting during repairs. Repetitive and static work can lead to a high risk of REPETITIVE STRESS INJURIES in the neck, shoulder, arm, hand, or fingers.

See also PERSONAL PROTECTIVE EQUIPMENT.

pianists' injuries See KEYBOARD INJURIES; PERFORMING ARTS MEDICINE.

pilots and flight attendants See AEROSPACE MEDICINE; CONFINED SPACES.

plant closings See CORPORATE BUYOUT; DOWNSIZING; LAYOFFS; MERGERS.

plants in the workplace See ASSOCIATED LANDSCAPE CONTRACTORS OF AMERICA.

plasterers See BRICKLAYERS, CEMENT WORKERS, AND PLASTERERS; CONSTRUCTION; LADDERS; SCAFFOLDING.

plastic molding See CADMIUM; FORMALDEHYDE.

plastic products See RUBBER PRODUCTS.

plastics See CADMIUM.

pleural mesothelioma See MESOTHELIOMA.

plumbers Plumbing work includes opening clogged drains, mending burst pipes, replacing washers in leaky faucets, securing pipes and fixtures with brackets, clamps, and hangers, cutting openings in walls and floors to accommodate pipes and fittings, and often using hand and power tools. Plumbing also includes assembling and installing valves, joining pipes with screws, bolts, or solder, and installing and repairing fixtures such as sinks, commodes, and hot water tanks.

Plumbers face many accident hazards, such as falling from ladders, scaffolds, and roofs, and slips and falls on wet and slippery surfaces. They face hazards of cuts, stabs, pinches, bruises, and finger crushing from hand tools and machinery, and blows on the head from pipes or overhead bars, particularly in confined spaces or in low-ceilinged basements and passageways. Foreign particles may get in their eyes, and they may have foot injuries from falling tools or pipe sections. They may have burns from hot or corrosive liquids emitted from burst pipes, and burns from portable blowtorches used for soldering and brazing.

Additional hazards come from electric shock and electrocution from portable lamps and electric tools, fires, and explosions as a result of using mobile electric lamps or tools in confined spaces, and drowning in accidental flooding of work areas.

Poisoning by phosgene released from chlorinated solvents at high temperature can occur, particularly in confined spaces. Toxic gases (such as sulfur dioxide and hydrogen sulfide) released in the sewage system can be poisonous.

Chemical hazards to plumbers include contact dermatitis from exposure to various components of draining and sewage liquids or from exposure to solvents and other components of cleaning fluids, irritation of the respiratory system and eyes from exposure to acids, alkalis, and various corrosive liquids used to unclog piping, oxygen deficiency or exposure to asphyxiant gases when working in confined spaces, irritation to the respiratory tract and possible damage to the lungs from exposure to ASBESTOS, mineral fibers, and other aerosols or fibers when applying or dismantling piping insulation or asbestos pipes.

Plumbers are also exposed to biological hazards, such as a wide variety of microorganisms, parasites, in sewage, stagnant water, and sanitary installations. Additionally, they are exposed to excessive damp, cold, and heat and may experience wrist problems due to overexertion during threading and cutting work or calluses on the knees (plumber's knee) because of prolonged kneeling.

Plumbers who work in laboratories in the chemical industry, in sewage systems, or in welding, brazing, or soldering operations, are exposed to all the chemical and biological hazards relevant for those workplaces.

See also CHEMICAL TOXICITY; CONFINED SPACES; ELECTRICITY RELATED INJURIES; HAND PROTECTION; PARASITES; PERSONAL PROTECTIVE EQUIPMENT; SLIPS, TRIPS AND FALLS; SOLDERING; WELDING.

Mager-Stillman, Jeanne, ed. *Encyclopaedia of Occupational Health and Safety.* 4th ed. vol. 4. Geneva: International Labor Organization, pp. 103.27–103.28.

plumber's knee   See BURSITIS.

plutonium   See NUCLEAR WEAPONS WORKERS.

pneumatic tools   See RIVETERS; REPETITIVE STRESS INJURIES; VIBRATION; VIBRATION WHITE FINGER.

pneumoconiosis, coal workers'   See BLACK LUNG DISEASE.

pneumocystic carinii pneumonia (PCP)   See ACQUIRED IMMUNODEFICIENCY SYNDROME.

poison ivy   The most common cause of allergic reactions in the United States. Poison ivy, poison sumac, and poison oak can cause severe skin rashes. It affects 10 million to 50 million Americans every year. People who work in landscape and gardening professions are particularly vulnerable to this discomfort.

Sufferers experience itching and a burning sensation on their skin. The colorless or slightly yellow oil, called urushiol, that oozes from any cut or crushed part of the plant is easily spread. Sticky and virtually invisible, it can be carried on the fur of animals, on garden tools and sports equipment, or on any objects that have come into contact with a crushed, cut, or broken plant. The effect on the skin can be neutralized by water.

Once the urushiol touches the skin, it penetrates in a few minutes. In those who are sensitive, a reaction appears in the form of a line or streak of rash, sometimes resembling insect bites, within 12 to 48 hours. Blisters and severe itching follow redness and swelling. The rash can affect almost any part of the body, especially areas where the skin is thin; the soles of the feet and palms of the hands are thicker and less susceptible.

First-aid treatment includes thorough cleansing of the infected area, sponging with alcohol, and applying calamine lotion. Severe reactions should be reported to a physician who may prescribe corticosteroid drugs to be taken by mouth or injection.

For information:

American Academy of Dermatology (AAD)
P.O. Box 4014
Schaumburg, IL 60168-4014
(847) 330-0230
(847) 330-0050 (fax)
www.aad.org

See also ALLERGIES; GARDENERS.

police   Law enforcement officers' jobs are inherently dangerous. They face unique hazards and are more likely than other workers to die violently. According to authors Cindy Clarke and Mark Zak, their risk of suffering a fatal incident is three times greater than for all other workers.

According to the Bureau of Labor Statistics' Census of Fatal Occupational Injuries (CFOI), more than 1,100 law enforcement personnel and firefighters were killed in the line of duty between 1992 and 1997. Most of the 887 police fatalities occurred during pursuit of criminals; some police officers were shot and others were fatally injured in highway crashes.

Police officers patrol designated areas to preserve peace and prevent crime. They perform a range of duties, from apprehending criminals to issuing traffic citations. Detectives may work as plainclothes investigators, collect evidence for criminal cases, and participate in raids and arrests.

Special agents are employed by federal government agencies and conduct complex criminal investigations, surveillance of criminals, infiltrate illicit drug organizations using undercover techniques, and apprehend violators of federal laws.

Injuries and fatalities can be prevented by good training, teamwork, and special equipment, such as bullet-resistant vests and helmets. Law enforcement officers must guard against the risks of assault while conducting drug raids, responding to calls reporting robberies or other felonies, serving arrest warrants and answering domestic disputes. Quick response time often requires traveling at high speed in police cruisers. Directing traffic and issuing traffic summonses exposes police officers to the dangers of working near speeding motor vehicles.

FATALITIES INCURRED BY LAW ENFORCEMENT PERSONNEL BY EVENT OR EXPOSURE, 1992–1997

Event or Exposure	Number	Percent
Total	**887**	**100**
Assaults and violent acts	449	51
Homicides	403	45
Transportation incidents	384	43
Highway	272	31
Falls	19	2
Exposure to harmful substances or environments	15	2
Contact with objects and equipment	12	1
Other	8	1

Source: *Compensation and Working Conditions,* Summer 1999, p. 4.

For further information:

Office of Safety, Health and Working Conditions
Bureau of Labor Statistics
2 Massachusetts Avenue, NE
#4130
Washington, D.C. 20212
691-6304
(202) 691-6196 (fax)

See also VIOLENCE.

Clarke, Cindy, and Mark J. Zak. "Fatalities of Law Enforcement Officers and Firefighters, 1992–1997." *Compensation and Working Conditions* (summer 1999): 3–7.

Pollution Standard Index (PSI)   See ENVIRONMENT.

polybrominated biphenyls (PBBs) and polybrominated diphenyl ethers (PBDEs)   Manufactured chemicals found in plastics used in a variety of products, including computer, monitors, television sets, textiles, and plastic foams, to make them difficult to burn. The manufacture of PBBs was discontinued in the United States in 1976, but the production of PBDEs continues.

Employees risk exposure to PBDEs if they work in a confined space where plastics and foam products are recycled or computers are repaired. Exposure to higher levels of PBDEs can occur in workers who produce or manufacture PBDE-containing products.

There are no federal guidelines or recommendations for protecting human health from exposure to these substances. The Environmental Protection Agency requires companies that transport, store, or dispose of these compounds to follow the rules and regulations of the federal hazardous waste management program. There is no definite information on health effects of PBDEs, although there is some evidence that PBBs may have caused skin problems, such as acne, in some people who ate contaminated food. Workers exposed to PBBs by breathing and skin contact for days to months also developed acne.

See also AGENCY FOR TOXIC SUBSTANCES AND DISEASE REGISTRY; DERMATITIS.

polychlorinated biphenyls (PCBs)   A group of manufactured organic chemicals that contain 209 individual chlorinated chemicals known as congeners. PCBs are either oily liquids or solids and are colorless to light yellow in color.

PCBs are good insulating material and do not burn easily. They have been used widely as coolants and lubricants in transformers, capacitors, and other electrical equipment. The manufacture of PCBs stopped in the United States in 1977 because of evidence that they build up in the environment and cause harmful effects. Products containing PCBs include old fluorescent lighting fixtures, electrical appliances containing PCB capacitors, and hydraulic fluids.

PCBs can be released in the environment from hazardous waste sites that contain PCBs, illegal or improper dumping of PCB wastes, and leaks from electrical transformers containing PCBs. Workers repairing or maintaining PCB transformers are exposed to PCBs and may experience irritation of the nose and lungs, and skin irritations, such as acne and rashes.

The Department of Health and Human Services (DHHS) has determined that PCBs may reasonably be anticipated to be carcinogens. The Environmental Protection Agency has set a maximum contaminant level of PCBs for drinking water and requires that spills or accidental releases into the environment of one pound or more of PCBs be reported.

For further information:

Agency for Toxic Substances and Disease Registry
Division of Toxicology
1600 Clifton Road, NE
Mailstop E-29
Atlanta, GA 30333
(888) 422-8737
(404) 498-0057 (fax)
www.atsdr.cdc.gov

See also AGENCY FOR TOXIC SUBSTANCES AND DISEASE REGISTRY; CHEMICAL TOXICITY; HAZARDOUS WASTE; ENVIRONMENTAL PROTECTION AGENCY; SKIN OR SENSE ORGAN TOXICITY.

polycyclic aromatic hydrocarbons (PAHs) A group of more than 100 different chemicals that are formed during the incomplete burning of coal, oil and gas, garbage, or other organic substances such as tobacco or charbroiled meat. PAHs are usually found as a mixture of compounds, such as soot.

Manufactured PAHs are found in coal tar, crude oil, creosote, and roofing tar, but a few are used in medicines or to make dyes, plastics, and pesticides.

PAHs enter the air mostly as releases from burning coal, volcanoes, forest fires, and automobile exhaust, and can occur in air attached to dust particles. Breathing the air containing PAHs in the workplace of coking, coal-tar, and asphalt production plants, smokehouses, and municipal trash incineration facilities can be a health hazard.

The Department of Health and Human Services (DHHS) has determined that some PAHs may reasonably be expected to be carcinogens. Some workers who have breathed or touched mixtures of PAHs and other chemicals for long periods of time have developed cancer. The Occupational Safety and Health Administration (OSHA) has set a limit of 0.2 milligram of PAHs per cubic meter of air. The OSHA permissible exposure limit (PEL) for mineral oil mist containing PAHs is 5 milligrams per cubic meter averaged over an eight-hour exposure period. The National Institute for Occupational Safety and Health (NIOSH) has also made recommendations regarding average workplace air levels for coal tar products.

For further information:

Agency for Toxic Substances and Disease Registry
Division of Toxicology
1600 Clifton Road NE
Mailstop E-29
Atlanta, GA 30333
(888) 422-8737
(404) 498-0057 (fax)
www.atsdr.cdc.gov

See also AGENCY FOR TOXIC SUBSTANCES AND DISEASE REGISTRY; CHEMICAL TOXICITY; HAZARDOUS WASTE; ENVIRONMENTAL PROTECTION AGENCY; NATIONAL INSTITUTE FOR OCCUPATIONAL SAFETY AND HEALTH; PERMISSIBLE EXPOSURE LIMITS; SKIN OR SENSE ORGAN TOXICITY.

post-traumatic stress disorder (PTSD) An anxiety disorder produced by an unusual and extremely stressful event, such as an airplane crash, explosion, shooting, rape, assault or other act of violence or physical injury. Historically, PTSD has been referred to as battle fatigue or shell shock when it resulted from military combat. Many workers who survived or witnessed the terrorist attack on the World Trade Center in New York on September 11, 2001, experienced symptoms of PTSD.

Often PTSD surfaces several months or even years later, although symptoms can occur soon after the event. Sufferers characteristically reexperience the trauma in painful recollections or recurrent dreams or nightmares. Some have diminished emotional responsiveness ("numbing"), feelings of estrangement from others, insomnia, disturbed sleep, difficulty in concentrating or remembering, GUILT about surviving when others did not, avoidance of activities that cause recollection of the traumatic event, and intense thoughts related to the event. Avoidance behavior also affects sufferers' relationships with others, because they often avoid close emotional ties with family, colleagues, and friends.

Sometimes the reexperience comes as a sudden, painful rush of emotions such as ANGER or intense fear that seem to have no cause. Some PTSD sufferers endure anxiety and PANIC ATTACKS as a result.

Overcoming PTSD

Individuals who have PTSD can learn to work through the trauma and pain and resolve their anxieties. Individual psychotherapy is one of many useful therapies. PTSD results, in part, from the difference between the individual's personal values and the reality of what was witnessed or experienced during the traumatic event. Psychotherapy helps the individual examine his/her values and behavior with the goal of resolving the conscious and unconscious conflicts that were created. Additionally, the individual works to build SELF-ESTEEM and SELF-CONTROL, develops a reasonable sense of personal accountability, and renews a sense of integrity and personal pride.

After major disasters, such as a the World Trade Center disaster or school shootings, therapists are provided to survivors and witnesses to encourage a therapeutic sharing of experiences and reactions.

For further information:

U.S. Veterans Administration
Mental Health and Behavioral Sciences Services
810 Vermont Avenue, NW
Room 915
Washington, DC 20410
(202) 389-3416

See also ANXIETY DISORDERS; COMMUNICATION; CONTROL; COPING; DEPRESSION; LISTENING; MENTAL HEALTH; NATIONAL INSTITUTE OF MENTAL HEALTH; PSYCHOTHERAPIES; SELF-ESTEEM; STRESS.

Kahn, Ada P., and Jan Fawcett. *The Encyclopedia of Mental Health*. 2d ed. New York: Facts On File, Inc., 2001.

poultry processing An industry that the U.S. Department of Labor Occupational Safety and Health Administration suggests dividing into two stages, each with its particular hazards. The first stage is the raising of live birds to the desired weight, delivery to the processing plant and preparing the live birds for slaughtering. The second stage is the slaughtering, processing, and packaging of the birds.

Major hazards to workers in the first stage are generally respiratory problems resulting from exposure to organic dusts (litter, manure, dander) and ammonia. These are controlled using ventilation and PERSONAL PROTECTIVE EQUIPMENT (PPE). Additional hazards include those associated with agricultural machinery, feed delivery systems, waste removal systems, and ergonomic hazards, particularly as birds are prepared for slaughtering. A potentially significant hazard is the presence of microbiologicals and endotoxins in the organic dusts.

In the second stage, common elements in an effective safety and health program include control of ergonomic hazards to prevent cumulative trauma disorders, machine guarding and PPE to prevent cuts, care of walking/working surfaces to reduce trips and falls, design and maintenance of electrical systems, and lockout/tagout procedures to prevent accidental startup of machinery.

See also BUTCHERS AND MEAT, POULTRY, AND FISH CUTTERS; CARPAL TUNNEL SYNDROME; DUST; ERGONOMICS; LOCKOUT/TAGOUT; REPETITIVE STRESS INJURIES; SLIPS, TRIPS, AND FALLS.

powerlessness The state of lacking the authority or capacity to act. It is an awkward situation for people in the workplace because they feel that they lack CONTROL and know that they cannot significantly affect the outcome of a situation.

For some people, feelings of powerlessness underlie DEPRESSION, suspiciousness, and aggressive behavior. Powerlessness is also associated with withdrawal, passivity, submissiveness, apathy, increased frustration, agitation, anxiety, AGGRESSION, acting-out behavior, and even violence. A person who feels powerless may be unable to set goals or follow through on activities relating to work assignments.

See also AUTONOMY; COPING; MENTAL HEALTH; SELF-ESTEEM.

McFarland, Gertrude K., and Mary Durand Thomas. *Psychiatric Mental Health Nursing.* Philadelphia: J. B. Lippincott Company, 1991.

printing plants/printing inks   Several categories of printing processes (flexography, gravure, letterpress, lithography, and screen printing) carry specific hazards. Hazards are related to the types of printing inks used, the likelihood of inhalation of mists or solvent fumes, and penetrable skin contact from the process and cleaning activities used.

According to the *Encyclopaedia of Occupational Health and Safety,* exposure of workers in the printing industry to organic solvents (for instance, toluene and turpentine), pigments, dyes, chromates, and cyanates has been markedly reduced in recent decades because of computer technologies, automated processes, and changes in materials. In 1996 the International Agency for Research on Cancer (IARC) concluded that occupational exposures in the printing process are possibly carcinogenic to humans. However, the IARC's conclusion was based on historical exposures, which are markedly different today. According to the encyclopedia, reports of malignant melanoma have suggested risks about twice the expected rate. Lung cancer rates were highest in newspaper pressmen.

See also ALLERGIES; CANCER; CHEMICAL TOXICITY; GRAPHIC ARTS; HAND TOOLS; LOCKOUT/TAGOUT; HEADACHES; SKIN OR SENSE ORGAN TOXICITY; SLIPS, TRIPS, AND FALLS; SOLVENTS.

Mager-Stillman, Jeanne. *Encyclopaedia of Occupational Health and Safety.* Vol. 3. Geneva: International Labour Organisation, 1998, pp. 85.9–85.10.

private industry: workplace injury and illness incidence   A total of 5.7 million injuries and illnesses occurred in private industry workplaces during 1999, resulting in a rate of 6.3 cases for every 100 equivalent full-time workers. According to the Bureau of Labor Statistics, U.S. Department of Labor, this was the lowest rate recorded.

progressive muscle relaxation   A STRESS MANAGEMENT technique in which individuals learn to make heightened observations of what goes on under their skin. They learn to control all of the skeletal muscles so that any portion can be systematically relaxed or tensed by choice. Many employee fitness programs include progressive muscle relaxation as part of their activities.

First, there is recognition of subtle states of tension. When a muscle contracts (tenses), waves of neural impulses are generated and carried to the brain along neural pathways. This muscle-neural phenomenon is an observable sign of tension.

Next, having learned to identify the tension sensation, the individual learns to relax it. Relaxation is the elongation (lengthening) of skeletal muscle fibers, which then eliminates the tension sensation. This general procedure of identifying a local state of tension, relaxing it away, and making the contrast between the tension and ensuing relaxation is then applied to all of the major muscle groups.

As a stress management technique, progressive relaxation is effective only when individuals have the ability to selectively elongate their muscle fibers on command. They can then exercise the self-control required for progressive relaxation and more rationally deal with a stressful situation.

See also BIOFEEDBACK; COMPLEMENTARY THERAPIES; RELAXATION; STRESS; WORKSITE WELLNESS PROGRAMS.

Jacobsen, E. *Progressive Relaxation.* 2d ed. Chicago: University of Chicago Press, 1983.
———. "The Origins and Development of Progressive Relaxation." *Journal of Behavior Therapy and Experimental Psychiatry* 8 (1977): 119–123.
Lehrer, Paul M., and Robert L. Woolfolk, eds. *Principles and Practice of Stress Management.* 2d ed. New York: Guilford Press, 1993.

propellants   See AEROSPACE MEDICINE.

protective clothing   See COLD ENVIRONMENTS; EYE INJURIES/PROTECTION; FOOT PROTECTION; PERSONAL PROTECTIVE EQUIPMENT.

psychiatrist   A medical doctor who specializes in the diagnosis and treatment of mental, emotional, or behavioral problems; some psychiatrists do research in the field of mental health. Many employed people who cannot cope with the stresses in their lives seek help from psychiatrists. Psychiatrists trace the patient's personal and family history to seek possible causes of a problem. A psychiatrist can prescribe counseling, individually or in groups, and medications and, if necessary, can admit patients to hospitals. In many cases, an EMPLOYEE ASSISTANCE PROGRAM will refer an employee to a psychiatrist.

Psychiatrists are trained in a variety of diagnostic techniques and therapies. There is a strong medical emphasis because of the development of techniques of psychopharmacology which require a knowledge of pharmacology, physiology, cardiology, and endocrinology. Recent advances in neuroscience as it relates to behavior have provided a strong medical and psychosocial focus for psychiatry.

See also DEPRESSION; MENTAL HEALTH; PSYCHOTHERAPIES.

National Institute of Mental Health. *Mental Health, United States, 1990.* Manderscheid, R. W., and Sonnenschein, M. A., eds. DHHS Pub. No. (ADM) 90-1708. Washington, D.C.; Supt. of Docs., U.S. Government. Printing Office, 1990.

psychoanalysis The mode of treatment for mental health disorders developed by Sigmund Freud and his followers at the beginning of the 20th century. He believed that mental disorders were a result of the failure of normal emotional development during childhood. While many employees are now referred to counselors by EMPLOYEE ASSISTANCE PROGRAMS for mental health concerns, few are encouraged to begin psychoanalysis.

Features of free association, dream analysis, and the development and working through of transference or distortions are used in the relationship with the analyst. Sessions are usually held four or five times a week and a completed analysis may take three to five years, but length of treatment varies considerably with the nature of the problems being treated. The therapy aims to help the patient understand his or her emotional development and to make appropriate adjustments in particular situations.

Psychoanalysis is practiced by clinicians who have undergone specialized training after resi-

dency. Individuals who practice psychoanalysis are usually medical doctors, but not necessarily so. Those who are not must pass certain examinations given by an accredited institute of psychoanalysis. Psychoanalysts must undergo psychoanalysis themselves to resolve their own emotional problems before they start their practice.

See also DEPRESSION; MENTAL HEALTH; PSYCHOTHERAPIES.

psychodrama An adjunct to MENTAL HEALTH therapy in which one acts out certain roles or incidents; this can be useful for individuals trying to overcome serious stresses in their lives. An example of the use of psychodrama may be when an individual has a major issue in getting along with a supervisor. The purpose of psychodrama is to bring out hidden concerns and to allow expression of the person's feelings. Therapeutic value comes from the release of pent-up emotions and from insights into the way other people feel and behave. Psychodrama is often carried out with a partner or in a group. In many cases, use of music, dance, and pantomime may be included.

The technique was developed by J. L. Moreno, a Viennese psychiatrist, in 1921. Psychodrama is considered an early form of group psychotherapy.

See also COMPLEMENTARY THERAPIES; PSYCHOTHERAPIES.

psychologist A nonmedical specialist in diagnosing and treating MENTAL HEALTH concerns such as difficulties in coping with STRESS in the workplace. In most states, a psychologist has a Ph.D. degree from a graduate program in psychology. Licensed psychologists receive insurance reimbursement, have hospital privileges, and act as expert witnesses in court cases. Many EMPLOYEE ASSISTANCE PROGRAMS refer employees to a psychologist for help in dealing with a problem in the workplace or in their personal lives.

Psychology has many subspecialties, including industrial, school, child, developmental, clinical, and social. Some psychologists have private practices, are employed by health care facilities, or teach in universities.

Psychologists cannot prescribe medications; they refer patients requiring medication to a physician.

See also BEHAVIOR THERAPY; PSYCHIATRIST; PSYCHOTHERAPIES.

psychotherapies Treatment for mental and emotional concerns by psychological methods. In psychotherapy, a therapeutic relationship between the patient and the psychotherapist is established. The relationship focuses on the patient's symptoms. Patterns of behavior—inability to deal with coworkers, mood swings, or low self-esteem—can be improved or altered from this interaction between patient and therapist. EMPLOYEE ASSISTANCE PROGRAMS refer workers for psychotherapy in many different settings.

There are many types of psychotherapists. When choosing a therapist, check out credentials. Know whether the therapist is a PSYCHIATRIST, PSYCHOLOGIST, or psychiatric social worker. Determine where the person received training and check with that institution. Also, because there are professional societies for many specialties, check with the appropriate organization to see that the therapist has appropriate accreditation.

Choosing a Psychotherapist

People seeking help may be faced with the question of who to choose. If they recognize what their problems are and have only occasional periods of feeling moody, a psychiatrist may not be needed. Guidelines for selecting a nonmedical therapist rather than a psychiatrist include:

The end of the stressful problem is in sight, but the individual just can't get there alone.
The individual realizes that symptoms are of short duration and that the stress that brought them on can be identified.

However, a person who has not found relief with a therapist may need a psychiatrist. Psychiatrists are the only mental health therapists who can prescribe medications. For certain emotional illnesses, medications may be helpful. If the individual has incapacitating or debilitating symptoms or other medical problems for which care and medications are being received, or if there is a history of mental illness in the family (if other family members have ever been hospitalized for mental illness) or requires hospitalization, a psychiatrist may be needed.

Group Therapy

Group therapy is treatment of emotional or psychological problems in groups of employees or in self-help support groups led by a mental health professional. These groups attract individuals with similar concerns. For example, such groups may be for people who have witnessed a tragedy, such as the terrorist attack on the World Trade Center on September 11, 2001, or a school shooting, or for people suffering from DEPRESSION or those concerned with OBESITY.

Therapy groups include from three to 40 people but work best with 10 to 12 participants who meet for an hour or more, once or twice a week. There is therapeutic interaction among the individuals in the group; members may find that others share their feelings and experiences and this may help them feel less alone and less helpless.

Group therapy is sometimes useful for people who have personality problems, alcoholism, drug dependency, EATING DISORDERS, and ANXIETY DISORDERS.

Family Therapy

Family therapy is a form of psychotherapy that focuses on the family unit, rather than separate treatment of one or more family members. It is based on the theory that an individual who is troubled or is mentally ill should not be seen in isolation from the family unit. Family members become aware of how they deal with each other and are encouraged to communicate more openly with each other. The discussions and confrontations can lead to greater understanding.

Family therapy usually focuses on immediate stresses and their practical solutions. It can be helpful when at least one member has a relatively serious problem such as recurrent depression or needs ongoing assistance in coping with outbursts of anger and emotional withdrawal, for instance.

Family therapy has become increasingly popular for dealing with problems of children and adolescents. In many cases, the child is brought to a mental health professional because of difficulties in school, such as exhibiting aggressive behavior or cutting classes.

See also COMMUNICATION; LISTENING; MENTAL HEALTH; SUPPORT GROUPS.

Public Citizen   See HEALTH RESEARCH GROUP.

public speaking   The art of making a speech to an audience. People in the workplace can experience STRESS relating to public speaking that may range from mild apprehension to true phobic reactions. The anticipation of giving a speech in public may arouse only a mild form of anxiety, which might be considered normal, to feelings of rapid heartbeat, faintness, dizziness, nausea, or other symptoms of PHOBIA.

An individual may suffer a mild degree of stress as a common reaction to being asked to give the speech, preparing it, and finally getting up in front of people to give it. The speaker may be apprehensive about appearance or voice and what people will think about the speech. All these apprehensions, however, could spur the individual to doing the best possible presentation.

A truly social phobic person who is phobic about public speaking probably would not accept such an invitation; nor would an individual who has an extreme fear of failure.

People who manage to give a speech in public but are extremely uneasy often exhibit behaviors such as shuffling the feet, pacing, lack of eye contact, facial tics or grimaces, moistening the lips and clearing the throat frequently, and noticeably perspiring.

Issues of self-confidence and SELF-ESTEEM are involved in the stress of public speaking. People who have given many speeches and feel confident about the subject matter, as well as their appearance, will probably experience only a mild degree of stress.

See also ANXIETY; PERFORMANCE ANXIETY; SOCIAL-PHOBIA; STAGE FRIGHT.

pulmonary dysfunction   See PERFORMING ARTS MEDICINE.

pulmonary rehabilitation   A multidisciplinary component of the medical management of individuals who have severe lung diseases, such as chronic obstructive pulmonary disease (COPD), asthma, bronchitis, and emphysema. The goal of pulmonary rehabilitation programs is to control and reduce symptoms of respiratory impairment and enable the individual to maintain and function at a maximum level of independence. Programs are usually individually tailored depending on the individual's level of disease. Outcomes sought include increases in exercise endurance, improving breathing capacity and reducing health-related costs by reducing need for hospitalization.

Rehabilitation programs generally include patient education regarding nutrition and exercise and psychological support and therapeutic components such as ventilatory therapy, breathing training, chest physical therapy, and instruction in use of medications.

See also ASTHMA, OCCUPATIONAL; BRONCHITIS; CHRONIC OBSTRUCTIVE PULMONARY DISEASE; EMPHYSEMA.

pulmonary tuberculosis   See TUBERCULOSIS.

pulp, paper, and paperboard mills   Hazardous places to work due to massive weights and falling, rolling, and or sliding pulpwood loads. According to the U.S. Department of Labor, Occupational Safety and Health Administration (OSHA), workers may be struck by loads, crushed by loads, or suffer lacerations from the misuse of equipment, particularly when machines are used improperly or without proper safeguards.

Also, there are many environmental hazards in this industry. In 1997 the U.S. Environmental Protection Agency (EPA) issued a "cluster rule" for the pulp and paper industry to protect human health and the environment by reducing toxic pollutant releases into the air and water. The rule regulates toxic air pollutants in 155 of the 565 pulp, paper, and paperboard mills in the United States and it regulates toxic water discharges from 96 of the 155 mills.

The technology standards in the rule cut toxic air pollutant emissions by almost 60 percent and virtually eliminate all dioxin discharged from pulp, paper, and paperboard mills into rivers and other surface waters. Specifically, the EPA requires mills to capture and treat toxic air pollutant emissions occurring during the cooking, washing, and bleaching stages of the pulp manufacturing process. Further, EPA sets effluent limits for toxic pollutants in the wastewater discharge during the bleaching process and in the final discharge from the mills. These limits are based on substituting chlorine dioxide for chlorine in the bleaching process.

Environmental benefits from this regulation include reduction of odor causing pollutants, volatile organic compounds, emissions of PARTICU-LATE MATTER, chloroform discharges to water, and dioxin and furan discharges.

See also CONFINED SPACES; CHEMICAL TOXICITY; ENVIRONMENT; ENVIRONMENTAL PROTECTION AGENCY; LOCKOUT/TAGOUT; OCCUPATIONAL SAFETY AND HEALTH ADMINISTRATION; PERSONAL PROTECTIVE EQUIPMENT; SLIPS, TRIPS, AND FALLS.

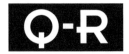

quarrying See EXTRACTIVE INDUSTRIES.

radiation See NUCLEAR WEAPONS WORKERS; OCCU-PATIONAL LUNG DISEASE.

Radiation Exposure Compensation Act See ENERGY EMPLOYEES OCCUPATIONAL ILLNESS COMPENSATION PROGRAM.

radioactive materials See NUCLEAR WEAPONS WORKERS; URANIUM MINERS/URANIUM EXPOSURE.

radionuclides See AIR POLLUTION.

radon A colorless, odorless, tasteless, radioactive gaseous element produced by the radioactive decay of radium. Radon has three naturally occurring isotopes that disintegrate with the emission of radiation to form solid radioactive materials. In addition to radon's naturally occurring radioisotopes, more than a dozen artificial ones have been produced.

Sources of radon occur naturally in many materials, such as soil, rock, and building materials, and the gas is released continually into the atmosphere. As a result, radon makes the largest single contribution to radiation doses received by humans from naturally radioactive materials. Some researchers suggest that radon may be a significant causative factor in some cases of cancer, particularly lung cancer; this claim has not yet been tested scientifically. Uranium miners and uranium workers are particularly exposed to radon.

See also CANCER; URANIUM MINERS/URANIUM EXPOSURE.

Clayman, Charles B., ed. *American Medical Association Encyclopedia of Medicine*. New York: Random House, 1989.

railroad work Although safety in the U.S. railroad industry has improved since 1980, the number of injuries and accidents in railroad yards exceeded the number of injuries and accidents in other aspects of the industry, according to the Federal Railroad Administration (FRA), part of the U.S. Department of Transportation. Almost half of all train accidents and a large proportion of employee injuries occurred in railroad yards in 1998. According to the Transportation Research Board, job injuries cost American railroads more than $1 billion annually.

Analysis of railroad yard worker injury data revealed that 8 percent of injuries involved one or more lost workdays (a lost workday is either a worker completely absent from the job or working with restricted duty). Sprains and strains accounted for more than half of the injuries; slips, trips, and falls were the most common trigger; and walking, running, or stepping were the leading physical acts leading to these injuries. Most lost workday injuries occurred between 10 A.M. and 12 P.M.

Analysis of human factor–attributed train accidents in railroad yards revealed that more accidents occurred during extremely cold or hot temperatures than during milder weather. Most of these accidents occurred between 2 A.M. and 4 A.M. and between 4 P.M. and 6 P.M.

For information:

Federal Railroad Administration
Office of Research and Development
1120 Vermont Ave. NW-Mail Stop 20
Washington, DC 20590
(202) 493-6356 (fax)
www.fra.dot.gov

random drug testing See DRUG TESTING.

rashes See DERMATITIS; SKIN OR SENSE ORGAN TOXICITY.

Raynaud's disease See VIBRATION WHITE FINGER.

recommended exposure limits (RELs) Exposure limits at the workplace protect workers from excessive exposure to toxic chemicals. Limits have been designed for healthy adults, usually for an exposure duration of eight hours. RELs are set by the National Institute for Occupational Safety and Health (NIOSH), which is part of the Department of Health and Human Services. Based on studies, NIOSH scientists recommend exposure limits to Occupational Safety and Health Administration (OSHA). NIOSH publishes criteria documents that include data related to each standard as well as sampling techniques and control measures. A useful publication is the *NIOSH Pocket Guide to Chemical Hazards.*

See also CHEMICAL TOXICITY; NATIONAL INSTITUTE FOR OCCUPATIONAL SAFETY AND HEALTH; *NIOSH POCKET GUIDE TO CHEMICAL HAZARDS;* OCCUPATIONAL SAFETY AND HEALTH ADMINISTRATION; PERMISSIBLE EXPOSURE LIMITS.

recycling facilities See WASTE INDUSTRY.

reflexology A form of body therapy based on the theory that every part of the body has a direct line of communication to a reference point on the foot, hand, and ear. By massaging these reference points, professional reflexologists say they can help the corresponding body parts to heal. Through improved circulation, elimination of toxic by-products, and overall reduction of stress, the body responds and functions better because it is more relaxed. Reflexology is one of many COMPLEMENTARY THERAPIES included in some employee wellness and fitness programs.

**USING REFLEXOLOGY
TO REDUCE WORKPLACE STRESS**

- Choose a quiet place.
- Apply a few drops of a light, absorbent, greaseless lotion to your feet and massage them, continuing until the lotion is totally absorbed.
- Grasp the ankle, heel, or toes of one foot firmly in one hand, place the thumb of your other hand on the sole of your foot at the heel and apply steady, even pressure with the edge of your whole thumb.
- Keep your thumb slightly bent at the joint and use a forward, caterpillar-like motion. This is called thumb-walking; press one spot, move forward a little, press again, etc.
- When you reach the toes, start again at a new spot on the heel. Continue until the entire bottom of the foot has been worked. Then fingerwalk the top of the foot. Work your entire foot twice this way.

See also BODY THERAPIES.

Kahn, Ada P. *Stress A–Z: A Sourcebook for Facing Everyday Challenges.* New York: Facts On File, Inc., 1998.

refuse collection See WASTE INDUSTRY.

refuse truck drivers See WASTE INDUSTRY.

relationships Relationships are formed between individuals connected by affinity. These relationships include the associates in the workplace, the family, spouse, or lovers. Good relationships are healthy and nurturing and act as a buffer against outside sources of stress. However, even the most meaningful relationships can at times be nonsupportive and stressful.

**HOW TO HAVE
A HEALTHY RELATIONSHIP WITH COWORKERS**

- Realism: openness and honesty with each other
- Trust: sharing feelings
- True friendship: having no hidden motives
- Forgiveness: accepting one another as they are
- Security: knowing that coworkers can count on one another
- Vulnerability: exposing weaknesses that allow the relationship to grow

---

Relationships and Health

Good friends fit this category: they are on the same wavelength with you and understand your personal situations, such as dealing with a difficult boss or overbearing parent; they appreciate and admire you, even if there is not always agreement on what is being done or said; they make you feel important; they are very much like you and share the same values and belief systems.

Socially isolated people may be more likely to adopt self-destructive health habits and may get depressed and become suicidal or accident-prone. "All diseases are 'social diseases,'" says Dennis Jaffe, author of *Healing from Within.* "It's as though a breakdown in the social support structure precipitates a breakdown in the body's immune system."

This breakdown in the body's immune system resembles the body's stress response. People who lack outlets for stress release are susceptible to a list of stress-related illnesses. Having one or two close friends with whom they feel free to say anything is invaluable. When they are overwhelmed, they do not trust their own judgment and an objective view from a friend can help.

Relationships and Support Groups

A lack of connections with other people can be detrimental to health, says Dr. Andrew Weil, author of *Spontaneous Healing.* "Surrounding yourself with supportive people is an important step for any healing you need to do. Whenever I take a family history from a patient, I always ask about people who are helping or hindering someone's illness. For example, sometimes a friend or family member who means well only makes matters worse, maybe by not wanting the patient to express sadness about being sick or show discomfort from pain."

In terms of building relationships through support groups, Dr. Weil urges people to find and develop relationships with others who have the same conditions who have improved rather than simply join a support group. "I find that some support groups can be counterproductive and cause more stress for the individual," he says. "For example, some patients with cancer are horrified and extremely stressed when they see another person with a more advanced form of the disease. There is

a similar phenomenon with chronic fatigue syndrome."

See also BODY LANGUAGE; COMMUNICATION; LISTENING; SUPPORT GROUPS.

Gilbert, Roberta M. *Extraordinary Relationships: A New Way of Thinking About Human Interactions.* Minneapolis: Chronimed Publishing, 1992.

Jaffe, Dennis T. *Healing from Within.* New York: Knopf, 1980.

Weil, Andrew. *Spontaneous Healing: How to Discover and Enhance Your Body's Natural Ability to Maintain and Heal Itself.* New York: Knopf, 1995.

relaxation   A feeling of freedom from anxiety and tension in which internal conflicts and disturbing feelings of STRESS are absent. Relaxation also refers to the return of a muscle to its normal state after a period of contraction. Many EMPLOYEE WELLNESS PROGRAMS include courses in relaxation among their offerings.

People who are very tense and anxious can learn to relax using relaxation training, a form of BEHAVIOR THERAPY, or alternative therapy. Relaxation techniques are methods used to unconsciously release muscular tension and achieve a sense of mental calm. Historically, relaxation techniques have included MEDITATION, T'AI CHI, MASSAGE THERAPY, YOGA, and music. More modern developments include PROGRESSIVE MUSCLE RELAXATION, hypnosis, BIOFEEDBACK, and aerobic exercise.

Many of these techniques were developed to help people cope with the challenges of life. They are different approaches to bringing about generalized physical as well as mental relaxation. Relaxation techniques have in common the production of the relaxation response as one of their stress-relieving actions. Additionally, relaxation may counter some of the immunosuppressing effects of stress and may actually enhance the activity of the immune system.

What Is the "Relaxation Response"?

In the 1970s, Herbert Benson, M.D., a cardiologist at Harvard Medical School, studied the relationship between stress and hypertension. In stressful situations, the body undergoes several changes, including rise in blood pressure and pulse and faster breathing. Dr. Benson reasoned that if stress could bring about this reaction, another factor might be able to turn it off. He studied practitioners of TRANSCENDENTAL MEDITATION (TM) and found that in their meditative states, some could willfully reduce their pulse, blood pressure, and breathing rate. Dr. Benson named this "the relaxation response." He explained this procedure in his book (written with Miriam Z. Klipper) *The Relaxation Response* (1976).

Applications of the Relaxation Technique

Relaxation training can be particularly useful for individuals before a job interview, a performance review, or when they have to make a speech in public. It is also useful for people who have "white coat hypertension," which means that their blood pressure is high only when facing certain situations, such as having a medical examination or visiting a dentist. It can also help reduce hostility and anger, which in turn affect the body and the individual's physical responses to stress. Anxieties can lead to panic attacks, nausea, or gastrointestinal problems.

There are many applications for relaxation training to help individuals learn control over their mental state and body and in treating conditions as diverse as high blood pressure, cardiac arrhythmia, chronic pain, insomnia, premenstrual syndrome, and side effects of cancer treatments. Relaxation training is an important part of childbirth classes to help women cope with labor.

In a training program, individuals are instructed to move through the muscle groups of the body, making them tense and then completely relaxed. Through repetitions of this procedure, individuals learn how to be in voluntary control of their feelings of tension and relaxation. Some therapists provide individuals with instructional audiotapes for use during practice, while other therapists go through the procedure repeatedly with their clients.

To determine the effectiveness of relaxation training, some therapists use biofeedback as an indicator of an individual's degree of relaxation and absence of anxiety.

See also BENSON, HERBERT; COMPLEMENTARY THERAPIES; EXERCISE; GUIDED IMAGERY; KABAT-ZINN, JON; MIND/BODY CONNECTIONS.

Benson, Herbert. *The Relaxation Response.* New York: Avon Books, 1975.
———. *Beyond the Relaxation Response.* New York: Berkeley, 1985.
Lehrer, Paul M., and Robert L. Woolfolk, eds. *Principles and Practice of Stress Management.* New York: Guilford Press, 1993.
Locke, Steven, and Douglas Colligan. *The Healer Within.* New York: New American Library, 1984.

relocation The transfer to a new company location as part of a promotion or lateral career move. Transfers sometimes also become necessary due to reorganizations and MERGERS. A fact of life for many working people and their families today, relocation may mean losing a SUPPORT GROUP (friends and/or relatives), finding a new residence and new community resources (places to worship, schools, doctors, dentists, and so on), handling the move (packing and unpacking), and, in the case of dual careers, the need for one spouse to find new employment and the possible financial impact of that.

Frequent transfers can be hard on all members of the family. Frequent moves have been known to trigger a group of reactions called the mobility syndrome which can include DEPRESSION, deterioration of health, dependency on one's own family for emotional satisfaction, reclusiveness, a high rate of alcoholism and drug dependency, and marital discord that often leads to divorce. There is an increase of acting-out behavior on the part of children and teenagers. Many of these reactions require professional help.

Many people have begun to assess the viability of a transfer not only in terms of careers and the financial and housing implications of the move, but in terms of the quality of life for themselves and their families. Since relocation often becomes a primary part of a promotion, it is important to see if it matches family values and priorities as well as the individual's career plan. Whatever the decision, applying constructive coping techniques and strategies is necessary to handle the resulting stress.

See also ACCULTURATION; COPING; GENERAL ADAPTATION SYNDROME.

repeated trauma disorders See CARPAL TUNNEL SYNDROME; REPETITIVE STRESS INJURIES.

repetitive stress injuries (RSI) Injuries that result from repetitive motions, such as using a computer or certain types of factory work. As people spend more time at computers, sitting at a desk, looking at a screen, and typing, they become more and more susceptible to repetitive stress injuries. Human beings are not meant to do repetitive motions all day in workspaces not set up to accommodate either the equipment or their bodies. The result is damage to muscles in the fingers, wrists, hand, arms, neck, head, and back.

The rate of RSIs is increasing as more Americans use computers at work and at home. RSIs are affected by the individual's work pacing, work stress, environment, and personality traits.

The kinds of problems computer users report include shooting pains in the arms, acute pain or stiffness in the arms, neck, shoulders and/or back, acute wrist or finger pain, numbness or tingling in the fingers, hands, arms, or shoulders, and chronic pain in the neck, shoulders, or back.

A specific type of repetitive stress injury relating to wrist-and-hand disorders is CARPAL TUNNEL SYNDROME. It has been identified as one of the fastest growing occupational illnesses. Carpal tunnel syndrome is the result of inflamed tendons in the wrist.

AVOIDING REPETITIVE STRESS OF COMPUTER USE

- Select chairs and desks that can be adjusted for maximum work comfort (feet should be flat on the floor).
- Support your back with a pillow to keep posture correct and relieve strain.
- Be sure your keyboard and mouse are at a comfortable level; raise or lower if necessary.
- Avoid flexing wrists; use a contoured wrist-support device.
- Take work breaks—stretch, roll the neck, and do hand squeezing exercises; stand up and walk about.
- Keep monitor at arm's length (24 inches) from face.
- If pain persists, see a doctor. Workspace or work-habit changes, physical therapy, special exercises, medication, braces, or surgery may be recommended.

For information:

Association for Repetitive Motion Syndrome
P.O. Box 471973
Aurora, CO 80047
(303) 369-0803
http://www.certifiedpst.com/arms

See also PERFORMING ARTS MEDICINE; VIDEO DISPLAY TERMINALS.

reproductive toxicity Adverse effects on the male and female reproductive systems that result from exposure to chemical substances. There may be alterations in sexual behavior, decreases in fertility, or miscarriage. A reproductive toxicant may interfere with the sexual functioning or reproductive ability of exposed individuals from puberty throughout adulthood.

Toxicants can disrupt a woman's ability to successfully reproduce. Toxicants can cause changes in sexual behavior, bring about onset of puberty or premature menopause, and affect fertility, gestation time, pregnancy outcome, and lactation. Exposure to lead, for example, can result in menstrual disorders and infertility. The toxicants carbon disulfide, MERCURY, and POLYCHLORINATED BIPHENYLS (PCBs) have been shown to cause irregularities in the menstrual cycle. An increased rate of spontaneous abortion has been found in hospital workers exposed to ETHYLENE OXIDE.

In males, toxicants can affect sperm count or shape, alter sexual behavior, and/or increase infertility. Carbon disulfide and the pesticides CHLORDECONE (Kepone), ethylene dibromide (EDB), and dibromochloropropane (DBCP) are examples of chemicals known to disrupt male reproductive health. Occupational exposure to DBCP has caused azoospermia (the total absence of sperm in the semen) and sterility.

See also CHEMICAL TOXICITY; CHLORDECONE.

Dixon, R. "Toxic Responses of the Reproductive System." Chap. 16 in *Casarett and Doull's Toxicology,* edited by C. Klaasen, M. Amdur, and J. Doull. New York: Pergamon Press, 1996.

rescue workers See FIREFIGHTERS AND RESCUE WORKERS.

respiratory protection See BORON; PERSONAL PROTECTIVE EQUIPMENT; RESPIRATORS.

respirators Devices designed to protect the wearer from inhalation of hazardous or toxic materials. Respirators are approved by the National

Institute for Occupational Safety and Health (NIOSH) and the Mine Safety and Health Administration (MSHA). Standards are also set by the American National Standards Institute.

TYPES OF RESPIRATORS

Atmosphere-supplying units provide breathing air from a source independent of the surrounding atmosphere.

- Air line or air-supplied respirators are connected to a stationary source of compressed breathing air by a hose.
- Self-contained breathing apparatus (SCBA); air is supplied from a compressed cylinder, usually through a full-face mask which is worn on the back. It gives greater movement than an air line respirator, but the air supply is limited.
- Combination respirators have a small, auxiliary self-contained air supply that can be used if the primary supply fails.

Air-purifying respirators, which contain an air-purifying filter, cartridge, or canister that removes specific air contaminants by passing ambient air through the air-purifying element

- Types of air-purifying respirators include particulate respirators used to mechanically remove particulate matter such as dusts. Not to be used to remove particulates or vapors. Gas and vapor respirators (or chemical cartridge respirators) use chemicals such as activated charcoal to remove specific gases and vapors from the air. Combination respirators have filters for both particulates and vapors.
- Powered air-purifying respirators (PAPR) use a blower to force the ambient air through air-purifying elements to the inlet covering.

Respirators should be used for protection only when engineering controls, such as ventilation and substitution of less toxic materials, have been shown to be infeasible for the control of the hazard or during the interim period when engineering controls are being installed.

Respirators provide adequate protection only if employers ensure that they are properly fitted and worn. Proper fitting may be conducted by a trained professional and may require employees to shave facial hair. Routine use of respirators requires regular medical examinations, fit testing, training, and purchasing expensive equipment. Employers should contract appropriate local, state, and federal agencies concerning use of respirators.

For information on respirators, contact Occupational Safety and Health Administration (OSHA) or American National Standards Institute (ANSI).

See also AMERICAN NATIONAL STANDARDS INSTITUTE; ASTHMA; DUST AND DEBRIS; NATIONAL INSTITUTE FOR OCCUPATIONAL SAFETY AND HEALTH; OCCUPATIONAL SAFETY AND HEALTH ADMINISTRATION; PERSONAL PROTECTIVE EQUIPMENT; RESPIRATORY TOXICITY.

respiratory toxicity Adverse effects on the structure or functioning of the respiratory system resulting from exposure to chemical substances. The respiratory system consists of the nasal passages, pharynx, trachea, bronchi, and lungs. The chief function of the respiratory system is to ensure the efficient exchange of oxygen and carbon dioxide between the blood and the air. Respiratory toxicants can produce a variety of acute and chronic pulmonary conditions, including local irritation, bronchitis, pulmonary edema, emphysema, and cancer.

Pulmonary fibrosis is a serious lung disease in which airways become restricted or inflamed, leading to loss of elasticity and difficulty in breathing. It can be caused by exposure to COAL DUST, aluminum, BERYLLIUM, and carbides of tungsten. EMPHYSEMA, a degenerative and potentially fatal disease, is characterized by the inability of the lungs to fully expand and contract. The most common cause of emphysema is heavy cigarette smoking, but the disease can be induced by exposure to aluminum, CADMIUM oxide, ozone, and nitrogen oxides. Several toxicants are known to cause respiratory cancer, including ASBESTOS, ARSENIC, and nickel.

See also ASTHMA.

@2001 Environmental Defense. Used by permission. Scorecard is available at: www.scorecard.com

Menzel, D. B., and M. Amdur. "Toxic Responses of the Respiratory System." Chap. 15 in *Casarett and Doull's Toxicology,* edited by C. Klaasen, M. Amdur, and J. Doull. New York: Pergamon Press, 1996.

Vallyathan, V., and X. Shi. "The Role of Oxygen Free Radicals in Occupational and Environmental Lung Disease." *Environmental Health Perspectives* 105 (Supplement 1) (1997): 165–177.

restaurants and cooks See COOKS; ERGONOMICS AND ERGONOMICS REGULATIONS; FOOD SERVICE INDUSTRY; HOT ENVIRONMENTS; SLIPS, TRIPS, AND FALLS.

retail   See VIOLENCE.

retirement   Retirement usually means that the individual is withdrawing from the work force of his or her own free will. It generally occurs when people are about age 65 (or older), but in times of economic problems due to DOWNSIZING, LAYOFFS, and MERGERS, it can occur earlier.

Retirement, highly desired by some, produces stresses, including ANXIETY, BOREDOM, and feelings of lack of productivity and loss of SELF-ESTEEM for others. Some retired people feel that they are not contributing members of society and become depressed and withdrawn. Some miss the identity and the prestige they formerly received from their position at work.

Those who adjust the best to retirement and experience the least stress seem to be the people who participate in new activities and make new acquaintances. Most retired people enjoy having more time for family and friends, for travel, for continuing their education, and for pursuing hobbies.

People who have planned ahead for their retirement generally start an interest or hobby before stopping work. For example, some individuals start to learn a musical instrument while others pursue a woodworking or sewing hobby. Many do volunteer work. In most of the big cities in the United States, there are "job corps" of senior citizens willing to donate their time and use their knowledge in business and industry.

Continuing education classes at local colleges and universities are targeted to retired people who enjoy learning. Many of these people participate in Elderhostel activities, where they travel to college campuses all over the world to study.

Retirement and Second Careers

Retirement is no longer a once-in-a-lifetime occurrence. Some individuals who retire go back to paid positions in an area in which they already have an expertise; some to an entirely different area. Researchers at the University of Southern California tracked 2,816 American men who turned 55 between 1966 and 1976. Approximately one-third went back to work for an average of two more years after they retired. Other significant findings indicated that the average American male retires between age 61 and 62, that white-collar workers stay on the job about two years longer than blue-collar workers, and that blue-collar workers spend an average of 10 years in retirement; white collar workers, 12.

Wives of retired men are sometimes affected by their mates' retirement. A study reported in *Modern Maturity* (December 1991–January 1992) indicated that most women polled reported satisfaction with their husbands' retirement. Effects of retirement on 413 upper-middle-class women married to men retired an average of 16 years were examined. More than one-third of the women had no problems with their husbands' retirement, and two-thirds said they were fully prepared for it. Only 12 percent said they felt stressed by some loss of personal freedom, and 5 percent to 6 percent reported an increase in household chores. Among those who said they would have done things differently, the majority mentioned the need to be better prepared financially for their later years.

Planning Ahead for Retirement

Relieving some of the stresses of retirement depends largely on preretirement planning and the retirement process itself. A variable in life satisfaction during retirement is socioeconomic status. According to the College of Family Physicians of Canada, those with middle and upper incomes report a higher degree of adaptation. In retirement, household income drops drastically, often by one-half to one-third. Many retirees experience poverty for the first time. Financial problems are the major reasons for stress and dissatisfaction with retirement.

Actual financial hardship may differ from perceived financial hardship. Strategies to cope with the stress of reduced income include expenditure reduction, rearrangement of assets, or continued activity in the labor force. Education is the most influential factor related to successful coping with reduced income.

In the early 2000s, many financial institutions and retirement funds suffered serious losses, causing retirement funds for many to diminish and cause concern for many anticipating retirement.

See also AGING; HARDINESS.

Dennis, Helen, and John Migliaccio. "Redefining Retirement: The Baby Boomer Challenge." *Generations: Journal of the American Society on Aging* 21, no. 2 (Summer 1997): 45.

Godin, Seth. *If You're Clueless About Retirement and Want to Know More.* Chicago: Dearborn Financial, 1997.

Manchester, Joyce. "Aging Boomers and Retirement: Who Is at Risk?" *Generations: Journal of the American Society on Aging* 21, no. 2 (Summer 1997): 19.

right sizing   See DOWNSIZING; LAYOFFS, MERGERS.

riveters   Workers who join together structural members, fixtures, parts of machines, or other items, by means of rivets. The terms *pneumatic tool worker* (any industry) and *air hammer operator* are synonymous with riveter. The occupation is common in machine-building, aerospace, automotive, garment, footwear, and other manufacturing industries and also in repair and servicing workshops. Riveters assemble parts of aircraft, missiles, space vehicles, and railroad cars using portable riveting, dimpling, and operation sheets. Riveters remove temporary bolts or fasteners and insert rivets in predrilled holes.

Riveters use vibrating tools, and the effect of VIBRATION on their body (hands, fingers, and so on) may be seriously harmful. Riveting is very noisy, which may badly affect their hearing and general health. Also, riveters may suffer eye injuries caused by flying pieces of metal. The work is usually physically hard and involves handling heavy loads, uncomfortable postures, and repetitive movements. This may cause trauma (including falls) and back, arm, and hand pains.

HAZARDS RELATED TO RIVETERS' WORK

Accident hazards
- Injuries as a result of carrying or lifting dies or riveting equipment
- Falls from ladders or scaffolding
- Burns on the skin from hot rivets
- Eye injuries from pieces of metal flying in the air, from drilling of dies, and from flying chips due to riveting operation
- Hand and finger injuries as a result of cuts and/or smashing of fingers in between dies

Physical hazards
- Exposure to high levels of noise during riveting process
- Exposure to excessive heat due to hot rivets
- Exposure to excessive whole body vibration from pneumatic riveting equipment

Chemical hazards
- Potential exposure to metal fumes from hot rivets

Ergonomic factors
- Back pain and other musculoskeletal problems as a result of overexertion and wrong postures due to lifting and carrying of equipment, bending, kneeling, pushing, and repetitive hand movements
- Segmental or hand-arm vibration leading to Raynaud's syndrome or vibration white finger, carpal tunnel syndrome, peripheral nerve damage, or debilitating joint injuries

---

PREVENTIVE MEASURES FOR RIVETERS AT WORK

Inspect ladder before climbing. Never climb on a shaky ladder or a ladder with slippery rungs.

Wear appropriate eye protection; consult a safety supervisor or a supplier.

Wear hearing protection appropriate for the noise levels and type of noise; consult the supplier or an expert.

Install air conditioning in premises to prevent heat stress and other adverse effects of heat.

Learn and use safe lifting and moving techniques for heavy or awkward loads; use mechanical aids to assist in lifting.

Use tools which reduce vibration strain by proper design of the mechanism. Use tools with vibration-absorbing handles.

See also CARPAL TUNNEL SYNDROME; ERGONOMICS; EYE INJURIES/PROTECTION; NOISE; REPETITIVE STRESS INJURIES; SLIPS, TRIPS, AND FALLS; VIBRATION WHITE FINGER.

robots, industrial   Programmable, multifunctional mechanical devices designed to move material, parts, tools, or specialized devices through variable programmed motions to perform a variety of tasks. Robots are generally used to perform unsafe, hazardous, highly repetitive, and unpleasant tasks. They have many different functions such as material handling, assembly, welding, machine tool load and unload functions, painting, spraying, and other uses.

According to the Occupational Safety and Health Administration, studies indicate that many robot accidents do not occur under normal operating conditions. They occur during programming, program touch-up or refinement, maintenance, repair, testing, setup, or adjustment. During many of these operations the operator, programmer, or corrective maintenance worker may temporarily be within the robot's working "envelope," where unintended operations may result in injuries.

See also Occupational Safety and Health Administration.

rocket propellants   See AEROSPACE MEDICINE.

rock musicians   See HEARING PROTECTION; NOISE; NOISE-INDUCED HEARING LOSS; PERFORMING ARTS MEDICINE.

Rolfing   One of many contemporary BODY THERAPIES used to relieve stress and improve emotional and physical health. A form of deep tissue massage, it is a combination of Eastern philosophical systems and practices and Western knowledge of muscular and skeletal structure. Some employee health programs refer employees for this therapy.

The technique, which is often combined with other body therapy techniques, was developed by Ida Rolf (1986–79), an American biochemist. As a young woman, she had an accident and was successfully treated by both an osteopathic physician and a yoga instructor. She combined these two techniques with the medical system of homeopathy, a practice that calls upon the patient's own healing powers rather than merely treating symptoms. The therapy gained recognition through Rolf's work at the Esalen Institute in California during the 1960s. Formerly considered fringe or one of many COMPLEMENTARY THERAPIES, rolfing and other body therapies entered the mainstream of mental and physical treatments in the late 1900s.

Rolfing focuses on the network of connective tissue—fascia, tendons, and ligaments—that contains the muscles and links them to the bones. Whenever connective tissue fails to work effectively, pain can result. For many, Rolfing helps to heal the body by bringing it into proper alignment and proper relationship to the forces of gravity. A Rolfing practitioner puts pressure on certain areas of the patient's connective tissue to improve the structure of the body. Certified Rolfers have had training in human anatomy, physiology, kinesiology, and various massage techniques.

Locating a Rolfing Therapist

The Rolf Institute, headquartered in Boulder, Colorado, has produced Rolfers since 1972. There are more than 600 practitioners across the United States and in 23 other countries. The institute provides a complete listing of its graduates, their addresses, and telephone numbers. The Institute also has a free pamphlet that lists books, videotapes, and audio-visual information currently available about Rolfing.

For information:

The Rolf Institute
205 Canyon Boulevard
Boulder, Colorado 80302
(800) 530-8875 (toll free)
(303) 449-5903
(303) 449-5978 (fax)
http://www.rolf.org

See also MASSAGE THERAPY.

Rolf, Ida P. *Rolfing: Reestablishing the Natural Alignment and Structural Integration of the Human Body for Vitality and Well Being.* Rochester, Vt.: Healing Arts Press, 1989.

roofing, siding, and sheet metal work   More than 25,000 roofing, siding, and sheet metal contractors employ approximately 300,000 workers for exterior construction work. These workers work on several types of structures, such as office buildings and houses.

According to author M. E. Personick, injury and illness rates for roofing and sheet metal work date back to the mid-1970s when the industry was one of five targeted for special study by the Occupational Safety and Health Administration (OSHA). Although roofing injury and illness rates have dropped slightly since then, compared with all construction, working in roofing remains relatively hazardous.

Falls, especially from rooftops, ladders, and other elevations, have been the leading category under type of accident or exposure. Overexertion (commonly resulting in sprains and strains from lifting objects) ranked second among major accident types, accounting for almost one-fourth of the roofing injury case total. Eye injuries were also common. Other major types of accidents included being struck by falling or flying objects and being splashed or burned by or contacting hot asphalt or coal tar.

Working conditions in these industries are monitored by OSHA and the National Institute for Occupational Safety and Health (NIOSH).

See also ASBESTOS; CONFINED SPACES; CONSTRUCTION; EYE INJURIES/PROTECTION; LADDERS; OCCUPATIONAL SAFETY AND HEALTH ADMINISTRATION; NATIONAL INSTITUTE FOR HEALTH AND SAFETY; SLIPS, TRIPS, AND FALLS.

Personick, Martin E. "Profiles in Safety and Health: Roofing and Sheet Metal Work." *Monthly Labor Review,* September 1990, pp. 27–32.

rotator cuff injuries The rotator cuff is a reinforcing structure around the shoulder joint composed of four muscle tendons that merge with the fibrous capsule enclosing the joint. The rotator cuff may be torn as the result of overuse or a fall. A partial tear may cause pain when the arm is lifted in a certain way from the body. A complete tear seriously limits the abilities to raise the arm.

These injuries are fairly common among professional athletes, particularly baseball pitchers, tennis players, and swimmers. However, they are also common in people whose jobs involve overhead lifting or reaching, such as carpenters and painters. Carrying something heavy or lifting, especially overhead lifting, can strain or tear tendons and muscles. Repeated overhead movement of the arms can stress the rotator cuff muscles and tendons, causing inflammation and, eventually, tearing. Falling on or breaking a fall with the arm can bruise or tear a rotator cuff's tendon or muscles.

See also SPORTS MEDICINE.

"Rotator Cuff Injuries." *Postgraduate Medicine Online* 104, no. 7, July 1998.

rubber products Rubber products such as automobile tires, automotive and appliance moldings, rubber bands, rubber gloves, and prophylactics are an integral part of modern life. However, according to the National Institute for Occupational Safety and Health (NIOSH), production of these items involves subjecting heterogeneous mixtures of hundreds of chemicals to heat, pressure, and catalytic action during a variety of manufacturing processes. As a result, the work environment may be contaminated with dusts, gases, vapors, fumes, and chemical by-products. Workers may be exposed to these hazards through inhalation and skin absorption during rubber processing and product manufacturing. Physical hazards such as noise, repetitive motion, and lifting are also common.

The rubber industry in 1989 employed approximately 54,600 U.S. workers in tire and inner tube production and 132,500 workers in the manufacture of nontire rubber products. (This is the most recent statistic available.)

Because the field is so diverse and the types of work are so varied, many types of injuries are common. According to the Rubber Industry Advisory Committee (RUBIAC) in England, manual handling resulting in sprain and strain injuries accounted for more than 40 percent of reported accidents in the industry in England. Many of these injuries lead to long-term disability and loss of earning capacity. To combat these injuries, RUBIAC recommends following the manual-handling guide published by RUBIAC, improved risk assessment of the basic requirements of health and safety, and accident investigation.

Historically, according to NIOSH, cancer has been the chronic disease most frequently reported in studies of rubber product workers. In the late 1940s British rubber workers were reported to be at increased risk of bladder cancer from exposure to a specific antioxidant. In the United States, investigations in 1968 revealed excess cancer deaths among a group of Ohio rubber products workers in 1938 and 1939. In 1970 the United Rubber, Cork, Linoleum, and Plastic Workers of America joined with six major American rubber companies to establish a joint occupational health program. A contract was negotiated with the schools of public health at Harvard University and the University of North Carolina to conduct epidemiological studies of rubber workers that emphasized cancer incidence and mortality. Many published and unpublished reports were produced as a result of these studies until the program was discontinued in 1980. The principal adverse health effects reported were cancer and respiratory effects such as reductions in pulmonary function, chest tightness, shortness of breath, and other respiratory symptoms.

According to NIOSH, currently the risks for cancer and other chronic diseases in rubber products workers are unknown because of the lack of substantial epidemiological and industrial hygiene research in the past decade. Toxicity data are also lacking for many chemical formulations found in tire and nontire manufacturing.

However, the U.S. Bureau of Labor Statistics (BLS) has included several categories of frequent injuries in its reports. "Disorders associated with repeated trauma is a broad BLS category that includes noise, hearing loss, synovitis, tenosynovitis, carpal tunnel syndrome, and other conditions resulting from repeated motion, vibration, or pressure." The overall incidence of injuries in 1991 was 80.5 cases per 10,000 fulltime workers, according to the BLS.

SAMPLE LIST OF RUBBER COMPOUNDING ADDITIVES WHICH MAY BE HAZARDOUS

Accelerators
Antioxidants
Antiozonants
Antitack agents
Chemical by-products
Curing fumes
Extenders
Fillers
Oils (process and extenders)
Organic vulcanizers
Pigment blends
Plasticizers
Reinforcing agents
Resins
Solvents

Source: National Institute of Safety and Health

Machinery accidents are a major cause of serious injuries to workers in the rubber industry, where in common with many other industries, much of the machinery used is extremely powerful, with the potential to inflect disfigurement or death. According to the RUBIAC, such accidents most commonly result in fractures and bruising of the hand, wrist, and arm, though in many cases far more serious injuries result. Estimates are that 40 percent of major injuries involve amputation.

Some design-related methods of prevention recommended by the RUBIAC include:

• Increasing the gap (trapping point) between adjacent conveyor systems
• Reducing the speed, pressure, and/or torque
• Easily identifiable emergency top buttons
• Clear operating controls
• Shrouding start buttons and pedals
• Avoid excessive noise, heat, and vibration to reduce stress on the operator
• Arranging for machines to be fed and cleaned automatically
• Providing fixed guards wherever possible, otherwise interlocking guards
• Use of pressure mats and photoelectric devices where fixed guards are not practical

NIOSH recommends that epidemiological toxicology and industrial hygiene studies are needed to assess the risk of cancer and other diseases from current occupational exposures. Detailed analyses of worker injuries are also needed to identify areas for training workers and other preventive measures. Results of future studies should be closely monitored to determine where recommendations to federal regulatory agencies should be developed for the rubber products manufacturing industry.

The Rubber Manufacturers Association (RMA) is the national trade association representing the U.S. tire and rubber products manufacturing industry, its suppliers, and manufacturers of a diverse array of finished rubber products, including industrial and automatic hoses and belts, automatic sealing systems, gaskets and oil seals, as well as industrial roll coverings, sheet rubber, roofing, flooring materials, and consumer products.

For information:

Rubber Manufacturers Association
Environmental Health and Safety Programs
1400 K Street, NW
Suite 900

Washington, DC 20005
(202) 682-4800
(202) 682-4854 (fax)
www.rma.org

For a copy of the Health Safety Committee's Rubber Advisory Committee's "Be On Your Guard—A Risk Assessment Approach to Machinery Safety in the Rubber Industry" contact:

HSE Books
P.O. Box 1999
Sudbury, Suffolk CO10 6FS
United Kingdom
017887 881165

See also HOT ENVIRONMENTS; LOCKOUT/TAGOUT; NOISE; SOLVENTS; VIBRATION (HAND/ARM).

S

safety Safety measures are the most effective ways of preventing injuries and illnesses in the workplace. A wide range of safety measures are employed, some general and some specific to certain industries and occupations.

General industry standards apply to manufacturing, wholesale, and retail businesses, as well as to work in any industry, including construction, maritime, and agriculture. Particular industry standards take priority over general safety standards. General safety measures include accident prevention, fire prevention, appropriate signage regarding use of materials and machines, use of personal protective equipment, protection against hot and cold environments, vehicle safety, protection against inhaling toxic substances, avoidance of alcohol use, and appropriate rest for workers.

Laws have been established to keep workplaces safe and to eliminate or reduce injuries and illnesses. These laws consist mainly of federal and state statutes; federal laws and regulations preempt state laws where they overlap or contradict one another. The Occupational Safety and Health Act is the main statute protecting the safety and health of workers. The act requires the U.S. secretary of labor to promulgate regulations and safety and health standards to protect employees and their families.

Safety in the workplace is necessary to prevent injuries to employees as well as to avoid incurring monetary penalties for failing to comply with federally mandated safety requirements. The NATIONAL INSTITUTE FOR OCCUPATIONAL SAFETY AND HEALTH (NIOSH) provide various types of consultation services to help employers comply with standards and set up safety and health programs.

Orient New Employees

New employees may be the most susceptible to injury during their first month at work. That is why basic safety training information should be provided to new employees as soon as possible. As a manager, take time to welcome them to the organization before assigning tasks. Walk them around the facility and introduce them to coworkers. Encourage experienced employees to help newer workers feel at ease.

New hires need to be made aware of how serious safety training is from the beginning. In your first meeting, reinforce the need for caution and appropriate protective equipment for each task. Emphasize that all unsafe conditions, accidents and near misses must be reported immoderately. Show them what equipment they can and cannot operate without authorization.

SAFETY BASICS TO REVIEW WITH NEW HIRES

Procedure to follow after an accident or injury
Location of emergency equipment and first-aid supplies
Reporting emergencies
Reporting accidents and near misses
Reporting a workers' compensation injury and file a claim
Location of material safety data sheets (MSDSs)
Use of personal protective equipment and how to care for it
Use of tools, machinery, or hazardous processes
Housekeeping and personal cleanup rules to follow

See also CONSTRUCTION; ERGONOMICS; FIRE SAFETY/FIRE PREVENTION; HAZARD COMMUNICATION; MATERIAL SAFETY DATA SHEETS; NATIONAL SAFETY COUNCIL; OCCUPATIONAL SAFETY AND HEALTH ADMINISTRATION; PERSONAL PROTECTIVE EQUIPMENT; SLIPS, TRIPS, AND FALLS; SOCIETY OF FIRE PROTECTION ENGINEERS; WORKERS' COMPENSATION.

safety glasses   See EYE INJURIES/PROTECTION; PERSONAL PROTECTIVE EQUIPMENT.

sales occupations   See CENSUS OF FATAL OCCUPATIONAL INJURIES.

"sandwich" generation   The so-called sandwich generation includes working people in midlife who have responsibilities for taking care of elderly parents as well as their own almost adult or adult children. Stresses abound because of the multiple and sometimes conflicting roles. Stressors include time constraints, living arrangements, and financial constraints, as many midlife couples are still working. Being in this situation often causes people to miss time from work or make many phone calls from the workplace just to keep their home situation going smoothly.

To improve such situations, open COMMUNICATION between all parties is essential. Young people need to realize that their concerns must be balanced with the concerns of the elderly, to reduce some of the stress on the middle generation. Those caught in the middle need to take time for themselves and their own interests. RELAXATION techniques can also be helpful.

See also DAY CARE; LISTENING; WORKING MOTHERS.

sanitarians   Workers in this job category may be sanitary inspectors, supervisors, pollution control technicians, environmental engineers, food and drug inspectors, public health inspectors, or other designations; sometimes exterminators or mosquito sprayers are referred to as sanitarians. The work of sanitarians may involve planning, developing, and executing environmental health programs, conducting training programs in environmental health practices for schools and other groups, setting health and sanitation standards and enforcing regulations concerned with food processing and serving, collection and disposal of solid wastes, sewage treatment and disposal, vector control, and other tasks.

Further, sanitarians may confer with community, industrial, government, and private organizations to promote environmental health programs, and collaborate with other health personnel in epidemiological investigations and control.

Because of the nature of their work, sanitarians face many health hazards. They may experience SLIPS, TRIPS, AND FALLS from ladders and elevated platforms during inspection visits in manufacturing plants or fall into open pits and manholes while inspecting water and sewage systems.

Poisoning is a hazard from gases such as sulfur dioxide and hydrogen sulfide during inspection and cleaning of sewage systems. Poisoning can also result from operation and handling of drinking water and swimming pool chlorination and bromination equipment and containers, or from use of various pesticides, insecticides, herbicides, fungicides, and other chemicals. Sanitarians may also experience skin disorders from working with these substances, or burns resulting from garbage-burning operations and from operating incinerators. They have a relatively high risk of being involved in road accidents as a result of extensive and frequent driving on all types of roads. They may experience electrical shock from work with electrical equipment, or be involved in fires or explosions caused by flammable and explosive substances such as SOLVENTS and gasoline.

Sanitarians are exposed to excessive NOISE in many situations, to ionizing and non-ionizing radiation, and to extreme climatic conditions while working in the field. Further, they are exposed to various microorganisms while working with liquid or solid waste, bites and stings by various insects, snakes, rodents during field and laboratory work, and they risk contracting infectious diseases while working in hospitals.

Finally, sanitarians may experience physical and or verbal assault while carrying out sanitary inspections.

See also AGGRESSION; ALLERGIES; ASBESTOS; BENZENE; CARBON MONOXIDE; DERMATITIS; FORMALDEHYDE; FUNGICIDES; CHEMICAL TOXICITY; HOSPITAL WORKERS; SKIN AND SENSE ORGAN TOXICITY.

Mager-Stillman, Jeanne, ed. *Encyclopedia of Occupational Health and Safety.* 4th ed. Vol. 4. Geneva: International Labour Organisation, 1998, p. 103.29–103.30.

sawmills   See LOGGING; PULP, PAPER, AND PAPERBOARD MILLS.

scaffolding According to the Occupational Safety and Health Administration (OSHA) an estimated 2.3 million CONSTRUCTION workers, or 65 percent of the construction industry, frequently work on scaffolds. Protecting these workers from scaffold-related accidents could prevent 4,500 injuries and 50 deaths every year, at a saving for American employers of $90 million in workdays not lost.

In a recent Bureau of Labor Statistics study, 72 percent of workers injured in scaffold accidents attributed the accident either to the planking or support giving way, or to the employee slipping or being struck by a falling object. OSHA reports that these accidents can be controlled by compliance with OSHA standards and following an effective safety and health program.

See also ELECTRICITY-RELATED INJURIES; LADDERS; PERSONAL PROTECTIVE EQUIPMENT; SLIPS, TRIPS, AND FALLS.

scuba diving See COMMERCIAL DIVING.

seasonal affective disorder (SAD) A form of mild depression resulting from not seeing much sunshine or daylight for months at a time. It is characterized by severe mood swings corresponding to the change of seasons. Depression usually becomes more prevalent during the winter months, and mood improves with the coming of spring. Some workers who seem lethargic or forgetful, or are late or absent, may suffer from SADs.

The incidence of SADs, which an estimated 35 million Americans suffer from, rises with geographic latitude, affecting only 1.4 percent of Floridians but almost 10 percent of the population of New Hampshire.

Role of Genetics

People who eat more, sleep more, and are more depressed during the winter months may have family members experiencing similar changes, according to an article in the *Archives of General Psychiatry* (January 1996). Researchers from Washington University School of Medicine surveyed 4,639 adult twins from Australia to determine if there is a biological predisposition to seasonal rhythms in mood and behavior (seasonality). Two types of seasonality were described: one characterized by a winter pattern and a second by a summer pattern of depressive mood disturbance. The researchers found that winter was much more likely than summer to provoke changes in mood, energy, social activity, sleep, appetite, and weight. They also found a "significant genetic influence" on those changes; 17 percent reported that they felt worse during the winter and eight percent reported that they experienced a summer pattern of worsening in mood.

Role of Light Therapy

Therapy for SADs includes use of specially made bright lights that extend the hours of illumination during short winter days and help reset the body's CIRCADIAN RHYTHMS. In some cases, medication and psychotherapy are useful.

See also PSYCHOTHERAPIES.

Anderson, Janis L., and Gabrielle I. Weiner. "Seasonal Depression." *Harvard Health Letter* 21, no. 4 (February 1996).

Madden, Pamela A. F. "Seasonal Changes in Mood and Behavior." *Archives of General Psychiatry,* January 1996.

Rae, Stephen. "Bright Light, Big Therapy." *Modern Maturity,* February–March 1994.

secondary depression Depression occurring in an individual who has another illness, either mental or physical, preceding the depression. For example, depression may accompany conditions such as obsessive-compulsive disorder, alcoholism and ALCOHOL DEPENDENCY (most common); depression may occur after or together with a medical illness. Careful evaluation of secondary depression by a physician is essential to determine the cause and course of treatment to help the individual recover. Referral to an EMPLOYEE ASSISTANCE PROGRAM is a good first step.

See also DEPRESSION; MENTAL HEALTH.

security guards See VIOLENCE.

self-esteem Accepting oneself, liking oneself, and appreciating one's self-worth. A high degree of self-esteem is a major characteristic of people who are successful on their jobs. Low self-esteem can lead to lateness, ABSENTEEISM, mental and physical disorders such as DEPRESSION, poor appetite, HEADACHES, insomnia, and in extreme cases, suicide.

Many people become stressed when they compare themselves with others or use their own unrealistic standards and standards set for them by others. Those who think they do not measure up have low self-esteem. In contrast, individuals with high self-esteem feel confident and capable. People with low self-esteem often become workaholics and depend on outside approval from others.

In a Gallup poll in 1992, 612 adults were interviewed and asked about situations that would make them feel very bad about themselves. Situations included losing a job, not being able to pay bills, being tempted into doing something immoral, having an abortion, getting a divorce, being noticeably overweight, doing something embarrassing in public, and being criticized by someone they admired. People over age 50 were more likely to feel bad about these situations than younger people.

See also CRITICISM; OBESITY; RELATIONSHIPS.

Hazelton, Deborah M. *Solving the Self-Esteem Puzzle.* Deerfield Beach, Fla.: Health Communications, 1991.
Hillman, Carolynn. *Recovery of Your Self-Esteem.* New York: Simon and Schuster, 1992.
Kahn, Ada P., and Sheila Kimmel. *Empower Yourself: Every Woman's Guide to Self-Esteem.* New York: Avon Books, 1997.

Self-Help for Hard of Hearing People (SHHH)

The largest international organization devoted to serving the interests of people with hearing loss through self-help, advocacy, and education. Founded in 1979, SHHH is a nonprofit membership association with more than 250 chapters throughout the United States. Publications include information on the Americans with Disabilities Act, employment, travel, hearing aids and cochlear implants, assistive listening devices, parenting, medical research, psychological stress, and telephone and television strategies. SHHH publishes *Hearing Loss: The Journal of Self-help for Hard of Hearing People.*

For information:

Self-Help for Hard of Hearing People
7910 Woodmont Avenue
Suite 1200
Bethesda, MD 20814
(301) 657-2248; 657-2249
(301) 913-9413 (fax)
www.shhh.org

See also AMERICANS WITH DISABILITIES ACT; BETTER HEARING INSTITUTE.

self-help groups The concept behind self-help groups is sharing feelings, perceptions, and concerns with others who have had or still have the same experience. A self-help group in the workplace may focus on alcoholism or dealing with aging parents. According to the American Medical Association, self-help groups typically exhibit the following characteristics and benefits:

Common problem: Members immediately identify with one another.
Mutual aid/helper therapy: Members benefit as much from giving help as from receiving it.
Network for support: Members provide a network of emotional and social support through regular and special gatherings, telephone calls, newsletters, visits, and computers.
Unconditional acceptance: Members are usually encouraged to share personal situations in a nonjudgmental, caring environment.
Shared information: Through the group process and written material, members capture and share their successful techniques for coping.
Low cost: Expenses are shared through collections at meetings, minimal membership dues, or fund-raising projects.

The self-help movement, with growing strength and visibility, has led to increased openness and understanding of many problems, such as ANXIETY DISORDERS and chronic illness. Such groups help many people develop better COPING skills to meet the challenges they face.

Self-Help Techniques

Self-help groups utilize group discussions as well as audio and video tapes. Self-help can work if the individual is motivated to make it work. In fact, even with psychotherapy, much of the improvement in a person's ability to cope with difficult situations actually comes from self-help.

Many individuals join SUPPORT GROUPS to learn self-help techniques for particular situations. These include MEDITATION and RELAXATION.

For further information:

National Self-Help Clearinghouse (NSHC)
365 Fifth Avenue
Suite 3300
New York NY 10016
(212) 817-1822
(212) 817-2290 (fax)
http://www.selfhelpweb.org

See also ANXIETY; COMPLEMENTARY THERAPIES; STRESS; WORKSITE WELLNESS PROGRAMS.

Selye, Hans   An Austrian-born Canadian endocrinologist and psychologist (1907–82), well known for his work in stress research. He introduced the concept of stress during the early 1940s. He is the author of *The Stress of Life* (1956) and *Stress without Distress* (1974).

He defined stress as "the nonspecific response of the body to any demand made upon it. It is more than merely nervous tension." He categorized more than 1,000 physiological occurrences related to stress and adaptation. His theory is a description of what people may expect with chronic exposure to stressors, and the body's attempts to adapt and return to its normal state.

In 1950, Selye coined the term GENERAL ADAPTATION SYNDROME (GAS). Selye borrowed the term *stress* from physics, and applied it to the mutual actions of forces that take place across any section of the body to threaten homeostasis. Although not all states of stress are harmful, according to Selye, he held that the more severe, protracted, and uncontrollable situations of psychological and physical distress led to disease states. His concept of GAS focused on the reaction of the body to illness or foreign substances as opposed to concentrating on specific illnesses and their treatment.

Although his work was controversial during his time, mental health disciplines profited from his groundbreaking work in stress research. His concept of stress opened new avenues of treatment through the discovery that hormones participate in the development of many degenerative diseases, including coronary thrombosis, hardening of the arteries, high blood pressure, arthritis, peptic ulcers, and even cancer.

Selye received his medical degree and his Ph.D. from the German University in Prague. He did most of his innovative research on the effects of stress in Montreal at McGill University and the Institut de Médicine et de Chirurgie Experimentales de l'Université de Montréal, of which he was director for many years. Selye earned doctorates in medicine, philosophy, and science, as well as at least 19 honorary degrees from universities around the world. He authored more than 32 books and more than 1,500 technical articles.

See also DIS-STRESS; EUSTRESS; STRESS; STRESS MANAGEMENT.

Selye, Hans. *The Stress of Life.* New York: McGraw-Hill, 1956.
———. *Stress without Distress.* Philadelphia: J. B. Lippincott Company, 1974.

semiconductor industry   The semiconductor industry is relatively new, having come into existence after 1960. Because of rapid changes in this industry, manufacturing processes and associated hazardous substances change frequently. This makes assessment of hazards difficult to keep current. Workers in this industry should be aware of the known hazards and the possibility of additional hazards, and use the best available measures to reduce these hazards. The Occupational Safety and Health Administration has not issued any standards specific to the semiconductor industry. The industry is regulated as a general industry and is subject to OSHA standards that address hazards found in specific workplaces.

See also OCCUPATIONAL SAFETY AND HEALTH ADMINISTRATION.

serotonin   A neurotransmitter found in the central nervous system, blood, nerve cells, and other tissues. Serotonin was identified during the 1950s as 5-hydroxytryptamine (5-HT). It is also known as hydroxytryptamine. Serotonin is involved in circuits that influence sleep and emotional arousal and is indirectly involved in the psychobiology of DEPRESSION. One theory suggests low levels of serotonin as a factor causing depression. Some antidepressant drugs increase the levels of serotonin, norepinephrine, and other neurotransmitters.

See also DEPRESSION; MENTAL HEALTH.

sexism   An attitude or belief that one sex is superior to the other in certain situations. The term often refers to male attitudes about women, such as "women in public office might cry if they are upset," or "a woman shouldn't be trained for a highly paying job because she will leave to have children." The women's liberation movement of the 1970s raised awareness of and fought to overcome sexism.

See also SEXUAL HARASSMENT.

sexual harassment   Unwelcome and unwanted sexual attention, usually in the workplace. The harassment may involve men toward women, women toward men, or people of the same sex; it may include jokes, remarks, and questions about the other's sexual behavior, "accidental" touching, and repeated and unwanted invitations for a date or for a sexual relationship. It can be verbal, visual, physical, or written.

Sexual harassment is defined in terms of its effect on the recipient. This means that behavior meant to be humorous or well-intentioned is sexual harassment if it is offensive to the individual at the receiving end. It is not the intent of the sender of the behavior that counts because what one person may view as harmless can be objectionable to others.

According to the Human Resource Department of Rush North Shore Medical Center, in Skokie, Illinois, 90 percent of harassment is stopped by a request from the victim. In 76 percent of cases where victims ignored the harassment, it continued. When propositioned, 67 percent of men are flattered and 83 percent of women are not. Equally important, 63 percent of women and 15 percent of men are insulted.

In the late 1990s, cases of sexual harassment in the military services were uncovered. Stresses arose when enlisted men and women felt obligated to follow requests of their superiors. Disciplinary charges in many cases led to discharges of those accused.

EXAMPLES OF SEXUAL HARASSMENT

- Dirty jokes or sexually oriented language
- Nude or seminude photos, posters, calendars or cartoons
- Obscene gestures, lewd actions, or leering
- Introduction of sexual topics into business conversations
- Requests for dates or sexual favors which are not mutually acceptable
- Unwelcome hugging, patting, or touching

SEXUAL HARASSMENT IN THE WORKPLACE: WHAT TO DO

- Tell the offender promptly and clearly that the conduct is unwelcome and unacceptable. Do this verbally, in writing, or both.
- Document in writing every incident, with specific details of the offensive behavior and your response.
- Do not feel guilty. Sexual harassment is not your fault. By clearly voicing your expectations, you force the offender to choose whether to change the unwelcome behavior, or to purposely continue it.
- If the problem continues, tell your supervisor. If your supervisor is the harasser, talk to another executive or report it to the department of human resources.

Sexual Harassment in the Federal Government: An Update. Washington, D.C.: U.S. Merit Systems Protection Board, June 1988.
"Sexual Harassment: What Am I Supposed to Do?" Skokie, Ill.: Rush North Shore Medical Center, 1995.

sharp injuries   See also HEALTH CARE WORKERS: HOSPITAL HAZARDS; NEEDLESTICK INJURIES AND PREVENTION.

sheep shearers   See CATTLE, SHEEP, AND GOAT WORKERS.

sheet metal   See ROOFING, SIDING, AND SHEET METAL WORK.

shell shock   See POST-TRAUMATIC STRESS DISORDER.

sheriffs/bailiffs   See POLICE VIOLENCE.

shiatsu   Shiatsu, a form of massage, is considered a COMPLEMENTARY THERAPY and may be useful for some individuals to prevent or relieve the effects of workplace stress. The technique is used by some massage therapists who visit workplaces.

According to practitioners, shiatsu is a specific method for manipulating *tsubos* (points along the meridians where the flow of energy may become blocked). The manipulation may occur through pressing with the fingers and hands, or through the use of elbows, knees, and feet. The points that are manipulated are known as acupressure or acupuncture points. Manipulation of the body's approximately 360 *tsubos* is thought to release the flow of energy (*chi*).

See also BODY THERAPIES; WORKSITE WELLNESS PROGRAMS.

McCarty, Patrick. *A Beginner's Guide to Shiatsu: Using Finger Pressure for the Relief of Headaches, Back Pain, and Hypertension.* Garden City Park, N.Y.: Avery Publishing Group, 1995.

shift work   Working a series of hours earlier or later in the day than the more usual 9 A.M. to 5 P.M. routine. Some work an afternoon shift, from 4 P.M. to 11 P.M.; others work at night shift, from 11 P.M. to 7 A.M. People who do shift work experience many unique stresses. How well people adapt to shift work depends on how well they handle the interruption of the body's CIRCADIAN RHYTHMS. The break in circadian rhythm can affect mental ability, alertness, and temperament. Thus some night shift workers experience anxiety and lapses in memory as a result of sleep deprivation.

Individuals who do shift work also suffer social stresses. For example, many people function on a 9 A.M. to 5 P.M. schedule, with most socialization occurring after work and on weekends. Night shift workers thus must schedule creatively. Spouses and children of shift workers also experience stress because of this schedule.

A study of 79,000 nurses published in *Circulation* indicated that those who worked irregular shifts for more than six years had a moderately higher risk of suffering a heart attack than did coworkers on regular shifts.

How Night Shift Workers Can Be More Productive

"The best strategy is to stay on one shift as long as possible. You'll have the best chance of getting restful sleep that way; you'll be more alert and potentially safer," says Rebecca Smith-Coggins, M.D., a Stanford University emergency medicine physician who studies what happens when people's sleep habits change.

"People who work random shifts in a 24-hour work environment suffer in their ability to perform specific physical tasks and to make decisions. Other studies have shown that when workers are shifted forward rather than randomly, they perform better and have fewer sick days. However, it still takes two weeks to get used to a night shift after a day shift," Smith-Coggins said.

Workers new to the night shift can help themselves adjust by knowing that they will not get a full six or eight hours' sleep in one stretch immediately. To help make the change, Smith-Coggins advises that new night workers take a three-hour nap before starting work, then sleep again after their shift. "Studies as well as our own experience among emergency department workers point to this double sleep pattern as the easiest ways to switch over," she says.

Eventually most shift workers will find themselves sleeping longer after they get home and napping less before they start work. Ultimately, a full "night's" sleep in the morning after working the night shift is possible.

Changing Work Shifts

For people who must change shifts, the healthiest approach seems to be to start the new shift later in the day. For example, it is easier on sleep and rest patterns to change from an eight-hour shift starting at 7 A.M. to one starting at 3 P.M. rather than the reverse. Moving forward is better because most humans operate on a 25-hour sleep-wake cycle. "Our body temperature and other natural functions rotate as if the day were 25 hours long. You can see how that works by studies that place people in darkened settings with no clues about time.

They develop a natural tendency to get up one hour later every day, a clear indication that we are on a forward rather than back or static cycle," Smith-Coggins explained.

Other ways for night workers to get more efficient rest include darkening the bedroom as much as possible or using a sleep mask. Ear plugs or so-called white noise, such as a humming sound from a fan or air conditioner, can help. It is also helpful to maintain the same bedtime rituals, such as relaxing with a book or television show, particularly if the material is not unsettling.

See also SLEEP.

Smith-Coggins, Rebecca. "Night Shifts Can Be Easier." *Circulation,* December 1, 1995.
Hurley, Margaret, and Elizabeth A. Neidlinger. "To Shift of Not to Shift." *Schumpert Medical Quarterly* 9, no. 2 (October 1991).

shipbuilding and repair   This industry includes the manufacture, repair, and maintenance of ships. Several types of hazards are common in this industry, including chemical (asbestos, welding fumes, solvents, paints, fumes), physical (noise, heat stress), safety (fire, confined spaces, falls, heavy equipment), as well as others.

According to the U.S. Department of Labor, shipyard work has traditionally been hazardous, with an injury-accident rate more than twice that of construction and general industry. Related processes include dry docking and launching, surface preparation and descaling, and tank cleaning.

See also ASBESTOS; CONFINED SPACES; MESOTHELIOMA; HOT ENVIRONMENTS; PERSONAL PROTECTIVE EQUIPMENT; SLIPS, TRIPS AND FALLS; SOLVENTS; WELDING.

shock rescue procedures   See ELECTRICITY-RELATED INJURIES.

short term psychotherapy   See DEPRESSION; MENTAL HEALTH; PSYCHOTHERAPIES.

sick building syndrome   Illnesses caused by working or living in modern buildings. Symptoms may be caused by air-conditioning systems, fluo-

rescent lighting, and not enough ventilation. Modern buildings are tighter in construction and depend on air circulators, as opposed to outside air from windows, for ventilation. A contemporary personal and societal source of stress, "sick building syndrome" was once known as "building-related illness." Symptoms may include HEADACHES, itchy eyes, nose, and throat, dry cough, diminished mental acuity, sensitivity to odor, and tiredness.

Additionally, stressful symptoms may be caused by the FRUSTRATION of feeling closed in and not being able to control the amount of heat or light in the immediate environment. Thus the stress of the syndrome is also related to feelings of lack of personal CONTROL.

A ripple effect sometimes occurs when one employee in such a building begins complaining of illness. Soon others believe that they, too, have headaches as a result of the workplace. An outbreak of Legionnaire's disease, a form of pneumonia, from bacteria in the air conditioning system was first identified among American Legion conventioneers in a Philadelphia hotel during the 1970s, and outbreaks of Legionnaire's disease occurred as recently as 1995. Organisms responsible for the disease as a contaminant of water systems had been responsible for earlier epidemics of pneumonia, although the cause had not been known.

The influence of sick building syndrome as a source of employee stress was recognized on a large scale when complaints of sick building syndrome to the U.S. Occupational Safety and Health Administration (OSHA) doubled between 1980 and 1981. Recognized by insurance industry under the name "tight building syndrome," Fireman's Fund Insurance Company established its own "tight building syndrome" laboratory in late 1983, after investigating 48 buildings in the United States and discovering that about one-third presented health hazards from indoor air pollution.

Relief from Sick Building Syndrome

Individuals who believe they are being made ill by their building should consult their department of human resources. Reports should be filed in a timely way so that investigations can be made. Removal of the pollutant, if possible, is essential.

There may be possibilities to improve air balance and adjustment, including percentage of outside air being circulated. All humidifiers, filters, and drip pans must be checked. Overall maintenance of the building should be evaluated, and cleaning materials, air fresheners, and moth repellents should be selected carefully. New carpeting should be installed on a Friday, allowing ventilation of the building over the weekend.

Additionally, individuals should determine if there are any possible steps they can take to relieve their symptoms. These may include moving to another part of the building or bringing a small electric fan or heater to work. If necessary, a short vacation away from the pollutants may be helpful.

For information:

National Safe Workplace Institute (NSWI)
P.O. Box 2481
Monroe, NC 28111
(704) 282-1111
(704) 550-5857 (fax)
www.safespaces.com

See also ALLERGIES; INDOOR ENVIRONMENT.

Griffin, Katherine. "When Your Office Calls in Sick." *Health*, January/February 1993.

silica See SILICOSIS.

silicosis A disabling, nonreversible, and sometimes fatal lung disease caused by overexposure to respirable crystalline silica. More than 1 million U.S. workers are exposed to crystalline silica, and each year more than 250 die from silicosis.

Sandblasters and exposed coworkers are particularly at risk. The silica sand used in abrasive blasting typically fractures into fine particles and becomes airborne. Inhalation of such silica appears to produce a more severe lung reaction than silica that is not freshly fractured. This factor may contribute to the development of acute and accelerated forms of silicosis among sandblasters.

According the U.S. Department of Labor, there is no cure for the disease but it is preventable if employers, workers, and health professionals work together to reduce exposures.

Workers may develop any one of three types of silicosis:

- Chronic silicosis, which usually occurs after 10 or more years of exposure to crystalline silica at relatively low concentrations

- Accelerated silicosis, which results from exposure to high concentrations of crystalline silica and develops five to 10 years after the initial exposure

- Acute silicosis, which occurs where exposure concentrations are the highest and can cause symptoms to develop within a few weeks to four or five years after the initial exposure

Acute silicosis is less common today than it was in the 1930s because engineering controls are used to reduce exposure to respirable crystalline silica and because the use of alternative abrasives is increasing.

Silicosis (especially the acute form) is characterized by shortness of breath, fever, and cyanosis (bluish skin); it may often be misdiagnosed as pulmonary edema (fluid in the lungs), pneumonia, or tuberculosis.

See also BLACK LUNG DISEASE; CONSTRUCTION; PERSONAL PROTECTIVE EQUIPMENT.

single (specific) phobia An intense, irrational fear that persists and compels one to avoid one specific situation or object. Almost any situation or object, such as heights, bridges, dogs, or cats can become a specific phobia. A specific phobia can be a hindrance in the workplace, particularly if it involves taking elevators, escalators, being on a high floor, or using particular kinds of machinery. This kind of fear is an intense source of suffering for the individual. Help can be obtained with BEHAVIOR THERAPY.

See also ANXIETY DISORDERS; MENTAL HEALTH; PHOBIAS.

skin cancer See CANCER; CARCINOGENS; SKIN OR SENSE ORGAN TOXICITY.

skin diseases/disorders/infections See DERMATITIS.

skin or sense organ toxicity   Adverse effects on the skin or sense organs that result from exposure to chemical substances. The senses of smell, vision, hearing, and taste are referred to as the special senses. Sense organs may be injured by a variety of physical, chemical, and biological agents. The sense of smell can become impaired, for example, as a result of occupational exposure to the metals CAD-MIUM and nickel. A variety of chemicals that act both locally and systemically in the body can affect vision. Airborne chemicals such as inorganic irritant gases and vapors (AMMONIA, CHLORINE GAS, hydrogen sulfide, and sulfur dioxide), FORMALDE-HYDE, and many organic solvents can cause external eye irritation, including conjunctivitis and keratitis, in some cases reducing visual acuity. Chemical substances can also induce auditory dysfunction. Occupational exposure to lead, for example, is associated with hearing loss.

The skin provides the body with a protective barrier, contains the nerves that support the sense of touch, and participates in the exchange of gases and liquids. When the skin is exposed to irritant compounds, symptoms of skin injury may occur; redness, inflammation, burning, and itching. Acute and chronic skin diseases and conditions that may result from contact with toxic agents include DER-MATITIS, PHOTOSENSITIZATION, CHLORACNE, urticaria, and CANCER.

One of the most common chemically induced skin disorders is contact dermatitis, an inflammatory reaction of the skin that is usually restricted to the exposed areas. Clinical signs may include reddening, edema, itching, or a burning sensation. Strongly alkaline and acidic substances, such as sodium hydroxide, sulfuric acid, and hydrofluoric acid, are some of the irritants that can cause contact dermatitis and related disorders.

A number of skin toxicants produce photosensitization, an abnormal reaction to ultraviolet and/or visible radiation. Known photosensitizers include anthraquinone dyes, sulfanilamide, and COAL TAR derivatives (anthracene, pyridine, acridine, and phenanthrene). Chloracne is a severe and unusual form of acne that can be triggered by exposure to certain halogenated aromatic compounds, such as polychlorinated dibenzo furans and dioxins. Addi-tionally, ARSENIC, coal tars, creosote oils and ultraviolet light have been shown to induce skin cancer.

Emmett, E. A. "Toxic Responses of the Skin." Chap. 15 in *Casarett and Doull's Toxicology,* edited by C. Klaasen, M. Amdur, and J. Doull. New York: Pergamon Press, 1996.

Potts, A. "Toxic Responses of the Eye." Chap. 17 in *Casarett and Doull's Toxicology,* edited by C. Klaasen, M. Amdur, and J. Doull. New York: Pergamon Press, 1996.

@2001 Environmental Defense. Used by permission. www.scorecord.org

slaughterhouses   See BUTCHERS AND MEAT, POUL-TRY, AND FISH CUTTERS.

sleep   Recurring periods of relative physical and psychological disengagement from one's environment. Sleep is a necessary activity that provides a restorative function. Lack of adequate sleep may make one feel nervous and jumpy, affect judgment and decision-making abilities, slow reaction times, reduce on-the-job efficiency and productivity, and contribute to accidents. Nodding off at work is not just unproductive; in the worst cases, it can cause serious industrial accidents. The 1989 *Exxon Valdez* Alaskan oil spill, for example, was reportedly due at least in part to the severe fatigue of the tanker's sleep-deprived third mate.

During sleep, daily bodily functions such as digestion and waste removal have a chance to rest and recharge. An evolutionary theory regarding sleep suggests that sleep originally allowed humans and other diurnal animals to conserve energy during the dark hours, when it was less practical to hunt for food and harder to escape from danger.

The average adult needs about eight hours of sleep per 24 hours; the need for sleep seems to decrease as the person ages. Individual sleep patterns vary. An average person may go through a sleep cycle about four to six times each night. A sleep cycle consists of stages (known as Stages I, II, III, and IV) in a cycle lasting about 90 minutes, followed by a period of rapid-eye-movement (REM) sleep for about 10 minutes. With each cycle, REM periods lengthen. During the last cycle, REM sleep may continue for 30 to 60 minutes. Dreaming is most likely to occur during REM sleep. This period is characterized by extensive muscular inhibition; most of the voluntary muscles in the body take on a paralyzed state and there are bursts of rapid movements of the eye, under the closed eyelid.

"People don't respect sleep enough," according to Daniel O'Hearn, a sleep disorders specialist at Johns Hopkins University. "They feel they can do more—have more time for work and family—by allowing themselves less time for sleep. But they do sleep; they sleep at work, or driving to work."

Aside from people with an unintentional inability to sleep, millions more Americans undersleep by choice, burning the candle at both ends because of work and family schedules. Recent surveys show that American sleep seven hours each night on average, down from nine hours in 1910 when, without electricity, people generally went to sleep as darkness fell.

Falling Asleep at the Wheel

The National Highway Traffic Safety Administration estimates that more than 200,000 crashes each year involve drivers falling asleep at the wheel, and thousands of Americans die in such accidents annually. Some of these accidents are caused by drivers suffering from sleep deprivation brought about by lack of sleep or by sleep apnea. Sleep apnea is a condition characterized by brief periods of ceasing to breathe. There may be at least 250,000 people in the United States who cease breathing so often or for such long periods of time at night that they are tired all day and are likely to drift off into sleep at any moment. Sleep apnea causes snoring. A diagnosis of sleep apnea can be made from a tape recording at the bedside of the snorer.

Ongoing research may result in inventions that can reduce the problem of sleepy truck drivers and other motorists. Australian researchers are developing a cap to be worn by drivers that reads brain waves and warns drivers when they are about to fall asleep. For tractor trailers, "black boxes," or onboard computers, could be programmed to warn drivers of fatigue, drowsiness, or approaching danger. A black box similar to that used in airplanes might track miles driven and rest stops made by long distance truck drivers.

**BE MORE PRODUCTIVE AT WORK:
GET A GOOD NIGHT'S SLEEP**

It takes most people about 15 minutes or less to fall asleep. If you have trouble getting to sleep and staying asleep long enough to feel good throughout the workday, try some of these suggestions:

- Try not to think about work you left undone. If you brought work home, do not do it just before going to bed.
- Drink a cup of warm milk before bedtime. Eat a light snack. Avoid stimulating beverages that contain caffeine, such as coffee, cola beverages, and chocolate.
- Take a warm, relaxing bath.
- Relax in bed and read something you enjoy, not work-related material. As your mind becomes engrossed, your muscles will relax. When your body is relaxed, you are likelier to become sleepy and ready for sleep. Watching television may have the same effect.
- Read something you find very dull. When your mind cannot handle what you present, your internal coping mechanism of falling asleep may take over. Watching television may have the same effect.
- Experiment by changing your environment. Make the room warmer or colder. Use different combinations of covers. Some people like the weight of many blankets, while others do not. If you like warmth without weight, use an electric blanket. Some have dual controls so that each bed partner can have individual arrangements.
- Avoid stressful situations before bedtime. Postpone discussions of work or personal problems until morning, whenever possible. Avoid lengthy telephone conversations, particularly about work, that may upset you before bedtime.
- If you have an argument or tension-filled discussion late at night, do not go to bed mad.
- If you are alone and feel hostile, call a friend and talk. Venting may help you unload and you will sleep better.
- Avoid using sleeping pills. People build up a tolerance to them and some have daytime hypnotic effects. Some pills induce sleep apnea.
- If you must take a sleeping pill during times of extreme stress, such as after the death of a loved one, after surgery, or during extreme jet lag, take short-acting sleeping medications.
- Nightly use of a sleeping medication may not be effective after a while. If you have to use them at all, use them only every other night, or every third night.
- Avoid taking naps during the day; go to bed a little later each night.

See also RELAXATION; SHIFT WORK; STRESS.

Kahn, Ada P., and Jan Fawcett. *Encyclopedia of Mental Health.* 2d ed. New York: Facts On File, Inc., 2001.

slips, trips, and falls   Possibly the single most common cause of injuries in the workplace, particularly in the manufacturing and service industries. More than a third of all nonfatal injuries reported each year are caused as a result of a slip, trip, or fall, either on level ground or from a height. These events are costly to employers in lost production and other costs.

Employers can help reduce slip-and-trip hazards through good safety arrangements. A good system will help workers identify problem areas, decide what to do, act on decisions made, and check that steps taken have been effective.

Slip-and-Trip Risks

Look for slip-and-trip hazards around the workplace such as uneven floors, trailing cables, and areas that are sometimes slippery due to spills (including outdoor areas). This is particularly important in the food service industry, in food processing plants, and in the meat industry. Determine who might be harmed and how. Know who comes into the workplace. Consider the risks and determine if the precautions already taken are enough to deal with the

risks. Record findings and regularly review the assessment. If any significant changes take place, make sure the precautions are still adequate to deal with the risks. Consider employees who work off-site. Look at hazards and risks they may encounter; provide proper training and equipment.

Maintenance: Preventing Slips and Falls

Maintenance should be done regularly. Maintenance includes inspection, testing, adjustment, and cleaning. Records should be kept so that the routine can be checked. Lighting should enable people to see obstructions and potentially slippery areas so they can work safely. Replace, repair, or clean lights before levels become too low for safe work. Floors should be checked for loose finishes, holes, and cracks, worn rugs and mats, and the like. Obstructions and objects left lying around can easily go unnoticed and cause a trip. Keep work areas tidy, and if obstructions cannot be removed, warn people using signs or barriers. Footwear can play an important part in preventing slips and trips.

When conditions are optimal, preventing slips and falls will be easier. Employers should be sure to use only suitable floor surfaces, provide adequate lighting levels, and plan pedestrian and traffic routes to avoid overcrowding. All work areas, pas-

REDUCE RISK OF SLIPS, TRIPS, AND FALLS	
Hazard/Risk Factor	**Precaution**
Spillage of wet and dry substances	Clean spills up immediately. If a liquid is greasy, be sure to use a suitable cleaning agent.
Trailing cables	Position equipment to avoid cables crossing pedestrian routes; use cable covers to securely fix to surfaces; restrict access to prevent contact.
Miscellaneous rubbish, such as plastic bags	Keep areas clear; remove rubbish. Do not allow it to build up.
Rugs/mats	Be sure mats are securely fixed and do not have curling edges.
Slippery surfaces	Assess the cause and treat accordingly.
Changing from wet to dry floor surfaces	Wear suitable footwear; warm employees of risks by using signs; locate doormats where these changes are likely.
Poor lighting	Improve lighting levels and placement of light fixtures to assure more even lighting of all floor areas.
Changes of level	Improve lighting; and appropriate floor treads.
Slopes	Improve visibility; provide hand rails, use floor markings.
Smoke/steam obscuring view	Eliminate or control by redirecting it away from risk area; improve ventilation and provide warnings.
Unsuitable footwear	Be sure workers choose suitable footwear, particularly with the correct type of sole.

sageways, staircases, and means of access must be unobstructed and free from tripping hazards. Stock must be properly stored and not left on floors; waste must not be allowed to accumulate and must be properly disposed of. Workers should be trained in the correct use of any safety and cleaning equipment provided. Cleaning methods and equipment must be suitable for the type of surface being treated. Care should be taken not to create additional slip-or-trip hazards while cleaning and maintenance work is being done. Notices and barriers must be used to prevent unauthorized persons from entering areas being cleaned or where spills have occurred. Openings in floors, on edges of balconies, platforms, or mezzanines must be adequately fenced to prevent falls. Temporary openings must be fenced and appropriate signs used to make people aware of their location. Ladders and scaffolding must be of suitable for their intended use and must be properly erected, made secure, and checked before access, if permitted. High openings must be securely fenced when not in use and adequate handrails must be provided at either side when goods are being raised or lowered. Access to high storage must be from suitable steps, and shelving should never be used for climbing.

See also BUTCHERS AND MEAT, POULTRY, AND FISH CUTTERS; CONSTRUCTION; FOOT PROTECTION.

smoking   Inhaling and exhaling smoke by using cigarettes, cigars, and pipes. A major public health problem in the United States, smoking is a source of stress for nonsmokers as well as smokers. Only in the late 1990s did cigarette companies reluctantly admit that the nicotine contained in cigarettes is habit-forming and addictive. Many smokers say they want to quit but cannot.

Smoking became a major workplace issue during the 1990s when many areas and sometimes whole buildings were designated as nonsmoking areas.

Effects of Smoking

Nicotine affects the central nervous system through routes that differ from other drugs but it produces very similar results, such as euphoria, dependency, and withdrawal symptoms when stopped suddenly. Smokers who quit may experience genuine physical discomfort and cravings. Withdrawal symptoms

from nicotine include HEADACHES, irritability, upset stomach, breathing and circulation problems, trouble sleeping, dizziness, and numbness.

The actual physiological effects of smoking are somewhat at odds with the sensations that smokers report. When nicotine enters the bloodstream, it raises the heart rate, blood pressure, and dilates the arteries. It also raises the level of glucose in the blood. However, smokers report a sense of relief from stress despite the stimulating effects of nicotine. Smokers claim it improves short-term memory, intellectual performance, and concentration.

While most smokers do not resort to deviant behaviors to maintain their habit, participants in the Stop Smoking Clinics in Evanston, Illinois, admitted going through ashtrays, garbage cans, and gutters looking for butts that may still have a salvageable few puffs if their own supplies are depleted. These recovered smokers are repulsed to think that they ever performed such acts.

Conflicts between Smokers and Nonsmokers

While scientists have documented harmful effects of smoking, many smokers still believe that it is their right to smoke when and where they want to. Antismoking laws were enacted in the United States during the 1980s and early 1990s, and there have been occasional incidents of anger and hostility between smokers and nonsmokers. Nonsmokers maintain they have a right to clean air. Increasingly, workplaces are becoming entirely smoke-free and are designating outdoor smoking areas. In the large cities of America, most restaurants have nonsmoking areas. For asthmatics and those with other respiratory disorders, smoke in the air is more than an annoyance; being forced to breathe secondhand smoke can make them physically ill.

Eventually the United States may become a smokeless society. However, in many developing-world countries, the numbers of smokers are unfortunately increasing and cigarette consumption is rising.

Consequences of Smoking

The main harmful components of cigarette smoke are tar, nicotine, and carbon monoxide. The lungs retain 70 percent to 90 percent of these chemicals after inhalation. Tarry substances clog the lungs and affect breathing. Carbon monoxide decreases the ability of red blood cells to carry oxygen throughout the body.

Smoking lowers the resistance to infection and ulcerative diseases. It also increases the risk of bad breath, severe gum diseases, tooth loss, and premature aging of the skin. Pregnant women who smoke have higher rates of miscarriage, stillbirth, premature birth, and complications of pregnancy, and have a greater chance of bearing a low-birth-weight baby. Smoking is credited as a factor in nearly 500,000 deaths per year, representing more Americans than die from accidents, infectious diseases, murders, suicides, diabetes, and cirrhosis combined.

The disease most often associated with cigarette smoking is lung cancer. This disease, which as recently as the 1950s was almost unheard of, is now the leading cause of cancer deaths in men and women. Lung cancer, once believed to be predominantly a disease of males, in the mid-1980s overtook breast cancer to become the number one cause of cancer deaths for women. More than 85 percent of those who die of lung cancer could have avoided the disease completely if they did not smoke. For this reason, coping with their deaths may be doubly stressful for their family members.

ENCOURAGEMENT FOR THOSE WHO ARE QUITTING SMOKING

- List your reasons for wanting to stop and wanting to continue smoking.
- Note when and where you smoke the most.
- Set a date for quitting; tell your family and friends.
- Remove cigarettes, ashtrays, and matches from your home, car, and workplace.
- Minimize stressful situations and other occasions where you might crave a cigarette.
- Spend time where smoking is prohibited.
- Reach for high-fiber, low-calorie snacks, such as vegetables or fruits when you have the urge to smoke.
- Talk to someone who is supportive until the urge to smoke passes.
- Increase aerobic exercise such as walking or biking.
- Use relaxation techniques such as meditation or guided imagery.
- Reward yourself for quitting smoking.

Stop Smoking Programs for Employees

Many stop-smoking programs exist to help cigarette addicts. However, for programs to be helpful,

individuals must attend regularly and follow the rules. For many, unfortunately, this is easier said than done. When one stops smoking, nicotine dependency may cause some unpleasant sensations. For example, one may temporarily experience withdrawal symptoms such as DEPRESSION, irritability, anxiety, restlessness, trouble concentrating, headache, drowsiness, gastrointestinal disturbances, increased coughing, or difficulty sleeping. All these factors can affect an employee's productivity in the workplace.

For information:

American Cancer Society
1599 Clifton Road, NE
Atlanta GA 30329
(800) 227-2345
(404) 315-9348 (fax)
www.cancer.org

American Heart Association (AHA)
7272 Greenville Avenue
Dallas, TX 75231-4596
(800) 242-USA1 (toll-free)
(214) 373-6300
(214) 987-4334 (fax)
www.americanheart.org

American Lung Association
1740 Broadway
New York, NY 10019
(800) LUNGUSA (toll-free)
(212) 315-8700
(212) 315-8872 (fax)
www.lungusa.org

National Cancer Institute (NCI)
NCI Public Inquiries Office
Suite 3036A
6116 Executive Boulevard
MSC 8322
Bethesda, MD 20892-8322
(301) 435-3848
www.nci.nih.gov

See also ADDICTIONS; CANCER; EMPHYSEMA; EMPLOYEE ASSISTANCE PROGRAMS; WORKSITE WELLNESS PROGRAMS.

Hammond, S. Katharine. "Environmental Tobacco Smoke Presents Substantial Risk in Workplaces." *The Journal of the American Medical Association,* September 26, 1995.

Spitzer, Joel. "Medical Implications of Smoking," Evanston Department of Health, Evanston, Illinois, 2002.

soccer injuries (professional)   Injuries sustained during professional soccer games can be severe. Some are incurred by head banging with an opponent while trying to get to the ball, sometimes resulting in a concussion. Soccer players can also break noses, cheekbones, or jaws from clashing in the air over the ball. Knocking heads can also cause cuts and bruises.

The repeated trauma from heading the ball may lead to subtle brain damage similar to that seen in boxers. According to a study of former Norwegian soccer players, 30 percent showed signs of minor brain damage, including headaches, dizziness, and neck pains. A player can head the ball several thousand times in a season. The Norwegian players averaged more than 5,000 headers per season over their 15-year careers.

Other injuries from soccer include "soccer shoulder" (dislocated shoulder), pulled leg muscles, knee injuries, broken and bruised legs, Achilles tendon ruptures, and ankle sprains. Soccer played on an artificial surface can lead to a sprained big toe, or turf toe, due to the stress of running on a hard surface.

Goalie Injuries

Goalies have problems peculiar to their position. When diving to stop shots, goalies often land on their hips and suffer cuts, scrapes, and bruises over the hipbones. Because they dive so often, goalies have much higher incidence of partial and full shoulder dislocations. They also dislocate and break fingers from the impact of the ball coming at them at high speed. Landing on the point of the elbow can leave a goalie with "Popeye elbow," a form of bursitis that causes little knobs to swell up behind the elbow.

See also BURSITIS; SPORTS MEDICINE; SPRAINS.

social phobia   Irrational fear and avoidance of being in a situation in which one's activities can be observed by others. It involves a fear of being embarrassed, humiliated, criticized, censured, or in some way evaluated in social settings. The most common social phobia is fear of speaking in public, whether in front of a large audience or in front of a small group, such as during a party. Other common social phobias include blushing, eating, drinking, writing, urinating, or vomiting in the presence of others. Some social phobics fear that their hands will tremble or shake as they eat or write and tend to avoid restaurants, banks, and other public places. They often avert their eyes when talking to another person. Some social phobics have been known to cross the street to avoid greeting people they know, and social phobics are fearful of attending parties, particularly with people they do not know. Holding a job in a workplace is difficult for a socially phobic person for these reasons.

Usually social phobias begin after puberty and peak after the age of 30 but social phobics have had lifelong shyness and introverted habits. Both men and women suffer from social phobias and may have more than one at a time. Also, many agoraphobics have social phobias, and many social phobics have some agoraphobic symptoms.

See also ANXIETY DISORDERS; MENTAL HEALTH; PHOBIAS; STRESS.

Kahn, Ada P., and Jan Fawcett. *Encyclopedia of Mental Health.* 2d ed. New York: Facts On File, Inc., 2001.

Kahn, Ada P., and Ronald M. Doctor. *Facing Fears: The Sourcebook for Phobias, Fears, and Anxieties.* New York: Checkmark Books, 2000.

Marshall, John R. *Social Phobia: From Shyness to Stage Fright.* New York: Basic Books, 1994.

social support system   An individual's relationships with others, including coworkers, significant others, friends, as well as material resources. An individual with a mental health concern may have an inadequate social support system because others do not understand his/her circumstances and thus may not offer the assistance or encouragement that could be helpful.

Individuals with good social support systems seem to have better work attendance records and better recoveries from illness and surgeries than those without such support.

See also SELF-HELP GROUPS; SUPPORT GROUPS.

social workers Social workers have been major providers of mental health services since the early 1920s, when they were an integral part of the beginning of the child guidance movement. Social workers are trained to have expertise concerning community resources available for various types of support and therapy, as well as to intervene when the individual and the environment, such as the workplace, do not mesh smoothly, causing discomfort or disruption for the individual, workplace, or family.

Social workers work in the public and private sectors; many work in publicly funded health and mental health clinics and in schools, family agencies, clinics, hospitals, and private practice. Some work in EMPLOYEE ASSISTANCE PROGRAMS (EAPs), and alcohol and chemical dependency programs.

For information:

National Association of Social Workers (NASW)
750 First Street, NE
Suite 700
Washington, DC 20002-4241
(800) 638-8799
(202) 408-8600
(202) 336-8312 (fax)
http://naswdc.org

See also MENTAL HEALTH; PSYCHOTHERAPIES.

Manderscheid, R. W., and M. A. Sonnenschein, eds. *Mental Health, United States, 1990.* Washington, D.C.: Supt. of Docs., U.S. Govt. Printing Office, National Institute of Mental Health. DHHS Pub. No. (ADM) 90-1708, 1990.

Society for Chemical Hazards Communication (SCHC) A professional society of individuals engaged in the business of designing, preparing, distributing, and evaluating labels and MATERIAL SAFETY DATA SHEETS (MSDSs) for hazardous chemicals. The SCHC has compiled and posted a list of references that can be used in the preparation of HAZARD COMMUNICATION documents.

See also CHEMICAL TOXICITY.

Society of Fire Protection Engineers (SFPE) An international professional organization, the SFPE seeks to advance the level of fire safety for the protection of life and property through the application of sound engineering principles and to encourage related disciplines to apply these principles. SFPE provides a source of specialized knowledge in fire protection engineering, how the profession interacts with allied disciplines, and how to gain recognition for work in the field of fire safety.

For information:

Society of Fire Protection Engineers (SFPE)
7315 Wisconsin Avenue
Suite 1225W
Bethesda, MD 20814
(301) 718-2910
(301) 718-2241 (fax)
www.sfpe.org

See also FIRE SAFETY/FIRE PROTECTION; SAFETY.

soft drink industry See BOTTLING INDUSTRY.

solderers/braziers Workers who join metal parts by means of a fusible alloy. Manual soldering processes include electric-iron, glass-flame, torch, chemical cartridge, and gas-heated iron soldering. Solderers work in electrical and electronic manufacturing, dental laboratories, air conditioning and refrigeration, and radiator manufacturing and repair, and may repair storage tanks and containers, gas and chemical supply lines, or artwork.

Hazards at work for solderers include being hit by falling pipe and other work pieces, and cuts and stabs, particularly on the fingers, from sharp edges or protrusions during the preparation of work for soldering and during the cleaning of the soldered product. Eye damage can result from penetration of solid particles, molten metal, or droplets of cleaning solutions in the eyes. Eye damage can also occur because of exposure to strong light emitted during certain high-temperature soldering processes. Irritation of the eyes, mucous membranes, and respiratory tract results from exposure to the aerosols and gases in acid cleaning processes, such as nitrogen oxides. These workers may experience electric shock when using electrical soldering equipment, and skin burns from contact with hot surfaces, flames, or splashes of hot soldering material. Heat rashes can result from continuous exposure of the skin to heat from the soldering process.

Fires can occur as a result of ignition of flammable solvents and other substances, as well as by the soldering flame or sparks. Fire and explosions can occur, particularly when using air propane and other blowtorch processes. Skin burns from contact with hot surfaces, flames, or splashes of solder are another hazard. Skin ALLERGIES, rashes, and dermatitis occur as a result of exposure to solvents and other activators used in soldering flux. Ulceration and other dermatological problems, particularly of the fingertips, occur due to the handling of metal pieces and exposure to flux.

Chemical burns can occur as a result of splashes of corrosive chemicals used in metal cleaning, particularly strong acids or mixtures of acids and oxidizing solutions. Poisoning can occur from phosgene and other poisonous gases formed from chlorinated solvents in contact with a high temperature source. Poisoning can result from exposure to many different poisonous metals present in the solder, primarily lead, CADMIUM, zinc, ANTIMONY, and their fumes released during the soldering. There may be adverse coronary effects as a result of chronic inhalation of small amounts of CARBON MONOXIDE in certain flame soldering operations.

Workers may suffer heat stress in a hot environment, muscular pains due to repetitive work, and leg fatigue because of standing and working long hours.

See also CHEMICAL TOXICITY; DERMATITIS; ELECTRICITY-RELATED INJURIES; FIRE SAFETY/FIRE PROTECTION; PERSONAL PROTECTIVE EQUIPMENT; SKIN AND SENSE ORGAN TOXICITY; SOLVENTS; WELDING.

Mager-Stillman, Jeane. *Encyclopaedia of Occupational Health and Safety.* 4th ed. Vol. 4. Geneva: International Labor Organization, 1998, pp. 103.31–103.32.

solvents   Ingredients used in nearly every phase of electronics and other manufacturing fields. They are used primarily for cleaning and degreasing, and for thinning plastics, resins, glues, inks, paints and waxes. There is a wide range of organic solvents, some very toxic and others only mildly toxic.

Millions of workers are exposed to solvents on a daily basis. Health hazards associated with solvent exposure include toxicity to the nervous system, reproductive damage, liver and kidney damage, respiratory impairment, cancer, and dermatitis.

The aromatic compounds and the chlorinated hydrocarbons may be the most harmful groups of solvents, as many of them are known to cause cancer and other serious diseases. Other examples of solvents include acetone, carbon disulfide, carbon tetrachloride, carbon tetrafluoride, chlorobenzene, chloroform, chlorotoluene, ethyl acetate, ethyl benzene, heptane, hexane, kerosene, naphtha, pentane, petroleum spirits, phenol, styrene, toluene, freons, turpentine, and xylene.

See also CANCER; DERMATITIS; DRY CLEANING; GASTROINTESTINAL OR LIVER TOXICITY; NEUROTOXICITY; OCCUPATIONAL SAFETY AND HEALTH ADMINISTRATION; REPRODUCTIVE TOXICITY; U.S. DEPARTMENT OF LABOR.

Special Exposure Cohort   Employees with specified cancers who worked at three U.S. Department of Energy facilities, or who participated in certain nuclear weapons tests and meet other requirements. These employees' cancers are presumed to be radiation-related for compensation purposes under the ENERGY EMPLOYEES OCCUPATIONAL ILLNESS COMPENSATION PROGRAM.

Employees include those who worked at gaseous diffusion plants in Paducah, Kentucky, Portsmouth, Ohio, or Oak Ridge, Tennessee for a total of at least 250 days before February 1, 1992, and were monitored for radiation exposure with dosimetry badges or had jobs with similar exposures to those monitored; or worked before January 1, 1974, on Amchitka Island, Alaska, and were exposed to radiation related to the Long Shot, Milrow or Cannikin underground nuclear tests.

Employees or their survivors are eligible for benefits if, after beginning covered employment they contracted bone cancer, leukemia, lung cancer or multiple myeloma, lymphomas (other than Hodgkin's disease) or one of many primary cancers, provided that the onset was at least five years after the first exposure.

spill exposure   See CHEMICAL SPILLS.

sports medicine   A field of medical care concerned with assessing and improving fitness as well as with prevention and treatment of injuries specific to professional and amateur athletes. There are various types of sports medicine practitioners, including orthopedic surgeons, podiatrists, chiropractors, physical therapists, and primary care physicians. A sports medicine clinic may offer a team approach to care for an injured athlete, in which several types of sports medicine specialists work together.

Sports medicine physicians advise athletes about exercises to improve strength, endurance, and flexibility. They may offer nutritional advice to help athletes improve performance and provide on-site medical care at sports events.

Many sports injuries can also occur in workplace situations. Such injuries include fractures, head injuries, muscle tears, ligament sprains or tears, tendinits, tendon rupture, joint dislocation or subluxation (partial dislocation), or injuries to a specific organ, such as eye injuries.

See also BASEBALL INJURIES/BASEBALL FINGER; BASKETBALL INJURIES (PROFESSIONAL); FOOTBALL INJURIES (PROFESSIONAL); SOCCER INJURIES; SPRAINS; TENDINITIS.

Clayman, Charles B. *The American Medical Association Home Medical Encyclopedia.* New York: Random House, 1989.
Levy, Allan M., and Mark L. Fuerst. *Sports Injury Handbook.* New York: John Wiley & Sons, 1993.

sprains   A sprain is a tearing or stretching of ligaments that hold bone ends together in a joint, following a violent or sudden twist or stretch that causes the joint to move out of its usual range of movement. The most common sprains occur in joints of the ankles and knees, and the arch of the foot. Sprains can result from a fall, a stumble, or sudden turning motion.

The injured person may experience rapid swelling, possible discoloration of the skin, impaired joint function, and pain and tenderness in the affected area. Emergency medical care should be sought if there is difficulty in using the joint after the injury.

See also BRICKLAYERS, CEMENT WORKERS AND PLASTERERS; CARPENTERS; CONSTRUCTION; PHYSICAL LOAD; SLIPS, TRIPS, AND FALLS; SPORTS MEDICINE.

stage fright   A feeling of nervous anticipation that some people experience before giving a speech or making an appearance on a stage. Stage fright is a workplace issue because many people must speak up at meetings, give presentations to coworkers, or make requests to boards of directors.

For some individuals, the uncomfortable feeling occurs before they approach the platform or stage, while others experience it just as they walk onstage. Anyone who has been in theatrical productions, plays a musical instrument, sings publicly, or been videotaped probably has experienced this feeling at some time. People who experience a high level of anxiety because of stage fright may view the audience as an adversary ready to judge them personally without regard to the content or message of their presentation.

Because of the stress caused by intense stage fright, some people go out of their way to avoid public speaking and public appearances and may actually develop a phobia. Some people actually turn down job advancements because they fear that speaking in front of an audience will be part of their new assignment.

Common symptoms of stage fright include dizziness and nausea, sweaty palms, weak knees, rapid heartbeat, and difficulty breathing. These symptoms may occur for only a few moments, but for many people, as soon as they are onstage their nervousness disappears and they focus all of their attention and energy on their performance.

Many successful public figures have overcome stage fright. Some lose their fear by systematically becoming accustomed to appearing in front of people. BEHAVIOR THERAPY and RELAXATION techniques can help people overcome stage fright. Physical relaxation involves exercises to eliminate nervousness and anxiety and can lead to physical ease and calmness. Mental and psychological relaxation involves exercises to develop objectivity, awareness, mental clarity, and a positive attitude.

Overcoming stage fright depends on the individual's developing confidence in his or her ability to speak or perform. Knowing the material well, whether it is a musical performance or a public speech, helps relieve stress. Confident individuals learn to convert their stress into positive energy.

See also ANXIETY; ANXIETY DISORDERS; COMPLEMENTARY THERAPIES; MENTAL HEALTH; PERFORMANCE ANXIETY; SOCIAL PHOBIA; PUBLIC SPEAKING; STRESS.

Desberg, Peter. *Controlling Stage Fright: Presenting Yourself to Audiences From One to One Thousand.* Oakland, Calif.: New Harbinger Publications, 1988.

stone workers   See BRICKLAYERS, CEMENT WORK-ERS, AND PLASTERERS; CONFINED SPACES; CONSTRUC-TION; LADDERS; SCAFFOLDING.

stress   The response of the body and mind to strains or burdens that demand adaptation; any hindrance that disturbs an individual's mental and physical well-being. These interferences may range from an impending performance review to life-threatening situations. Stress in the workplace may be caused by BOREDOM, poor communication with coworkers and superiors, FRUSTRATION, BULLYING by superiors or coworkers, or many other reasons.

From a scientific perspective, stress causes an imbalance in an individual's equilibrium. Control-ling stress is essential for wellness because contin-ued exposure can lead to symptoms such as HEADACHES or more serious conditions such as high blood pressure and DEPRESSION. Research has shown that stress also affects the IMMUNE SYSTEM and causes it to be less efficient in fighting off diseases.

What Are Stressors?

Stress is an internal response to circumstances known as stressors. Stressors may be internal situ-ations, such feelings of insecurity or frustration, or external events, such as a bad review at work, or cancellation of an airplane flight.

Stressors can also be reactions to happy events as well as unhappy events; these are good stressors derived from satisfying personal and professional events. For example, good personal stressors may include getting married, having a baby or moving to a new house; good work stressors may include landing a new job or getting a promotion. Unpleas-ant stressors may include being fired, marital diffi-culties, or illness. HANS SELYE, pioneer in stress research, and author of *Stress without Distress* and *The Stress of Life,* termed the good events that cause stress EUSTRESS and those that caused unpleasant effects DIS-STRESS. Both types of stress cause physi-ological responses, including activation of the ner-vous system and of the fight or flight response.

That is why, during stressful times, people may notice that they have faster heartbeats and sick feelings in their stomachs; it is difficult to work or function efficiently at such times.

Stressors often represent significant changes in one's life or habits. How individuals accommodate change influences the extent of stress they experi-ence. Selye used the term GENERAL ADAPTATION SYN-DROME to explain how individuals cope with stressors. He suggested that individuals experience events in different ways; what results in emotional strain and ANXIETY for one person may not bring about those reactions in others. Also, in the same individual, adaptations that are tolerated well at one time may not be handled so well at another.

Chronic stress results in ongoing wear and tear on the body's organs and systems, making them more susceptible to illness. When symptoms show up, many individuals begin to seek medical or psy-chological help. According to Herbert Benson, M.D., a Harvard cardiologist and author of *The Relaxation Response,* more than 80 percent of visits to physicians' offices may result from stress in patients' lives. "Physicians are aware of stress as a factor in diagnosing and treating many common health concerns. For example, many people seek help for gastrointestinal symptoms, an inability to sleep, headaches, depression, and chronic fatigue. They may have high blood pressure."

Sources of Stress

Stress can come from an individual's workplace, family, or community connections. Stress within a family causes tension and difficulties in communi-cating effectively. There may be intergenerational conflicts or situations arising from assisting elderly parents, for example. In a family, several people may be trying to cope with their own stress as well as the stress of others about whom they care. For example, when a husband loses his job, he may try to console his wife, even when struggling with his own emotions.

Stress that starts within the family can affect work, and the reverse is also true. Family problems can make a person irritable on the job, distrustful of coworkers, and prone to mistakes and accidents. Likewise, a difficult day at the office can make a person short-tempered and hostile at home. Workplace factors that contribute to stress include lack of autonomy, lack of satisfaction, and feeling bored, underpaid, or overworked.

While stress can be physiologically devastating to many people, others find that stress actually raises their energy level and helps them focus their mind better on their work, family, or social activities. Some thrive on such stressors as COMPETITION. People who do are often attracted to high-stress occupations and professions, or do well at competitive games and sports.

Sources of Occupational Stress

Work involves human interactions, and whenever these occur, stress is a possibility. A group of authors has identified four major job stressors that they say can affect workers' health and productivity. According to authors Daniel A. Girdano, George S. Everly, and Dorothy E. Dusek, in their book *Controlling Stress and Tension: A Holistic Approach,* major factors are work overload, lack of control, being underqualified, and job interference with interpersonal affairs. Other stressors include job ambiguity and role conflict, stifled communications, discrimination, bureaucracy, inactivity and boredom, poor financial rewards, and lack of career guidance, promotion, and reorganization.

Employees who are highly satisfied with most aspects of their work will often overlook low pay, but low pay and lack of job satisfaction represent a bad combination that contributes to stress. Aspects of career development are important components of the working environment and can contribute to job satisfaction and prevent occupational frustration. Workers want to fully use their occupational skills, develop new or expanded skills, and have career counseling available to facilitate career decisions.

Promotion is a source of adaptive stress. Although promotion is a good stressor, individuals who are promoted experience significant changes in job function, increased responsibility subordinates, production, and money, and changes in social role. Certain social obligations, such as entertaining clients, may cause social or financial stress.

Departmental or organizational restructuring can bring about feelings of insecurity and apprehension, in addition to fears about and job security.

Adjusting to RETIREMENT is a source of stress. The association between self-esteem and job is significant. Many people tend to replace their identity in terms of broad personal characteristics with job-related characteristics and role. When some workers retire, particularly if they are forced to retire from a very rewarding job, results typically include a sense of worthlessness and loss of self-esteem, lack of motivation in general, and increased cardiovascular complaints. Factors that increase the stressfulness of retirement, according to Girdano, Everly, and Dusek, include many years on the job; lack of interests outside the job, such as hobbies and social involvement; lack of preparation for retirement, such as retirement counseling or just informal mental preparation; lack of alternative sources of income; and lack of alternative sources of ego gratification.

SELF-TEST: HOW STRESSFUL IS YOUR JOB?

During the typical course of your work, if these situations occur often, you may be suffering from job stress. Do you often:

- Face important time deadlines that you have difficulty meeting?
- Feel less competent than you think you should?
- Wish your work could be less complex?
- Feel overwhelmed by your job?
- Feel as though you're in the wrong job?
- Feel frustrated by "red tape"?
- Think of yourself as lost in bureaucracy?

Other factors that lead to stress:

- Do you feel guilty for taking time off from work?
- Do you have a tendency to rush into work that needs to be done before knowing the correct procedure to complete the job?
- Do you attempt to complete two or more tasks at once?

If you answer yes to most of these questions, seek out more stress-reducing activities.

Learning to Manage Stress

"Stressors cannot be eliminated, so our goal should be to control and manage stress," says Elaine Shepp, M.S.W., a psychotherapist on the staff at Rush North Shore Medical Center, in Skokie, Illinois. She adds, "It is possible to neutralize the toxic effects of unrelenting stress. People who cope well with stress put their personal and professional lives into perspective. They may experience a constantly high level of pressure and unrealistic demands at work but develop their own ideals of conduct and test themselves by their own standards. They are able to prioritize their work and enjoy family life as well as their chosen recreational activities."

Experiencing stress is part of human nature. In his book *Why Zebras Don't Get Ulcers,* Robert M. Sapolsky looks at how wild animals process stress and explains what humans can learn from them. "The key thing with humans is, we're all going to have a bit of stress response. It's part of life. Three minutes or three hours [of stress response] is no problem, but do it chronically, and you're up a creek. The stress response increases blood pressure, which can led to a stroke. It also shuts down digestion, which can lead to ulcers."

In explaining why zebras do not get ulcers, Sapolsky said: "Because they don't have computers, they don't worry about mortgages, blind dates, or Social Security. They worry about lions, and with lions, it's all taken care of in three minutes, or it's all over in three minutes. No stress."

Relieving Stress: An Individual Matter

Avenues toward relieving stress are personal matters. Many people find that regular exercise helps them overcome a stressful day and get ready to effectively face tomorrow's challenges. Using muscles is a way to use up some of the "fight or flight" readiness in the body.

A healthy diet with three meals a day is a basic for wellness and can also help prevent and relieve stress. Well-balanced meals provide a slow release of necessary nutrients throughout the day. For some people, too much CAFFEINE causes additional stress by bringing on symptoms of anxiety. "Crash diets" or "fad diets" can lead to anxiety, depression, and an inability to maintain an appropriate weight. Acceptance of one's body image and a good sense of SELF-ESTEEM will encourage people to maintain good nutrition as well as good health.

People use many COMPLEMENTARY THERAPIES to relieve stress. These include MEDITATION, PROGRESSIVE MUSCLE RELAXATION, and YOGA. Some use MASSAGE THERAPY or listen to music to relieve stress. However, what allows one person to relax may

actually cause stress for another. An example is noise level in the workplace or at home. Each individual should try to create an environment in which to work and live that is the least stressful in order to focus on reaching his or her peak performance and a feeling of well-being.

Hobbies outside work help many people combat stress. Participating in an activity, no matter what, simply for the enjoyment of it can reduce stress level. Choices of hobbies are as diverse as human nature.

A good SOCIAL SUPPORT SYSTEM is important too. Many people find relief from stress in talking with their coworkers who share the same job. When they are able to talk about their issues, problems, and concerns and get FEEDBACK from trusted friends, people get an enlightened perspective that often helps them to lighten their stress load.

When Professional Help May Be Necessary

There are times when reactions to stress detract from the energy necessary for productive work and effective personal functioning. At these times, when talking to a friend just is not enough, professional assistance is available. Those who seek professional help to overcome effects of extreme stress should not consider themselves "weak," says Shepp. "Seeking help is an intelligent way of using available tools to increase one's level of functioning. Counseling can help prevent burnout and assist in dealing with life situations requiring the input of a noninvolved, knowledgeable person."

If you find yourself feeling totally overwhelmed and decide to seek professional help, how should you select a psychotherapist and choose from a myriad of PSYCHOTHERAPIES? You may want to talk with a close relative, colleague, or friend who has experienced psychotherapy. However, if confidentiality is important to you, find a mental health professional or social worker in a hospital or community agency who can help direct you. The psychotherapist should be someone you feel comfortable with, who understands your particular stressors, and who can suggest practical ways for you to handle your stress. Find a therapist who is multifaceted in his or her approach to problems and knowledgeable about many options available to treat particular problems. Look for one who is open to consulting with other professionals who have additional expertise.

RECOGNIZE SIGNALS OF STRESS AT WORK AND AT HOME

Each person has unique sources of stress as well as personal symptoms of stress. Sources of stress come from within oneself (personal), from family life, from the workplace, and from community activities. Some common sources of stress and personal symptoms are listed below.

SOURCES OF STRESS

Workplace
- Difficulties with boss or coworkers
- Threatened layoffs
- Boredom; not enough work
- Overwork; underpayment
- Lack of autonomy
- Automation in the workplace

Personal
- Aging
- Feeling unattractive or insecure
- Achievement or success problems
- Change in habits
- Relationship concerns
- Inability to pay bills or mortgage

Family
- Death, illness, or injury of a family member
- Divorce; remarriage
- Marital or sexual difficulties
- Holidays, vacations
- Problems with children
- Young adult leaving home or returning home
- Lack of privacy
- Not enough time

PERSONAL SYMPTOMS OF STRESS

- Irritability or bad temper
- Headaches; stomachaches; digestive problems
- Inability to sleep
- Grinding teeth
- High blood pressure
- Lethargy; inability to work; finger-tapping
- Depression; panic or anxiety
- Fatigue; restlessness; accident proneness
- Sexual difficulties

CHECKLIST: COPING WITH STRESS

- Identify external stress-producing factors over which you may have little or no control, such as on your job.

- Identify internal factors such as perfectionism and unrealistic self-expectations.
- Recognize your personal signs of stress, such as:
    Increased irritability with family members or coworkers
    Headaches; stomachaches; digestive disorders
    Overeating; increased alcohol consumption
    Sleeplessness; chronic fatigue
    Depression; feelings of hopelessness
- Separate your problems at home from your work concerns, and vice versa.
- Be realistic in your daily outlook; do not expect too much of yourself or others.
- Prioritize your responsibilities; learn to occasionally say no to requests you consider unreasonable.
- Maintain a healthy lifestyle by eating a well-balanced diet and exercising.
- Reduce your consumption of caffeinated beverages: cut down on coffee, tea, and cola, which can increase your heart rate and your irritability level.
- Develop a regular habit of exercising; a 20-minute walk each day can be effective in fighting muscle tension.
- Develop a sense of humor; increase your ability to see humor in sometimes intolerable situations.
- Learn some relaxation techniques that work for you, such as deep breathing or listening to your favorite music.
- Seek professional help if you feel overwhelmed.

See also ANGER; BEHAVIOR THERAPY; BENSON, HERBERT; ERGONOMICS; EXERCISE; KABAT-ZINN, JON; MIND/BODY CONNECTIONS; NUTRITION; RELATIONSHIPS; RELAXATION; SLEEP; SUPPORT GROUPS.

Benson, Herbert. *The Relaxation Response.* New York: Avon Books, 1975.
———. *Beyond the Relaxation Response.* New York: Berkeley Press, 1985.
Benson, Herbert, and Eileen M. Stuart. *The Wellness Book: The Comprehensive Guide to Maintaining Health and Treating Stress-Related Illness.* New York: Carol, 1992.
Carey, Benedict. "Don't Face Stress Alone." *Health,* April 1997.
DeMarco, Tom. *Slack: Getting Past Burnout, Busywork, and the Myth of Total Efficiency.* New York: Broadway Books, 2001.
Field, Tiffany, Olga Quintino, et al. "Job Stress Reduction Therapies." *Alternative Therapies* 3, no. 4 (July 1997).
Girdano, Daniel A., George S. Everly, and Dorothy E. Dusek. *Controlling Stress and Tension: A Holistic Approach.* 3d ed. Englewood Cliffs, N.J.: Prentice Hall, 1990.

Hornig-Rohan, Mady. "Stress, Immune Mediators, and Immune-Mediated Disease." *Advances: The Journal of Mind-Body Health* 11, no. 2 (spring 1995).

Kahn, Ada P. *Stress A–Z: A Sourcebook for Facing Everyday Challenges.* New York: Facts On File, Inc., 1998.

"Women and Stress." *Sacramento Medicine,* September 1995.

———. "Win the Case against Stress." *Chicago Bar Association Record,* May 1994.

———. *Stress.* Chicago: Mental Health Association of Greater Chicago, 1989.

Pelletier, Kenneth R. *Sound Mind, Sound Body: A Model for Lifelong Health.* New York: Simon and Schuster, 1994.

———. *Healthy People in Unhealthy Places: Stress and Fitness at Work.* New York: Delacorate Press, 1984.

Sapolsky, Robert M. *Why Zebras Don't Get Ulcers.* New York: W. H. Freeman and Co., 1994.

Selye, Hans. *Stress without Distress.* Philadelphia: J. B. Lippincott Company, 1974.

———. *The Stress of Life.* Rev. ed. New York: McGraw-Hill, 1978.

stress management   Stress management refers to an individual's personal COPING skills for dealing with stress. It also refers to a multibillion-dollar industry that includes programs, products, services, and techniques to help people reduce stress on an individual or group basis. For example, stress management programs offer help to people interested in overcoming stress-related disorders ranging from EATING DISORDERS to issues of SELF-ESTEEM. Programs may include use of many COMPLEMENTARY THERAPIES.

Many stress management programs are offered in the workplace and address such problems as alcoholism and other ADDICTIONS, finances, nutrition, and other employee concerns.

See also EMPLOYEE ASSISTANCE PROGRAMS; MENTAL HEALTH; STRESS; PSYCHOTHERAPIES; WORKSITE WELLNESS PROGRAMS.

Murphy, Lawrence R. "Stress Management in Work Settings: A Critical Review of the Health Effects." *American Journal of Health Promotion* 11, no. 2 (November/December 1996): 112–135.

student's elbow   See BURSITIS.

sulfanilamide   See SKIN OR SENSE ORGAN TOXICITY.

sulfur dioxide   See AIR POLLUTION; ASTHMA; COMBUSTION POLLUTANTS; SKIN OR SENSE ORGAN TOXICITY.

sulfuric acid   See SKIN OR SENSE ORGAN TOXICITY.

Superfund   Another name for the COMPREHENSIVE ENVIRONMENTAL RESPONSE, COMPENSATION, AND LIABILITY ACT of 1980 (CERCLA), which created the AGENCY FOR TOXIC SUBSTANCES AND DISEASE REGISTRY.

superiority complex   A person with a superiority complex has an unrealistic and exaggerated belief that he or she is better than others. When a supervisor or manager has such a complex, it is difficult for coworkers to be productive and have good morale. Such a complex is a source of stress for the individual as well as others. In some people, this is a compensation mechanism for unconscious feelings of low SELF-ESTEEM or inadequacy. For example, bullies who treat coworkers badly may do so because they have low self-esteem.

See also MENTAL HEALTH; STRESS.

support groups   Individuals with the same experience or specific concern who join together to help each other by sharing experiences and advice and providing emotional support. Many employee groups support each other regarding issues such as alcoholism, smoking, or elder care.

Many EMPLOYEE ASSISTANCE PROGRAMS recommend that people join support groups because sharing with others can be effective and augment medical therapies. An additional benefit of belonging to a support group is than one can stay up-to-date on progress as researchers work toward better treatments or legislators work on the issues. Many groups circulate articles from popular and scientific publications and bring in experts to discuss their latest findings.

See also DEPRESSION; STRESS.

Kreiner, Anna. *Everything You Need to Know about Creating Your Own Support System.* New York: Rosen Publishing Group, 1996.

Locke, Steve, and Douglas Colligan. *The Healer Within.* New York: New American Library, 1986.

surgeons   See MUSIC IN THE WORKPLACE.

Survey of Occupational Injuries and Illnesses   A U.S. federal/state program in which reports are collected from approximately 250,000 private-sector establishments. These reports are processed by agencies cooperating with the Bureau of Labor Statistics. The survey measures nonfatal injuries and illnesses only. The survey excludes the self-employed, farms with fewer than 11 employees, and employees in federal, state, and local government agencies.

The Census of Fatal Occupational Injuries (CFOI), part of the survey programs uses diverse data sources to identify, verify, and profile fatal work injuries. Information about each workplace fatality is obtained by cross-referencing source documents such as death certificates, workers' compensation records, and reports to federal and state agencies.

See also BUREAU OF LABOR STATISTICS; CENSUS OF FATAL OCCUPATIONAL INJURIES; NONFATAL WORKPLACE ILLNESS BY CATEGORY.

For information:

U.S. Bureau of Labor Statistics
2 Massachusetts Avenue, NE
Washington, DC 20212-0001
(202) 691-7800
(202) 691-7797 (fax)
http://www.bls.gov

tai chi A physical, mental, and spiritual practice that uses movement to balance energy, and aims to help achieve and maintain harmony within the self. Those who practice tai chi say that it aids them to develop more mental and spiritual energy, feel more overall vitality, and obtain relief from workplace stresses. Many employee wellness programs include training in tai chi.

Tai chi is an outgrowth of Chinese martial arts, spirituality, and Chinese medicine, and has been practiced for more than 2,000 years. As a martial art and a popular meditative practice, it is often called MEDITATION in motion. According to Chinese philosophy, to do tai chi is to connect the individual with nature through movement. It is considered "great shadow boxing" which draws on Taoist beliefs in the interdependence of the body and the mind. In the open spaces and parks of China today, millions of young and old people practice tai chi, gently swaying, gliding and stepping.

Tai Chi and Productivity

Practitioners of tai chi usually experience deep and restful sleep. Their nervous system is soothed and calmed. The gentle movements of tai chi ensure that they do not suffer strains and other muscular injuries, but instead develop greater strength, flexibility, and suppleness. Some athletes use tai chi as a way of warming up.

People who perform tai chi move all their joints and exert more energy than they appear to. Through the use of slow breathing, individuals can pace some of the systems of their body. They can stabilize their heartbeat, the exchange of oxygen and carbon dioxide, and the secretion and absorption of endocrine fluids. The movements also improve health by assisting the flow of blood, creating tranquility for the entire nervous system, and

through deep concentration, fostering deep peace of mind.

Tai Chi Classes

Books and videos on tai chi are available, but the best way to learn tai chi is in classes held in tai chi studios, adult education courses at high schools and colleges, YMCAs and YWCAs, or senior centers. Many people combine tai chi with other forms of exercise. Some workplaces are said to bring a tai chi instructor to their sites to provide instruction.

See also COMPLEMENTARY THERAPIES; MEDITATION; HEALTH PROMOTION; RELAXATION.

Kahn, Ada P., and Jan Fawcett. *Encyclopedia of Mental Health.* 2d ed. New York: Facts On File, Inc., 2001.

tanning Workers involved in the leather tanning industry may include those in leather and leather products, boot and shoe bindings, footwear (except rubber), leather gloves and mittens, luggage and handbags, and other personal leather goods.

Hazards in this work involve possible release of poisonous gases during the tanning process. Exposure to dust and to hazardous chemicals in processing baths may cause skin rashes, and irritation of the eyes and respiratory tract. Tending moving machinery, including rotating drums and pulleys, may cause entanglement and crushing of limbs. Slips and falls on wet or cluttered floors are a common hazard; a major hazard is posed by falls into vats and pits. Cuts and other injuries by sharp and or mechanized tools may occur.

Fatigue and back pain may result from working for long hours standing up or in a semibending posture, and handling heavy and bulky loads, such as hides, skins, leather or other bundles, and containers of chemicals.

See also ALLERGIES; BACK PAIN; CONFINED SPACES; ELECTRICITY-RELATED INJURIES; HOT ENVIRONMENTS; PERSONAL PROTECTIVE EQUIPMENT; SLIPS, TRIPS, AND FALLS.

taxicab drivers/chauffeurs See CHAUFFEURS; VIOLENCE.

teenage workers Employed youths under the age of 20. Every year about 70 teens die from work injuries in the United States. Another 70,000 get hurt badly enough that they go to a hospital emergency room.

According to the National Institute of Occupational Safety and Health (NIOSH), teens are often injured on the job due to unsafe equipment, stressful conditions, and working too fast. Also, teens may not receive adequate safety training and supervision.

By law, an employer must provide a safe and healthful workplace, safety and health training, including providing information on chemicals that could be harmful to health. As an employee, a teenage worker has the right to report safety problems to the Occupational Safety and Health Administration (OSHA), work without racial or sexual harassment, refuse to work if the job is immediately dangerous to life or health, and to join or organize a union.

HAZARDS FOR TEENAGE WORKERS

Type of Work	Type of Hazard
Janitor/clean-up	Toxic chemicals in cleaning products
	Blood on discarded needles
Food service	Slippery floors
	Hot cooking equipment
	Sharp objects
Retail/sales	Violent crimes
	Heavy lifting
Office/clerical	Stress
	Harassment
	Poor computer workstation design

Source: NIOSH

Federal child labor laws protect younger teens from working too long, too late, or too early. Some states have laws restricting the hours that older teens may work. The table below shows the hours

14- and 15-year-olds may work (with exceptions for students in some work experience programs).

WORK HOURS FOR TEENS (AGE 14 AND 15)

• Work hours	Not before 7 A.M. or after 7 P.M. between Labor Day and June 1 Not during school hours 7 A.M.–9 P.M. between June 1 and Labor Day
• Maximum hours when school is in session	18 hours a week but no more than 2 hours a day on school days 8 hours a day Saturday, Sunday, and holidays
• Maximum hours when school is not in session	40 hours a week 8 hours a day

See also CHILD LABOR; FAIR LABOR STANDARDS ACT.

telecommunications A field of employment that includes workers in such areas as telephone work, electronics, and numerous related technical fields and manufacturing. Hazards of the field include ELECTRICITY-RELATED INJURIES, SLIPS, TRIPS, AND FALLS, and effects of hot or cold environments. Telecommunications workers work outdoors and indoors, and some may climb poles. Telecommunications workers often work during several shifts. Some workers must work long hours, often through nights, when there are breakdowns in systems.

See also ARSENIC; COLD ENVIRONMENTS; HOT ENVIRONMENTS; LADDERS; MANUFACTURING; SHIFT WORK.

temporomandibular joint disorder (TMJ disorder) A problem commonly encountered by violinists and violists as a result of displacing the left side the jaw against the instrument's chin rest, thus stressing the right TMJ. Musicians must be alert to the problem because it can become highly symptomatic or do permanent damage to the integrity of the joints. The approach to treatment is generally dual: a technical approach by reducing the pressure and the displacement of the instrument against the jaw, and a dental approach through the use of a splinting device and exercise.

See also MUSICIANS' INJURIES; PERFORMING ARTS MEDICINE.

tendinitis   An inflammation or irritation of a tendon (a thick fibrous cord that attaches muscle to bone or muscle to muscle), usually caused by an injury. A common form of tendinitis is known as painful arc syndrome, which causes pain in the shoulder when the arm is raised above a certain angle. Working in an awkward position or being in poor physical condition can result in development of tendinitis.

According to the American College of Rheumatology, overuse during work or athletic activities is the most common cause.

For information:

American College of Rheumatology
1800 Century Place
Suite 250
Atlanta, GA 30345
(404) 633-3777
(404) 633-1870 (fax)
acr@rheumatology.org

See also BURSITIS; ERGONOMICS; REPETITIVE STRESS INJURIES.

teratogens   Chemicals, drugs, and other substances that are known or suspected to cause physical defects in the developing human embryo.

See REPRODUCTIVE TOXICITY.

terrorism   Terrorism has been defined as "The unlawful use or threat of violence against persons or property to further political or social objectives. It is usually intended to intimidate or coerce a government, individuals or groups to modify their behavior or politics."

Terrorists are usually young men who are fanatical about their cause to the extent that they have no concern for their victims or for their own lives. Some terrorists have been as young as 14 or 15. Some terrorist groups are self-supporting through activities such as bank robbery or selling drugs, but most are supported by governments who find terrorism effective and inexpensive in comparison to the costs of conventional military force.

Since September 11, 2001, the threat of terrorism affects all aspects of society, including workplaces. More than 3,000 working people lost their lives in the terrorist acts on the World Trade Center in New York that day, more than 350 workers at the Pentagon in Washington, DC, and others on several airplanes besieged by terrorists, many of whom were en route to a work assignment.

Many working people, as well as airline employees, who must travel for their jobs have become more concerned with airline safety, as have commercial airlines and airports.

Employers as well as employees are concerned with security at the workplace. Additional security measures add tremendous costs to employers' budgets, but these steps are considered essential to guard workers' safety and peace of mind. Many employers have instituted elaborate identification systems for entering the worksite, posted guards at entrances and exits, and now screen delivery personnel who enter the premises.

Mental Health Effects of Terrorism Threats

According to the NATIONAL MENTAL HEALTH ASSOCIATION (NMHA), emotional responses to perceived or real threats of terrorism may include working slowly, missing deadlines, calling in sick frequently, irritability and anger, difficulty concentrating and making decisions, and difficulty with changing routines.

Many employees who survived the September 11, 2001, attacks suffer from POST-TRAUMATIC STRESS DISORDER (PTSD) and experience flashbacks when hearing explosions or sirens or smelling smoke. Many employers have provided mental health counseling for survivors of the attacks.

The NMHA recommends providing resources about EMPLOYEE ASSISTANCE PROGRAMS, allowing people to break from work periodically to talk with each other about their mutual concerns, consider bringing a professional counselor/facilitator to the site to identify and get help for those who need it. Further, employers might allow people to take time off beyond the usual to donate blood, take part in community activities, and address personal needs. Employers should make it clear that hostility directed at coworkers will not be tolerated, that supervisors will challenge discriminatory remarks or acts or any form of harassment, and that disciplinary action will be taken.

Employers should create or review the organization's emergency plan to address any situations that might arise. Employees should be reminded of emergency procedures; feeling prepared will help ease their anxiety.

The threat of terrorism comes from sources outside as well as inside the United States, but there have always been random acts of violence at workplaces, many involving disgruntled former or current employees and mentally impaired workers who have access to guns and other weapons.

See also ABSENTEEISM; ANTHRAX; ANXIETY; BULLYING; DISCRIMINATION; DOMESTIC VIOLENCE; MENTAL HEALTH; STRESS; VIOLENCE.

For information:

National Mental Health Association
2001 N. Beauregard Street
12th Floor
Alexandria, VA 22311
(703) 684-7722
(800) 969-NMHA (toll-free)
(703) 684-5968 (fax)
www.nmha.org

textile workers   These are employees engaged in diverse operations including fiber synthesis, weaving, manufacturing, dyeing, and finishing. These workers face many health and safety issues, including chemical exposure from the processing and dyeing of materials, exposure to cotton dust and other organic dusts, musculoskeletal stresses, and noise exposure.

During the handling and processing of cotton, cotton dust is a hazard as it may contain mixtures of many substances, including ground-up plant matter, fiber, bacteria, fungi, soil, pesticides, noncotton matter, and other contaminants.

See also COTTON DUST AND TEXTILE INDUSTRY; ERGONOMICS; FORMALDEHYDE; NOISE; SOLVENTS.

theater (actors) injuries   Hazards facing stage actors include physical hazards, such as falling or tripping onstage during stunts or active scenes, falling into the orchestra pit, being hit with falling props from overhead riggings, inhaling theatrical smoke, fire hazards from special effects, or heat stress due to stage lights and confining costumes. Psychological hazards include fearing loss of memory for lines and PERFORMANCE ANXIETY. Actors must cope with STRESS when auditioning or looking for jobs in a highly competitive field. Voices can be damaged by frequent loud talking onstage. Further physical hazards include wearing costumes near open flames onstage and allergic reactions to theatrical makeup.

See also ALLERGIES; BELTING (VOCAL); PERFORMING ARTS MEDICINE.

timber cutters   See CENSUS OF FATAL OCCUPATIONAL INJURIES; LOGGING.

tobacco   A native American plant that is cultivated for its leaves, which are harvested, dried, and smoked. The active ingredient in tobacco is nicotine, which is addictive. It affects the central nervous system through routes that differ from other drugs, but it produces very similar results, such as euphoria, dependency, and withdrawal symptoms when stopped suddenly.

Nicotine acts as both a stimulant and a depressant. Shallow puffs seem to increase alertness, but deep ones are relaxing. Smokers sense their nicotine levels and tend to self-regulate them by varying inhalation patterns, as well as their frequency of smoking. In regular smokers, nicotine improves short-term memory, intellectual performance, and concentration. Although smoking speeds up the heart rate and raises blood pressure, it also seems to relieve stressful feelings for some smokers. Nicotine consumption also appears to control weight to some extent, probably by lowering circulating insulin levels and thus decreasing the smoker's craving for sweets and tendency to store fat. This particular aspect of nicotine makes smoking appeal to those who do not wish to gain weight.

Smokers who quit may experience genuine physical discomfort and cravings. Withdrawal symptoms from nicotine include headaches, irritability, upset stomach, breathing and circulation problems, trouble sleeping, dizziness and numbness. Smoking causes lung cancer.

See also ADDICTIONS; HEALTH PROMOTION; SMOKING.

toluene disocyant **(TDI)** See GLUERS; IMMUNOTOXICITY.

toxic air pollutants See AIR POLLUTION.

toxic hepatitis See HEPATITIS C.

toxicology reports and fatal injuries Abuse of drugs and alcohol is a serious workplace concern; many fatal injuries can be traced to recent use of drugs and alcohol. Attempts have been made to correlate drug and alcohol use with deaths resulting from fatal occupational injuries. An analysis of fatal occupational injuries and toxicology reports submitted to the BUREAU OF LABOR STATISTICS (BLS) for the CENSUS OF FATAL OCCUPATIONAL INJURIES (CFOI) was completed for the reporting years 1993 and 1994.

The CFOI is the primary source of information on fatal work injuries in the United States. Various data sources are used to compile comprehensive information on each occupational fatality, including industry, occupation, type of event, equipment involved, demographic characteristics, and circumstances. For this study, a variety of sources provided toxicology results: police accident reports, medical examiner and coroner reports, autopsy reports, and followup questionnaires. In addition to unintentional fatal injuries such as falls and motor vehicle crashes, the study also covered intentional injuries such as suicides and homicides that occurred when the victim was at work.

For a fatality to be included in the census, the decedent must have been employed at the time of the event, working for pay, compensation, or profit; performing a legal work activity; and present at the site of the incident as a requirement of his or her job. Fatalities that occurred during a person's commute to or from work are excluded from census counts.

As reported in *Compensation and Working Conditions* (fall 1999), during 1993 and 1994, 6,331 and 6,632 fatal occupational injuries, respectively, were reported nationwide. Toxicology reports were available for approximately one-fourth of the occupa-

tional fatalities in the study periods. About one-fifth of the toxicology reports showed positive readings for alcohol or one or more drugs. This is about 5 percent of total fatal work injuries. (See Table 1 below.)

TABLE 1. TOXICOLOGY REPORTS FOR WORKPLACE DEATHS, 1993–94

Toxicology Reports	1993	1994
States providing toxicology reports	32	23
Total fatalities	6,331	6,632
Percent of total fatalities involving positive toxicology reports	4.4	5.1
Toxicology reports reviewed	1,899	1,242
Positive toxicology reports	277	339
Percent of reviewed toxicology reports that were positive	14.6	27.3

Of substances identified in the toxicology reports, alcohol was the most common substance found in deceased individuals. In 1993, 47 percent of the 277 positive toxicology cases indicated the presence of alcohol, compared to 44 percent of the 339 positive toxicology cases in 1994. (See Table 2.)

TABLE 2. SUBSTANCES IDENTIFIED IN POSITIVE TOXICOLOGY REPORTS FOR DECEASED INDIVIDUALS, 1993–94

Substances Identified	1993		1994	
	NUMBER	PERCENT	NUMBER	PERCENT
Positive toxicology reports:	277	100.0	339	100.0
Alcohol	130	46.9	150	44.2
Opiates	35	12.6	39	11.5
Benzodiazepines	24	8.7	22	6.5
Antihistamines	3	1.1	10	2.9
Cocaine	42	15.2	51	15.0
THC	42	15.2	44	13.0
Amphetamine/ Methamphetamine	18	6.5	12	3.5
Barbiturates	6	2.2	16	4.7
Other substances: PCP, benzene, methaqualone, propoxyphene, methanol	3	1.1	6	1.8

Note: Due to the presence of more than one substance in some of the decedents, components do not equal totals.

Among occupations, construction trade workers, truck drivers, and farmers accounted for almost two-thirds of the positive cases. (See table 3 below.)

The percentage of positive test results by gender closely approximates that of occupational fatalities by gender (see table 4.)

For both years, motor vehicle incidents, homicides, and falls were the leading events for all fatal work injuries. Likewise, the leading events contributing to job-related fatalities with positive test results for each reporting year were motor vehicle incidents, homicides, and falls (See table 5.)

See also ADDICTIONS; COCAINE; FATAL INJURIES; WOMEN AND JOB-RELATED INJURIES.

TABLE 3. PERCENT DISTRIBUTION OF POSITIVE TOXICOLOGY REPORTS BY OCCUPATION, 1993–94

Occupation	1993	1994
Total fatalities	6,331	6,632
Positive toxicology reports	277	339
Percent	100	100
Construction trade	25	22
Truck drivers	18	19
Farmers	17	15
Sales	13	10
Mechanics	8	10
Laborers	6	10
Fishers	6	8
Police	5	4
Health care workers	2	2

TABLE 4. OCCUPATIONAL FATALITIES AND NUMBER AND PERCENT OF POSITIVE TOXICOLOGY REPORTS BY GENDER, 1993–94

Gender	Fatalities		Positive Toxicology Reports	
	NUMBER	PERCENT	NUMBER	PERCENT
1993				
Male	5,842	92	263	95
Female	489	8	14	5
1994				
Male	6,104	92	319	94
Female	528	8	20	6

Adapted with permission from Greenberg, Michael, Richard Hamilton, and Guy Toscano. "Analysis of Toxicology Reports from the 1993–1994 Census of Fatal Occupational Injuries." *Compensation and Working Conditions,* fall 1999, pp. 16–28.

tractor-related injuries   See FARMING.

transcendental meditation (TM)   One of the oldest and most scientifically documented techniques known to elicit the RELAXATION response. TM is a revised and simplified form of YOGA and is the method on which most other MEDITATION techniques are based. Many employee wellness programs include classes in TM to help employees cope with stress.

TABLE 5. PERCENT DISTRIBUTION OF FATALITIES AND POSITIVE TOXICOLOGY REPORTS BY EVENT AND EXPOSURE, 1993–94

	1993		1994	
Event or Exposure	FATALITIES	POSITIVE TOXICOLOGY REPORTS	FATALITIES	POSITIVE TOXICOLOGY REPORTS
Total	6,331	277	6,632	339
Percent	100	100	100	100
Highway crashes	20	22	20	18
Homicides	17	10	16	12
Falls	10	8	10	6
Electrocutions	5	7	5	5
Struck by vehicle	6	7	6	6
Struck by object	9	6	9	5
Other or unknown	33	40	34	48

Developed by Maharishi Mahesh Yogi, TM is based on ancient Hindu writings. It was introduced to the United States in the early 1960s by Herbert Benson, M.D. who studied people who practiced TM and developed his own methods for eliciting relaxation. His method is described in his book *The Relaxation Response.*

Typically, a TM meditator spends two 20-minute periods a day sitting quietly with eyes closed, and attention focused totally on the verbal repetition of a special sound, or mantra. Repetition of the mantra blocks distracting thoughts. The effect achieved is better relaxation and relief from stress.

See also BENSON, HERBERT; COMPLEMENTARY THER-APIES.

Mahesh Yogi, Maharishi. *Science of Being and Art of Living: Transcendental Meditation.* New York: Meridian, 1995.

traumatic injury   According to the Bureau of Labor Statistics of the U.S. Department of Labor, a traumatic injury is any unintentional or intentional wound or damage to the body resulting from acute exposure to energy, such as heat, electricity, or kinetic energy from a crash, or from the absence of such essentials as heat or oxygen caused by a specific event, incident, or series of events within a single workday or shift.

See also BUREAU OF LABOR STATISTICS; OCCUPATIONAL ILLNESS; WORK RELATIONSHIP CRITERIA.

trench foot   See COLD ENVIRONMENTS.

trenching and excavation   See CONSTRUCTION.

trichlorethane   See VINYL CHLORIDE.

trichloroethylene (TCE)   See KIDNEY TOXICITY; NEUROTOXICITY; VINYL CHLORIDE.

trimellitic anhydride   A chemical known to cause asthma.

See also ASTHMA; CHEMICAL TOXICITY; OCCUPATIONAL LUNG DISEASE.

truck drivers   Workers who drive large or small delivery trucks to transport materials and goods to and from specified destinations, or who drive for specific purposes, such as fighting fires or installing and repairing utility company lines.

Truck drivers may also have to prepare receipts for loads, collect payments, maintain telephone or radio contact with supervisors, load and unload the truck, inspect the equipment and perform emergency roadside repairs.

Drivers are at high risk of road accidents due to possible loss of control while driving heavily loaded trucks on steep or slippery roads, and overturning of a heavily loaded truck due to mechanical failure. There may be accidents because of lengthy driving periods, night driving, driving under unfavorable weather conditions or on bad roads, and driving at high speeds due to the lure of bonus payments. Because of long hours, drivers may suffer physical and mental fatigue, drowsiness, and poor or irregular meals. They are exposed to NOISE and may suffer delayed hearing loss; extremes of heat and cold, which may result in heat stress or frostbite; and vibrations of their body, which may result in musculoskeletal problems. They may have low back pain and pains in their arms and legs caused by prolonged driving, sitting in uncomfortable seats, vibration or inadequate vehicle suspension, or visual discomforts and eye problems caused by inadequate illumination and eyestrain.

They may have accidents while changing tires, unfastening tight bands and ropes, lifting heavy items, and using various maintenance and repair tools such as wrenches and jacks. They may encounter acute poisoning by exhaust gases, including CARBON MONOXIDE. There are fire hazards resulting from spills and leaks of inflammable materials that may ignite on contact with an open flame, electric sparks, or as a result a road collision or overturning.

Further, according to the fourth edition of the *Encyclopaedia of Occupational Health and Safety* truck drivers are exposed to CHEMICAL TOXICITY because of hauling toxic and radioactive substances, skin diseases and conditions caused by exposure to chemicals such as cleaning compounds, brake fluids, gasoline diesel oil, and chronic effects caused by inhaling gasoline or diesel fuel fumes and exhaust gases containing carbon monoxide, nitrogen oxides, and hydrocarbons.

Truck drivers may have deterioration of their health due to smoking inside the cabin of the truck, and may be victims of violent crime because some aspects of organized crime may be attracted to valuable cargo in their trucks.

See also FIRE SAFETY/FIRE PROTECTION; SKIN AND SENSE ORGAN TOXICITY; SLEEP; SMOKING; VIBRATION; VIOLENCE.

Mager-Stillman, Jeanne, ed. *Encyclopaedia of Occupational Health and Safety.* 4th ed. Vol. 4. Geneva: International Labour Organisation, 1998, pp. 103.18–103.19.

tuberculosis   Tuberculosis is a treatable, communicable disease that has two general states: latent infection and active disease. With few exceptions, only those who develop active tuberculosis in the lungs or larynx can infect others, usually by coughing, sneezing, or otherwise expelling tiny infectious particles that someone else inhales. Although the occupational risk of tuberculosis has declined in recent years, vigilance is still necessary in certain workplaces, particularly institutional settings such as hospitals and prisons.

Unlike occupational health problems such as those involving hazardous chemicals or dust exposures, the occupational risk of tuberculosis is closely connected with the risk of tuberculosis in the surrounding community. Historically, health care workers were at higher risk from tuberculosis than others in the community. However, in recent years, effective treatment has drastically cut tuberculosis case rates and consequently reduced health care workers' occupational risk of tuberculosis. Also, lower community case rates also mean that prison, jail, homeless shelter, and other workers are less likely to be exposed to tuberculosis than in the past.

After World War II, there was a striking reduction in the disease because of more effective treatments. Complacency led to disinterest in the goal of tuberculosis elimination and to the dismantling of tuberculosis control programs. Basic public health measures were neglected, including surveillance activities, contact tracing, outbreak investigations, and case management services to ensure completed treatment of latent infection and active disease. This led to the resurgence of tuberculosis in the 1980s when new circumstances emerged, particu-larly the HIV and AIDS epidemic, the increase in the rate of multidrug-resistant disease (largely due to incomplete treatment), and expanded immigration from areas with high rates of tuberculosis.

The Institute of Medicine (IOM), in a report issued in 2001, indicated that where basic infection control measures are in place, the risk to health care workers approaches community levels. The major risk to workers now comes from patients, inmates, or others with unsuspected and undiagnosed infectious tuberculosis. Workers in communities with high rates of tuberculosis are at particular risk.

Risks to Health Care Workers
In the mid-1980s and early 1990s, a number of high-profile outbreaks of tuberculosis, including cases of multidrug-resistant disease, were documented in hospitals, nursing homes, prisons, homeless shelters, and other settings. Most outbreaks were linked to lapses in infection control practices, delays in diagnosis and treatment of infectious individuals, and the presence of high-risk populations, including people with HIV infection or AIDS and recent immigrants from countries with high rates of tuberculosis.

In 1999, the U.S. Congress requested that the National Academy of Sciences undertake a study of occupational tuberculosis. The study focused on questions regarding risk of infection to health care workers and selected other workers, whether the risk of occupational exposure can be quantified for different work environments and different job classifications, results of implementation and effects of the 1994 Centers for Disease Control and Prevention (CDC) guidelines for the prevention of tuberculosis in health care facilities, and how the Occupational Safety and Health Administration (OSHA) standard to protect workers from occupational exposure to tuberculosis will affect the disease.

Conclusions of the IOM Study
Conclusions of the study reflected the changing epidemiology of tuberculosis, continuing geographic variation in tuberculosis case rates, evolving institutional and public responses to tuberculosis in the workplace and the community, and ongoing risk from people with undiagnosed infectious tuberculosis.

REGULATING OCCUPATIONAL EXPOSURE TO TUBERCULOSIS: SELECTIVE CHRONOLOGY OF EVENTS

1950s	Health care workers' risk of tuberculosis accepted by most experts
1953	National reporting of tuberculosis cases initiated
1953–1984	Consistent declines in tuberculosis cases and deaths reported
1982	CDC issues guidelines on preventing tuberculosis transmission in health care facilities
1985–1986	First increase in numbers of tuberculosis deaths (1985) and cases (1986) since national data reporting began
1990	CDC issues new tuberculosis prevention guidelines for health care settings with specific focus on those with HIV infection and AIDS
1991	Outbreak of multidrug-resistant tuberculosis in a New York State prison results in the deaths of seven inmates and one correctional officer
1992	CDC advisory committee presents recommendations to prevent and control tuberculosis among homeless persons
1992	National Institute for Occupational Safety and Health recommends that health care workers in contact with tuberculosis patients wear industrial-type powered air purifying respirators
1992	Labor Coalition to Fight TB in the Workplace requests OSHA enforcement actions
1993	OSHA issues nationwide enforcement procedures related to occupational exposure to tuberculosis
1993	CDC issues draft revised guidelines on preventing tuberculosis transmission in health care facilities
1993	Decline in tuberculosis cases recorded, reversing 1986–1992 trend
1994	OSHA announces initiation of rulemaking process but declines request for an emergency temporary standard
1994	CDC issues revised and expanded guidelines for health care facilities
1995	OSHA meets with "stakeholder groups" to discuss workplace tuberculosis standard; seeks peer review of its risk assessment; publishes tuberculosis training and resource guide for field inspectors
1995	NIOSH issues revised certification procedures for nonpowered air-purifying personal respirators
1995	CDC initiates demonstration project to improve skin test surveillance for health care workers
1996	CDC advisory committee presents recommendations for correctional facilities
1997	OSHA issues proposed standard on workplace tuberculosis and provides for comment period and hearings
1998	OSHA conducts public hearings in Washington, New York, Chicago, and Los Angeles
1999	OSHA reopens comment period on the proposed rule with focus on issues related to homeless shelters, risk assessment, and other matters
1999	Continued decrease in tuberculosis cases and case rates
2000	CDC begins reexamination of 1994 guidelines

Source: Institute of Medicine, Committee on Regulating Occupational Exposure to Tuberculosis.

Available data suggest that where tuberculosis is uncommon or where basic infection control measures are in place, occupational risk to health care workers of tuberculosis infection now approaches the level in their community of residence. Tuberculosis risk in communities has declined since 1993. Overall, rates of active tuberculosis among health care workers are similar to those reported for other employed workers. However, whatever the origins of their disease, health care workers and others with compromised immune systems are at higher risk of death if they contract multidrug-resistant tuberculosis.

The potential for exposure to tuberculosis in health care and other facilities varies within and across communities. Where the disease is more common, health care and other workers are at higher risk of coming into contact with people who have infectious tuberculosis. However, the population in the United States is very mobile, and visitors and new residents can bring tuberculosis with them into communities where the disease is rare. When a hospital or other worker encounters such a person, she or he may be at higher risk than colleagues in high-prevalence inner cities, who are more likely to be familiar with and alert to the signs and symptoms of tuberculosis.

The occupational risk of exposure to tuberculosis varies with job category and work environment. Only some health care, correctional, and other workers are reasonably anticipated to have contact with people with tuberculosis, even in facilities that treat or admit such individuals. Although data are not completely consistent, the risk tends to be higher for those who work on wards where patients with suspected or confirmed tuberculosis are admitted and for those whose jobs involve aerosol-generating procedures, such as bronchoscopies. For these workers in particular, effective workplace tuberculosis control measures are essential.

Workers at particular risk from occupationally acquired tuberculosis infection include those with HIV infection or AIDS or other conditions associated with suppression of normal functioning of the immune system.

CDC Guidelines and OSHA Regulations

Since the early 1990s, both the CDC and OSHA have issued control guidelines and enforcement procedures based on respiratory protection regulations and on statutory requirements that employers provide a safe workplace. In general, guidelines and proposed rules focus their respirator use provisions on the worker's reasonably anticipated risk of exposure rather than the facility's risk category.

The IOM committee concluded that standards can have a positive effect if three basic conditions are met. They:

1. Are consistent with tuberculosis control measures that appear to be effective.
2. Sustain or increase the level of compliance with these measures.
3. Allow employers appropriate flexibility to adopt control measures that are matched to the level of risk facing their workers.

The IOM report included some suggestions for ending neglect and stresses better methods for identifying people with recently acquired tuberculosis infection, stronger efforts to effectively treat those who could benefit from treatment of infection, research to develop effective vaccines, more active product development initiatives focused on diagnostic and treatment technologies, and research on the problem of patient and provider failure to follow treatment recommendations.

See also IMMUNE SYSTEM; LUNG DISEASES, OCCUPATIONAL.

Field, Marilyn J., ed. *Tuberculosis in the Workplace.* Washington, D.C.: National Academy Press, 2001.

turf toe   See BASEBALL INJURIES (PROFESSIONAL).

Type A personality   A designation that usually relates to lifestyle and style of work and performance, characterized by competitive feelings, drive, ambition, impatience, goal orientation, anxiety, worry, or hostility. Type A employees worry about problems they cannot solve, a self-destructive type of behavior that can lead to FRUSTRATION and BURNOUT.

Many of these individuals neglect family responsibilities in favor of working and tending to business interests. They tend to feel guilty if not working and take little pleasure in other activities. They may take on multiple commitments and become preoccupied with meeting deadlines. Some researchers believe that Type A people have traits that set them apart from others, tend to be suspicious, and lack the emotional support that comes from close relationships.

The Type A personality pattern was found to double the risk of developing heart disease, particularly in men under the age of 60. The power of the Type A behavior pattern to predict heart disease has been shown in many countries, with data from Belgium, China, India, Japan, and Lithuania. Even when account is taken of other heart disease risk factors such as cigarette smoking, high blood pressure, and elevated serum cholesterol, the Type A pattern appears to contribute a further risk in many, but not all, people.

Researchers are studying the relationship of Type A behavior to other health outcomes. In a U.S. study of air traffic controllers, Type A personalities experienced 38 percent more mild and moderate illnesses from all causes than their colleagues. Furthermore, Type A personalities had a frequency of injury three and half times higher than those with other behavior patterns. The important information from this study is the knowledge that risks can be measured quantitatively and that recommendations can be made to change people's behavior patterns and thus lower risks of both heart attacks and injuries.

Many individuals make efforts to change their personality traits after a serious illness, and as a result, relax more and take advantage of their leisure in enjoyable ways. Studies involving Type A individuals show that they can change their behavior by learning RELAXATION techniques, developing a sense of HUMOR and making other lifestyle changes, thus, becoming a combination of the Type A and the TYPE B PERSONALITY.

A study reported by psychologist D. Ariel Kerman, Ph.D., in her book, *The H-A-R-T Program: Lower Your Blood Pressure without Drugs,* indicated that researchers at Duke University found that when Type A personalities participated in a walking/jogging program (three miles per day, three days a week), their Type A characteristics became less dominant.

See also ANGER; HOSTILITY; TYPE C PERSONALITY.

Kerman, D. Ariel. *The H-A-R-T Program: Lower Your Blood Pressure without Drugs.* New York: HarperCollins, 1992.

Type B personality
Personality traits that enable an individual to enjoy activities that are not competitive. Type Bs are not particularly goal oriented, do not constantly worry about work, and, when they are working, do so without the agitation or sense of urgency, as do people with a Type A personality.

Successful executives are often people who can move back and forth between the Type A and Type B characteristics, depending on the situation. These combined personality types are distributed fairly evenly among top and middle management.

For optimal coping with workplace challenges, a combination of Types A and B may be best. People with this combination can enjoy a balanced life with aspects of work, family, love, friends, and fun.

See also TYPE A PERSONALITY; TYPE C PERSONALITY.

Type C personality
Individuals who have Type C personalities refuse to let any negative feeling show. They usually seem happily in CONTROL and do not express emotion, especially ANGER, fear, sadness, or even joy.

Type Cs tend to be patient, cooperative, and are highly focused on meeting other people's needs while showing little or no concern for their own. Usually, Type Cs tend to stay in stressful situations, such as bad marriages or frustrating jobs, longer than other people. They do not recognize their emotions and may not even realize when they are under stress. However, their bodies produce stress hormones, including cortisol, which has been known to suppress the immune system.

Because they do not express emotions, Type C people do not produce natural opiates, the brain chemicals that have a painkilling effect similar to drugs such as morphine. This, too, reduces the overall effectiveness of their immune system.

According to psychologist Lydia Temoshok, Ph.D., author of *The Type C Connection: The Behavioral Link to Cancer and Your Health,* Type C personalities often are more likely to relapse than recover, compared to individuals in other personality categories.

WORKPLACE TIPS FOR TYPE C PERSONALITIES

- Be aware of your emotions; get psychotherapeutic help if necessary.
- Be able to express your anger in a constructive way.
- Become more assertive; learn how to say no when you want to.
- Develop effective relaxation techniques.

See also ASSERTIVENESS TRAINING; CODEPENDENCY; DEPRESSION; RELAXATION; SELF-ESTEEM; STRESS; TYPE A PERSONALITY; TYPE B PERSONALITY.

Temoshok, Lydia. *The Type C Connection: The Behavioral Link to Cancer and Your Health.* New York: Random House, 1992.

ultraviolet light See SKIN AND SENSE ORGAN TOXI-CITY.

unemployment Unemployment relates to all people who want to work but have been unable to find jobs—those who have worked but are laid off, recent high school and college graduates, people with disabilities, the poor and uneducated, women returning to the workplace after child rearing, and retirees who need additional income and/or stimulation. Because unemployment often means financial hardship, it can cause STRESS not only for the people directly involved but for their spouses, children, parents, and friends.

Unemployment is also a source of stress for those who have jobs but are constantly threatened with losing them. However, in a 1995 poll conducted by Towers Perrin, a management consulting firm, most workers are "amazingly stress hardy, pragmatic and coping with the uncertainties of corporate America." The poll also showed that one measure of a worker's adjustment to today's climate of job instability is that less than half of the workers surveyed expect to spend their entire careers with one company. Among those under age 34, only one-third counted on retiring from their present employer.

According to authors Leana and Feldman in their 1992 book *Coping with Job Loss,* "Unemployment as a fact of life will continue, if not worsen. Current statistics on unemployment and layoffs underestimate the dimensions of the problem. Even with unemployment at six percent, there would still be seven million people out of work. Because government statistics do not include the discouraged job seekers (individuals who have stopped applying for new positions) and those who

have joined the expanding ranks of the permanently unemployed, these figures vastly underrepresented the number of people actually out of work."

Leana and Feldman also reported that among the many situational factors influencing how a person reacts to a stressful life event such as losing a job, perception of unemployment levels has a "substantial influence." They write, "The higher workers perceive the unemployment rates in their communities and/or professions to be, the more pessimistic they will be about the prospects for finding new jobs, especially ones at equal pay."

Fran Lowry, in *Canadian Medical Association Journal,* says, "Now, when unemployment is still an important problem in many parts of the country [Canada], idle hands are making more work for physicians. People who are out of work make more visits to their physicians for a variety of complaints. Areas of high unemployment also report a higher incidence of alcohol use, and more marital and family abuse and violence. Because unemployment causes stress, it can have bad health consequences not only for the unemployed but also for the people who are closest to them."

In June 2003, according to a U.S. Department of Labor report, the unemployment rate rose to a nine-year high of 6.4 percent. The report indicated that businesses had cut payrolls by a total of 30,000 that month, the fifth straight month of unemployment losses.

Leana, Carrie R., and Daniel C. Feldman. *Coping with Job Loss: How Individuals, Organizations and Communities Respond to Layoffs.* New York: Lexington Books, 1992.
Lowry, Fran. "Larger Private Sector Role in Health Care Needed Now." *Canadian Medical Association Journal* (February 1995) 154, no. 4: 549–551.

See also GENERAL ADAPTATION SYNDROME; HARDI-
NESS; LAYOFFS; LIFE CHANGE SELF-RATING SCALE;
MERGERS; STRESS.

unions See AMERICAN FEDERATION OF LABOR-CON-
GRESS OF INDUSTRIAL ORGANIZATIONS; INTERNATIONAL
BROTHERHOOD OF TEAMSTERS; INTERNATIONAL LADIES
GARMENT WORKERS UNION.

unipolar depression See DEPRESSION.

UNITE! See INTERNATIONAL LADIES' GARMENT
WORKERS UNION (ILGWU).

uranium miners/uranium exposure In addition
to the usual risks of mining, uranium miners have
experienced a higher incidence of lung cancer
and other lung diseases than others. Studies have
also indicated an increase of skin cancer, stomach
cancer, and kidney disease among uranium miners.
Many research studies of hard rock miners
exposed to radon in the United States, Canada, and
Europe, show increased lung cancer rates. The
amount of cancer depends on the radiation exposure of the miners. Higher exposure is equated
with higher numbers of cancer deaths. Increases in
lung cancer due to radiation have been noted in
both smokers and nonsmokers.

In the early 1980s an independent study on the
risks for uranium miners was published by the
Atomic Energy Control Board (AECB), the organization that sets standards for radiation exposure in
Canada. This study concluded that risks are very
high. If uranium miners worked at AECB's maximum permissible level over their entire working
lifetime, the report found that the lung cancer incidence would likely quadruple. Instead of 54 lung
cancer deaths per 1,000 males, the Ontario average,
there could be close to 200 lung cancers per 1,000.

See also CANCER; CONFINED SPACES; ENERGY
EMPLOYEES COMPENSATION PROGRAM; NUCLEAR
WEAPONS WORKERS.

urethane See GASTROINTESTINAL OR LIVER TOXICITY.

**U.S. Agency for Toxic Substances and Disease
Registry** See AGENCY FOR TOXIC SUBSTANCES AND
DISEASE REGISTRY (ATSDR).

vacation Time off from the workplace, often on a paid basis. Typical paid vacation time for many American workers is two weeks per year; some executives and others have more time off. According to Emrika Padus, author of *The Complete Guide to Your Emotions and Your Health,* "getting away from it all—breaking free from routine—can bring a new perspective to old dilemmas and put a positive charge in your mental outlook. You will get to know yourself a little better. And when you come home, you'll be happier, healthier, and much more effective in coping with stress."

The book offers healthy reasons for taking a vacation, with concurrence by Edward Heath, Ph.D., professor in the Department of Recreation, Park and Tourism Sciences at Texas A&M University, and Richard I. Curtis, author of *Taking Off.* These reasons include:

Getting away from the daily routine
Relaxing
Seeing new sights
Opening up to different experiences
Making new friends
Sharing an event
Learning new skills
Participating in an adventure
Enjoying beauty
Anticipating pleasure
Remembering the joy

Dr. Heath says, "The major goal of a vacation is happiness. You leave your troubles behind you. . . . return refreshed and renewed. You should like your life a little better after a vacation."

However, vacations do not always result in stress reduction. Vacations themselves can add to stress. First there is the choice of how to travel, by car, train, ship, or plane. Dealing with reservations can be stressful. Packing and preparing those left behind, in the case of families, can be difficult, especially when parents leave young children. When grandparents take on the responsibilities of caring for the children, intergenerational conflicts may result.

Delays of trains and planes, missed connections, and accommodations not up to one's expectations can be stressful. Bad weather can do more than dampen one's spirits; weather affects enjoyment of many sites. Additionally, interpersonal relationships can be put to the test on vacations, when friends, couples, or other groupings are in close quarters together every day. Many people are happy to go back to work after their vacations for these reasons.

See also RETIREMENT.

Kahn, Ada P. *Stress A–Z: A Sourcebook for Facing Everyday Challenges.* New York: Facts On File, Inc., 2000.
Padus, Emrika. *The Complete Guide to Your Emotions and Your Health.* Emmaus, Pa.: Rodale, 1992.
Curtis, Richard I. *Taking Off.* New York: Harmony Books, 1981.

ventilation See INDOOR ENVIRONMENT.

veterinarians See ANIMAL HANDLERS; ASTHMA.

vibration (hand/arm) Over a prolonged period, hand/arm vibration can damage bones and joints. The best-known resulting condition is VIBRATION WHITE FINGER. This is extremely painful and can be disabling. The cause of such injury is usually the long-term use of handheld power tools, chain saws, or devices used in mining.

Whole body vibration can impair working efficiency and even cause serious injury if the body is subjected to accelerations. The most common

315

symptom of whole body vibration is probably travel sickness, but longer-term effects can be caused by agricultural machinery or movement that tends to throw people about. Selections of tools and systems of work that avoid long periods of repetitive activity without breaks are important considerations.

See REPETITIVE STRESS INJURIES.

vibration white finger (VWF)   A condition caused by continuous working with vibrating machinery such as chain saws and drills. VWF causes the fingers to become numb and begin turning white.

Symptoms include tingling and numbness in the fingers, which often continue after the machinery has been switched off. One fingertip temporarily turns white and may start aching. The finger turns white with increasing frequency. Other fingers begin turning white, but the thumb is usually not affected. After several fingers turn white, the disease may be irreversible. Eventually, the person may lose fingers. This only happens in extreme cases, for example, when people are working with vibrating machinery in very cold conditions. It is most common in the forestry industry and people working with chain saws.

The condition is one form of Raynaud's disease. Raynaud's is caused by a restriction in the blood supply to the extremities, usually the fingers and toes. With vibration white finger, the fingers may go into spasm, due to an intermittent lack of blood supply to the fingers.

See also CHAIN SAWS/CHAIN SAW INJURIES; VIBRATION (HAND/ARM); REPETITIVE STRESS INJURIES.

vinyl chloride   A colorless, flammable gas at normal temperatures with a mild, sweet odor. It is a manufactured substance used to make polyvinyl chloride (PVC), which is used to make a variety of plastic products, including pipes, wire and cable coatings, and furniture upholstery.

Vinyl chloride also results from the breakdown of other substances, such as trichloroethane, trichloroethylene, and tetrachloroethylene. Vinyl chloride is also known as chloroethene, chloroethylene, and ethylene monochloride.

Workers are exposed to vinyl chloride by breathing contaminated air from plastic industries, haz-ardous-waste sites, and landfills, or are when it contacts their skin or eyes in the workplace.

Breathing high levels of vinyl chloride can cause people to feel dizzy or sleepy. Breathing very high levels can cause one to pass out, and breathing extremely high levels can cause death. Most of the studies on long-term exposure (365 days or longer) to vinyl chloride involve workers who make or use vinyl chloride. They were exposed to much higher levels of vinyl chloride in the air than is the general population.

People who breathe vinyl chloride for long periods of time have experienced changes in the structure of their livers, or developed nerve damage and immune reactions. Other workers have developed problems with the blood flow in their hands; the tips of their fingers turn white and hurt when they are in cold temperatures. Sometimes the bones in the tips of their fingers have broken down.

The Department of Health and Human Services has determined that vinyl chloride is a known human carcinogen; vinyl chloride exposure results in liver cancer.

The Environmental Protection Agency (EPA) requires that spills or accidental releases into the environment of one pound or more of vinyl chloride be reported to the EPA. The Occupational Safety and Health Administration (OSHA) has set the maximum allowable level of vinyl chloride in workroom air during an eight-hour workday in a 40-hour workweek as one part vinyl chloride per million parts of air (1 ppm).

See also CARCINOGENS; CARDIOVASCULAR OR BLOOD TOXICITY; ENVIRONMENTAL PROTECTION AGENCY; GASTROINTESTINAL OR LIVER TOXICITY; OCCUPATIONAL SAFETY AND HEALTH ADMINISTRATION; SKIN OR SENSE ORGAN TOXICITY.

Agency for Toxic Substances and Disease Registry
1600 Clifton Road, NE
Atlanta, GA 30333
(888) 422-8737 (toll-free)
(404) 498-0057 (fax)
http://www.atsdr.cdc.gov

violence in the workplace   Murders, shootings, knifings, beatings, rape, and other aggressive assaults on fellow employees, employers, or members of the public in a workplace.

According to the National Institute for Occupational Safety and Health (NIOSH), homicide is the second leading cause of death on the job (second only to motor vehicle crashes). Homicide is the leading cause of death for workers under 18 years of age. Homicide is the leading cause of workplace death among females. However, men are at a three times higher risk of becoming victims of workplace homicides than women. The majority of workplace homicides are related to robberies (71 percent), with only nine percent committed by coworkers or former coworkers. Seventy-six percent of all workplace homicides are committed with a firearm.

NIOSH reported 1,071 workplace homicides in 1994. Victims included 179 supervisors or proprietors of retail sales, 105 cashiers, 86 taxicab drivers, 49 managers in restaurants or hotels, 70 police officers or detectives, and 76 security guards. An additional 1 million workers are victims of nonfatal assaults each year. These figures indicate that an average of 20 workers are murdered and 18,000 are assaulted each week while at work or on duty.

Researchers report a difference between the circumstances of workplace violence and those of other types of homicides. While most workplace homicides are robbery-related, less than 10 percent of homicides in the general population occur during a robbery. Also, about 50 percent of all murder victims in the general population were related to their assailants, whereas the majority of workplace homicides are believed to occur among people who do not know each other.

Nonfatal workplace assaults result in more than 876,000 lost workdays and $16 million in lost wages. NIOSH reports that most nonfatal workplace assaults occur in settings such as hospitals, nursing homes, and social service agencies. Forty-eight percent of nonfatal assaults in the workplace are committed by a health care patient. Nonfatal assaults occur among men and women at an almost equal rate.

Predicting Violence at Work

A predictor of workplace violence, according to Barling, is the development of a profile of a potentially violent or disgruntled employee. This person may be male, white, age 20–33, a loner, probably an alcohol abuser, who has a fascination with guns. Personal factors outside the workplace may also contribute to violence at work. Such factors may include low self-esteem, alcohol abuse, or a history of aggression in the family.

Other factors leading to on-the-job aggression and violence may include stress, feelings of job insecurity, perceptions that management and supervision policies are harsh and unjust, electronic monitoring, perceived crowding, and extreme heat and noise.

**FACTORS PLACING WORKERS
AT RISK OF VIOLENCE AT WORK**

Interacting with the public
Exchanging money
Having a mobile workplace, such as a taxicab or police
    cruiser
Delivering services or goods
Working late at night or during early morning hours
Working alone or in small numbers
Working in high crime areas
Guarding valuable goods or property
Dealing with unstable people
Working with volatile persons in health care, social ser-
    vice, or criminal justice settings

Source: NIOSH

Risks of violence are higher in certain occupations than others, although anyone can become the victim of a workplace assault. Occupations with the highest homicide rates are taxicab drivers/chauffeurs, sheriffs/bailiffs, police, gas station/garage workers, and security guards. Taxicab drivers face the highest risk, at 41.4 per 100,000, nearly 60 times the national average of .70 per 100,000. The taxicab industry is followed by liquor stores (7.5), detective/protective services (7.0), gas service stations (4.8), and jewelry stores (4.7).

The majority of nonfatal assaults occurred in the service and retail trade industries. Specifically, 27 percent occurred in nursing homes, 13 percent in social services, 11 percent in hospitals, 6 percent in grocery stores, and 5 percent occurred in eating and drinking places.

According to NIOSH research, the risk of workplace victimization is related more to the task performed than to the demographic characteristics of the person performing the job. Factors related to an increased risk for workplace victimization include routine face-to-face contact with large numbers of people, the handling of money, and jobs that required routine travel or did not have a single worksite.

A recent Bureau of Labor Statistics report indicated that nearly half of workplace assaults were described as incidents involving hitting, kicking, or beating; there were also cases of squeezing, pinching, scratching, biting, stabbing, and shooting, as well as rapes and threats of violence. The median days away from work as the result of the assault were five, but this figure varied by type of assault.

VIOLENT ACTS RESULTING IN DAYS AWAY FROM WORK, 1992, BY INDUSTRY

Industry	Violent Acts Resulting in Days Away from Work (% of total)
Services	64
Nursing homes	27
Social services	13
Hospitals	11
Other services	13
Retail trades	21
Grocery stores	6
Eating and drinking places	5
Other retail	10
Transportation/communication/ public utilities	4
Finance/insurance/real estate	4
Other	4
Manufacturing	3

Source: Bureau of Labor Statistics, 1994.

TYPES OF VIOLENT ACTS RESULTING IN DAYS AWAY FROM WORK: PRIVATE INDUSTRY

Type of Violent Act	Number of Cases	Median Days Away from Work
Hitting, kicking, beating	10,425	5
Squeezing, pinching, scratching, twisting	2,457	4
Biting	901	3
Stabbing	598	28
Shooting	560	30
All other specified acts (e.g., rapes, threats)	5,157	5

Source: Bureau of Labor Statistics, 1994.

Relationship of the Victim to the Offender

The Bureau of Justice Statistics (BJS) analyzed the relationship of the victim to the offender for violent acts by gender. Female workers appeared to be most likely to be attacked by someone they knew, although only 5 percent of victimizations were attributed to an intimate (defined as a husband, ex-husband, boyfriend, or ex-boyfriend; see chart). (The BJS suggests that a customer, client, or patient with whom the victim had an ongoing professional relationship would have been attributed to the acquaintance or well-known person category.)

U.S. WORKPLACE VICTIMIZATION BY VICTIM-OFFENDER RELATIONSHIP AND SEX, 1987–1992.

Victim-Offender Relationship	% of Workplace Victimizations	
	MALE WORKERS	FEMALE WORKERS
Stranger	58	40
Acquaintance	30	35
Well-known person	10	19
Relative	1	1
Intimate (spouse, ex-spouse)	1	5

Source: NIOSH

Prevention of Violence

NIOSH suggests that while no single strategy is appropriate for preventing violence in all workplaces, all workers and employers should assess the risk of violence in their workplaces and take appropriate action to reduce those risks. A number of environmental, administrative, and behavioral strategies may reduce the risk of workplace violence. These include good visibility and lighting within and outside the workplace, cash handling policies, staffing patterns, physical separation of workers from customers or clients, security devices, and employee training.

Further, NIOSH suggests that a workplace violence prevention program include a system for documenting incidents, procedures to be taken when incidents occur, and open communication between employers and workers. Policies and procedures for assessing and reporting threats allow employers to track and assess threats and violent incidents. Such policies clearly indicate a zero tolerance of violence and provide mechanisms by which incidents can be reported and handled. Additionally, such information allows employers to assess whether prevention strategies are appropriate and effective. Policies should also include education, training, and guidance on recognizing the potential for violence, methods for defusing or de-escalating potentially violent situations, and instructions about the use of security devices and protective equipment. Procedures for obtaining medical care and psychological support following violent incidents should also be addressed. Appropriate referrals to EMPLOYEE ASSISTANCE PROGRAMS or local mental health services may be appropriate for debriefing sessions after critical incidents.

See also AGGRESSION; FATAL INJURIES; HEALTH CARE WORKERS; HOSPITAL HAZARDS; LOST WORKDAYS; NATIONAL INSTITUTE OF OCCUPATIONAL SAFETY AND HEALTH; OCCUPATIONAL SAFETY AND HEALTH ADMINISTRATION; STRESS.

Barling, Julian. "Workplace Violence." *Encyclopaedia of Occupational Health and Safety.* 4th ed. Geneva: International Labour Organisation, 1998.
National Institute of Occupational Safety and Health. *Current Intelligence Bulletin 57: Violence in the Workplace: Risk Factors and Prevention* Strategies, (DHHS [NIOSH] Publication No. 96-100).

voice disorders   See BELTING; PERFORMING ARTS MEDICINE.

volatile hydrocarbons   See INDOOR ENVIRONMENT.

volunteer workers   See WORK RELATIONSHIP CRITERIA.

waste industry   Because of the character of the work, hazards abound for refuse collectors, refuse and recycling truck drivers and other waste industry workers. In the 1992–97 period, refuse collectors were identified as holding one of the most dangerous jobs in the United States.

The waste industry accounted for 499 (1.3 percent) of the 37,875 occupational fatalities reported to the Bureau of Labor Statistics' (BLS) Census of Fatal Occupational Injuries (CFOI) since its inception in 1992.

Refuse systems involving trucking without storage can involve recycling, refuse collection, and disposal. Several aspects of the industry, including wholesale durable scrap, recovery of nonferrous metals from scrap metal and dross (the waste industry aspect of secondary smelting and refining) almost exclusively involve recycling.

The following table shows the distribution of fatality cases for 1992–97 within the recycling industry.

RECYCLING FATALITIES

Industry	Number of Fatalities
Total fatalities	499
Secondary smelting and refining of nonferrous metals	25
Local trucking without storage	64
Refuse systems	223
Wholesale durable scrap and waste materials	187

Refuse Systems

This aspect of the waste industry primarily involves collection and disposal of refuse by processing or destruction, or in the operation of incinerators, waste treatment plants, landfills, or other disposal sites.

From 1991 through 1997, nearly three-quarters of the 223 refuse systems workers suffering fatal job injuries were either refuse collectors (69 fatalities), truck drivers (63 fatalities), or nonconstruction laborers (30 fatalities).

Refuse collection often involves jumping off and on trucks, carrying trash containers, and walking on streets, alleys, and parking lots. Collectors often have to collect from both sides of a street and near vehicles that stop and start frequently. Sometimes vehicles obscure approaching traffic. Vehicles inflict most fatal injuries involving refuse collectors; for example, collectors may be run over by the refuse truck or struck by a passing vehicle, sometimes after falling from the truck.

FATALITIES AMONG REFUSE WORKERS

Event	Number of Fatalities	Percent
Total	223	100
Workers struck by vehicle, mobile equipment	66	30
Highway transportation crashes and other incidents	58	26
Caught in or compressed by equipment or objects	25	11
Other	74	33

Not all injuries are fatal. The Bureau of Labor Statistics' Annual Survey of Occupational Injuries and Illnesses, which excludes government employees and self-employed individuals, estimates that an average of 2,162 refuse collectors suffered nonfatal job injuries and illnesses each year from 1992 through 1997. Cuts, lacerations, punctures, bruises, and contusions account for 18 percent of all cases involving refuse collectors during this time span. Fractures accounted for 3 percent of such cases. Sprains, strains, and muscle tears accounted for 48 percent of cases.

Overexertion, predominantly in lifting, is the leading cause of nonfatal injury or illness for refuse collectors, followed by being struck by, striking against, or being compressed in equipment or objects.

See also AGENCY FOR TOXIC SUBSTANCES AND DISEASE REGISTRY; BUREAU OF LABOR STATISTICS; DEATHS IN THE WORKPLACE; HAZARDOUS WASTE; NONFATAL OCCUPATIONAL ILLNESS BY CATEGORY.

Drudi, Dino. "Job Hazards in the Waste Industry," Office of Safety, Health and Working Conditions, Bureau of Labor Statistics.

weekend depression   A type of DEPRESSION that some individuals experience when away from their work. Particularly for some individuals who live alone, facing solitude creates a stressful situation.

To overcome the stresses of being alone, as well as the change in mood from the workweek when one is surrounded by people, individuals can schedule pleasurable activities with friends or like-minded others so that they will not spend the entire weekend alone. Weekend depression should be distinguished from chronic depression and from seasonal affective disorder, which strikes some individuals during winter months.

See also MENTAL HEALTH; SEASONAL AFFECTIVE DISORDER.

Kahn, Ada P. *Stress A–Z: A Sourcebook for Facing Everyday Challenges.* New York: Facts On File, Inc., 1998.

weight management   See OBESITY; WORKSITE WELLNESS PROGRAMS.

welding   Work involving joining metal parts by various processes. In most cases the surface layers of the metals are heated to fusion, with or without pressure. Welders adjust valves or electric switches to control flow of gases and electric current. They ignite or extinguish gas flames and other sources of heat.

Physical hazards to welders include exposure to excessive NOISE levels, exposure to excessive heat or cold, particularly in CONSTRUCTION work, chronic damage to eyes, and skin drying and other skin problems as a result of exposure to strong light and heat.

Chemical hazards include exposure to welding fumes, chronic poisoning as a result of exposure to zinc or cadmium in fumes when welding zinc or cadmium-plated parts or to polychlorinated biphenyls from the decomposition of anticorrosion oils, or to constituents of thermal decompositions products from paints during welding of painted pieces, or to asbestos when flame-cutting asbestos insulated pieces. Welders may experience siderosis (a type of pneumoconiosis) as a result of inhaling iron oxides, damage to the central nervous system, lungs and liver as a result of inhalation of phosphine. Additionally, they may experience respiratory disease, due to high concentrations of carbon dioxide in the air and the related oxygen deficiency, particularly in poorly ventilated places, irritation of the eyes and the pulmonary system by nitrogen oxides and or ozone, and carbon monoxide poisoning.

ACCIDENT HAZARDS FACING WELDERS

- Falls from heights, particularly in construction work
- Blows from falling metal parts or gas cylinders
- Cuts and stabs from sharp metal objects
- Burns from hot metal surfaces, flames, flying sparks
- Foreign particles in the eye
- Dust explosions during welding in places where flour or grain dust are present
- Ignition and explosion of hydrogen (produced by corrosion processes and various residual combustible gases in mixtures with air in closed containers)
- Poisoning by phosgene formed from chlorinated hydrocarbons used to clean the metal or as paint, glue and other SOLVENTS, or by hazardous gases generated during welding, particularly ozone, CARBON MONOXIDE and nitrogen oxide
- Electrocutions or electric shocks
- Ignition or trapping of clothing
- Fires and explosions

See also CHEMICAL TOXICITY; CONFINED SPACES; ELECTRICITY RELATED INJURIES; EYE PROTECTION; FALLS; FIRE SAFETY; PERSONAL POLYCHLORINATED BIPHENYLS; PNEUMOCONIOSIS; REPETITIVE STRESS INJURIES; SKIN AND SENSE ORGAN TOXICITY.

Encyclopaedia of Occupational Health and Safety, 4th ed. Geneva: International Labor Organization, 1998. Vol. IV, p. 103.33–103.34.

Wellness Councils of America (WELCOA) An organization devoted to promoting, building, and sustaining corporate wellness programs. WELCOA has partnered with corporations, hospitals, universities, and governmental agencies to design and deliver comprehensive wellness initiatives that address employee health and well-being, productivity, safety, and work and family issues. WELCOA has developed a systemic blueprint that companies can follow in designing and implementing a worksite wellness program. With more than 2,000 member organizations located throughout North American and locally affiliated community wellness councils, WELCOA is highly regarded for its innovative and results-oriented approach to worksite wellness.

For organizations that have adhered to the well workplace process, WELCOA presents Well Workplace Awards to recognize quality and excellence in worksite health promotion. Known as the Well Workplace/Well City initiatives, there are three levels of designations to employers: Bronze, Silver, and Gold. More than 400 companies and three cities nationwide have met a rigid set of criteria and received Well Workplace and Well City awards.

For further information:

Wellness Councils of America
9802 Nicholas Street
Suite 315
Omaha, NE 68114
(402) 827-350
(402) 827-3594 (fax)
http://www.welcoa.org

See also WORKSITE NEWS; WORKSITE WELLNESS PROGRAMS.

Well Workplace Awards See WELLNESS COUNCILS OF AMERICA.

Western blot A blood test for HIV (human immunodeficiency virus). The first-line serum test used to detect HIV is known as the enzyme-linked immunosorbent assay (ELISA). If the result is positive, the serum is then subjected to the more accurate Western blot test, because false positives may occur with ELISA. Persons should not be notified of a positive result until the Western blot test has been performed. In some states, all positive results are reported to public health authorities.

See also ACQUIRED IMMUNODEFICIENCY SYNDROME; ELISA TEST.

wheezing Coughing and shortness of breath, usually related to ASTHMA. Often workers can readily identify a specific chemical compound, dust, or fume that causes coughing, shortness of breath, or wheezing. If something unique to a workplace causes coughing or wheezing, the diagnosis may be asthma or occupational bronchitis.

In classic allergic occupational asthma, a specifically inhaled substance from the workplace sensitizes the worker's airways. Later exposure to the same vapor, dust, or fume can cause coughing, wheezing, or difficulty in breathing, all symptoms of an asthma attack.

Many workers who inhale organic dusts are exposed to many types of microbes and other substances associated with plants, trees, animals, and crops. Some workers experience asthma symptoms, while other symptoms mimic pneumonia, with fever and shortness of breath. Most of the organic-dust reactions are allergic in nature and only affect some of the exposed population. Large amounts of inhaled dust are more likely to cause actual irritation of the lung passages. Genetic and additional environmental risk factors also play a part.

Some 250 substances in the workplace can cause occupational respiratory disorders, including chemicals, enzymes, animal proteins, and plant allergens.

According to Brobson Lutz in *New Orleans Magazine*, treatment of the wheezing of asthma is the same whether it is work related or not. It is best for workers to avoid fumes and dusty areas as much as possible. For continuous exposures, workplace modifications and engineering controls are more practical than masks and respirator equipment.

For those affected with occupational lung allergies, the consequences from persistent exposure range from chronic cough to permanent lung damage. If it is not possible to avoid or safely reduce exposure to an asthma-causing dust or fume, a job change may be the only alternative.

See also AIR CONDITIONER LUNG; ALLERGIES; BIRD FANCIER'S LUNG; CHEMICAL TOXICITY; DUST; FARMER'S LUNG; RESPIRATORY TOXICITY.

Lutz, Brobson. "Wheezing While You Work: Occupational Allergies Are Nothing to Sneeze At." *New Orleans Magazine,* December 2001, p. 2.

whole body vibration   See BACK INJURIES/BACK PAIN; RIVETERS.

wind instrumentalists' injuries   See CLARINETIST'S CHEILITIS; MUSICIANS' INJURIES; PERFORMING ARTS MEDICINE.

wine industry   Workers in this industry face common risks from wet and slippery floors and the quality of illumination and ventilation. Hazards include exposure to vapors and gases released during the various stages of the wine-making processes, particularly straining, fermentation, and the use of disinfectants and other products intended to guarantee the hygienic condition and quality of the wine. Refrigerant gases such as ammonia may cause toxic and explosive risks. Adequate ventilation and strict maintenance to prevent leakage are essential.

The vapors from alcohol and carbon dioxide released by fermentation processes can cause asphyxiation, particularly when liquids are transported and decanted into reservoirs or CONFINED SPACES with inadequate ventilation.

SUBSTANCES USED IN WINE-MAKING AND POSSIBLE HARMFUL EFFECTS

Substance	Possible Harmful Effects
Metabisulphite	In concentrated solution, is irritating to the skin and the mucous membranes
Tartaric acid	Although considered nontoxic, can be slightly irritating in very concentrated solutions
Sulfur dioxide	Intense irritation of the eyes and the respiratory tract
Tannins	Can dry a worker's skin and cause it to lose pigmentation
Disinfectants and detergents for washing storage tanks	Dermatitis

Protecting Workers

Because of the humidity of several processes, protecting electrical equipment is necessary and, where possible, low voltages should be used, particularly for inspection lamps and portable equipment. Ground fault circuit interrupters should be installed where necessary. In the vicinity of distillation plants, electrical equipment should be flameproof.

Bottling and Other Hazards

The hazards associated with bottling come from handling of glass. Risks vary according to whether the bottles to be washed are new or returned, and according to the products used, such as detergents, and the techniques, such as hand washing or machine washing. Other hazards depend on the shape of the bottles, how the filling is done (manually or with a machine), the process of corking, the system of stacking, and how boxes are placed in boxes or crates.

Other risks come from the filling of containers with liquids. The worker's hands are constantly wet. If the bottles break, the glass particles and liquid can cause injuries.

See also BREWING INDUSTRY; SKIN OR SENSE ORGAN TOXICITY; SLIPS, TRIPS, AND FALLS.

Durao, Alvaro. "Wine Industry." *Encyclopaedia of Occupational Health and Safety.* 4th ed. Vol. 3. Geneva: International Labour Organisation, 1998, pp. 65.1–65.12.

wood dust   A potential health problem when wood particles from processes such as sanding and cutting become airborne. Breathing of these particles may cause allergic respiratory effects, mucosal and nonallergic respiratory effects, and cancer. In addition to the health effects of wood dust, airborne dust can create the potential for an explosion.

According to the U.S. Department of Labor, Occupational Safety and Health Administration (OSHA), hardwoods are more hazardous to human health than softwoods. There are exceptions. In particular, western red cedar, a softwood, is usually identified as one of the most hazardous to human health. The health effects appear to be related to the concentration of tannin and similar compounds in the wood.

The health effects associated with wood dust come not only from the wood dust itself but also biological organisms such as MOLD and FUNGI which grow on the wood, and chemicals such as FORMALDEHYDE, copper naphthanate, and pentachlorophenol used in the processing of some woods.

Engineering controls and PERSONAL PROTECTIVE EQUIPMENT (PPE) are two methods used for controlling wood dust exposure. Engineering controls, the preferred approach, typically include an exhaust ventilation system with collectors placed at points where dust is produced. PPE is another short-term solution to wood dust exposure. Respirators may be worn to remove hazardous particulates (dusts) and gases.

Wood dust is classified by OSHA as a hazardous chemical. In December 2002, the Department of Health and Human Services released a report listing wood dust created when machines and tools cut, shape, and finish wood as a known carcinogen.

See also CARCINOGENS; WOOD PRODUCTS INDUSTRY.

wood products industry

wood products industry Working in a sawmill is one of the most dangerous occupations in the United States. Massive weights and falling, rolling, or sliding logs can be very dangerous. Sawmill equipment also can be hazardous, particularly when workers use machines improperly or without proper safeguards.

The wood products industry includes many operations, including LOGGING, sawmills, planning mills, manufacturing plywood and reconstituted wood products such as particleboard and fiberboard, woodworking in wood shops, cabinet shops, the prefabricated wood buildings/mobile home industry, and pulp, paper, and paperboard mills.

See also ERGONOMICS; HAZARD COMMUNICATIONS; NOISE; PERSONAL PROTECTIVE EQUIPMENT; RESPIRATORY PROTECTION; WOOD DUST.

woodworker's lung

woodworker's lung See WHEEZING.

women and job-related injuries and deaths

women and job-related injuries and deaths According to a 1998 U.S. Department of Labor, Bureau of Labor Statistics Census, women experience fewer job-related injuries and deaths than

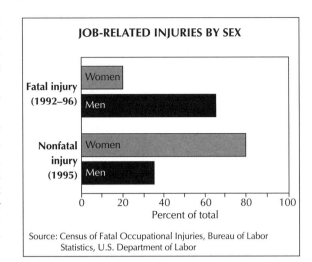

JOB-RELATED INJURIES BY SEX

Source: Census of Fatal Occupational Injuries, Bureau of Labor Statistics, U.S. Department of Labor

men. Women incurred less than one-tenth of the job-related fatal injuries and about one-third of the nonfatal injuries and illnesses that required time off to recuperate in 1991–96. During this period, women accounted for just under 50 percent of the nation's workforce.

One explanation for this discrepancy is that women are employed in relatively less dangerous jobs. Few women work in high-risk jobs where work is generally performed outdoors. However, as more women enter high-risk occupations, their risk of injury or death may increase.

Fatal Injuries

Of the 32,000 job-related fatalities that occurred during 1991–96, slightly more than 2,500 victims (8 percent) were women. Two-thirds of these work injury deaths were attributed to homicides and highway incidents. (See chart.)

Homicides. Women were 20 percent of victims in all job-related homicides in 1991–96. Most homicide victims were shot; women were strangled or beaten to death relatively more often than men. Two-thirds of the homicides occurred in the retail and service industries.

About one-third of the women who were murdered on the job worked in sales occupations either as cashier, supervisor, proprietor, or clerk. Robbery was the primary motive for these fatal assaults. More than 25 percent of the female victims of job-related homicides were assaulted by people they knew (coworkers, clients, spouses, or friends). About 16 percent of murders of women resulted from domestic disputes that spilled over into the workplace.

Highway vehicle crashes. Job-related highway incidents claimed the lives of 650 women during 1992–96, a little over 2 percent of all fatalities during the period. Health care and social service workers accounted for almost 20 percent of these deaths, about the same number as motor vehicle operators, such as truck and bus drivers and driver-sales workers.

Other causes of fatalities. About 15 percent of the fatal injuries to women resulted from other transportation-related incidents, such as aircraft crashes or being struck by a vehicle. Falls accounted for 5 percent of the job-related fatalities among women, compared with 11 percent for men. Another 5 percent of female workers' fatalities resulted from contact with objects and equipment, such as being crushed in running machinery or struck by a falling object. Exposure to harmful substances or environments, such as electrocutions, drownings, and the inhalation of chemicals, accounted for 4 percent of the fatalities among women workers. Fires and explosions claimed the lives of 2 percent of the women killed at work.

Comparison of occupational fatality rates. In addition to incurring fewer fatal work injuries than men, women have much lower fatality rates than men. Employed women had a fatality rate of less then one fatal injury per 100,000 in 1996, compared with employed men, who had eight fatal work injuries per 100,000 for the same period of time.

Nonfatal Injuries and Illnesses

Women incurred slightly over a third of the 2 million cases of work-related injuries and illnesses resulting in days away from work that occurred among private-sector wage and salary workers in 1995.

Sprains and strains among women accounted for 45 percent of their job-related injury and illness cases, compared to 42 percent among men. Women accounted for more cases than men of carpal tunnel syndrome, tendinitis, respiratory system diseases, infectious and parasitic diseases, and disorders resulting from anxiety or stress.

Almost half of the female workers' injuries and illnesses resulted from bodily reaction or exertion, such as overexertion in lifting or pushing and repetitive grasping of hand tools. Falls, primarily on the same level, and contact with objects (such as being struck by falling objects, striking against objects, or getting caught in running equipment) each accounted for about 20 percent of the job-related injuries among women.

Women were more likely to be assaulted than men and accounted for about 65 percent of the nearly 123,000 reported assault-related injuries. The manner in which women were assaulted varied. About 70 percent resulted in days away from work and occurred in the service industries, such as

JOB-RELATED FATALITIES BY EVENT OR EXPOSURE, 1992–96

Event or Exposure	Women		Men	
	NUMBER	PERCENT	NUMBER	PERCENT
Total	2,506	100	29,061	100
Homicides	973	39	4,173	14
Highway crashes	650	26	5,764	20
Struck by vehicle	156	6	1,683	6
Falls	137	5	3,081	11
Aircraft crashes	128	5	1,536	5
Contact with objects	125	5	4,862	17
Harmful exposures	102	4	2,868	10
Other	235	9	5,094	18

Source: U.S. Department of Labor, Bureau of Labor Statistics, Census of Fatal Occupational Injuries, 1992–96

nursing homes, social services, and hospitals. Another 20 percent occurred in retail industries, the most vulnerable workers being female stock handlers who incurred about 25 percent of those assaults.

For additional information:

U.S. Department of Labor
Bureau of Labor Statistics
Postal Square Building, Rm. 2850
2 Massachusetts Avenue, NE
Washington, DC 20212-0001
(202) 691-7800
(202) 691-7797 (fax)
http://stats.bls.gov/oshhome.htm
cfoistaff@bls.gov

See also VIOLENCE.

U.S Department of Labor, Bureau of Labor Statistics, Summary 98-8, July 1998.

workers' compensation   Laws designed to assure that employees who are injured or disabled on the job are provided with fixed monetary awards, eliminating the need for litigation. According to Joseph B. Treaster, in a *New York Times* article, when workers' compensation began in the United States in the early 1900s it was intended to largely eliminate the need for litigation. However, researchers now say that the workers' compensation system is such a dense patchwork of rules and regulations that seriously injured workers require the guidance of a lawyer. These laws also provide benefits for dependents of workers who are killed because of work-related accidents or illnesses. Some laws also protect employers and coworkers by limiting the amount an injured employee can recover from an employer and by eliminating coworkers' liability in most accidents. State workers compensation statutes establish this framework for most employment. Federal statutes are limited to federal employees or those workers employed in some significant aspect of interstate commerce.

The Federal Employment Compensation Act provides workers' compensation for nonmilitary federal employees. Many of its provisions are typical of most worker compensation laws. Awards are limited to disability or death sustained while in the performance of the employee's duties but not caused willfully by the employee or by intoxication. The act covers medical expenses due to the disability and may require the employee to undergo job retraining. A disabled employee receives two-thirds of his or her normal monthly salary during the disability and may receive more for permanent physical injuries or if he or she has dependents. The act provides compensation for survivors of employees who are killed. The act is administered by the Office of Workers' Compensation Programs (OWCP).

The OWCP administers four major disability compensation programs that provide wage replacement benefits, medical treatment, vocational rehabilitation, and other benefits to federal workers or their dependents who are injured at work or acquire an occupational disease.

The Energy Employees Occupational Illness Compensation Program, the Federal Employees' Compensation Program, the Longshore and Harbor Workers' Compensation Program, and the Black Lung Benefit Program serve the specific employee groups who are covered under the relevant statutes and regulations by mitigating the financial burden resulting from workplace injury.

The Federal Employment Liability Act (FELA), while not a workers' compensation statute, provides that railroads engaged in interstate commerce are liable for injuries to their employees if they have been negligent.

The Merchant Marine Act (the Jones Act) provides seamen with the same protection from employer negligence as FELA provides railroad workers.

Congress enacted the Longshore and Harbor Workers' Compensation Act (LHWCA) to provide workers' compensation to specified employees of private maritime employers. The OWCP administers the act.

The Black Lung Benefits Act provides compensation for miners suffering from black lung (pneumoconiosis). The act requires liable mine operators to pay disability payments and establishes a fund administered by the secretary of labor providing disability payments to miners where the mine operator is unknown or unable to pay. The OWCP regulates administration of the act.

The Worker's Compensation Act in California provides an example of a comprehensive state compensation program. It is applicable to most employers. The statute limits the liability of the employer and fellow employees. California also requires employers to obtain insurance to cover potential workers' compensation claims, and sets up a fund for claims that employers have illegally failed to insure against.

In spring 2003 Robert P. Hartwig, chief economist at the Insurance Information Institute, a New York trade group, reported that the average cost of workers' compensation insurance had risen 50 percent in the previous three years.

For further information:

Legal Information Institute
Cornell Law School
Myron Taylor Hall
Ithaca, NY 14853

See also ENERGY EMPLOYEES OCCUPATIONAL ILLNESS COMPENSATION PROGRAM; LONGSHORE WORKERS OCCUPATIONAL ILLNESS COMPENSATION PROGRAM.

Treaster, Joseph B. "Cost of Work Injuries Soars Across U.S." *New York Times*, June 23, 2003.
Adapted from: Legal Information Institute, "Worker's Compensation: An Overview."

working mothers Women who balance workplace duties with responsibilities of caring for children under the age of six are nearly three times as likely as other women to suffer work-related injuries, according to a study from the UCLA School of Public Health. Caring for young children seemed to have a pronounced impact on working mothers in their 30s, who were nearly five times as likely as other women to suffer workplace injuries, according to the study published in the March 1995 issue of the journal *Epidemiology*. "These findings have particular relevance because working mothers make up the fastest growing segment of the work force," said Dr. Amy Rock Wohl, primary author of the study. While just 12 percent of mothers with preschool-age children were employed outside the home in 1950, 52 percent of that group was in the workforce in 1990. The study examined 1,400 women in manufacturing jobs at a large aerospace company in Southern California during 1989. The women comprised one-third of the company's manufacturing workforce. Researchers identified 156 cases of traumatic workplace injuries, mostly strains, cuts, and bruises. Repetitive motion injuries were excluded. For each woman who was injured, researchers found two uninjured controls of the same age who worked in the same department. The study compared working women with children under age six to women who had no children and to women who had older children. Working mothers in their 20s who had preschool children were 1.2 times as likely to be injured than other women, while the risk for mothers in their 30s was 4.7 times that of other women. Mothers in their 40s were 1.6 times as likely to be injured. Mothers in their 50s were 7.5 times as likely to be injured, but researchers cautioned that the finding may not be valid because it is based on a very small sample.

Married women with young children had about the same accident rate as their single counterparts with young children. Researchers also found little evidence that years of work experience, the number of children at home or ethnicity had an effect on workplace injuries. Researchers did not study what may be responsible for the injuries among working mothers, but they suspected that it is linked to the fatigue caused by raising young children. Other authors involved in the study were Jess Kraus and Hal Morgenstern of the UCLA School of Public Health.

An Issue for Employers

Working mothers are a major issue for employers. At the end of the 1990s, about half of the total work force was female. Almost 60 percent of all women 16 years and older held down jobs. On a national level, women earned 71.6 percent of men's wages, according to a 1994 study by Women Employed.

Because there are so many working mothers and because child rearing is widely assumed to be the mother's responsibility, DAY CARE facilities have become widespread. For many women, placing children in day care is stressful and guilt-inducing and they must work through it to come to terms with the reality of trying to remain in the workforce as well as raise a family.

In 1995 *Working Mother* magazine released its 10th annual list of the nation's top 100 companies for working mothers. The rankings indicate "family friendly" characteristics of many employers, including provision of day care, summer camps, scholarships, flexible work hours, and care for a child's special needs. However, for many who work at less enlightened companies, the workplace remains a difficult and stressful place when it comes to balancing family and careers. Even at companies that make a major commitment to family issues, there is a point beyond which few businesses are willing to go.

According to Anne Ladky, executive director of Women Employed, a Chicago-based advocacy group, if a parent has to leave work on time a certain number of nights a week to pick up a child, there is still some bias against him or her. Additionally, when companies add family benefits, they do so because either the field or the geographical area is competitive when it comes to hiring and retaining employees.

A conference on work, stress, and health held in 1995, sponsored by the American Psychological Association, the National Institute of Occupational Safety and Health, the U.S. Office of Personnel Management, and the U.S. Department of Labor's Occupational Safety and Health Administration, focused on issues relating to working mothers. Research reported at that conference pointed to two competing hypotheses, according to Nancy L. Marshall of Wellesley College's Center for Research on Women. One is the "scarcity hypothesis," which presumes that people have a limited amount of time and energy that women with competing demands suffer from overload and inter-role conflict. The other, the "enhancement hypothesis," theorizes that the greater self-esteem and social support people gain from multiple roles outweigh the costs.

Results of other studies were cited. Theorists suggested that having children gives working women a mental and emotional boost that childless women lack. However, having children also increases work and family stress, and indirectly may increase symptoms of DEPRESSION.

According to Ulf Lundberg of the University of Stockholm, the "total workload scale" leads to the conclusion that women typically spend much more time working at paid and unpaid tasks than men.

Age and occupational level do not make much difference in terms of women's total workload. What matters is whether they have children. In families without children, men and women both work about 60 hours a week. However, as soon as there is a child in the family, total workload increases rapidly for women. In a family with three or more children, women typically spend 90 hours a week in paid and unpaid work, while men typically spend only 60, according to Lundberg.

Lundberg's research indicated that women's stress is determined by the interaction of conditions at home and at work, whereas men respond more selectively to situations at work and they seem to be able to relax more easily once they get home.

Many working mothers experience role conflicts between home and employment responsibilities. Despite these conflicts, they have feelings of self-fulfillment and realize economic advantages. Many find cooperation from their husbands or other family members helpful.

TIPS FOR WORKING MOTHERS TO BE MORE EFFECTIVE PARENTS AND EMPLOYEES

- Prioritize your home and work projects.
- Develop realistic expectations for yourself and others.
- Delegate projects to others in the family.
- Know that you have choices.
- Identify your key stressors and ways to reduce them.
- Learn to say no to excessive demands at home or at work.
- Ask for help when you need it.
- Realize that perfection is not a realistic goal.
- Make time for your own physical, emotional, and spiritual needs.
- Find humor in everyday situations; learn to laugh more.

See also "HAVING IT ALL"; MENTAL HEALTH; STRESS.

Kahn, Ada P. *Stress A–Z: The Sourcebook for Facing Everyday Challenges.* New York: Facts On File, Inc., 1998.
Lev, Michael, and Bonnie Rubin. "For Some Working Mothers, Some Improvement," *Chicago Tribune,* September 12, 1995.

workplace fatalities See TOXICOLOGY REPORTS AND FATAL INJURIES.

work relationship criteria According to the Bureau of Labor Statistics, U.S. Department of

Labor, a work relationship exists if an event or exposure results in the fatal injury or illness of a person: (1) on the employer's premises and the person was there to work; or (2) off the employer's premises and the person was there to work, or the event or exposure was related to the person's work or status as an employee.

The employer's premises include buildings, grounds, parking lots, and other facilities and property used in the conduct of business. Work is defined as duties, activities, or tasks that produce a product or result; that are done in exchange for money, goods, services, profit, or benefit; and, that are legal activities in the United States.

Following are clarifications of the Census of Fatal Occupational Injuries (CFOI) as compiled by the Bureau of Labor Statistics:

Volunteer workers. Fatalities to volunteer workers who are exposed to the same work hazards and perform the same duties or functions as paid employees and that meet the CFOI work relationship criteria are in scope.

Institutionalized persons. Fatalities to institutionalized persons, including inmates or penal and mental institutions, sanitariums, and homes for the aged, infirm and needy, are out of the scope of the CFOI unless they are employed off the premises of their institutions.

Suicides and homicides. Those that meet the CFOI work relationship criteria are in scope.

Fatal heart attacks and strokes. These are in scope if they occurred on or off the employer's premises and the person was there to work. Those fatal heart attacks and strokes that occurred under other circumstances are out of scope, unless work relationship is verified.

Recreational activities. Fatal events or exposures that occurred during a person's recreational activities, that were not required by the person's employer, are out of scope.

Travel status. Fatal events or exposures that occurred when a person was in travel status are in scope if the travel was for work purposes or was a condition of employment.

Commuting. Fatal events or exposures that occurred during a person's commute to or from work are out of scope.

For further information:

U.S. Bureau of Labor Statistics
OCWC/OSH
Suite 318
2 Massachusetts Avenue, NE
Washington, DC 20212-0001
(202) 691-7800
(202) 691-7797 (fax)
http://www.bis.gov/IIF

Worksite News   A news magazine focusing on occupational safety, health and environmental issues for the industrial and commercial sectors across North America. General themes include safety/loss control, transportation safety, environmental controls, air quality controls, waste management, ergonomics, first aid, and emergency planning and preparedness. *Worksite News* details the cooperative effort among Canada, the United States and Mexico to create and maintain common occupational safety, health, and environmental standards, as called for in the North American Free Trade Agreement (NAFTA).

See also HEALTH PROMOTION; WORKSITE WELLNESS; WORKSITE WELLNESS COUNCILS OF AMERICA.

worksite wellness programs   Wellness promotion, through organized programming at the workplace, that encourages voluntary behavior changes in employees. Worksite wellness activities are designed to reduce health risks and improve individual productivity. Wellness programs can help employees choose to live a more successful physical, emotional, psychological, and occupational existence. According to the Wellness Councils of America, worksite wellness initiatives have the power to change lives and transform organizations. Since the late 1980s, the Wellness Councils of America has dedicated its efforts to helping member companies build and sustain wellness programs. Since then, much has been learned about worksite health promotion. From improving health and well-being to demonstrating cost benefit, worksite health promotion has rapidly gained acceptance among a variety of constituents, including business and industry, health care, education, and government.

About half of companies with more than 750 employees offer a comprehensive employee health promotion program, according to the National Worksite Health Promotion Survey from 1999, the most recent year such a survey was done. According to the Wellness Councils of America and Canada, more than 81 percent of America's businesses with 50 or more employees have some form of health promotion program. The most popular are exercise, weight loss programs, stop-smoking classes, back care programs, and stress management.

Health Promotion: Controlling Health Care Costs

Health promotion is important to employers because health care costs continue to be an issue of major concern. More than $1 trillion are spent in the United States alone on health care, more than any other nation in the world. The average annual health care cost per person in the United States far exceeds $3,000. Lifetime costs per person are in the area of $225,000.

Because much of these costs are linked to health habits, it is possible for employers to take action toward reducing health care utilization and containing costs by providing health promotion activities.

A factor in rising health costs is Americans' growing tendency toward obesity. According to David Hunnicutt, president of the Wellness Councils of America, "the vast majority of Americans spend the majority of time at work. And it's sedentary." Health experts say it is incumbent on employers to find ways to get workers to exercise and become more concerned about their health. A National Center for Health Statistics report released in April 2002 said seven in 10 adults do not exercise regularly and nearly four in 10 are not physically active at all. Meanwhile, a federal government survey in 2000 found that 56.4 percent of Americans are overweight. Obesity can result in higher health insurance claims and employee absenteeism.

Companies say wellness programs have proven effective, with reductions in blood pressure, smoking, and cholesterol levels. For instance, about 1,000 people participated in Cigna's weight management program in 2001, and the average weight loss was 10 to 15 pounds, according to Catherine

Hawkes, assistant vice president of the insurer's employee health and work-life programs. Autoworkers at General Motors Corp. relax and stretch with yoga and tai chi classes offered just floors above the assembly lines in Flint, Michigan. Union Pacific Railroad employees can use a fitness center at many remote spots; the company used to have traveling fitness railcars before workers started staying in hotels. Chrysler Group offers incentives for its employees to use its programs, giving out "well bucks" that can be redeemed for gym bags, golf balls, and other gear. Employees earn the well bucks if they get a health screening, check out a book or video from the company health library, or get a workplace massage.

Increased Technology: A Threat to Good Health

People are working harder than they ever have before. The typical American now works 47 hours a week. Because of modern conveniences such as laptop computers, modems, fax machines, e-mail, and cellular phones, traditional boundaries of work have been erased. Despite the conveniences of these advances, they become a threat to good health because they use up time people might have devoted to exercise or recreational activities. Progressive health promotion programs at the worksite can help alleviate some of these concerns.

Additionally, increased reliance on technology has ushered in many new health concerns including repetitive stress injuries, low back problems, and compromised vision. Because almost one-third of the workforce now spends most of the day seated at computers, sedentary lifestyles have become a concern to employers.

Stress

The pace of technological change and the challenge of information management has increased the level of stress for both employers and employees. According to the Wellness Councils of America, a recent nationwide poll indicated that 78 percent of Americans describe their jobs as stressful. High levels of organizational stress exact a toll on business. From increased accidents to reduced productivity, to unnecessary absenteeism, to increased medical care costs, the impact of stress is devastating.

Increasingly, more business leaders and health promotion practitioners look to health promotion programs as a means of reducing, managing and in some instances, even eliminating harmful sources of stress. By implementing a comprehensive stress management intervention, it is possible to successfully combat prevalent stressors in the workplace.

Examples of stress reduction techniques include teaching employees stress management skills, implementing flexible work schedules, increasing the quality and quantity of social interaction, and increasing participation in the company decision-making process.

Increasing Diversity in the Workforce

Because of increasing diversity in the workforce, there is a need to address many health and wellness issues to keep employees healthy and productive. For example, jobs generated by small firms are more likely to be filled by younger workers, older workers, and women. According to recent statistics obtained from the Small Business Administration, the number of women-owned firms and firms owned by people of color has increased significantly. Between 1987 and 1992, the number of women-owned businesses rose approximately 43 percent. In 1996 nearly 8 million women-owned firms provided jobs for 18.5 million persons, more people than are employed in the Fortune 500.

Data on black-owned businesses revealed an increase of 46 percent. Hispanic-owned businesses proved to be one of the fastest-growing segments, increasing 82.7 percent between 1987 and 1992. Businesses owned by Asian-Americans, American Indians, Alaskan natives and Pacific Islanders increased 87.2 percent between 1987 and 1992.

With increasing diversity comes the challenge of being responsive to many additional health concerns. Because health promotion programs help pinpoint specific health issues of most concern, such initiative can be used to identify and address a variety of diverse health issues.

Health Promotion Helps Avoid Illnesses

Many causes of illnesses are preventable. Estimates are that preventable illnesses make up approximately 70 percent of the entire burden of illness and associated costs in the United States. Preventable factors include tobacco use, high-risk alcohol consumption, sedentary lifestyle, and poor nutritional habits. By offering a health promotion initiative, employers can take important steps toward preventing unnecessary sickness and death.

For further information:

Wellness Councils of America
9802 Nicholas Street
Suite 315
Omaha, NE 68114
(402) 827-3590
(402) 827-3594 (fax)
http://www.welcoa.org

See also ABSENTEEISM; DISABILITIES; HEALTH INSURANCE; LOST WORKDAYS; REPETITIVE STRESS INJURIES; STRESS; WORKERS' COMPENSATION; *WORKSITE NEWS.*

Moses, Alexandra R. "Wellness Programs a Fit for Bottom Lines." *Chicago Tribune,* April 28, 2002, Sec. 5, p. 9.

workstation   See COMPUTERS; ERGONOMICS; PERSONAL SPACE.

World Trade Center   See DUST AND DEBRIS; FIREFIGHTERS AND RESCUE WORKERS.

writer's block   An obstacle to the free expression of a writer's ideas on paper; there is an interruption in the flow between the thought and the recording of it. When a block occurs, the writer may feel stressed and frustrated. Unable to go on while waiting for an inspiration, the writer may have doubts about his or her capabilities to do his or her job appropriately, hopes for advancement, and even future in the chosen field.

Many writers suffer from writer's block at some time. The block may involve an inability to get started with a project or to set words down on paper; it may occur in the middle of a project or before starting. The block may occur in writing a report, a request, or a proposal. Writers may be concerned about the validity of their topic or premise, ability to communicate on paper, and acceptance by supervisors or readers.

Too much stress can paralyze the writer, and too little stress can lead to apathy. The ideal state of mind, the one that unblocks, was called "eustress," or good stress, by HANS SELYE, the Canadian author of *The Stress of Life* (1956) and *Stress Without Distress* (1974). That middle point in the stress spectrum is the state of relaxed concentration accompanied by energy. Because writing can be hard work, one must be in the right mental framework to take risks and have confidence and SELF-ESTEEM regarding one's own abilities.

Overcoming Writer's Block

Writing usually involves several steps: incubation, planning, research, organization, first draft, revision, and final draft. Before starting, the writer develops ideas and insights for the written material; this is the important incubation process. To bring these ideas out of the mind and onto paper, and thus break writer's block, he or she must reach a state of relaxed, energized concentration, in which self-criticism is set aside, leaving room for creative thoughts.

There are a number of exercises one can perform to help reach the state of energized relaxation. Physical exercise energizes and is conducive to a relaxed state of mind. MEDITATION and imagery exercises are also very useful in reducing stress and minimizing the self-doubt that obstructs expression. Proper nutrition and enough sleep are similarly important to the writer.

Another way to avoid writer's block is to avoid people who are critical in the early stage of the project. While criticisms may be helpful later, early in the project criticism may be stifling.

See also CREATIVITY; FRUSTRATION; STRESS.

Kahn, Ada P. *Stress A–Z: A Sourcebook for Facing Everyday Challenges.* New York: Facts On File, Inc., 1998.

Sloane, Beverly LeBov. "Creativity." *Town Hall of California Reporter,* March-April 1987, pp. 6–7.

yoga A method of attaining a higher level of consciousness that can help eliminate anxiety-producing thought patterns. Yoga is a mental and physical discipline intended to help one get in touch with one's true nature and mystical feelings outside of everyday existence and improve mental health. Many workplace wellness programs include yoga classes for employees.

There are several types of yoga practice and varying emphasis on physical, mental, and social activity. Some yoga disciplines are more spiritual and metaphysical. The most commonly practiced yoga in the West is hatha yoga; it concentrates on spiritual improvement through the practice of physical postures called asanas. Mantras, or sacred sounds, are used in mantra yoga. Still another branch of yoga concentrates on the kundalini, or serpent power, which is thought to lie at the base of the spine and which can be released through postures, mantras, and meditation. In some yoga practices, various forms are combined.

Yoga is an ancient practice that influenced and was in turn influenced by Brahminism, Jainism, Buddhism, and Hinduism. Yoga practice started to move westward as a result of the Muslim invasions of India, but only the colonial expansion of the British brought Europeans in contact with yoga.

Critics of yoga say that it can be physically dangerous if practiced without supervision and that it may lead to introversion or a hedonistic philosophy. The degree to which adherents depend on their teacher or guru may decrease a sense of independence in the student and may give the teacher too strong a sense of his or her own power.

Choice of an instructor for a worksite yoga program is important. Appropriate credentialing and training as well as an ability to communicate with employees is essential.

See also EXERCISE; MENTAL HEALTH; WORKSITE WELLNESS PROGRAMS.

Kahn, Ada P., and Jan Fawcett. *Encyclopedia of Mental Health.* 2d ed. New York: Facts On File, Inc., 2001.
Guiley, Rosemary Ellen. *Harper's Encyclopedia of Mystical and Paranormal Experience.* San Francisco: HarperSan Francisco, 1991.

younger workers See TEENAGE WORKERS.

youth-related injuries See TEENAGE WORKERS.

Z

zoonoses   Diseases that are contractible by workers from animals. Good animal health and personal hygiene programs can help workers avoid risks from zoonoses. Most zoonoses are avoidable and treatable if diagnosed correctly at an early stage. Incidence of allergy-related illness is high and is best treated by avoiding the irritant when it is identified. Chemicals used to clean animal cages and areas may be irritating to some workers and lead to respiratory or mucus membrane discomfort. Some diseases are potentially lethal, such as rabies.

Routine prophylaxis against tetanus and hepatitis may be appropriate for many workers. Clothing worn by animal handlers should be chosen carefully, avoiding floppy materials; gloves may protect and reduce some injuries.

See also ALLERGIES; ANIMAL HANDLERS; CATTLE, SHEEP and GOAT WORKERS; CHEMICAL SENSITIVITY; HAND PROTECTION; PERSONAL PROTECTIVE EQUIPMENT:

Mager-Stillman, Jeanne, ed. *Encyclopaedia of Occupational Health and Safety.* 4th ed. Volume 3, p. 96.40 Geneva: International Labor Organization, 1998.

APPENDIXES

APPENDIX I
ASBESTOSIS MORTALITY RATES

ASBESTOSIS: PROPORTIONATE MORTALITY RATIO (PMR) BY USUAL INDUSTRY, RESIDENTS AGE 15 AND OVER, SELECTED STATES AND YEARS, 1987–1996

CIC	Industry	Number of Deaths	PMR	95% Confidence interval	
				LCL	UCL
360	Ship and boat building and repairing	195	33.95	29.27	39.29
262	Miscellaneous nonmetallic mineral and stone products	67	24.97	19.06	32.14
502	Lumber and construction materials	18	11.33	6.70	17.90
192	Industrial and miscellaneous chemicals	105	8.32	6.76	10.12
200	Petroleum refining	32	5.85	3.95	8.36
211	Other rubber products, and plastics footwear and belting	34	5.48	3.70	7.83
282	Fabricated structural metal products	35	5.26	3.65	7.32
272	Primary aluminum industries	18	5.11	3.02	8.07
462	Electric and gas, and other combinations	12	4.98	2.57	8.69
420	Water transportation	25	4.51	2.91	6.65
180	Plastics, synthetics, and resins	13	4.48	2.38	7.66
521	Hardware, plumbing and heating supplies	11	4.31	2.15	7.71
060	Construction	638	4.21	3.90	4.56
460	Electric light and power	45	4.08	2.98	5.46
210	Tires and inner tubes	15	3.66	2.04	6.04
881	Membership organizations	14	3.13	1.71	5.25
181	Drugs	11	3.05	1.52	5.46
472	Not specified utilities	7	3.03	1.22	6.25
250	Glass and glass products	21	2.95	1.82	4.51
400	Railroads	81	2.79	2.21	3.47
050	Nonmetallic mining and quarrying, except fuel	7	2.62	1.05	5.40
212	Miscellaneous plastics products	7	2.60	1.04	5.36
350	Not specified electrical machinery, equipment, and supplies	12	2.10	1.08	3.66
580	Lumber and building material retailing	13	2.06	1.10	3.52
160	Pulp, paper, and paperboard mills	23	1.97	1.25	2.96
270	Blast furnaces, steelworks, rolling and finishing mills	44	1.61	1.15	2.19
392	Not specified manufacturing industries	66	1.60	1.22	2.06

CIC - Census Industry Code   n.e.c. - not elsewhere classified   LCL - lower confidence limit   UCL - upper confidence limit
Source: National Center for Health Statistics multiple cause of death data.

**ASBESTOSIS: PROPORTIONATE MORTALITY RATIO (PMR) BY USUAL INDUSTRY,
RESIDENTS AGE 15 AND OVER, SELECTED STATES AND YEARS, 1987–1996** *(continued)*

CIC	Industry	Number of Deaths	PMR	95% Confidence interval	
				LCL	UCL
593	Insulation workers	124	192.27	160.23	229.99
643	Boilermakers	61	44.69	34.11	57.52
585	Plumbers, pipefitters, and steamfitters	237	19.98	17.37	22.94
646	Layout workers	8	18.20	7.84	35.83
653	Sheet metal workers	55	13.54	10.03	17.86
058	Marine and naval architects	5	12.26	3.97	28.64
584	Plasterers	9	11.20	5.14	21.25
534	Heating, air conditioning, and refrigeration mechanics	17	9.86	5.73	15.78
575	Electricians	106	7.60	6.18	9.25
829	Sailors and deckhands	10	6.90	3.32	12.68
544	Millwrights	25	6.67	4.30	9.84
757	Separating, filtering, and clarifying machine operators	13	6.02	3.20	10.29
783	Welders and cutters	73	5.96	4.66	7.53
224	Chemical technicians	5	5.68	1.84	13.27
759	Painting and paint spraying machine operators	13	5.42	2.88	9.26
555	Supervisors, electricians and power transmission installers	6	5.38	1.97	11.72
547	Specified mechanics and repairers, n.e.c.	21	5.37	3.31	8.21
518	Industrial machinery repairers	27	3.90	2.57	5.68
849	Crane and tower operators	14	3.80	2.08	6.38
876	Stevedores	5	3.66	1.18	8.55
507	Bus, truck, and stationary engine mechanic	14	3.64	1.99	6.11
696	Stationary engineers	23	3.52	2.23	5.29
056	Industrial engineers	9	3.25	1.49	6.17
057	Mechanical engineers	15	3.18	1.78	5.25
756	Mixing and blending machine operators	7	3.15	1.27	6.49
563	Brickmasons and stonemasons	21	3.10	1.91	4.74
567	Carpenters	97	3.01	2.43	3.70
549	Not specified mechanics and repairers	17	2.86	1.66	4.58
856	Industrial truck and tractor equipment operators	13	2.82	1.50	4.82
766	Furnace, kiln, and oven operators, except food	10	2.75	1.32	5.06
516	Heavy equipment mechanics	9	2.70	1.24	5.12
503	Supervisors, mechanics and repairers	12	2.63	1.36	4.59
558	Supervisors, construction, n.e.c.	35	2.63	1.83	3.66
637	Machinists	67	2.60	1.98	3.35
777	Miscellaneous machine operators, n.e.c.	41	2.55	1.82	3.47
779	Machine operators, not specified	52	2.47	1.83	3.26
579	Painters, construction and maintenance	26	2.37	1.55	3.48
633	Supervisors, production occupations	72	2.31	1.80	2.92
365	Stock and inventory clerks	13	2.15	1.14	3.68
869	Construction laborers	48	1.83	1.34	2.45
453	Janitors and cleaners	67	1.52	1.16	1.96

CIC - Census Industry Code   n.e.c. - not elsewhere classified   LCL - lower confidence limit   UCL - upper confidence limit
Source: National Center for Health Statistics multiple cause of death data.

APPENDIX II
ABSENTEEISM STATISTICS

ABSENCES FROM WORK OF EMPLOYED FULL-TIME WAGE AND SALARY WORKERS BY AGE AND SEX (NUMBERS IN THOUSANDS)

Age and Sex	Total Employed	2001					
		Absence Rate[1]			Lost Worktime Rate[2]		
		Total	Illness or Injury	Other Reasons	Total	Illness or Injury	Other Reasons
Total, 16 years and over	99,508	3.6	2.5	1.0	1.9	1.3	0.5
16 to 19 years	2,179	3.4	2.5	.9	1.5	1.1	.4
20 to 24 years	9,429	3.5	2.3	1.2	1.7	1.0	.7
25 years and over	87,899	3.6	2.6	1.0	1.9	1.4	.5
25 to 54 years	76,680	3.5	2.5	1.1	1.9	1.3	.6
55 years and over	11,220	3.8	3.1	.8	2.2	1.8	.4
Men, 16 years and over	55,931	2.6	2.0	.6	1.4	1.1	.3
16 to 19 years	1,274	2.6	2.0	.6	1.2	.9	.3
20 to 24 years	5,279	2.5	1.8	.6	1.1	.9	.2
25 years and over	49,378	2.6	2.0	.6	1.4	1.2	.3
25 to 54 years	43,121	2.5	1.9	.6	1.4	1.1	.3
55 years and over	6,257	3.2	2.6	.6	1.9	1.6	.2
Women, 16 years and over	43,576	4.8	3.2	1.6	2.6	1.7	.9
16 to 19 years	905	4.4	3.2	1.2	2.1	1.3	.7
20 to 24 years	4,150	4.9	2.9	2.0	2.6	1.3	1.3
25 years and over	38,521	4.8	3.2	1.6	2.6	1.7	.9
25 to 54 years	33,559	4.8	3.2	1.6	2.6	1.6	.9
55 years and over	4,963	4.7	3.6	1.0	2.5	2.0	.5

[1] Absences are defined as instances when persons who usually work 35 or more hours a week worked less than 35 hours during the reference week for one of the following reasons: Own illness, injury, or medical problems; child-care problems; other family or personal obligations; civic or military duty; and maternity or paternity leave. Excluded are situations in which work was missed due to vacation or personal days, holiday, labor dispute, and other reasons. For multiple jobholders, absence data refer only to work missed at their main jobs. The absence rate is the ratio of workers with absences to total full-time wage and salary employment. The estimates of full-time wage and salary employment shown in this table do not match those in other tables because the estimates in this table are based on the full CPS sample and those in the other tables are based on a quarter of the sample only.

[2] Hours absent as a percent of hours usually worked.

U.S. Bureau of Labor Statistics, Current Population Survey Website: www.bls.gov/cps/cpsaat46.pdf

U.S. EMPLOYEE ABSENCES BY INDUSTRY RANKED: 1997

Rank	Industry	Employees (000)	Absence Rate	Variance from Average
1	Agriculture	1,338	2.3%	−39.4%
2	Mining	583	2.5%	−34.2%
3	Wholesale trade	3,930	3.0%	−21.0%
4	Construction	5,276	3.4%	−10.4%
5	Finance, insurance, and real estate	6,204	3.5%	−7.8%
6	Wholesale and retail trade	16,314	3.5%	−7.8%
7	Retail trade	12,384	3.6%	−5.2%
8	Transportation and public utilities	6,267	3.7%	−2.5%
9	Communications and other public utilities	2,616	3.7%	−2.5%
10	Durable goods	11,491	3.7%	−2.5%
11	Transportation	3,651	3.7%	−2.5%
12	Manufacturing	19,012	3.8%	0.1%
13	Nondurable goods	7,521	3.9%	2.7%
14	Services	23,074	4.0%	5.4%
15	Government	15,357	4.7%	23.8%
	OVERALL AVERAGE	135,018	3.8%	0.0%

Source: Labor Market Reporter.

U.S. EMPLOYEE ABSENCES BY INDUSTRY: 1997

Industry	Employees (000)	Absence Rate	Variance from Average
Agriculture	1,338	2.3%	−39.4%
Private Non-Agricultural	76,730	3.7%	−2.5%
Mining	583	2.5%	−34.2%
Construction	5,276	3.4%	−10.4%
Manufacturing	19,012	3.8%	0.1%
Durable goods	11,491	3.7%	−2.5%
Nondurable goods	7,521	3.9%	2.7%
Transportation and public utilities	6,267	3.7%	−2.5%
Transportation	3,651	3.7%	−2.5%
Communications and other public utilities	2,616	3.7%	−2.5%
Wholesale and retail trade	16,314	3.5%	−7.8%
Wholesale trade	3,930	3.0%	−21.0%
Retail trade	12,384	3.6%	−5.2%
Finance, insurance, and real estate	6,204	3.5%	−7.8%
Services	23,074	4.0%	5.4%
Government	15,357	4.7%	23.8%
OVERALL AVERAGE	135,018	3.8%	0.0%

Source: U.S. Department of Labor Bureau of Labor Statistics

APPENDIX III
NIOSH CARCINOGEN LIST

The following is a list of substances National Institute for Occupational Safety and Health (NIOSH) considers to be potential occupational carcinogens.

A number of the carcinogen classifications deal with groups of substances: aniline and homologs, chromates, dintrotoluenes, arsenic and inorganic arsenic compounds, beryllium and beryllium compounds, cadmium compounds, nickel compounds, and crystalline forms of silica. There are also substances of variable or unclear chemical makeup that are considered carcinogens, coal tar pitch volatiles, coke oven emissions, diesel exhaust and environmental tobacco smoke.

Some of the potential carcinogens listed in this index may be reevaluated by NIOSH as new data become available and the NIOSH recommendations on these carcinogens either as to their status as a potential occupational carcinogen or as to the appropriate recommended exposure limit may change.

Acetaldehyde
2-Acetylaminofluorene
Acrylamide
Acrylonitrile
Aldrin
4-Aminodiphenyl
Amitrole
Aniline and homologs
o-Anisidine
p-Anisidine
Arsenic and inorganic arsenic compounds
Arsine
Asbestos
Asphalt fumes
Benzene

Benzidine
Benzidine-based dyes
Beryllium
Butadiene
tert-Butyl chromate; class, chromium hexavalent
Cadmium dust and fume
Captafol
Captan
Carbon black (exceeding 0.1% PAHs)
Carbon tetrachloride
Chlordane
Chlorinated camphene
Chlorodiphenyl (42% chlorine); class polychlorinated biphenyls
Chlorodiphenyl (54% chlorine); class polychlorinated biphenyls
Chloroform
Chloromethyl methyl ether
bis(Chloromethyl) ether
B-Chloroprene
Chromium, hexavalent[Cr(VI)]
Chromyl chloride; class, chromium hexavalent
Chrysene
Coal tar pitch volatiles; class, coal tar products
Coke oven emissions
DDT (dichlorodiphenyltrichloroethane)
Di-2-ethylhexyl phthalate (DEHP)
2,4-Diaminoanisoleo
o-Dianisidine-based dyes
1,2-Dibromo-3-chloropropane (DBCP)
Dichloroacetylene
p-Dichlorobenzene
3,3'-Dichlorobenzidine
Dichloroethyl ether
1,3-Dichloropropene
Dieldrin

Diesel exhaust
Diglycidyl ether (DGE); class, glycidyl ethers
4-Dimethylaminoazobenzene
Dimethyl carbomoyl chloride
1,1-Dimethylhydrazine; class, hydrazines
Dimethyl sulfate
Dinitrotoluene
Dioxane
Environmental tobacco smoke
Epichlorohydrin
Ethyl acrylate
Ethylene dibromide
Ethylene dichloride
Ethylene oxide
Ethyleneimine
Ethylene thiourea
Formaldehyde
Gallium arsenide
Gasoline
Heptachlor
Hexachlorobutadiene
Hexachloroethane
Hexamethyl phosphoric triamide (HMPA)
Hydrazine
Kepone
Malonaldehyde
Methoxychlor
Methyl bromide; class, monohalomethanes
Methyl chloride
Methylhydrazine
Methyl iodide; class, monohalomethanes
Methyl hydrazine; class, hydrazines
4,"-Methylenebis (2-chloroaniline) (MBOCA)
Methylene chloride
4,4-Methylenedianiline (MDA)
a-Naphylamine
B-Naphylamine
Nickel, metal, soluble, insoluble, and inorganic;
    class, nickel, inorganic
Nickel carbonyl
Nickel sulfide roasting
4-Nitrobiphenyl
p-Nitrochlorobenzene
2-Nitronaphthalene
2-Nitropropane

N-Nitrosodimethylamine
Pentachloroethane; class, chloroethanes
N-Phenyl-b-naphthylamine; class, b-naphthalene
Phenyl glycidyl ether; class, glycidyl ethers
Phenylhydrazine; class, hydrazines
Propane Sultone
B-Propiolactone
Propylene dichloride
Propylene imine
Propylene oxide
Radon
Rosin core solder, pyrolysis products (containing
    formaldehyde)
Silica, crystalline cristobalite
Silica, crystalline quartz
Silica, crystalline tripoli
Silica, crystalline tridymite
silica, fused
Soapstone, toal dust silicates
Tremolite silicates
2,3,7,8-Tetrachlorodibenzo-p-dioxion (TCDD)
    (dioxin)
1,1,2,2-Tetrachloroethane
Tetrachloroethylene
Titanium dioxide
o-Tolidine-based dyes
o-Tolidine
Toluene diisocyanate (TDI)
Toluene diamine (TDA)
o-Toluidine
p-Toluidine
1,1,2-Trichloroethane; class, chloroethanes
Trichloroethylene
1,2,3-Trichloropropane
Uranium, insoluble compounds Uranium, soluble
    compounds
Vinyl bromide; class, vinyl halides
Vinyl chloride
Vinyl cyclohexene dioxide
Vinylidene chloride (1,1-dichloroethylene); class,
    vinyl halides)
Welding fumes, total particulates
Wood dust
Zinc chromate; class, chromium hexavalent

APPENDIX IV
ASTHMA MORTALITY RATES

ASTHMA: PROPORTIONATE MORTALITY RATIO (PMR) BY USUAL INDUSTRY, RESIDENTS AGE 15 AND OVER, SELECTED STATES AND YEARS, 1987–1996

CIC	Industry	Number of Deaths	PMR	95% Confidence interval	
				LCL	UCL
862	Child day care services	57	2.19	1.62	2.89
840	Health services, n.e.c.	133	1.60	1.33	1.91
592	Variety stores	34	1.54	1.04	2.20
790	Dressmaking shops	36	1.53	1.06	2.13
831	Hospitals	1,064	1.46	1.38	1.55
832	Nursing and personal care facilities	221	1.43	1.24	1.64
812	Offices and clinics of physicians	125	1.39	1.16	1.66
772	Beauty shops	172	1.36	1.16	1.59
922	Administration of human resources programs	88	1.32	1.05	1.64
761	Private households	648	1.31	1.21	1.42
961	Nonpaid worker or nonworker	9,107	1.29	1.26	1.32
771	Laundry, cleaning, and garment services	164	1.23	1.05	1.44
850	Colleges and universities	253	1.23	1.09	1.39
691	Not specified retail trade	264	1.20	1.06	1.36
591	Department stores	254	1.16	1.03	1.31
842	Elementary and secondary schools	1,220	1.15	1.10	1.22

CIC - Census Industry Code   n.e.c. - not elsewhere classified   LCL - lower confidence limit   UCL - upper confidence limit
Source: National Center for Health Statistics multiple cause of death data

APPENDIX V
BYSSINOSIS MORTALITY RATES

**BYSSINOSIS: MOST FREQUENTLY RECORDED INDUSTRIES ON DEATH CERTIFICATE,
RESIDENTS AGE 15 AND OVER, SELECTED STATES AND YEARS, 1987–1996**

CIC	Industry	Number	Percent
142	Yarn, thread, and fabric mills	56	56.6
961	Nonpaid worker or nonworker	8	8.1
041	Coal mining	3	3.0
060	Construction	3	3.0
050	Nonmetallic mining and quarrying, except fuel	2	2.0
351	Motor vehicles and motor vehicle equipment	2	2.0
392	Not specified manufacturing industries	2	2.0
831	Hospitals	2	2.0
	All other industries	19	19.2
	Industry not reported	2	2.0
	Total	99	100.0

CIC - Census Industry Code
Note: Percentages may not total 100% due to rounding. See appendices for source description, methods, ICD codes, industry and occupation
  codes, and list of selected states (and years) for which usual industry and occupation have been reported.
Source: National Center for Health Statistics multiple cause of death data.

APPENDIX VI
CHRONIC OBSTRUCTIVE PULMONARY DISEASE MORTALITY RATES

CHRONIC OBSTRUCTIVE PULMONARY DISEASE: PROPORTIONATE MORTALITY RATIO (PMR) BY USUAL INDUSTRY, RESIDENTS AGE 15 AND OVER, SELECTED STATES AND YEARS, 1987–1996

CIC	Industry	Number of Deaths	PMR	95% Confidence interval	
				LCL	UCL
041	Coal mining	9,454	2.40	2.35	2.45
050	Nonmetallic mining and quarrying, except fuel	955	1.64	1.55	1.75
271	Iron and steel foundries	1,273	1.56	1.49	1.65
040	Metal mining	1,076	1.53	1.44	1.63
261	Pottery and related products	582	1.51	1.39	1.65
252	Structural clay products	591	1.49	1.37	1.63
402	Taxicab service	1,041	1.45	1.37	1.54
410	Trucking service	11,642	1.44	1.41	1.47
751	Automotive repair and related services	6,128	1.40	1.37	1.44
060	Construction	45,201	1.38	1.35	1.41
760	Miscellaneous repair services	2,031	1.37	1.32	1.43
201	Miscellaneous petroleum and coal products	96	1.36	1.10	1.67
230	Logging	2,138	1.36	1.31	1.42
250	Glass and glass products	2,087	1.36	1.31	1.42
360	Ship and boat building and repairing	1,703	1.35	1.29	1.42
621	Gasoline service stations	2,182	1.34	1.29	1.40
232	Wood buildings and mobile homes	110	1.33	1.08	1.62
251	Cement, concrete, gypsum, and plaster products	930	1.33	1.25	1.42
262	Miscellaneous nonmetallic mineral and stone products	774	1.33	1.24	1.43
231	Sawmills, planning mills, and millwork	2,672	1.32	1.27	1.37
042	Oil and gas extraction	1,850	1.30	1.25	1.36
141	Carpets and rugs	403	1.30	1.18	1.43
270	Blast furnaces, steelworks, rolling and finishing mills	7,675	1.30	1.27	1.33
752	Electrical repair shops	564	1.28	1.17	1.40
290	Screw machine products	197	1.27	1.09	1.47
400	Railroads	8,358	1.27	1.25	1.30
031	Fishing, hunting, and trapping	394	1.26	1.14	1.40
331	Machinery, except electrical, n.e.c.	4,672	1.26	1.22	1.30
212	Miscellaneous plastics products	715	1.25	1.17	1.35
282	Fabricated structural metal products	1,790	1.25	1.19	1.31
320	Metalworking machinery	1,951	1.25	1.20	1.31
420	Water transportation	1,501	1.25	1.19	1.32
470	Water supply and irrigation	947	1.25	1.18	1.33
392	Not specified manufacturing industries	11,116	1.24	1.22	1.26

CHRONIC OBSTRUCTIVE PULMONARY DISEASE: PROPORTIONATE MORTALITY RATIO (PMR) BY
USUAL INDUSTRY, RESIDENTS AGE 15 AND OVER, SELECTED STATES AND YEARS, 1987–1996 *(continued)*

CIC	Industry	Number of Deaths	PMR	95% Confidence interval	
				LCL	UCL
502	Lumber and construction materials	428	1.24	1.13	1.37
801	Bowling alleys, billiard and pool parlors	1,157	1.24	1.17	1.32
942	Military	6,900	1.24	1.22	1.27
242	Furniture and fixtures	2,962	1.23	1.18	1.28
301	Not specified metal industries	426	1.23	1.12	1.36
351	Motor vehicles and motor vehicle equipment	7,779	1.22	1.20	1.25
030	Forestry	423	1.21	1.10	1.33
221	Footwear, except rubber and plastic	1,701	1.21	1.15	1.27
101	Dairy products	1,466	1.20	1.14	1.26
160	Pulp, paper, and paperboard mills	3,075	1.20	1.17	1.24
531	Scrap and waste materials	470	1.20	1.10	1.32
111	Bakery products	1,422	1.19	1.13	1.25
140	Dyeing and finishing textiles, except wool and knit goods	224	1.19	1.03	1.37
220	Leather tanning and finishing	187	1.19	1.03	1.38
280	Other primary metal industries	1,223	1.19	1.13	1.26
211	Other rubber products, and plastics footwear and belting	1,621	1.18	1.12	1.24
241	Miscellaneous wood products	688	1.18	1.09	1.28
312	Construction and material handling machines	1,421	1.18	1.12	1.24
332	Not specified machinery	420	1.18	1.07	1.30
401	Bus service and urban transit	1,579	1.18	1.12	1.24
562	Miscellaneous wholesale, nondurable goods	235	1.18	1.03	1.35
641	Eating and drinking places	12,679	1.18	1.16	1.20
120	Beverage industries	1,610	1.17	1.11	1.23
272	Primary aluminum industries	882	1.17	1.09	1.25
300	Miscellaneous fabricated metal products	1,689	1.17	1.11	1.23
461	Gas and steam supply systems	867	1.17	1.09	1.25
552	Petroleum products	1,252	1.17	1.11	1.24
560	Alcoholic beverages	194	1.17	1.01	1.35
612	Motor vehicle dealers	3,394	1.17	1.14	1.21
011	Agricultural production, livestock	5,970	1.16	1.14	1.19
281	Cutlery, hand tools, and general hardware	392	1.16	1.05	1.29
311	Farm machinery and equipment	591	1.16	1.06	1.27
010	Agricultural production, crops	24,290	1.15	1.13	1.17
110	Grain mill products	523	1.15	1.06	1.26
291	Metal forgings and stampings	529	1.15	1.06	1.26
340	Household appliances	1,174	1.15	1.08	1.22
620	Auto and home supply stores	1,178	1.15	1.08	1.22
672	Fuel dealers	681	1.15	1.06	1.25
020	Agricultural services, except horticultural	432	1.14	1.04	1.26
021	Horticultural services	1,268	1.14	1.09	1.21
310	Engines and turbines	640	1.14	1.06	1.24
352	Aircraft and parts	2,519	1.14	1.10	1.19
521	Hardware, plumbing and heating supplies	627	1.14	1.06	1.24
192	Industrial and miscellaneous chemicals	3,104	1.13	1.10	1.17
292	Ordnance	502	1.13	1.04	1.23
580	Lumber and building material retailing	1,580	1.13	1.08	1.19
471	Sanitary services	1,063	1.12	1.06	1.19
551	Farm-product raw materials	469	1.12	1.03	1.23
721	Advertising	626	1.12	1.04	1.21
741	Detective and protective services	682	1.12	1.04	1.21

CHRONIC OBSTRUCTIVE PULMONARY DISEASE: PROPORTIONATE MORTALITY RATIO (PMR) BY
USUAL INDUSTRY, RESIDENTS AGE 15 AND OVER, SELECTED STATES AND YEARS, 1987–1996 (continued)

CIC	Industry	Number of Deaths	PMR	95% Confidence interval	
				LCL	UCL
122	Not specified food industries	694	1.11	1.03	1.20
200	Petroleum refining	1,351	1.11	1.06	1.17
390	Toys, amusement, and sporting goods	375	1.11	1.00	1.23
100	Meat products	1,666	1.10	1.05	1.16
411	Warehousing and storage	539	1.10	1.01	1.20
460	Electric light and power	2,664	1.10	1.06	1.14
550	Groceries and related products	1,776	1.10	1.05	1.16
901	General government, n.e.c.	9,322	1.10	1.08	1.12
171	Newspaper publishing and printing	1,921	1.09	1.05	1.14
210	Tires and inner tubes	995	1.09	1.03	1.16
321	Office and accounting machines	462	1.09	1.00	1.20
802	Miscellaneous entertainment and recreation services	1,128	1.09	1.03	1.16
142	Yarn, thread, and fabric mills	13,353	1.08	1.06	1.10
350	Not specified electrical machinery, equipment, and supplies	1,324	1.08	1.03	1.14
611	Food stores, n.e.c.	872	1.07	1.00	1.15
780	Barber shops	1,077	1.07	1.01	1.14
791	Miscellaneous personal services	773	1.07	1.00	1.15
932	National security and international affairs	3,391	1.07	1.04	1.11
722	Services to dwellings and other buildings	1,339	1.06	1.01	1.12
750	Automotive services, except repair	1,376	1.06	1.01	1.12
601	Grocery stores	5,922	1.05	1.03	1.08
172	Printing, publishing, and allied industries, except newspapers	3,125	1.04	1.01	1.08
342	Electrical machinery, equipment, and supplies, n.e.c.	3,510	1.04	1.01	1.08
910	Justice, public order, and safety	4,960	1.04	1.01	1.07

CIC - Census Industry Code   n.e.c. - not elsewhere classified   LCL - lower confidence limit   UCL - upper confidence limit
Source: National Center for Health Statistics multiple causes for death data.

APPENDIX VII
COAL WORKERS'
PNEUMOCONIOSIS MORTALITY RATES

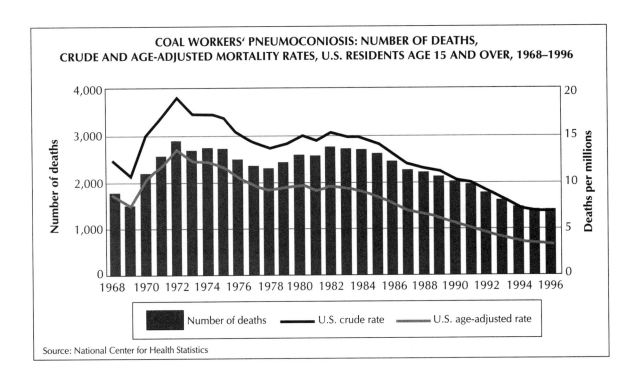

COAL WORKERS' PNEUMOCONIOSIS: NUMBER OF DEATHS,
CRUDE AND AGE-ADJUSTED MORTALITY RATES, U.S. RESIDENTS AGE 15 AND OVER, 1968–1996

Source: National Center for Health Statistics

APPENDIX VIII
FATAL INJURIES STATISTICS

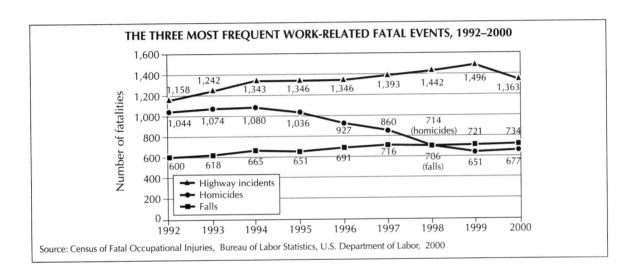

THE THREE MOST FREQUENT WORK-RELATED FATAL EVENTS, 1992–2000

Number of fatalities

Highway incidents: 1,158 — 1,242 — 1,343 — 1,346 — 1,346 — 1,393 — 1,442 — 1,496 — 1,363

Homicides: 1,044 — 1,074 — 1,080 — 1,036 — 927 — 860 — 714 (homicides) — 721 — 734

Falls: 600 — 618 — 665 — 651 — 691 — 716 — 706 (falls) — 651 — 677

Legend:
- Highway incidents
- Homicides
- Falls

Years: 1992, 1993, 1994, 1995, 1996, 1997, 1998, 1999, 2000

Source: Census of Fatal Occupational Injuries, Bureau of Labor Statistics, U.S. Department of Labor, 2000

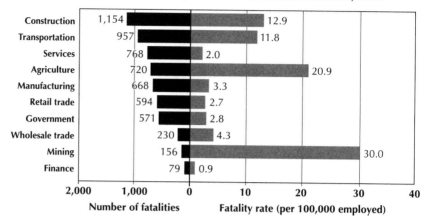

NUMBERS AND RATES OF FATAL OCCUPATIONAL INJURIES BY INDUSTRY DIVISION, 2000

Industry Division	Number of fatalities	Fatality rate (per 100,000 employed)
Construction	1,154	12.9
Transportation	957	11.8
Services	768	2.0
Agriculture	720	20.9
Manufacturing	668	3.3
Retail trade	594	2.7
Government	571	2.8
Wholesale trade	230	4.3
Mining	156	30.0
Finance	79	0.9

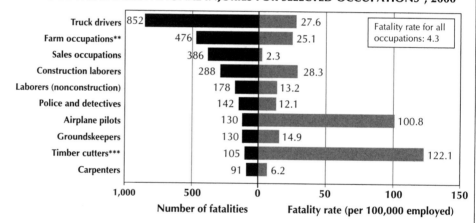

NUMBERS AND RATES OF FATAL OCCUPATIONAL INJURIES FOR SELECTED OCCUPATIONS*, 2000

Fatality rate for all occupations: 4.3

Occupation	Number of fatalities	Fatality rate (per 100,000 employed)
Truck drivers	852	27.6
Farm occupations**	476	25.1
Sales occupations	386	2.3
Construction laborers	288	28.3
Laborers (nonconstruction)	178	13.2
Police and detectives	142	12.1
Airplane pilots	130	100.8
Groundskeepers	130	14.9
Timber cutters***	105	122.1
Carpenters	91	6.2

*Selected occupations had a minimun of 40 fatalities and 45,000 employed workers in 2000.
**Farm occupations include the following: nonhorticultural farmers, nonhorticultural farm managers, farmworkers, and farmworker supervisors.
***Timber cutters include the following: timber cutting and logging occupations, supervisor, forestry, and logging workers.
Note: Rate = (Fatal work injuries/Employment) x 100,000 workers. Employment data extracted from the 2000 Current Population Survey.
The fatality rates were calculated using employment as the denominator: employment-based rates measure the risk for those employed during a given period of time regardless of exposure hours.
Source: Census of Fatal Occupational Injuries, Bureau of Labor Statistics, U.S. Department of Labor, 2000

APPENDIX IX
WORK-RELATED HOMICIDE STATISTICS

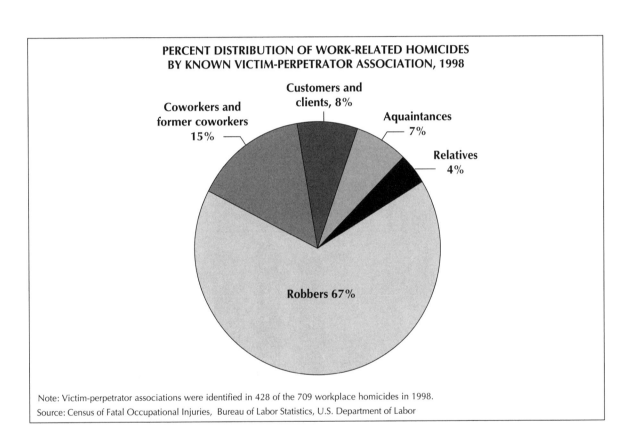

PERCENT DISTRIBUTION OF WORK-RELATED HOMICIDES BY KNOWN VICTIM-PERPETRATOR ASSOCIATION, 1998

Customers and clients, 8%

Coworkers and former coworkers 15%

Aquaintances 7%

Relatives 4%

Robbers 67%

Note: Victim-perpetrator associations were identified in 428 of the 709 workplace homicides in 1998.

Source: Census of Fatal Occupational Injuries, Bureau of Labor Statistics, U.S. Department of Labor

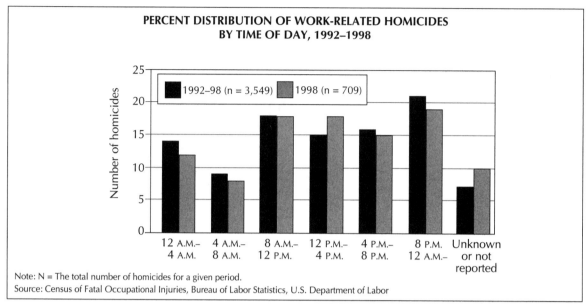

PERCENT DISTRIBUTION OF WORK-RELATED HOMICIDES
BY TIME OF DAY, 1992–1998

Note: N = The total number of homicides for a given period.
Source: Census of Fatal Occupational Injuries, Bureau of Labor Statistics, U.S. Department of Labor

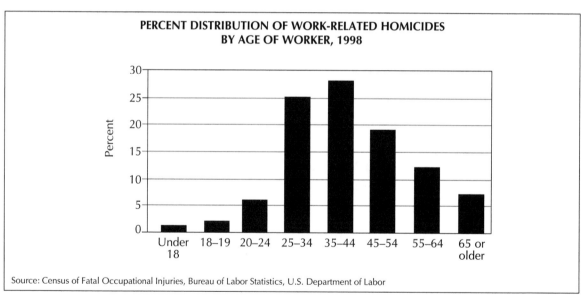

PERCENT DISTRIBUTION OF WORK-RELATED HOMICIDES
BY AGE OF WORKER, 1998

Source: Census of Fatal Occupational Injuries, Bureau of Labor Statistics, U.S. Department of Labor

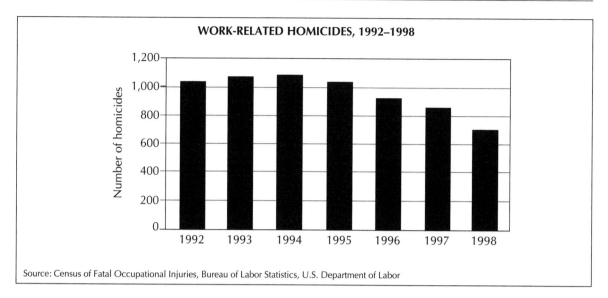

WORK-RELATED HOMICIDES, 1992–1998

Source: Census of Fatal Occupational Injuries, Bureau of Labor Statistics, U.S. Department of Labor

APPENDIX X
COAL WORKERS' PNEUMOCONIOSIS
BLACK LUNG BENEFITS RATES

FEDERAL BLACK LUNG PROGRAM: NUMBER OF BENEFICIARIES AND TOTAL PAYMENTS BY THE SOCIAL SECURITY ADMINISTRATION AND DEPARTMENT OF LABOR, 1980–1996

Year	Social Security Administration		Department of Labor		SSA and DOL
	Total Beneficiaries	Total Amount (dollars)	Total Beneficiaries	Total Amount (dollars)	Total Amount (dollars)
1980	399,477	1,032,000,000	139,073	813,205,000	1,845,205,000
1981	376,505	1,081,300,000	163,401	805,627,000	1,886,927,000
1982	354,569	1,076,000,000	173,972	784,085,000	1,860,085,000
1983	333,358	1,055,800,000	166,043	858,854,000	1,914,654,000
1984	313,822	1,038,000,000	163,166	873,932,000	1,911,932,000
1985	294,846	1,025,000,000	160,441	905,517,000	1,930,517,000
1986	275,783	971,000,000	156,892	629,075,000	1,600,075,000
1987	258,988	940,000,000	153,769	655,290,000	1,595,290,000
1988	241,626	904,000,000	150,123	656,689,000	1,560,689,000
1989	225,764	882,000,000	145,289	650,123,000	1,532,123,000
1990	210,678	863,400,000	139,854	626,521,000	1,489,921,000
1991	196,419	844,400,000	134,205	942,428,000	1,786,828,000
1992	182,396	822,500,000	128,761	973,636,000	1,796,136,000
1993	168,365	794,300,000	123,213	984,666,000	1,778,966,000
1994	155,122	751,900,000	117,569	994,655,000	1,746,555,000
1995	143,011	696,700,000	111,769	995,722.000	1,692,422,000
1996	131,143	654,600,000	105,923	992,128,000	1,646,728,000

Note: The Social Security Administration (SSA) was assigned initial responsibility for administering the black lung benefits program. The Department of Labor (DOL) assumed responsibility for processing and paying claims on July 1, 1973. Most claims filed prior to July 1, 1973 remain within the jurisdiction of SSA, which also continues to be responsible for processing and paying claims field by the survivors of these miners. The dollar amounts from the Department of Labor are for fiscal years. See appendices for source description.
Source: Social Security Bulletin Annual Statistical Supplement: 1998 and Black Lung Benefits Act Annual Report to Congress: FY 1996.

APPENDIX XI
COTTON DUST EXPOSURE RATES

**COTTON DUST: NUMBER AND PERCENT OF OSHA INSPECTOR SAMPLES,
PERCENT EXCEEDING THE PERMISSIBLE EXPOSURE LIMIT (PEL) AND
AVERAGE SEVERITY LEVEL, BY INDUSTRY, 1995–1996**

CIC	Industries Most Frequently Sampled, 1995–1996	Number of Samples	% of total Samples	% > PEL	Average Severity
142	Yarn, thread, and fabric mills	45	81.8	11.1	0.55
152	Miscellaneous fabricated textile products	6	10.9	0.0	0.09
150	Miscellaneous textile mill products	2	3.6	0.0	0.19
140	Dyeing and finishing textiles, except wool and knit goods	1	1.8	0.0	0.11
242	Furniture and fixtures	1	1.8	100.0	9.79
	Total	55	100.0	10.9	0.65

CIC - Census Industry Code.
Note: Percentage of total samples may not total 100% due to rounding. See appendices for source description, methods, ICD codes, industry codes, and agents.
Source: Occupational Safety and Health Administration: Integrated Management Information System.

APPENDIX XII
PULMONARY TUBERCULOSIS
MORTALITY RATES

PULMONARY TUBERCULOSIS: PROPORTIONATE MORTALITY RATIO (PMR) BY USUAL INDUSTRY, RESIDENTS AGE 15 AND OVER, SELECTED STATES AND YEARS, 1987–1996

CIC	Industry	Number of Deaths	PMR	95% Confidence interval LCL	UCL
040	Metal mining	21	2.51	1.55	3.84
130	Tobacco manufacturers	33	2.41	1.63	3.44
791	Miscellaneous personal services	26	2.35	1.54	3.45
262	Miscellaneous nonmetallic mineral and stone products	17	2.33	1.35	3.73
471	Sanitary services	32	2.32	1.57	3.31
050	Nonmetallic mining and quarrying, except fuel	16	2.29	1.31	3.72
030	Forestry	10	2.17	1.04	3.99
271	Iron and steel foundries	21	2.13	1.31	3.26
780	Barber shops	25	2.13	1.37	3.14
010	Agricultural production, crops	489	2.11	1.94	2.31
230	Logging	43	2.05	1.46	2.79
280	Other primary metal industries	24	1.95	1.25	2.90
951	Retired	18	1.86	1.10	2.94
041	Coal mining	80	1.76	1.40	2.19
420	Water transportation	24	1.69	1.08	2.51
620	Auto and home supply stores	23	1.68	1.06	2.52
762	Hotels and motels	67	1.66	1.27	2.14
360	Ship and boat building and repairing	24	1.59	1.02	2.37
231	Sawmills, planning mills, and millwork	37	1.48	1.03	2.06
060	Construction	676	1.47	1.36	1.59
761	Private households	164	1.37	1.17	1.60
410	Trucking service	145	1.29	1.09	1.52

CIC - Census Industry Code   n.e.c. - not elsewhere classified   LCL - lower confidence limit   UCL - upper confidence limit
Source: National Center for Health Statistics multiple cause of death data.

APPENDIX XIII
UNSPECIFIED/OTHER PNEUMOCONIOSES
MORTALITY RATES

UNSPECIFIED/OTHER PNEUMOCONIOSES: MOST FREQUENTLY RECORDED INDUSTRIES ON DEATH CERTIFICATE, RESIDENTS AGE 15 AND OVER, SELECTED STATES AND YEARS, 1987–1996

CIC	Industry	Number	Percent
041	Coal mining	694	50.3
060	Construction	99	7.2
270	Blast furnaces, steelworks, rolling and finishing mills	41	3.0
351	Motor vehicles and motor vehicle equipment	26	1.9
392	Not specified manufacturing industries	24	1.7
400	Railroads	21	1.5
010	Agricultural production, crops	20	1.5
192	Industrial and miscellaneous chemicals	17	1.2
262	Miscellaneous nonmetallic mineral and stone products	15	1.1
040	Metal mining	14	1.0
842	Elementary and secondary schools	14	1.0
961	Nonpaid worker or nonworker	14	1.0
	All other industries	339	24.6
	Industry not reported	41	3.0
	Total	1,379	100.0

CIC - Census Industry Code
Source: National Center for Health Statistics multiple cause of death data.

APPENDIX XIV
WORK-RELATED MUSCULOSKELETAL DISORDERS STATISTICS

NUMBER OF NONFATAL OCCUPATIONAL INJURIES AND ILLNESSES INVOLVING DAYS
AWAY FROM WORK[1] INVOLVING MUSCULOSKELETAL DISORDERS[2]
BY SELECTED WORKER AND CASE CHARACTERISTICS, 1999

Characteristic	All Events	Musculoskeletal Disorders
Total	1,702,470	582,340
Sex		
Men	1,129,243	359,661
Women	558,127	219,208
Age		
Under 14	–	–
14 to 15	866	225
16 to 19	58,206	13,548
20 to 24	197,841	58,122
25 to 34	457,555	159,845
35 to 44	483,545	180,739
45 to 54	310,502	111,888
55 to 64	138,391	43,614
65 and over	22,538	5,220
Occupation		
Managerial and professional	94,671	32,080
Technical, sales and administrative support	249,426	96,656
Service	289,479	101,707
Farming, forestry, and fishing	42,899	9,814
Precision production, craft, and repair	297,965	91,927
Operators, fabricators, and laborers	719,728	247,646
Length of service with employer		
Less than 3 months	229,969	59,805
3 months to 11 months	308,348	96,955
1 year to 5 years	549,718	193,687
More than 5 years	413,776	161,997
Not reported	200,660	69,897
Race or ethnic origin		
White, non-Hispanic	859,591	306,076
Black, non-Hispanic	155,149	50,818
Hispanic	182,896	46,047

Characteristic	All Events	Musculoskeletal Disorders
Race or ethnic origin *(continued)*		
Asian or Pacific Islander	25,328	7,073
American Indian or Alaskan Native	6,812	1,839
Not reported	472,693	170,489
Major industry division		
Agriculture, forestry, and fishing[3]	34,941	7,143
Mining[4]	11,318	3,326
Construction	193,765	48,810
Manufacturing	403,568	149,761
Transportation and public utilities[4]	196,725	66,569
Wholesale trade	136,110	50,653
Retail trade	291,648	90,904
Finance, insurance, and real estate	39,472	12,376
Services	394,922	152,797
Number of days away from work		
Cases involving 1 day	272,605	72,786
Cases involving 2 days	219,191	68,738
Cases involving 3-5 days	348,806	121,213
Cases involving 6-10 days	226,406	83,615
Cases involving 11-20 days	193,564	72,493
Cases involving 21-30 days	107,415	40,641
Cases involving 31 or more days	334,483	122,855
Median days away from work	6	7
Nature of injury, illness		
Sprains, strains	739,742	449,790
Carpal tunnel syndrome	27,922	27,832
Tendinitis	16,582	14,466
Soreness, Pain	109,257	52,752
Back pain	43,198	29,185
All other	808,967	37,501
Part of body affected		
Head	107,696	–
Eye	53,096	–
Neck	30,889	11,945
Trunk	631,173	417,324
Back	424,251	302,744
Shoulder	93,787	56,834
Upper extremities	397,118	87,956
Finger	149,475	4,449
Hand, except finger	70,809	5,827
Wrist	84,410	49,909
Lower extremities	350,202	40,038
Knee	127,953	25,547
Foot, toe	77,649	1,933
Body systems	21,910	–
Multiple	148,188	23,879
Source of injury, illness		
Chemicals, chemical products	28,773	137
Containers	244,574	172,265
Furniture, fixtures	58,537	24,220

**NUMBER OF NONFATAL OCCUPATIONAL INJURIES AND ILLNESSES INVOLVING DAYS
AWAY FROM WORK[1] INVOLVING MUSCULOSKELETAL DISORDERS[2]
BY SELECTED WORKER AND CASE CHARACTERISTICS, 1999**

Characteristic	All Events	Musculoskeletal Disorders
Source of injury, illness *(continued)*		
Machinery	114,183	24,510
Parts and materials	192,005	77,194
Worker motion or position	267,060	139,761
Floor, ground surfaces	272,026	2,432
Handtools	77,942	16,391
Vehicles	137,660	20,783
Health care patient	72,363	59,002
All other	237,346	45,645
Event or exposure:		
Bending, climbing, crawling, reaching, twisting	77,995	74,810
Overexertion	459,441	440,151
Overexertion in lifting	264,837	255,286
Repetitive motion	73,195	67,380

[1] Days away from work include those which result in days away from work with or without restricted work activity.

[2] Includes cases where the nature of injury is: sprains, strains, tears; back pain, hurt back; soreness, pain, hurt, except back; carpal tunnel syndrome; hernia; or musculoskeletal system and connective tissue diseases and disorders and when the event or exposure leading to the injury or illness is: bodily reaction/bending, climbing, crawling, reaching, twisting; overexertion; or repetition. Cases of Raynaud's phenomenon, tarsal tunnel syndrome, and herniated spinal discs are not included. Although these cases may be considered MSDs, the survey classifies these cases in categories that also include non-MSD cases.

[3] Excludes farms with fewer than 11 employees.

[4] Data conforming to OSHA definitions for mining operators in coal, metal, and nonmetal mining and for employees in railroad transportation are provided to BLS by the Mine Safety and Health Administration, U.S. Department of Labor; and the Federal Railroad Administration, U.S. Department of Transportation. Independent mining contractors are excluded from the coal, metal, and nonmetal mining industries.

Note: Because of rounding and data exclusion of nonclassifiable responses, data may not sum to the totals. Dashes indicate data that do not meet publication guidelines. The scientifically selected probability sample used in 1999 was one of many possible samples, each of which could have produced different estimates. A measure of sampling variability for each estimate is available upon request.

Source: Bureau of Labor Statistics, U.S. Department of Labor, March 2001.

APPENDIX XV
MULTIPLE WORK-RELATED RESPIRATORY CONDITIONS MORBIDITY RATES

ANNUAL AVERAGE EMPLOYMENT (IN THOUSANDS) BY MAJOR INDUSTRY DIVISION, 1992–1996

Year	Agriculture	Mining	Construction	Manufacturing	Transportation and Public Utilities	Wholesale and Retail Trade	Finance	Services	Total
1992	1,224	631	4,471	18,040	5,709	25,391	6,571	28,422	90,460
1993	1,224	599	4,574	17,802	5,708	25,856	6,604	29,544	91,932
1994	1,228	600	5,010	18,303	6,006	28,577	6,933	30,792	95,449
1995	1,641	582	5,088	18,473	5,858	27,564	6,617	30,920	96,886
1996	1,717	578	5,360	18,461	5,989	28,027	6,746	31,895	98,773

Note: The sum of individual industries may not equal yearly total due to rounding. See appendices for source description and methods.
Source: Bureau of Labor Statistics annual reports of occupational injuries and illnesses.

WORK-RELATED RESPIRATORY ILLNESSES (WITH DAYS AWAY FROM WORK): ESTIMATED NUMBER, BY INDUSTRY DIVISION, 1992–1996

Year	Agriculture	Mining	Construction	Manufacturing	Transportation and Public Utilities	Wholesale and Retail Trade	Finance	Services	Total
1992	100	100	300	1,300	300	700	200	1,100	3,900
1993	71	148	141	1,461	226	378	279	1,544	4,347
1994	27	87	237	1,303	248	504	122	1,140	3,668
1995	41	24	84	1,068	367	431	131	1,461	3,606
1996	-	15	178	840	503	589	161	1,365	3,665

- indicates no data reported or data that do not meet BLS publication guidelines.
Note: The sum of individual industries may not equal yearly total due to rounding. See appendices for source description and methods.
Source: Bureau of Labor Statistics annual reports of occupational injuries and illnesses.

WORK-RELATED RESPIRATORY ILLNESSES (WITH DAYS AWAY FROM WORK): RATE (PER 100,000 WORKERS), BY INDUSTRY DIVISION, 1992–1996

Year	Agriculture	Mining	Construction	Manufacturing	Transportation and Public Utilities	Wholesale and Retail Trade	Finance	Services	Total
1992	8.2	15.8	6.7	7.2	5.3	2.8	3.0	3.9	4.3
1993	5.8	24.7	3.2	8.2	4.0	1.5	4.2	5.2	4.7
1994	2.2	14.5	4.7	7.1	4.1	1.8	1.8	3.7	3.8
1995	2.5	4.1	1.7	5.8	6.3	1.6	2.0	4.7	3.7
1996	-	2.6	3.3	4.6	8.4	2.1	2.4	4.3	3.7

- indicate no data reported or data do not meet BLS publication guidelines.
Note: See appendices for source description and methods.
Source: Bureau of Labor Statistics annual reports of occupational injuries and illnesses.

OCCUPATIONAL RESPIRATORY CONDITIONS DUE TO TOXIC AGENTS: INDUSTRIES WITH THE HIGHEST REPORTED INCIDENCE RATES, U.S. PRIVATE SECTOR, 1992–1996

Year/Industry	SIC	Rate (per 10,000 full time workers)
1992		
Transportation equipment	37	15.2
Forestry	08	7.0
Primary metal industries	33	6.9
Instruments and related products	38	6.8
Museums, botanical, zoological gardens	84	6.6
Petroleum and coal products	29	6.6
Electronic and other electric equipment	36	6.5
Rubber and miscellaneous plastic products	30	6.3
Food and kindred products	20	6.1
Chemical sand allied products	28	5.7
Overall		**3.1**
1993		
Miscellaneous manufacturing industries	39	12.6
Transportation equipment	37	12.3
Primary metal industries	33	8.1
Food and kindred products	20	7.3
Fabricated metal products	34	6.6
Tobacco products	21	6.6
Agricultural production—livestock	02	6.5
Leather and leather products	31	6.5
Rubber and miscellaneous plastics products	30	6.3
Chemicals and allied products	28	6.0
Overall		**3.1**
1994		
Transportation equipment	37	20.4
Rubber and miscellaneous plastics products	30	8.2
Primary metal industries	33	7.8
Electric and other electric equipment	36	7.1
Museums, botanical, zoological gardens	84	7.0

Year/Industry	SIC	Rate (per 10,000 full time workers)
1994 *(continued)*		
Health services	80	6.0
Food and kindred products	20	5.7
Fabricated metal products	34	5.5
Instruments and related products	38	5.1
Chemicals and allied products	28	4.7
Overall		**3.1**
1995		
Transportation equipment	37	13.5
Primary metal industries	33	7.6
Electronic and other electric equipment	36	7.6
Health service	80	6.9
Rubber and miscellaneous plastic products	30	6.6
Food and kindred products	20	5.8
Apparel and other textile products	23	5.4
Transportation by air	45	4.8
Amusement and recreation services	79	3.9
Paper and allied products	26	3.9
Overall		**3.0**
1996		
Transportation equipment	37	11.2
Fishing, hunting, and trapping	09	7.4
Health services	80	6.9
Hotels and other lodging places	70	6.3
Food and kindred products	20	5.7
Primary metal industries	33	4.8
Communications	48	4.7
Fabricated metal products	34	4.7
Chemicals and allied products	28	4.5
Leather and leather products	31	4.5
Rubber and miscellaneous plastic products.	30	4.5
Overall		**2.6**

SIC - 1987 Standard Industrial Classification
Note: Respiratory conditions due to toxic agents include pneumonitis, pharyngitis, rhinitis or acute congestions due to chemicals, dusts, gases or
   fumes. See appendices for source description.
Source: Bureau of Labor Statistics annual reports of occupational injuries and illnesses.

**SILICOSIS: MOST FREQUENTLY RECORDED INDUSTRIES ON DEATH CERTIFICATE,
RESIDENTS AGE 15 AND OVER, SELECTED STATES AND YEARS, 1987–1996**

CIC	Industry	Number	Percent
060	Construction	114	10.8
040	Metal mining	105	10.0
041	Coal mining	68	6.5
270	Blast furnaces, steelworks, rolling and finishing mills	68	6.5
262	Miscellaneous nonmetallic mineral and stone products	65	6.2
050	Nonmetallic mining and quarrying, except fuel	59	5.6
271	Iron and steel foundries	53	5.0
392	Not specified manufacturing industries	43	4.1
331	Machinery, except electrical, n.e.c.	28	2.7
010	Agricultural production, crops	22	2.1
252	Structural clay products	22	2.1
261	Pottery and related products	22	2.1
961	Nonpaid worker or nonworker	22	2.1
	All other industries	334	31.7
	Industry not reported	29	2.8
	Total	1,054	100.0

CIC - Census Industry Code   n.e.c. - not elsewhere classified
Source: National Center for Health Statistics multiple cause of death data.

APPENDIX XVI
RESOURCES

Acoustical Society of America (ASA)
2 Huntington Quadrangle
Suite 1NO1
Melville, NY 11747-4502
(516) 576-2360
(516) 576-2377 (fax)
http://asa.aip.org

Agency for Toxic Substances and Diseases Registry (ATSDR)
1600 Clifton Road, NE
Atlanta, GA 30333
(888) 422-8737 (toll-free)
(404) 498-0057 (fax)
http://www.atsdr.cdc.gov/

AIDS Clinical Trials Information Service
PO Box 6421
Rockville, MD 20849-6421
(800) TRIALS-A (toll-free)
http://www.actis.org

AIDS Health Project
1930 Market Street
San Francisco, CA 94102
(415) 476-6430
http://www.ucsf-ahp.org

Al-Anon/Alateen Family Group Headquarters, World Service Office (AFG)
1600 Corporate Landing Parkway
Virginia Beach, VA 23454-5617
(800) 344-2666 (toll-free)
(800) 4AL-ANON (Toll-free)
(757) 563-1600
(757) 563-1655 (fax)
http://www.al-anon.alateen.org

Alcoholics Anonymous (AA)
A.A. World Services, Inc.
P.O. Box 459

Grand Central Station
New York, NY 10163
(212) 870-3400
(212) 870-3003 (toll-free)
http://www.aa.org

American Academy of Ophthalmology (AAO)
P.O. Box 7424
San Francisco, CA 94120-7424
(415) 561-8500
(415) 561-8533 (fax)
http://www.aao.org

American Association for CFS (AAFCFS)
c/o Harborview Medical Center
325 9th Avenue
Box 359780
Seattle, WA 98104
(206) 521-1932
(206) 521-1930 (fax)
E-mail: debrap@washington.edu

American Association of Naturopathic Physicians (AANP)
8201 Greensboro Drive
Suite 300
McLean, VA 22102-3814
(877) 969-2267 (toll-free)
(703) 610-9037
(703) 610-9005 (fax)
http://www.naturopathic.org

American Association of Occupational Health Nurses (AAOHN)
2920 Brandy Wine Road
Suite 100
Atlanta, GA 30341
(770) 455-7757
(770) 455-7271 (fax)
http://www.aaohn.org

American Association of Oriental Medicine (AAOM)
433 Front Street
Catasauqua, PA 18032-2506
(888) 500-7999 (toll-free)
(610) 266-1433
(610) 264-2768 (fax)
http://www.aaom.org

American Cancer Society (ACS)
1599 Clifton Road, NE
Atlanta, GA 30329
(800) 227-2345 (toll-free)
(404) 315-9348 (fax)
http://www.cancer.org

American Chemical Council
1300 Wilson Boulevard
Arlington, VA 22209
(703) 741-5000
(703) 741-6000 (fax)
http://americanchemistry.com

American Chemical Society (ACS)
1155 16th Street, NW
Washington, DC 20036
(800) 227-5558 (toll-free)
(202) 872-4600
(202) 872-4615 (fax)
http://www.acs.org

American Chiropractic Association (ACA)
1701 Clarendon Boulevard
Arlington, VA 22209
(800) 986-4636 (toll-free)
(703) 276-8800
(703) 243-2593 (fax)
http://www.amerchiro.org

American Civil Liberties Union AIDS Project
132 West 43rd Street
New York, NY 10036
(212) 944-9800

American College of Medical Toxicology (ACMT)
777 E. Park Drive
P.O. Box 8820
Harrisburg, PA 17105-8820
(888) 633-5784 (toll-free)
(717) 558-7846
(717) 558-7841 (fax)
http://www.acmt.net

American College of Toxicology (ACT)
c/o Secretariat
9650 Rockwell Pike
Bethesda, MD 20814
(301) 571-1840
(301) 571-1852 (fax)
http://www.actox.org

American College of Occupational and Environmental Medicine
1114 N. Arlington Heights Road
Arlington Heights, IL 60004-4770
(847) 818-1800 ext. 368
(847) 818-9266 (fax)
http://www.acoem.org

American Conference of Governmental Industrial Hygienists (ACGIH)
1330 Kemper Meadows Drive
Suite 600
Cincinnati, OH 45240
(513) 742-2020
(513) 742-6163
(513) 742-3355 (fax)
http://www.acgih.org

American Council of the Blind (ACB)
1115 15th Street, NW
Suite 1004
Washington, DC 20005
(800) 424-8666 (toll-free)
(202) 467-5081
(202) 467-5085 (fax)
http://www.acb.org

American Council on Science and Health (ACSH)
1995 Broadway
2nd floor
New York, NY 10023-5860
(212) 362-7044
(212) 362-4919 (fax)
http://acsh.acsh.org
acsh@acsh.org

American Diabetes Association (ADA)
1701 N. Beauregard Street
Alexandria, VA 22311
(800) DIABETES (toll-free)
(703) 549-1500
(703) 836-7439 (fax)
http://www.diabetes.org

American Environmental Health Foundation
8345 Walnut Hill Lane
Suite 225
Dallas, TX 75231
(800) 428-2343 (toll-free)
(214) 361-2534 (fax)
http://www.aehf.com

American Federation of Labor-Congress of Industrial Organizations
815 16th Street, NW
Washington, DC 20006
(202) 637-5000
(202) 637-5058 (fax)
feedback@aflcio.org

American Group Psychotherapy Association
25 East 21st Street
Sixth Floor
New York, NY 10010
(212) 477-2677
(212) 979-6627 (fax)
http://www.agpa.org
groupsinc@aol.com

American Headache Society (AHS)
19 Mantua Road
Mt. Royal, NJ 08061
(856) 423-0043
(856) 423-0082 (fax)
http://www.aashnet.org

American Healthcare Association
1201 L Street, NW
Washington, DC 20005-4014
(202) 841-4444
(202) 842-3860 (fax)
http://www.ahca.org

American Heart Association (AHA)
7272 Greenville Avenue
Dallas, TX 75231-4596
(800) 242 USA1 (toll free)
(214) 373-6300
(214) 987-4334 (fax)
http://www.americanheart.org

American Industrial Hygiene Association (AIHA)
2700 Prosperity Avenue
Suite 250
Fairfax, VA 22031
(703) 849-8888

(703) 207-3561 (fax)
http://www.aiha.org

American Lung Association
1740 Broadway
New York, NY 100019-4374
(800) LUNGUSA (toll-free)
(212) 315-8700
(212) 315-8872 (fax)
http://www.lungusa.org

American Massage Therapy Association (AMTA)
820 Davis Street
Suite 100
Evanston, IL 60201-4444
(888) 843-2682 (toll-free)
(847) 864-0123
(847) 864-1178 (fax)
http://www.amtamassage.org

American Mental Health Counselors Association
801 N. Fairfax Street
Suite 304
Alexandria, VA 22314
(800) 326-2642 (toll-free)
(703) 548-6002
(703) 548-4775 (fax)
http://www.amhca.org
vmoore@amhca.org

American National Standards Institute (ANSI)
1819 L Street, NW
#600
Washington, DC 20036
(202) 293-8020
(202) 293-9287 (fax)
http://www.ansi.org

American Nurses Association
600 Maryland Avenue, SW
Suite 100W
Washington, DC 20024-2571
(800) 274-4ANA (toll-free)
(800) 274-4262 (toll-free)
(202) 651-7000
http://www.nursingworld.org

American Petroleum Institute (API)
1220 L Street, NW
Washington, DC 2005-4070
(202) 682-8000
(202) 682-8029 (fax)
http://www.api.org

American Psychiatric Association
1400 K Street, NW
Washington, DC 20005
(202) 692-6850
http://www.psych.org
apa@psych.org

American Psychological Association
750 First Street, NE
Washington, DC 20002-4242
(800) 374-3120 (toll-free)
(202) 336-5700
(202) 336-5568 (fax)
http://apa.org
webmaster@apa.org

American Public Health Association (APHA)
800 I Street, NW
Washington, DC 20001-3710
(202) 777-2742
(202) 777-2534 (fax)
http://www.apha.org

American Red Cross National Headquarters (ARC)
431 18th Street, NW
Washington, DC 2006
(800) 797-8022 (toll-free)
(202) 639-3520
(202) 942-2024 (fax)
http://redcross.org

American Sleep Apnea Association
1424 K Street NW
Suite 302
Washington, DC 20005
(202) 293-3650
(202) 293-3656 (fax)
http://www.sleepapnea.org

American Society of Addiction Medicine (ASAM)
4601 N. Park Avenue Arcade
Suite 101
Chevy Chase, MD 20815
(301) 656-3920
(301) 656-3815 (fax)
http://www.asam.org

American Society of Safety Engineers
1800 E. Oakton Street
Des Plaines, IL 60018

(847) 699-2929
(847) 768-3434 (fax)
http://www.asse.org

Anorexia Nervosa and Related Eating Disorders (ANRED)
P.O. Box 5102
Eugene, OR 97405
(541) 344-1144
http://www.anred.com

Anxiety Disorders Association of America (ADAA)
8700 Georgia Avenue
Silver Springs, MD 20910
(240) 487-0120
http://adaa.org

Association for Advancement of Behavior Therapy
305 7th Avenue
16th Floor
New York, NY 10001-6008
(212) 647-1890
(212) 647-1865 (fax)
http://www.aabt.org
info@aabt.org

Association of Applied Psychophysiology and Biofeedback
12267 W. 44th Avenue
#304
Wheat Ridge, CO 80303
(303) 422-8436
(303) 422-8894 (fax)
http://www.aapb.org

Association of Occupational and Environmental Clinics (AOEC)
1010 Vermont Avenue NW
Suite 513
Washington, DC 20005-1503
(202) 347-4976
(202) 347-4950 (fax)
http://www.aoec.org

Better Hearing Institute (BHI)
P.O. Box 1840
Washington, DC 20013
(800) EAR WELL (toll-free)
(703) 684-6048 (fax)
http://www.betterhearing.org

Board of Certified Safety Professionals
208 Burwash Avenue
Savoy, IL 61874
(217) 359-9263
(217) 359-0055 (fax)
http://www.bcsp.org

**Bureau of Transportation Statistics
 (Transportation Dept.)**
400 Seventh Street, SW
#3103
Washington, DC 20590
(202) 366-3640
(202) 366-3640 (fax)
http://www.bts.gov

**CDC National Prevention Information Network
 (NPIN)**
Box 6003
Rockville, MD 20849-6003
(800) 458-5231 (toll-free)
(800) 243-7012 (toll-free)
(301) 562-1050 (fax)
http://www.cdcnpin.org

Census of Fatal Occupational Injuries (CFOI)
U.S. Bureau of Labor Statistics
OCWC/OSH
2 Massachusetts Avenue, NE
Suite 3180
Washington, DC 20212-0001
(202) 691-6170
(202) 691-6196 (fax)
http://www.bls.gov/iif

Center for Substance Abuse Prevention
5600 Fishers Lane, Rockwall II
Rockville, MD 20857
(301) 443-0365

CFIDS Association of America Inc.
P.O. Box 2203398
Charlotte, NC 29222-0398
(800) 442-3437 (toll-free)
(704) 365-9755 (fax)
http://www.cfids.org

**Chronic Fatigue Immune Dysfunction
 Syndrome Activation Network (CAN)**
P.O. Box 345
Larchmont, NY 10538
(212) 280-4266
(914) 636-6515 (fax)
cfidsnet@aol.com

Clean Air Trust
1625 K Street, NW
#790
Washington, DC 20006
(202) 785-9625
http://www.cleanairtrust.org

**Cocaine Anonymous World Services
 (CAWS)**
3740 Overland Avenue
Suite C
Los Angeles, CA 90034-6337
(800) 347-8998 (toll-free)
(310) 559-5833
(310) 559-2554 (fax)
http://www.ca.org

**Commission on Mental and Physical Disability
 Law**
American Bar Association
740 15th Street, NW
Washington, DC 20005
(202) 662-1570
(202) 662-1032 (fax)
http://www.abanet.org/disability
cmpdl@abanet.org

Communication Workers of America (CWA)
501 Third Street, NW
Washington, DC 20001-2797
(202) 434-1100
(202) 434-1279 (fax)
http://www.cwa-union.org

**Depression and Related Affective Disorders
 Association**
The Johns Hopkins Hospital
Meyer 3-181
600 North Wolfe Street
Baltimore, MD 21287-7381
(410) 955-4647
(410) 614-3241 (fax)
http://www.med.jhu.edu/drada
drada@jhmi.edu

Easter Seals National Headquarters
230 W. Monroe Street
Suite 1800
Chicago, IL 60606
(800) 221-6827 (toll-free)
(312) 726-6200
(312) 726-1494 (fax)
http://www.easter-seals.org

Eating Disorders Awareness and Prevention, Inc. (EDAP)
603 Stewart Street
Suite 803
Seattle, WA 98101
(800) 931-2237 (toll-free)
(206) 382-3587
(206) 292-9890 (fax)
http://www.edap.org
info@edap.org

Employee Assistance Professionals Association (EAPA)
2101 Wilson Boulevard
Suite 500
Arlington, VA 22201-3062
(703) 387-1000
(703) 522-4585 (fax)
http://www.eap-assn.com

Employment Law Center
1663 Mission Street
Suite 400
San Francisco, CA 94103
(415) 864-8848

Environmental Health Clearinghouse
Meridian Parkway
Suite 115
Durham, NC 27713
(800) 643-4794 (toll-free)
(919) 361-9408 (fax)
http://www.infoventures.com

Environmental Protection Agency
1200 Pennsylvania Avenue, NW
Washington, DC 20460
(202) 564-6953
(202) 501-1450 (fax)
http://www.epa.gov

Equal Employment Opportunity Commission
1801 L Street, NW
Washington, DC 20507
(202) 663-4001
(202) 663-4110 (fax)
http://www.eoc.gov

Federal Highway Administration (FHWA)
Transportation Department
400 Seventh Street, SW
#4218

Washington, DC 20590
(202) 366-0650
(202) 366-3244 (fax)
http://www.fhwa.dot.gov

Federal Railroad Administration
Transportation Department
1120 Vermont Avenue
Seventh Floor
Washington, DC 20590
(202) 493-6014
(202) 493-6009 (fax)
http://www.fra.dot.gov

Feldenkrais Guild of North America
c/o Ruth A. Hurst
3611 SW Hood Avenue
Suite 100
Portland, OR 97201
(800) 775-2118 (toll-free)
(503) 221-6612
(503) 221-6616 (fax)
http://www.feldenkrais.com

Gamblers Anonymous (GA)
P.O. Box 17173
Los Angeles, CA 90017
(213) 386-8789
(213) 386-0030 (fax)
http://gamblersanonymous.org

Health Research Group (HRG)
1600 20th Street, NW
Washington, DC 20009
(202) 588-1000
(202) 588-7796 (fax)
http://www.citizen.org/hrg

International Association of Eating Disorders Professionals (IAEDP)
P.O. Box 1295
Pekin, IL 61555-1295
(800) 800-8126 (toll-free)
(775) 239-1597 (fax)
http://www.iaedp.com

International Brotherhood of Teamsters (IBT)
25 Louisiana Avenue, NW
Washington, DC 20001
(202) 624-6800
(202) 624-8102 (fax)
http://www.teamster.org

International Foundation for Homeopathy (IFH)
P.O. Box 7
Edmonds, WA 98020
No Phone Listed
(425) 776-1499 (fax)
ifh@nwlink.com

International Labour Organisation—U.S.
1828 L Street, NW
Suite 600
Washington, DC 20036
(202) 653-7652
(202) 653-7687 (fax)
http://www.us.ilo.org

International Labour Organisation
4 Route des Morillons
CH-1211 Geneva 2
Switzerland
41 22 79888685 (fax)
http://www.ilo.org

International Occupational Hygiene Association
IOHA Secretariat
Suite 2, Georgian House
Great Northern Road
Derby
DE 1LT
United Kingdom
+44 1332 298101
+44 1332 298099 (fax)

International Safety Equipment Association (ISEA)
1901 N. Moore Street
Suite 808
Arlington, VA 22209-1762
(703) 525-1695
(703) 528-2148 (fax)
http://www.safetyequipment.org

International Union, United Automobile, Aerospace and Agricultural Implement Workers of America (UAW)
8000 E. Jefferson
Detroit, MI 48214
(800) 243-8829 (toll-free)
(313) 926-5000
(313) 823-6016 (fax)
http://www.uaw.org

International Union of Bricklayers, Allied Craft Workers & Plasterers
1776 I Street, NW

Washington, DC 20006
(202) 783-3788
http://www.bacweb.org

Judge David L. Bazelon Center for Mental Health Law
1101 15th Street, NW
Suite 1212
Washington, DC 20005-5002
(202) 467-5730
(202) 223-0409 (fax)
http://www.bazelon.org
bazelon@nicom.com

Mainstream, Inc.
6930 Carroll Avenue
Suite 240
Takoma Park, MD 20912
(301) 891-8777
(301) 891-8778 (fax)
info@mainstreaminc.org

Mine Safety and Health Administration
4015 Wilson Boulevard
#622
Arlington, VA 22203
(703) 235-1385
(703) 235-4369 (fax)
http://www.msha.gov

Narcolepsy Network
10921 Reed Hartman Highway
Cincinnati, OH 45242
(513) 891-3522
(513) 891-3836 (fax)
http://www.websciences.org/narnet

Narcotics Anonymous (NA)
P.O. Box 9999
Van Nuys, CA 91409
(818) 773-9999
(818) 700-0700 (fax)
http://www.wsoinc.com

National AIDS Hotline: (800) 342-2437 (toll-free)
TTY//TDD: (800) 243-7889 (toll-free)
English Hotline: (800) 342-AIDS (toll-free)
Spanish Hotline: (800) 344-SIDA (toll-free)

National Alliance for Hispanic Health
1501 Sixteenth Street, NW
Washington, DC 20036
(202) 387-5000
(202) 797-4353 (fax)
http://www.hispanichealth.org

National Alliance for Research on Schizophrenia and Depression
60 Cutter Mill Road
Suite 404
Great Neck, NY 11021
(800) 829-8289 (toll-free)
(516) 829-0091
(516) 487-6930 (toll-free)
http://www.narsad.org

National Alliance for the Mentally Ill
200 N. Glebe Road
Suite 1015
Arlington, VA 22203-3754
(800) 950-6264 (toll-free)
(703) 524-7600
(703) 524-9094 (fax)
http://www.nami.org

National Association of Anorexia Nervosa and Associated Disorders
P.O. Box 7
Highland Park, IL 60035
(847) 831-3438
(847) 433-4632 (fax)
http://www.anad.org
anad.20@aol.com

National Association of Cognitive-Behavioral Therapists
P.O. Box 2195
Weirton, WV 26062
(800) 853-1135 (toll-free)
(304) 723-3982 (fax)
http://www.nacbt.org
nacbt@nacbt.org

National Association of People with AIDS (NAPWA)
1413 K Street, NW
Washington, DC 20005-3442
(202) 898-0414
(202) 898-0435 (fax)
http://www.napwa.org

National Association of Protection and Advocacy Systems
900 Second Street, NE
Suite 211
Washington, DC 20002
(202) 408-9514
(202) 408-9520 (fax)
http://www.protectionandadvocacy.com
napas@vipmail.earthlink.net

National Association of Social Workers
750 First Street, NE
Suite 700
Washington, DC 20002-4241
(800) 638-8799 (toll-free)
(202) 408-8600
(202) 336-8310 (fax)
http://www.socialworkers.org

National Cancer Institute
NCI Public Inquiries Office
Suite 3036A
6116 Executive Boulevard
MSC 8322
Bethesda, MD 20892-8322
(800) 4-CANCER (toll-free)
(800) 422-6237 (toll-free)
(301) 435-3848
http://nci.nih.gov

National Center for Complementary and Alternative Medicine
National Institutes of Health (NIH)
31 Center Drive
Building 31
#2B11, MSC 2182
Bethesda, MD 20892-2182
(301) 435-5042
(301) 435-6549 (fax)
http://www.nccam.nih.gov

National Center for Farmworkers' Health
1770 FM 967
Buda, TX 78610-2884
(512) 312-2700
(512) 312-2600 (fax)
http://www.ncfh.org

National Center for Homeopathy (NCH)
801 North Fairfax Street
Suite 306
Alexandria, VA 22314
(703) 548-7790
(703) 548-7792 (fax)
http://www.homeopathic.org

National Chronic Fatigue Syndrome and Fibromyalgia Association (NCFSFA)
P.O. Box 18426
Kansas City, KS 64133
(816) 313-2000
(816) 524-6782 (fax)
http://www.ncfsfa.org

National Clearinghouse for Alcohol and Drug Information
11426 Rockville Pike
Rockville, MD 20852
(800) 729-6686 (toll-free)
http://www.health.org
info@health.org

National Council on Alcoholism and Drug Dependence (NCADD)
20 Exchange Place
Suite 3902
New York, NY 10005-3201
(800) 622-2255 (toll-free)
(212) 269-7797
(212) 269-7510 (fax)
http://www.ncadd.org

National Council on Problem Gambling
208 G Street, NE
2nd Floor
Washington, DC 20002
(202) 547-9204
(202) 547-9206 (fax)
http://www.ncpgambling.org

National Depressive and Manic-Depressive Association
730 N. Franklin Street
Suite 501
Chicago, IL 60610-3526
(800) 826-3632 (toll-free)
(312) 642-0049
(312) 642-7243 (fax)
http://www.ndmda.org

National Eating Disorders Association
603 Stewart Street
Suite 803
Seattle, WA 98101
(206) 382-3587
(206) 829-8501 (fax)
http://nationaleatingdisorders.org

National Fire Protection Association (NFPA)
1 Batterymarch Park
P.O. Box 9101
Quincy, MA 02269-9101
(800) 344-3555 (toll-free)
(617) 770-0700 (fax)
http://www.nfpa.org

National Foundation for Depressive Illness
P.O. Box 2257
New York, NY 10116
(800) 239-1265 (toll-free)
http://www.depression.org

National Headache Foundation
428 West St. James Place
2nd Floor
Chicago, IL 60614
(800) NHF-5552 (toll-free)
(773) 388-6399
(773) 525-7357 (fax)
http://www.headaches.org

National Heart, Lung and Blood Institute
9000 Rockville, Pike
Building 31
#5A52
Bethesda, MD 20891-2486
(301) 496-5166
(301) 402-0818 (fax)
http://www.nhlbi.nih.gov

National Highway Traffic Safety Administration Transportation Department
400 7th Street, SW
#5220
Washington, DC 20590
(202) 366-1836
(202) 366-2106 (fax)
http://www.nhtsa.dot.gov

National Institute for Allergy and Infectious Diseases
31 Center Drive
MSC-2520
Building 31
#7AO3
Bethesda, MD 20892-2520
(301) 496-2263
(301) 496-5717
(301) 496-5509 (fax)
http://www.niaid.nih.gov

National Institute for Occupational Safety & Health (NIOSH)
Centers for Disease Control and Prevention
200 Independence Avenue, SW
Washington, DC 20201
(202) 401-6997
(202) 260-4464 (fax)
http://www.cdc.gov/niosh

National Institute of Arthritis and Musculoskeletal and Skin Diseases
31 Center Drive
MSC-2350
Building 31
#4C32
Bethesda, MD 20892-2350
(301) 496-4353
(301) 496-8190
(301) 402-3607 (fax)
http://www.nih.gov/niams

National Institute of Environmental Health Sciences/NIH
Building 31
#B1CO2
31 Center Drive
MSC 2256
Bethesda, MD 20892-2256
(301) 496-3511
(301) 496-0563 (fax)
http://www.niehs.nih.gov

National Institute of Mental Health (NIMH)
6001 Executive Boulevard
Room 8184
Bethesda, MD 20892-9663
(800) 421-4211 (toll-free)
(301) 443-4513
(301) 443-4279 (fax)
http://www.nimh.nih.gov
nimhinfo@nih.gov

National Institute on Aging
31 Center Drive
MSC-2292
Building 31
#5C35
Bethesda, MD 20892-2292
(301) 496-9265
(301) 496-2525 (fax)
http://www.nih.gov/nia

National Institute on Alcohol Abuse and Alcoholism
6000 Executive Boulevard
Wilco Building
Bethesda, MD 20892-7003
(301) 496-4452
http://www.niaaa.nih.gov

National Institute on Disability and Rehabilitation Research
U.S. Department of Education
400 Maryland Avenue, SW
Washington, DC 20202-2572
(202) 732-1134
(202) 732-5079 (TDD)

**National Institute on Drug Abuse
National Institutes of Health**
6001 Executive Boulevard
Room 5213
Bethesda, MD 20892-9561
(800) 644-6432 (toll-free)
http://www.nida.nih.gov

National Institutes of Health
31 Center Drive
MSC-0148
Building 1
#126
Bethesda, MD 20892-0148
(301) 496-2433
(301) 402-2700 (fax)
http://www.nih.gov

National Mental Health Association
1021 Prince Street
Alexandria, VA 22314-2971
(800) 969-6642 (toll-free)
(703) 684-7722
(703) 684-5968 (fax)
http://www.nmha.org
infoctr@nmha.org

National Oceanic & Atmospheric Administration
U.S. Department of Commerce
14th Street & Constitution Avenue, NW
Room 6013
Washington, DC 20230
(202) 482-6090
(202(482-3154 (fax)
http://www.noaa.gov

National Safety Council
1121 Spring Lake Drive
Itasca, IL 60143-3201
(800) 621-7619 (toll-free)
(630) 285-1121
(630) 285-1315 (fax)
http://www.nsc.org

National Self-Help Clearinghouse (NSHC)
365 Fifth Avenue
Suite 3300
New York, NY 10016
(212) 817-1822
(212) 817-2990 (fax)
http://www.selfhelpweb.org

National Sleep Foundation
1522 K Street NW
Suite 500
Washington, DC 20005
(202) 347-3471
(202) 347-3472 (fax)
http://www.sleepfoundation.org

Obsessive Compulsive Foundation (OCF)
337 Notch Hill Road
North Branford, CT 06471
(203) 315-2190
(203) 315-2196 (fax)
http://ocfoundation.org

Occupational Safety & Health Administration (OSHA)
200 Constitution Avenue, NW
#52315
Washington, DC 20210
(202) 693-1900
(202) 693-2106 (fax)
http://www.osha.gov

Office of Minority Health
Public Health Service
U.S. Department of Health and Human Services
5515 Security Lane
#1000
Rockwall II Building
Rokville, MD 20852
(800) 444-6472 (toll-free)
(301) 443-5084
(301) 594-0767 (fax)
http://www.omhrg.gov

Office of Smoking and Health
Centers for Disease Control and Prevention
Mailstop K-50
4770 Buford Highway, NE
Atlanta, GA 30341-3724
(800) CDC-1311 (toll-free)
(770) 488-5705
(770) 488-5939 (fax)
http://cdc.gov/tobacco

Office of the Americans with Disabilities Act
U.S. Department of Justice
P.O. Box 66118
Washington, DC 20025-6118
(202) 514-0301
(202) 514-0383 (TDD)

Office of Work/Life Programs
U.S. Office of Personnel Management
Room 7425
Theodore Roosevelt Building
1900 East Street, NW
Washington, DC 20415-2000
(202) 606-5520
(202) 606-2091 (fax)
http://www.opm.gov/ehs/eappage.asp

Pan American Health Organization
525 23rd Street, NW
Washington, DC 20037
(202) 974-3000
(202) 974-3458
(202) 974-3663 (fax)
http://www.paho.org

President's Committee on Employment of People with Disabilities
1331 F Street, NW
3rd Floor
Washington, DC 20004
(202) 376-6200
(202) 376-6205 (TDD)

Project Inform (PI)
National HIV Treatment Line
205 13th Street
#2001
San Francisco, CA 94103
(800) 822-7422 (toll-free)
(415) 558-0684 (fax)
http://www.projectinform.org

Recovery, Inc.
802 N. Dearborn Street
Chicago, IL 60610
(312) 337-5661
(312) 337-5756 (fax)
http://www.recovery-inc.com

Registry of Toxic Effects of Chemical Substances (RETECS)
National Institute of Occupational Safety & Health
4676 Columbia Parkway

Cincinnati, OH 45226
(800) 356-4674 (toll-free)
http://www.cdc.gov/niosh/rtecs.html

Rehabilitation Services Administration
U.S. Department of Education
Mary E. Switzer Building
Room 3028
330 C Street, SW
Washington, DC 20202-2531
(202) 732-1282

Self-Help for Hard of Hearing People
7910 Woodmont Avenue
Bethesda, MD 20814
(301) 657-2248
(301) 657-2249
(301) 913-9413 (fax)
http://www.shhh.org

Skin Cancer Foundation
245 5th Avenue
Suite 1403
New York, NY 10016
(800) SKI-N490 (toll-free)
(212) 725-5751 (fax)
http://www.skincancer.org

Social Security Administration
Office of Disability
Room 545
Altimeyer Building
6401 Security Boulevard
Baltimore, MD 21235
(301) 965-3424

Society for Chemical Hazard Communication
P.O. Box 1392
Annandale, VA 22003-9392
(703) 658-9246
(703) 658-9247 (fax)
http://www.schc.org

Society of Environmental Toxicology and Chemistry (SETAC)
1010 N. 12th Avenue
Pensacola, FL 32501-3367
(888) 899-2088 (toll-free)
(850) 469-1500
(850) 469-9778 (fax)
http://www.setac.org

Society of Fire Protection Engineers (SFPE)
7315 Wisconsin Avenue

Suite 1225W
Bethesda, MD 20814
(301) 718-2910
(301) 718-2242 (fax)
http://www.sfpe.org

Society of Toxicology (SOT)
1767 Business Center Drive
Suite 302
Reston, VA 20190
(703) 438-3115
(703) 438-3113 (fax)
http://www.toxicology.org

Special Interest Group on Phobias and Related Anxiety Disorders (SIGPRAD)
245 E. 87th Street
New York, NY 10128
(212) 860-5560
http://www.cyberpsych.org/anxsig.htm

Substance Abuse and Mental Health Services Administration
Center for Mental Health Services
5600 Fishers Lane
Rockville, MD 20857
(800) 789-2647 (toll-free)
(301) 443-2792
http://www.samhsa.gov/cmhs/cmhs.html

Tire Industry Association (TIA)
11921 Freedom Drive
Suite 550
Reston, VA 20190
(800) 876-8372 (toll-free)
(703) 736-8020
(703) 904-4399 (fax)
http://www.tana.net

Unite! Union of Needletrades, Industrial and Textile Employees
1710 Broadway
New York, NY 10019
(212) 265-7000
(212) 315-3803 (fax)
http://www.uniteunion.org

United Food and Commercial Workers International Union (UFCW)
1775 K Street, NW
Washington, DC 20006
(202) 223-3111

(202) 466-1562 (fax)
http://www.ufcw.org

U.S. Department of Labor
U.S. Bureau of Labor Statistics
Postal Square Building
Room 2850
2 Massachusetts Avenue, NE
Washington, DC 20212-0001
(202) 691-7800
(202) 691-7797 (fax)
http://www.bls.gov

U.S. Nuclear Regulatory Commission
11555 Rockville Pike
MSO16C1
Rockville, MD 20852
(301) 415-1759
(301) 415-1757 (fax)
http://www.nrc.gov

U.S. Veterans Administration
Mental Health and Behavioral Sciences Services
810 Vermont Avenue, NW
Room 915
Washington, DC 20410
(202) 389-3416

Volunteer Management Associates
320 South Cedar Brook Road
Boulder, CO 80304-0468
(800) 944-1470 (toll-free)
(720) 304-3638
(720) 304-3638 (fax)
http://www.volunteermanagement.com

Wellness Councils of America
9802 Nicholas Street
Suite 315
Omaha, NE 68114
(402) 827-3590
(402) 827-3594 (fax)
http://www.welcoa.org
wellworkplace@welcoa.org

BIBLIOGRAPHY

Acquired Immunodeficiency Syndrome (AIDS)

Andriote, John-Manuel. *Victory Deferred: How AIDS Changed Gay Life in America.* Chicago: University of Chicago Press, 1999.

Banta, William F. *AIDS in the Workplace; Legal Questions and Practical Answers.* New York: Lexington Books, 1993.

Check, William A. *AIDS.* Philadelphia: Chelsea House, 1999.

Devita, Vincent T. *AIDS: Etiology, Diagnosis, Treatment, Prevention,* 4th ed. Philadelphia: Lippincott, 1997.

Dispezio, Michael A. *The Science, Spread, and Therapy of HIV Disease: Everything You Need to Know but Had No Idea Who to Ask.* Shrewsbury, Mass.: ATL Press, 1998.

Gedatus, Gustav Mark. *HIV and AIDS.* Mankato, Minn.: Lifematters, 2000.

Gifford, Allen. *Living Well with HIV & AIDS.* Palo Alto, Calif.: Bull Publishers, 2000.

Jenkins, Mark. *HIV/AIDS: Practical Medical, and Spiritual Guidelines for Daily Living When You're HIV-Positive.* Center City, Minn.: Hazelden Information & Educational Services, 2000.

Storad, Conrad J. *Inside AIDS: HIV Attacks the Immune System.* Minneapolis: Lerner Publications Co., 1998.

Ward, Darrell E. *The AmFAR AIDS Handbook: The Complete Guide to Understanding HIV and AIDS.* New York: W. W. Norton, 1999.

Addictions (See also ALCOHOLISM; SMOKING)

Carroll, Marilyn. *Cocaine and Crack.* Hillside, N.J.: Enslow Publishers, 1994.

Chopra, Deepak. *Overcoming Addictions: The Spiritual Solution.* New York: Harmony Books, 1997.

Ruden, Ronald A. *The Craving Brain: The Biobalance to Controlling Addictions.* New York: HarperCollins, 1997.

White, Robert K., and Deborah George Wright, eds. *Addiction Intervention: Strategies to Motivate.* New York: Haworth Press, 1998.

Affective Disorders
(See BIPOLAR DISORDER; DEPRESSION)

Agoraphobia (See also ANXIETY DISORDERS; PHOBIAS)

Ballenger, Janes C., ed. *Biology of Agoraphobia.* Washington, D.C.: American Psychiatric Press, 1984.

Frampton, Muriel. *Agoraphobia: Coming to Terms with the World Outside.* Wellingstorough, Northamptonshire, England: Turnstone Press, Ltd., 1984.

Goldstein, Alan J. *Overcoming Agoraphobia: Conquering Fear of the Outside World* New York: Viking, 1987.

Seagrave, Ann, and Faison Covington. *Free from Fears: A New Help for Anxiety, Panic and Agoraphobia.* New York: Poseidon Press, 1987.

Scrignar, Chester R. *From Panic to Peace of Mind: Overcoming Panic and Agoraphobia.* New Orleans, La.: Brunn Press, 1991.

Air Quality (See ENVIRONMENT)

Alcoholism (See also ADDICTIONS)

Barbour, Scott, ed. *Alcohol: Opposing Viewpoints.* San Diego: Greenhaven Press, 1998.

Cohen, S., and J. F. Callahan. *The Diagnosis and Treatment of Drug and Alcohol Abuse.* New York: Haworth Press, 1986.

Dick, R. *New Light on Alcoholism.* Corte Madera, Calif.: Good Book Publishing, 1994.

Helzer, J. E., G. J. Canino, E. K. Yeh, et al. "Alcoholism—North America and Asia: A Comparison of Population Surveys with the Diagnostic Interview Schedule," *Archives of General Psychiatry* 47 (1990):313–319.

Ketchum, Katherine, and William F. Asbury. *Beyond the Influence: Understanding and Defeating Alcoholism.* New York: Bantam Books, 2000.

O'Brien, Robert. *Encyclopedia of Understanding Alcohol and Other Drugs.* New York: Facts On File, Inc., 1999.

Powter, Susan. *Sober—and Staying That Way: The Missing Link in the Cure for Alcoholism.* New York: Simon & Schuster, 1997.

St. Clair, Harvey R. *Recognizing Alcoholism and Its Effects: A Mini-Guide.* New York: Karger, 1991.

Torr, James D., ed. *Alcoholism.* San Diego: Greenhaven Press, 2000.

Alternative Therapies
(See COMPLEMENTARY THERAPIES)

Americans with Disabilities Act

Allen, J. G. *Complying with the ADA: A Small Business Guide to Hiring and Employing the Disabled.* New York: John Wiley & Sons, 1993.

McCormick, J. A. *The Americans with Disabilities Act: A Manager's Guide.* New York: McGraw-Hill, 1994.

Schneid, T. D. *The Americans with Disabilities Act: A Practical Guide for Managers.* New York: Van Nostrand Reinhold, 1992.

Anorexia Nervosa (See EATING DISORDERS)

Anxiety and Anxiety Disorders
(See also PHOBIAS; OBSESSIVE-COMPULSIVE DISORDER; POST-TRAUMATIC STRESS DISORDER)

Barlow, D. H., and Michael Craske. *Mastery of Your Anxiety and Panic II.* Albany, N.Y.: Graywind Publications, 1994.

Bloomfield, Harold H. *Healing Anxiety with Herbs.* New York: HarperCollins, 1998.

Dattilio, Frank M., and Jesus A. Salas-Auvert. *Panic Disorder: Assessment and Treatment through a Wide-Angle Lens.* Phoenix, Ariz.: Zeig, Tucker & Co., 2000.

Doctor, Ronald M., and Ada P. Kahn. *The Encyclopedia of Phobias, Fears, and Anxieties.* 2d ed. New York: Facts On File, Inc., 2000.

———. *Facing Fears: The Sourcebook for Phobias, Fears, and Anxieties.* New York: Checkmark Books, 2000.

Feniger, Mani. *Journey from Anxiety to Freedom: Moving Beyond Panic and Phobias and Learning to Trust Yourself.* Rocklin, Calif.: Prima, 1997.

Marks, Isaac. *Living with Fear.* New York: McGraw-Hill, 1980.

———. *Fears, Phobias, and Rituals: Panic, Anxiety, and Their Disorders.* New York: Oxford University Press, 1987.

Root, Benjamin A. *Understanding Panic and Other Anxiety Disorders.* Jackson: University Press of Mississippi, 2000.

Ross, Jerilyn. *Triumph over Fear: A Book of Help and Hope for People with Anxiety, Panic Attacks, and Phobias.* New York: Bantam Books, 1994.

Swedo, Susan, and H. L. Leonard. *It's Not All in Your Head.* New York: HarperCollins, 1996.

Trickett, Shirley. *Panic Attacks: A Natural Approach.* Calif.: Ulysses Press, 1999.

Back Pain (See also INJURIES)

Churchill, Adams N. *The Psychophysiology of Low Back Pain.* New York: Livingstone, 1997.

Drukteinis, A. M. *The Psychology of Back Pain: A Clinical and Legal Handbook.* Springfield, Ill.: Charles C. Thomas, 1996.

Pope, M. H., G. B. U. Andersson, J. W. Frymoyer, et al. *Occupational Low Back Pain: Assessment, Treatment and Prevention.* St. Louis: Mosby-Year Book, 1991.

Behavior Therapy

Bellack, A. S., Hersen, M., eds. *Dictionary of Behavioral Therapy Techniques.* New York: Pergamon Press, 1985.

Hersen, M., ed. *Pharmacological and Behavioral Treatment: An Integrative Approach.* New York: John Wiley & Sons, 1986.

Boredom

Leckart, B., and L. G. Weinberger. *Up from Boredom, Down from Fear.* New York: Richard Marek Publishers, 1980.

Rediger, G. L. *Lord, Don't Let Me Be Bored.* Philadelphia: Westminster Press, 1986.

Savitz, J., and M. Friedman. "Diagnosing Boredom and Confusion," *Nursing Research* 30, no. 1 (1981): 16–19.

Burnout

Potter, Beverly. *Beating Job Burnout: How to Transform Work Pressure into Productivity.* Berkeley, Calif.: Ronin Publishing, 1994.

Stevens, Paul. *Beating Job Burnout: How to Turn Your Work into Your Passion.* Lincolnwood, Ill.: NTC Publishing Group, 1995.

Chronic Fatigue Syndrome/Fatigue

Brody, Jane E. "Chronic Fatigue Syndrome: How to Recognize It and What to Do about It," *New York Times,* July 28, 1988.

Fackelmann, K. A. "The Baffling Case of Chronic Fatigue," *Science News,* January 1989.

Feiden, Karyn. *Hope and Help for Chronic Fatigue Syndrome.* New York: Prentice Hall Press, 1990.

McGee-Cooper, Ann. *You Don't Have to Go Home from Work Exhausted: The New Energy Engineering Approach.* Dallas, Tex.: Bowen & Rogers, 1990.

Zoler, Mitchel L. "Chronic Fatigue: Taking the Syndrome Seriously," *Medical World News,* December 12, 1988.

Complementary Therapies
(See also MIND-BODY CONNECTIONS)

Eisenberg, D., et al. "Unconventional Medicine in the United States: Prevalence, Costs, and Patterns of Use." *New England Journal of Medicine* 328 (1993): 246–252.

Facklam, Howard. *Alternative Medicine: Cures or Myths?* New York: Twenty-First Century Books, 1996.

Gordon, James S. *Manifesto for a New Medicine: Your Guide to Healing Partnerships and Wise Use of Alternative Therapies.* Reading, Mass.: Addison-Wesley, 1996.

McGill, Leonard. *The Chiropractor's Health Book: Simple Natural Exercises for Relieving Headaches, Tension and Back Pain.* New York: Crown, 1995.

Morton, Mary, and Michael Morton. *5 Steps to Selecting the Best Alternative Medicine.* Novato, Calif.: New World Library, 1996.

Rondberg, Terry A. *Chiropractic First: The Fastest Growing Healthcare Choice before Drugs or Surgery.* Chandler, Ariz.: Chiropractic Journal, 1996.

Sachs, Judith. *Nature's Prozac: Natural Therapies and Techniques to Rid Yourself of Anxiety, Depression, Panic Attacks and Stress.* Englewood Cliffs, N.J.: Prentice Hall, 1997.

Computer-Related Injuries (See also INJURIES)

Brown, Stephanie. *Preventing Computer Injury: The Hand-Book with KeyMoves Software.* New York: Ergonome, 1993.

Galinsky, T., L. S. Schleifer, and C. S. Pan. "The Influence of Performance Standards and Feedback on Speed and Accuracy in an Electronically Monitored Data-Entry Task." *International Journal of Human-Computer Interaction* 7, no. 1 (1995): 25–36.

Godnig, E. D., and J. S. Hacunda. *Computers and Visual Stress.* Grand Rapids, Mich.: Abacus, 1991.

Hoekstra, E., J. Hurrell, and N. Swanson. "Evaluation of Work-Related Musculoskeletal Disorders and Job Stress among Teleservice Center Representatives." *Applied Occupational and Environmental Hygiene* 10, no. 10 (1995): 812–817.

Hurrell J. J., B. P. Bernard, T. R. Hales, et al. "Psychosocial Factors and Musculoskeletal Disorders; Summary and Implications of Three NIOSH Health Hazard Evaluations of Video Display Terminal Work." In *Beyond Biomechanics: Psychosocial Aspects of Musculoskeletal Disorders in Office Work,* edited by S. D. Moon and S. L. Sauter. Bristol, Pa.: Taylor & Francis, pp. 99–105.

Lim, S. Y., S. L. Sauter, and T. M. Schnorr. "Occupational Health Aspects of Work with Video Display Terminals." In *Environmental and Occupational Medicine.* 3d ed., edited by W. N. Rom. Philadelphia, Pa.: Lippincott-Raven Publishers, 1998, pp. 1333–1344.

Pan, C. S., and L. M. Schliefer. "An Exploratory Study of the Relationship between Biomechanical Factors and Right-Arm Musculoskeletal Discomfort and Fatigue in a VDT Data-Entry Task." *Applied Ergonomics* 27, no. 3 (1996): 195–200.

Schleifer, L. M., R. Ley, and C. Pan. "Breathing, Psychological Stress and Musculoskeletal Complaints in VDT Work." Proceedings of the HCI International '97 Conference on Human-Computer Interaction, San Francisco, Calif., pp. 545–550.

Swanson, N. G., T. L. Galinsky, L. L. Cole, et al. "The Impact of Keyboard Design on Comfort and Productivity in a Text-Entry Task." *Applied Ergonomics* 28, no. 1 (1997): 9–16.

Crisis Intervention (See also VIOLENCE)

Aguilera, D. C., and J. M. Messick. *Crisis Intervention: Theory and Methodology.* 5th ed. St. Louis: Mosby, 1986.

Dixon, S. L. *Working with People in Crisis: Theory and Practice.* St. Louis: Mosby, 1979.

Everstine, D. S., and L. Everstine. *People in Crisis.* New York: Brunner/Mazel, 1983.

Cumulative Trauma Disorders (See also COMPUTER-RELATED INJURIES; INJURIES)

Parker K. G., and H. R. Imbus. *Cumulative Trauma Disorders, Current Issues and Ergonomic Solutions: A Systems Approach.* New York: Lewis Publishers, 1992.

Rosenbaum, R. B., and J. L. Ochoa. *Carpal Tunnel Syndrome and Other Disorders of the Median Nerve.* Boston: Butterworth Heinemann, 1993.

Dance Injuries (Professional) (See PERFORMING ARTS MEDICINE)

Depression/Bipolar Disorder/Manic Depression

Baskin, Valerie D. *When Words Are Not Enough: The Women's Prescription for Depression and Anxiety.* New York: Broadway Books, 1997.

Fawcett, Jan, Nancy Rosenfeld, and Bernard Golden. *New Hope for People with Bipolar Disorder.* Roseville, Calif.: Prima Publishing, 2000.

Greist, John H., and James W. Jefferson. *Depression and Its Treatment: Help for the Nation's #1 Mental Problem.* Rev. ed. New York: Warner Books, 1992.

Healy, David. *The Anti-Depressant Era.* Cambridge, Mass.: Harvard University Press, 1997.

Kim, Henry H., ed. *Depression.* San Diego: Greenhaven Press, 1999.

Martin, Philip. *The Zen Path through Depression.* San Francisco: HarperSanFrancisco, 1999.

Quinn, Brian. *The Depression Sourcebook.* Los Angeles: Lowell House, 1997.

Reichenberg-Ullman, Judyth. *Prozac-free: Homeopathic Medications for Depression, Anxiety and Other Mental and Emotional Problems.* Rocklin, Calif.: Prima Health, 1999.

Sanders, Pete. *Depression and Mental Health.* Brookfield. Conn.: Copper Beech Books, 1998.

Turkington, Carol. *Making the Prozac Decision: A Guide to Antidepressants.* Los Angeles: Contemporary Books, 1997.

Eating Disorders

Cassell, Dana K. *Encyclopedia of Obesity and Eating Disorders.* New York: Facts On File, Inc., 1994.

Kinoy, Barbara P., ed. *Eating Disorders: New Directions in Treatment and Recovery.* New York: Columbia University Press, 1994.

Orbach, Susie. *Hunger Strike: An Anorexic's Struggle as a Metaphor for Our Age.* New York: Norton, 1986.

Sonder, Ben. *Eating Disorders: When Food Turns against You.* New York: Franklin Watts, 1993.

Environment

Bowker, Michael. *Fatal Deception: The Untold Story of Asbestos: Why It Is Still Legal and Still Killing Us.* Emmaus, Pa.: Rodale, 2003.

Fisk, W. J. "Estimates of Potential Nationwide Productivity and Health Benefits from Better Indoor Environments: An Update." In *Indoor Air Quality Handbook,* edited by J. Spengler, J. M. Samet, J. F. McCarthy. New York: McGraw-Hill, 2000, pp. 4.1–4.36.

Fisk W. J., and Rosenfeld, A. H. "Estimates of Improved Productivity and Health from Better Indoor Environments." *Indoor Air* 7 (1997): 158–172.

Kreiss, K. "The Epidemiology of Building-Related Complaints and Illness." *Occupational Medicine* 4 (1989): 1–18.

Mendell, Mark J., William J. Fisk, Kathleen Kreiss, et al. "Improving the Health of Workers in Indoor Environments: Priority Research Needs for a National Occupational Research Agenda. *American Journal of Public Health* 92, no. 9 (September, 2002): 1430–1440.

Mendell, M. J. "Non-Specific Symptoms in Office Workers: A Review and Summary of the Epidemiologic Literature." *Indoor Air* 3, no. 2 (1993): 227–236.

Rosenstock, L., C. Olenec, G. R. Wagner. "The National Occupational Research Agenda: A Model of Broad Stakeholder Input into Priority Setting." *American Journal of Public Health* 88 (1998): 353–356.

U.S. Environmental Protection Agency. *Building Air Quality: A Guide for Building Owners and Facility Managers.* EPA publication 400/1-91/033. Washington, D.C.: U.S. Environmental Protection Agency, 1991.

U.S. Environmental Protection Agency. *Building Air Quality Action Plan.* EPA publication 402-K-98-001. Washington, D.C.: U.S. Environmental Protection Agency, 1998.

Ergonomics

Chaffen, D. B., and G. B. J. Andersson. *Occupational Biomechanics.* New York: John Wiley & Sons, 1994.

Donkin, S. W. *Sitting On the Job.* Lincoln, Nebr.: Parallel Integration, 1986.

Kroemer, K. H. E. *Ergonomic Design of Material Handling Systems.* New York: Lewis Publishers, 1997.

Grandjean, E. *Fitting the Task to the Man: A Textbook of Occupational Ergonomics.* New York: Taylor & Francis, 1988.

———. *Ergonomics in Computerized Offices.* New York: Taylor & Francis, 1987.

Feminist Viewpoints on Working

Friedan, Betty. *The Feminine Mystique.* New York: W. W. Norton, 1963.

Fuller, Margaret. *Woman in the Nineteenth Century.* New York: W. W. Norton, 1971.

Goldman, Emma. *Red Emma Speaks: Selected Writings and Speeches by Emma Goldman.* New York: Random House, 1972.

Morgan, Robin, ed. *Sisterhood Is Powerful: An Anthology of Writings from the Woman's Liberation Movement.* New York: Vintage Books, 1970.

Rossi, Alice S., ed. *The Feminist Papers: From Adams to de Beauvoir.* New York: Bantam Books, 1976.

Steinem, Gloria. *Outrageous Acts and Everyday Rebellions.* New York: Holt, Rinehart and Winston, 1983.

Headaches

Diamond, Seymour. *The Hormone Headache: New Ways to Prevent, Manage, and Treat Migraines and Other Headaches.* New York: Macmillan, 1995.

Finnigan, Jeffrey. *Life beyond Headaches.* Olympia, Wash.: Finnigan Clinic, 1999.

Hartnell, Agnes. *Migraine Headaches and the Foods You Eat: 200 Recipes for Relief.* Minneapolis: Chronimed, 1997.

Inlander, Charles B., and Porter Shimer. *Headaches: 47 Ways to Stop the Pain.* New York: Walker and Company, 1995.

Kahn, Ada P. *Headaches.* Chicago: Contemporary Books, 1983.

Maas, Paula, and Deborah Mitchell. *The Natural Health Guide to Headache to Relief: The Definitive Handbook of Natural Remedies for Treating Every Kind of Headache Pain.* New York: Pocket Books, 1997.

Health and Well-being (See also HEALTH PROMOTION; WORKSITE WELLNESS)

Benson, Herbert. *The Wellness Book: The Complete Guide to Maintaining Health and Treating Stress-Related Illness.* Secaucus, N.J.: Carol Publishing Group, 1992.

Dychtwald, Ken. *Age Power: How the 21st Century Will Be Ruled By the New Old.* New York: J. P. Tarcher/Putnam, 1999.

Illich, Ivan. *Medical Nemesis: The Expropriation of Health.* New York: Pantheon, 1982.

Lesnoff-Caravaglia, Gari. *Health Aspects of Aging: The Experience of Growing Old.* Springfield, Ill.: C. C. Thomas, 2000.

Loverde, Joy. *The Complete Eldercare Planner: Where to Start, Which Questions to Ask, and How to Find Help.* New York: Times Books, 2000.

Pelletier, Kenneth R. *Sound Mind, Sound Body: A Model for Lifelong Health.* New York: Simon and Schuster, 1994.

Peterson, Christopher, and Lisa M. Bossio. *Health and Optimism.* New York: Macmillan, 1991.

Stutz, David, and Bernard Feder. *The Savvy Patient: How to Be an Active Participant in Your Medical Care.* Yonkers, N.Y.: Consumer Reports Books, 1990.

Weil, Andrew. *Eight Weeks to Optimum Health: A Proven Program for Taking Full Advantage of Your Body's Healing Power.* New York: Alfred A. Knopf, 1997.

Williams, R. W., and V. Williams. *Anger Kills: 17 Strategies for Controlling the Hostility That Can Harm Your Health.* New York: Times Books, 1993.

Wolinsky, Stephen. *Quantum Consciousness: The Guide to Experiencing Quantum Psychology.* Norfolk, Conn.: Bramble Books, 1993.

Health Care Workers

Arellano, R., J. Bradley, G. Sussman. "Prevalence of Latex Sensitization among Hospital Physicians Occupationally Exposed to Latex Gloves." *Anesthesiology* 77 (1992): 905–908.

Centers for Disease Control and Prevention. "Evaluation of Blunt Suture Needles in Preventing Percutaneous Injuries among Health Care Workers During Gynecologic Surgical Procedures. *Morbidity and Mortality Weekly Report* 46 (1997): 25–29.

Gershon, R. "Facilitator Report: Bloodborne Pathogens Exposure among Healthcare Workers." *American Journal of Industrial Medicine* 29 (1996): 418–420.

Institute of Medicine: *Nursing Staff in Hospitals and Nursing Homes: Is It Adequate?* Washington, D.C.: National Academy Press, 1996.

Sepkowitz, K. A. "Tuberculosis and Healthcare Workers: An Historical Perspective." *Annals of Internal Medicine* 120 (1994): 71–79.

Sepkowitz, K. A. "AIDS, Tuberculosis, and the Healthcare Workers." *Clinical Infectious Diseases* 20 (1995): 232–242.

Health Promotion
(See also HEALTH; WORKSITE WELLNESS)

Nemcek, M. A. "Research Trends in the Health Promotion of Well Adults," *AAOHN (American Association of Occupational Health Nurses) Journal* 34 (1986): 470–475.

Immune System (See also HEALTH)

Borysenko, M. "The Immune system: An Overview," *Annals of Behavioral Medicine* 9 (1987): 3–10.

Cohen, S., D. A. J. Tyrrell, and A. P. Smith. "Psychological Stress and Susceptibility to the Common Cold," *New England Journal of Medicine* 325 (1991): 606–612.

Herbert, Tracy B. "Stress and the Immune System." *World Health,* March-April 1994.

Locke, Steven, and Douglas Colligan. *The Healer Within.* New York: New American Library, 1986.

Indoor Workplace Environment (See ENVIRONMENT)

Injuries (See also BACK INJURIES/BACK PAIN)

CDT News, Inc. *Cumulative Trauma Disorders: A Legal Guide to CTD Prevention, Regulation* and *Liability.* Westtown, Pa.: Andrews Professional Books, 1994.

Kome, Penny. *Wounded Workers: The Politics of Musculoskeletal Injuries.* Toronto: University of Toronto, 1998.

Parker, K. B., and H. R. Imbus. *Cumulative Trauma Disorders, Current Issues and Ergonimic Solutions: A Systems Approach.* New York: Lewis Publishers, 1992.

Rosenbaum, R. B., and J. L. Ochoa. *Carpal Tunnel Syndrome and Other Disorders of the Median Nerve.* Boston: Butterworth Heinemann, 1993.

Legal Issues in the Workplace

Brakel, S. J., J. Parry, B. A. Waner. *The Mentally Disabled and the Law.* 3d ed. Chicago: American Bar Foundation, 1985.

Simon, J. T. *Clinical Psychiatry and the Law.* Washington, D.C.: American Psychiatric Press, 1987.

Men in the Workplace

Bednarik, Karl. *The Male in Crisis.* New York: Alfred A. Knopf, 1970.

Farrell, Warren. *Why Men Are the Way They Are.* New York: McGraw-Hill, 1986.

Mind/Body Connections
(See also COMPLEMENTARY THERAPIES)

Benson, Herbert. *The Relaxation Response.* New York: Avon Books, 1975.

———. *Beyond the Relaxation Response.* New York: Berkeley, 1985.

Borysenko, Joan. *Guilt Is the Teacher, Love Is the Lesson.* New York: Warner, 1991.

———. *Minding the Body, Mending the Mind.* New York: Bantam, 1988.

Chopra, Deepak. *Perfect Health.* New York: Harmony Books, 1990.

———. *Quantum Healing: Exploring the Frontiers of Mind/Body Medicine.* New York: Bantam Books, 1989.

Cousins, Norman. *Anatomy of an Illness as Perceived by the Patient.* New York: Norton, 1979.

———. *Head First: The Biology of Hope and the Healing Power of the Human Spirit.* New York: Viking Penguin, 1990.

———. *The Healing Heart.* New York: Norton, 1983.

Dienstfrey, Harris. *Where the Mind Meets the Body.* New York: HarperCollins, 1991.

Dossey, Larry. *Space, Time and Medicine.* Boston: Shambhala, 1982.

Moyers, B. *Healing and the Mind.* New York: Doubleday, 1993.

Pelletier, Kenneth R. *Mind as Healer, Mind as Slayer.* Rev. ed. New York: Delacorte, 1992.

———. *Sound Mind, Sound Body: A New Model for Lifelong Health.* New York: Simon & Schuster, 1994.

Siegel, Bernie. *Love, Medicine and Miracles.* New York: Harper and Row, 1986.

———. *Peace, Love and Healing.* New York: Harper and Row, 1989.

Musicians' Injuries (See PERFORMING ARTS MEDICINE)

Nutrition

Brody, Jane. *Jane Brody's Nutrition Book.* New York: W. W. Norton, 1981.

Brown, Judith E. *Everywoman's Guide to Nutrition.* Minneapolis: University of Minnesota Press, 1991.

Finn, Susan Calvert, and Linda Stern. *The Real Life Nutrition Book: Making the Right Food Choices without Changing Your Life-Style.* New York: Penguin Books, 1992.

Haas, Robert. *Eat Smart, Think Smart: How to Use Nutrients and Supplements to Achieve Maximum Mental and Physical Performance.* New York: HarperCollins, 1994.

Kotsanis, Frank N., and Maureen A. Mackey, eds. *Nutrition in the '90s: Current Controversies and Analysis.* Vol. 2. New York: Marcel Dekker, 1994.

Obsessive-compulsive Disorder
(See also ANXIETY DISORDERS)

DeSilva, Padmal. *Obsessive-Compulsive Disorder: The Facts.* New York: Oxford University Press, 1998.

Gravitz, Herbert L. *Obsessive Compulsive Disorder: New Help for the Family.* Santa Barbara, Calif.: Healing Visions Press, 1998.

Reyes, Karen. "Obsessive-Compulsive Disorder: There Is Help," *Modern Maturity,* November-December 1995.

Occupational Health
(See also HEALTH; INJURIES; WORKSITE WELLNESS)

Levy, B. S., and D. H. Wegman, eds. *Occupational Health: Recognizing and Preventing Work Related Disease.* 3d ed. Boston: Little Brown, 1995.

Sataloff, R. T., and J. Sataloff. *Occupational Hearing Loss.* 2d ed. New York: Marcel Dekker, 1993.

Panic Attacks and Panic Disorder
(See ANXIETY AND ANXIETY DISORDERS)

Performance Anxiety
(See also PERFORMING ARTS MEDICINE)

Dawson, William J. "Hand and Upper Extremity Problems in Musicians: Epidemiology and Diagnosis." *Medical Problems of Performing Artists* 3, no. 1 (March 1988): 19–22.

Dunkel, Stuart Edward. *The Audition Process: Anxiety Management and Coping Strategies.* Stuyvesant, N.Y.: Pendragon Press, 1989.

Estill, Jo. "Belting and Classic Voice Quality: Some Physiological Differences." *Medical Problems of Performing Artists* 3, no. 1 (March 1988): 37–43.

Fishbein, Martin, and Susan E. Middlestadt. "Medical Problems Among ICSOM Musicians: Overview of a National Survey." *Medical Problems of Performing Artists* 3, no. 1 (March 1988): 1–43.

Fry, Hunter J. H. "Occupational Maladies of Musicians: Their Cause and Prevention." *International Journal of Music Education* 2 (1984): 59–63.

Goodman, Glenn, and Sheryl Staz. "Occupational Therapy for Musicians with Upper Extremity Overuse Syndrome: Patient Perceptions Regarding Effectiveness of Treatment." *Medical Problems of Performing Artists,* 4, no. 1 (March 1989): 9–14.

Howse, J., and S. Hancock, eds. *Dance Technique and Injury Prevention.* New York: Theatre Arts Books, 1992.

Lederman, Richard. "An Overview of Performing Arts Medicine." *American Music Teacher* 40, no. 4 (February/March 1991): 12–70.

Middlestadt, Susan E., and Martin Fishbein. "The Prevalence of Severe Musculoskeletal Problems Among Male and Female Symphony Orchestra String Players." *Medical Problems of Performing Artists* 4, no. 1 (March 1989): 41–48.

Moss, Robert. "Stage Fright Is Actors' Eternal Nemesis." *New York Times,* January 6, 1992, E2.

Nolan, William B., and Richard G. Eaton. "Thumb Problems of Professional Musicians." *Medical Problems of Performing Artists* 4, no. 1 (March 1989): 20–24.

Ryan, A.J., and R. E. Stephens, eds. *Dance Medicine: A Comprehensive Guide.* Chicago: Pluribus Press, 1987.

Sataloff, Robert. "Arts Medicine: An Overview." *American Music Teacher* 50, no. 2 (October/November 2000): 33–38.

Sataloff, Robert Thayer, Alice G. Brandfonbrener, and Richard J. Lederman, eds. *Textbook of Performing Arts Medicine.* New York: Raven Press, Ltd., 1991.

Watkins, A., and P. M. Clarkson. *Dancing Longer, Dancing Stronger.* Princeton, N.J.: Princeton Book Co., 1990.

Wolfe, Mary L. "Correlates of Adaptive and Maladaptive Musical Performance Anxiety." *Medical Problems of Performing Artists* 4, no. 1 (March 1989): 49–56.

Phobias (See also ANXIETY DISORDERS)

Bourne, Edmund J. *The Anxiety & Phobia Workbook.* Oakland, Calif.: New Harbinger Publications, 1995.

Doctor, Ronald M., and Ada P. Kahn. *Encyclopedia of Phobias, Fears and Anxieties.* 2d ed. New York: Facts On File, Inc., 2000.

———. *Facing Fears: The Sourcebook for Phobias, Fears and Anxieties.* New York: Checkmark Books, 2000.

Marks, Isaac M. *Living with Fear.* New York: McGraw-Hill, 1980.

———. *Fears, Phobias, and Rituals.* New York: Oxford University Press, 1987.

Marshall, John R. *Social Phobia: From Shyness to Stage Fright.* New York: Basic Books, 1994.

Monroe, Judy. *Phobias: Everything You Wanted to Know, but Were Afraid to Ask.* Springfield, N.J.: Enslow Publishers, 1996.

Post-Traumatic Stress Disorder (See also ANXIETY DISORDERS)

Catherall, Donald Roy. *Back from the Brink: A Family Guide to Overcoming Traumatic Stress.* New York: Bantam Books, 1992.

Herman, Judith. *Trauma and Recovery.* New York: Basic Books, 1992.

Van der Kolk, B. A., ed. *Post-Traumatic Stress Disorder: Psychological and Biological Sequelae.* Washington, D.C.: American Psychiatric Press, 1996.

Psychology, Contemporary (See also COMPLEMENTARY THERAPIES; MIND/BODY CONNECTIONS)

Borysenko, Joan. *Guilt Is the Teacher, Love Is the Lesson.* New York: Warner Books, 1990.

Bradshaw, John. *Bradshaw On: The Family.* Deerfield Beach, Fla.: Health Communications, 1988.

———. *Healing the Shame That Binds You.* Deerfield Beach, Fla.: Health Communications, 1988.

Cousins, Norman. *The Healing Heart.* New York: Avon Books, 1984.

Csikzentmihalyi, Mihaly. *Flow: The Psychology of Optimal Experience.* New York: HarperCollins, 1991.

Peck, M. Scott. *The Road Less Traveled.* New York: Simon and Schuster, 1978.

Wolinsky, Stephen H. *Trances People Live: Healing Approaches in Quantum Psychology.* Norfolk, Conn.: Bramble Books, 1991.

Relaxation

Benson, Herbert. *Beyond the Relaxation Response.* New York: Berkeley Press, 1985.

———. *The Relaxation Response.* New York: Avon Books, 1975.

———. *Your Maximum Mind.* New York: Times Books, 1987.

Benson, Herbert, Eileen M. Stuart, and staff of the Mind/Body Medical Institute. *The Wellness Book: The Comprehensive Guide to Maintaining Health and Treating Stress-Related Illness.* New York: Carol, 1992.

Blumenfeld, Larry, ed. *The Big Book of Relaxation: Simple Techniques to Control the Excess Stress in Your Life.* Roslyn, N.Y.: Relaxation Company, 1994.

Davis, Martha, Elizabeth Robbins Eshelman, and Matthew McKay. *The Relaxation and Stress Reduction Workbook.* Oakland, Calif.: New Harbinger Publications, 1995.

Davis, M., and E. R. Eshelman, and M. McKay. *The Relaxation and Stress Reduction Workbook* Oakland, Calif.: New Harbinger, 1995.

Safety (See also INJURIES)

Baker, S. P., B. O'Neill, M. J. Ginsburg, et al. *The Injury Fact Book.* 2d ed. New York: Oxford University Press, 1992.

Geller, S. W. *The Psychology of Safety.* Radnor, Pa.: Chilton, 1996.

Kornerg, J. P. *The Workplace Walkthrough.* New York: Macmillan, 1993.

Self-esteem

Hillman, Carolynn. *Recovery of Your Self-Esteem.* New York: Simon & Schuster, 1992.

Johnson, Carol. *Self-Esteem Comes in All Sizes.* New York: Doubleday, 1995.

Kahn, Ada P., and Sheila Kimmel. *Empower Yourself: Every Woman's Guide to Self-Esteem.* New York: Avon Books, 1997.

Lindenfield, Gael. *Self-Esteem.* New York: HarperPaperbacks, 1997.

McKay, Matthew. *The Self-Esteem Companion: Simple Exercises to Help You Challenge Your Inner Critic and Celebrate Your Personal Strengths.* Oakland, Calif.: New Harbinger, 1999.

Steinem, Gloria. *Revolution from Within: A Book of Self-Esteem.* Boston: Little, Brown and Co., 1992.

Sleep

Knab, B., and R. Engle. "Perception of Waking and Sleeping: Possible Implications for Evaluation of Insomnia," *Sleep* 11 (1988): 265–272.

Ruler, A., and L. Lack. "Gender Differences in Sleep," *Sleep Research* 17 (1988): 244.

Smoking (See also ADDICTIONS)

Hammond, S. Katharine. "Environmental Tobacco Smoke Presents Substantial Risk in Workplaces." *The Journal of the American Medical Association,* September 26, 1995.

Liesges, Robert C., and Margaret DeBon. *How Women Can Finally Stop Smoking.* Alameda, Calif.: Hunter House, 1994.

Rogers, Jacquelyn. *You Can Stop Smoking.* New York: Pocket Books, 1995.

Sanders, Pete, and Steve Myers. *Smoking.* Brookfield, Conn.: Copper Beech Books, 1996.

Pietrusza, David. *Smoking.* San Diego: Lucent Books, 1997.

Social Phobias
(See ANXIETY and ANXIETY DISORDERS; PHOBIAS)

Social support, support groups, and self-help

Kahn, Ada P. "Psychosocial Support Influences Survival of Cancer Patients." *Psychiatric News,* October 1991.

Kreiner, Anna. *Everything You Need to Know About Creating Your Own Support System.* New York: Rosen Publishing Group, 1996.

Spiegel, David. *Living beyond Limits.* New York: Times Books, 1993.

White, Barbara J., and Edward J. Madara. *The Self-Help Sourcebook: Finding and Forming Mutual Aid Self-Help Groups.* Denville, N.J.: American Self-Help Clearinghouse, St. Clares–Riverside Medical Center, 1992.

Stress and Stress Management

Arrobe, Tanya. "Reducing the Cost of Stress: An Organizational Model" *Personnel Review* 19 (winter 1990).

Brammer, L. M. *How to Cope with Life Transitions: The Challenge of Personal Change.* New York: Hemisphere Publishing, 1991.

Colin, Stacey. "How to Find Your Stress Hot Spots." *McCall's* (September 1994).

Eliot, Robert S. *From Stress to Strength: How to Lighten Your Load and Save Your Life.* New York: Bantam Books, 1994.

Evans, Karin. "Is Stress Wrecking Your Mood?" *Health,* April 2000, p. 119–124.

Feder, Barnaby J. "A Spreading Pain, and Cries for Justice." *New York Times,* June 5, 1994.

Flint, Robert S. *From Stress to Strength: How to Lighten Your Load and Save Your Life.* New York: Bantam Books, 1994.

Gonthier, Giovinella, and Kevin Morrissey. *Rude Awakenings: Overcoming the Civility Crisis in the Workplace.* Chicago: Dearborn Trade, 2002.

Hafen, B. Q., K. J. Frandsen, K. J. Karren, and K. R. Hooker. *The Health Effects of Attitudes, Emotions and Relationships.* Provo, Utah: EMS Associates, 1992.

Kahn, Ada P. *The A–Z of Stress: A Sourcebook for Facing Everyday Challenges.* New York: Facts On File, Inc., 2000.

Lehrer, Paul M., and Robert L. Woolfolk, eds. *Principles and Practice of Stress Management.* 2d ed. New York: Guilford Press, 1993.

Maddi, Salvatore, and Suzanne Kobasa. *The Hardy Executive: Health under Stress.* Homewood, Ill.: Dow Jones–Irwin, 1984.

Murphy, Lawrence R. "Stress Management in Work Settings: A Critical Review of the Health Effects." *American Journal of Health Promotion.* 11, no. 2 (November/December, 1996).

Ornish, Dean. *Stress, Diet, and Your Heart.* New York: Holt, Rinehart and Winston, 1983.

Pelletier, Kenneth R. *Healthy People in Unhealthy Places: Stress and Fitness at Work.* New York: Delacorte Press, 1984.

Reinhold, Barbara Bailey. *Toxic Work: How to Overcome Stress, Overload and Burnout and Revitalize Your Career.* New York: Dutton, 1996.

Sapolsky, Robert M. *Why Zebras Don't Get Ulcers.* New York: W. H. Freeman & Company, 1994.

Selye, Hans. *Stress without Distress.* New York: Lippincott, 1974.

———. *The Stress of Life.* Rev. ed. New York: McGraw-Hill, 1978.

Shalowitz, Deborah. "Another Health Care Headache: Job Stress Could Strain Corporate Budgets." *Business Insurance* 25 (May 20, 1991).

Unions

Lorwin, L. L. *The Women's Garment Workers.* New York: Arno, 1969.

Stolberg, B. *Tailor's Progress: The Story of a Famous Union and the Men Who Made It.* Garden City, N.Y.: Doubleday, Doran and Company, 1944.

Danish, M. D. *The World of David Dubinsky.* Cleveland: World Publishing, 1957.

Tyler, G. *Look for the Union Label.* N.Y.: M. E. Sharpe, 1995.

Violence

Anfuso, D. "Deflecting workplace violence." *Personnel Journal* 73, no. 10 (1994).

Borwegen, W. "Violence as a preventable occupational hazard: a labor perspective." *New Solutions,* 1995, spring issue.

Capozzoli T., and R. S. McVey. *Managing Violence in the Workplace.* Delray Beach, Fla.: St. Lucie Press, 1996.

Fawcett, J., ed. *Dynamics of Violence.* Chicago: American Medical Association, 1972.

McCune, J. "Companies grapple with workplace violence." *Management Review* 83, no. 3, 1994.

Remsberg, Charles. *Tactics for Criminal Patrol: Vehicle Stops, Drug Discovery and Officer Survival.* Northbrook, Ill.: Calibre Press, 2000.

Shepherd, E., ed. *Violence in Health Care: A Practical Guide to Coping with Violence and Caring for Victims.* New York: Oxford University Press, 1994.

Voice Disorders (professional)
(See PERFORMING ARTS MEDICINE)

Women

Berg, Barbara J. *The Crisis of the Working Mother.* New York: Summit Books, 1986.

Cohen, Rona, and Marsha B. Mrtek. "The Impact of Two Corporate Lactation Programs on the Incidence and Duration of Breast-feeding by Employed Mothers." *American Journal of Health Promotion* 8, no. 6 (July/August 1994).

Cohen, Rona, Marsha B. Mrtek, and Robert B. Myrtek. "Breast-feeding in the workplace." *American Journal of Health Promotion* 10, no. 2. (November/December 1995).

Freudenberger, Herbert and Gail North. *Women's Burnout: How to Spot It, How to Reverse It, and How to Prevent It.* Garden City, N.Y.: Doubleday & Company, 1985.

Kahn, Ada P. "Women and Stress." *Sacramento Medicine,* September 1995.

Long, B. C., and C. J. Haney. "Coping Strategies for Working Women: Aerobic Exercise and Relaxation Interventions." *Behavior Therapy* (1988): 75–83.

Powell, J. Robin. *The Working Woman's Guide to Managing Stress.* Englewood Cliffs, N.J.: Prentice Hall, 1994.

Siress, Ruth Hermann. *Working Women's Communications Survival Guide: How to Present Your Ideas With Impact, Clarity, and Power and Get the Recognition You Deserve.* Englewood Cliffs, N.J.: Prentice Hall, 1994.

Workers' Compensation

Larson, Arthur. *Workmen's Compensation for Injuries and Death.* New York: Matthew Bender, 1991.

Workplace

DeMarco, Tom. *Slack: Getting Past Burnout, Busywork, and the Myth of Total Efficiency.* New York: Broadway Books, 2001.

Fraser, Jill Andresky. *White-Collar Sweatshop: The Deterioration of Work and Its Rewards in Corporate America.* New York: Norton, 2001.

Grappel, Jack L. *The Corporate Athlete: How to Achieve Maximal Performance in Business and Life.* New York: Wiley, 2000.

Karasek, Robert, and Tores Theorell. *Health Work: Stress, Productivity, and the Reconstruction of Working Life.* New York: Basic Books, 1990.

Lazear, Jonathon. *The Man Who Mistook His Job for His Life.* New York: Crown, 2001.

Leana, Carrie R., and Daniel C. Feldman. *Coping with Job Loss: How Individuals, Organizations and Communities Respond to Layoffs.* New York: Lexington Books, 1992.

Meyer, G. J. *Executive Blues: Down and Out in Corporate America.* New York: Franklin Square Press, 1997.

Paulsen, Barbara. "Work and Play: A Nation out of Balance." *Health,* October 1994.

Peterson, Michael. "Work, Corporate Culture, and Stress: Implications for Worksite Health Promotion." *American Journal of Health Behavior* 21, no. 4 (1997): 243–252.

Potter, Beverly. *Beating Job Burnout: How to Transform Work Pressure into Productivity.* Berkeley, Calif.: Ronin Publishing, 1993.

Rosch, Paul J. "Measuring Job Stress: Some Comments on Potential Pitfalls." *American Journal of Health Promotion* 11, no. 6 (July/August 1997).

Rosen, Robert. *The Healthy Company.* Los Angeles: Jeremy P. Tarcher, 1991.

Schor, Juliet. *The Overworked American: The Unexpected Decline of Leisure.* New York: Basic Books, 1991.

Shalowitz, Deborah. "Another Health Care Headache: Job Stress Could Strain Corporate Budgets." *Business Insurance* 25 (May 20, 1991).

Snyder, Don J. *The Cliff Walk: A Memoir of a Lost Job and a Found Life.* Boston: Little Brown, 1997.

Stevens, Paul. *Beating Job Burnout: How to Turn Your Work into Your Passion.* Lincolnwood, Ill.: NTC Publishing Group, 1995.

Terez, Tom. *22 Keys to Creating a Meaningful Workplace.* Holbrook, Mass.: Adams Media, 2000.

Worksite Wellness
(See also HEALTH; HEALTH PROMOTION)

Goetzel, Ron Z., ed. *"The Financial Impact of Health Promotion." American Journal of Health Promotion* 15, no. 5 (May/June 2001).

O'Donnell, Michael P., and Thomas H. Ainsworth. *Health Promotion in the Workplace.* New York: Wiley, 1984.

INDEX

M